Obesity: Causes, Consequences and Interventions

Obesity: Causes, Consequences and Interventions

Editor: Johnny Hendrix

FOSTER
ACADEMICS
www.fosteracademics.com

www.fosteracademics.com

FOSTER ACADEMICS

Cataloging-in-Publication Data

Obesity : causes, consequences and interventions / edited by Johnny Hendrix.
p. cm.
Includes bibliographical references and index.
ISBN 978-1-63242-645-1
1. Obesity. 2. Obesity--Etiology. 3. Obesity--Diagnosis. 4. Obesity--Treatment. I. Hendrix, Johnny.
RC628 .O24 2019
616.398--dc23

Foster Academics,
118-35 Queens Blvd., Suite 400,
Forest Hills, NY 11375, USA

ISBN 978-1-63242-645-1 (Hardback)

Printed and bound in China.

Contents

Preface

I am honored to present to you this unique book which encompasses the most up-to-date data in the field. I was extremely pleased to get this opportunity of editing the work of experts from across the globe. I have also written papers in this field and researched the various aspects revolving around the progress of the discipline. I have tried to unify my knowledge along with that of stalwarts from every corner of the world, to produce a text which not only benefits the readers but also facilitates the growth of the field.

A person may be said to be obese if he/she has a body mass index or BMI of over 30 kg/m^2. Obesity is detrimental to the overall health of the individual. It increases the likelihood of various diseases such as type 2 diabetes, cardiovascular diseases, obstructive sleep apnea, osteoarthritis, certain cancers and depression. It is a leading cause of death worldwide but it is largely preventable. It is generally caused due to a combination of excessive food intake, genetic susceptibility and lack of physical activity. Certain factors such as endocrine disorders, mental disorders, genes and medications may also influence its incidence. The management of obesity is generally done by making lifestyle and dietary changes. Reducing the consumption of fats and sugars, increasing dietary fiber intake and regular exercising are the most recommended strategies. Medication can also help decrease fat absorption in the body or reduce appetite. In some cases, a surgery may be performed as a potential intervention. This book is compiled in such a manner, that it will provide in-depth knowledge about obesity. The topics covered in this extensive book deal with the core aspects of the causative factors and consequences of obesity as well as the interventions aimed at its management. It will help the readers in keeping pace with the rapid changes in this field.

Finally, I would like to thank all the contributing authors for their valuable time and contributions. This book would not have been possible without their efforts. I would also like to thank my friends and family for their constant support.

Editor

1

The Effects of Food Labelling on Postexercise Energy Intake in Sedentary Women

Jacynthe Lafrenière,[1] Jessica McNeil,[1] Véronique Provencher,[2] and Éric Doucet[1]

[1]*Behavioural and Metabolic Research Unit, School of Human Kinetics, University of Ottawa, Ottawa, ON, Canada*
[2]*Institute of Nutrition and Functional Foods, Laval University, Quebec City, QC, Canada*

Correspondence should be addressed to Éric Doucet; eric.doucet@uottawa.ca

Academic Editor: Chris I. Ardern

Food labelling has been previously reported to influence energy intake (EI). Whether food labels influence postexercise EI remains to be determined. We assessed how food labelling and exercise (Ex) interact to influence food perception and postexercise EI. In this randomized crossover design, 14 inactive women participated in 4 experimental conditions: Ex (300 kcal at 70% of VO_{2peak}) and lunch labelled as low in fat (LF), Ex and lunch labelled as high in fat (HF), Rest and LF, and Rest and HF. The lunch was composed of a plate of pasta, yogurt, and oatmeal cookies, which had the same nutritional composition across the 4 experimental conditions. EI at lunch and for the 48-hour period covering the testing day and the following day was assessed. Furthermore, perceived healthiness of the meal and appetite ratings were evaluated. There were no effects of exercise and food labelling on EI. However, meals labelled as LF were perceived as heathier, and this label was associated with higher prospective food consumption. Initial beliefs about food items had a stronger effect on healthiness perception than the different food labels and explain the positive correlation with the amount of food consumed ($\rho = 0.34$, $P < 0.001$).

1. Introduction

To maintain stable body weight and composition in response to increases in energy expenditure (EE) from exercise, an equivalent increase in caloric intake and/or a decrease in the energy cost of daily activities must also occur [1]. This is defined as complete (100%) postexercise energy compensation. Numerous studies have evaluated the effects of exercise on energy intake (EI), but results are conflicting with studies reporting increases in EI following exercise [2–4], while others did not [5, 6].

The perception of food items is based on socially promoted preconceptions of their impacts on health and weight, and this can exert influence over food choices and ultimately on EI [7, 8]. Foods presented as low in fat or rich in nutrients often carry the reputation of being healthier regardless of the portion size presented [9, 10]. As presented by Chandon and Wansink [11], this cognitive bias is represented by a categorical classification of food items, which has been coined the "health halo" and can lead to overconsumption of foods perceived as healthy. Along these lines, Provencher et al. [12] showed that individuals consumed more cookies when they were described as a healthy snack as opposed to when they were presented as a gourmet treat. Initial knowledge and perception of food items could thus potentially alter projected feelings of fullness and, therefore, the amount of ingested food and consequently calories [13].

In parallel, it has also been reported that individuals overestimate the energy cost of exercise while underestimating the caloric content of ad libitum food intake [14]. According to Spence et al. [15], exercise could also be associated with "guiltless eating," a concept that refers to the prevalent belief that EE from exercise can offset the EI of a larger meal. As such, in addition to the labelling of food, the perception of EE derived from exercise could also impact postexercise EI, at least acutely.

Discrepant results in postexercise EI between studies could be partly explained by differences in the usual level of physical activity. High physical activity participation tends to be related to a relatively stable weight over time, meaning that EI is closely matched to EE from exercise in these individuals [16]. Moreover, active individuals seem to be more sensitive and responsive to appetite signals, which allow them to maintain energy balance throughout the day [17, 18]. Of interest to the study of postexercise EI is the observation that inactive women could be more prone to increasing food intake following a bout of exercise [4] and are also seemingly more responsive to food labelling [19, 20]. As such, investigating the effects of food labelling on postexercise EI in sedentary women is warranted.

The aim of this study was thus twofold. First, we wanted to determine whether food labelling interacts with exercise to influence EI, the perceived healthiness, and appetite both acutely and for a 48-hour period in sedentary women. Secondly, we aimed to assess whether variations in EI correlated with variations in health perception of the meals. First, we hypothesized that food presented as low in fat (LF) would (1) be consumed in larger amounts independently of exercise and (2) would be perceived as healthier. Second, it was hypothesized that an increase in EI would only be observed following the exercise session from the meal labelled as high in fat (HF) as a result of "guiltless eating" that contributes to partly explaining postexercise energy compensation. Third, it was hypothesized that a healthier perception rating would be associated with an increase in EI.

2. Experimental Methods

2.1. Participants. Twenty women aged between 18 and 40 years were recruited through ads posted on the University of Ottawa campus. In order to be included, they had to be premenopausal, free from metabolic disorders, and inactive (<150 minutes of moderate to vigorous physical activity/week, which is below the recommendations put forth by the Canadian Society for Exercise Physiology (CSEP)) [21]. Physical activity level was self-reported by participants. Irregular menstrual cycle was also an exclusion criterion given that all testing sessions were performed during the follicular phase of the menstrual cycle. This was done to minimize the impact of hormonal variations on appetite-related variables, since appetite, food intake, and frequency of food craving have been shown to fluctuate across the menstrual cycle [22, 23]. Moreover, participants were not included if they had variations in body weight of more than ±2 kg over the last 6 months. Candidates who smoked, consumed greater than 2 alcoholic drinks per day, took medication affecting food intake (e.g., corticosteroid), had food allergies, and were enrolled in a weight loss diet at the time of the study were also excluded from the study. All selected participants provided written informed consent. Of note is the fact that the true objectives of the study were only divulged when participants had completed all experimental sessions. None of the participants had identified the true objectives of the study. At the onset of the protocol, they were told that the objective was to evaluate variations in appetite and post-workout recovery according to the fat content of the meal. From the 20 participants who met the inclusion criteria, 14 completed all experimental sessions. Their results are presented hereafter. All procedures were approved by the University of Ottawa's ethics committee and are in accordance with the Declaration of Helsinki.

2.2. Procedures

2.2.1. Overall Experimental Design. Participants were first invited to a preliminary session during which descriptive data were collected. This study used a crossover design with the four experimental conditions, which were randomly assigned in a counterbalance order (Rest + Meal labelled LF; Rest + Meal labelled HF; Exercise + Meal labelled LF; and Exercise + Meal labelled HF).

2.2.2. Preliminary Session. During the preliminary session, the consent form was reviewed and signed by participants. At this time, anthropometric measurements were taken and maximal aerobic capacity was determined, as the intensity of exercise during the experimental session was set at 70% of each participant's maximal oxygen consumption (VO_{2peak}), which was determined using the VO_2 reserve method [24]. This is considered to be high intensity exercise [25] and was associated with postexercise energy compensation in women [3]. For VO_{2peak}, a progressive stress test to exhaustion was completed under the supervision of an exercise physiologist using the Canadian Society for Exercise Physiology protocol [26]. The grade on the treadmill was increased progressively every two-minute until exhaustion, whereas the speed was constant for the duration of the test. A Vmax 229 series metabolic cart (SensorMedics Corporation, Yorba Linda, CA) was used to collect breath-by-breath samples of expired air through a mouthpiece, from which VO_2 was obtained. Heart rate (Polar RS300X, Kempele, Finland), as well as perceived exertion assessed with the Borg scale [27, 28], was closely monitored throughout the test. Participants were then also asked to fill out the Three-Factor Eating Questionnaire (TFEQ) [29] to determine the level of dietary restraint, disinhibition, and hunger.

2.2.3. Experimental Sessions. Participants were asked to arrive at the laboratory following a 12-hour overnight fast and to avoid alcohol consumption, as well as intense physical activity participation (e.g., training, playing sports) for at least 24 hours prior to the start of each experimental session. These instructions were sent by e-mail before each session and compliance was confirmed on the morning of all 4 experimental sessions. For the first session only, participants were instructed to arrive at the laboratory at 7:00 a.m. following a 12-hour overnight fast for a measurement of resting metabolic rate (RMR) (Vmax Encore 29N metabolic cart (SensorMedics Corporation, Yorba Linda, CA)). Data were collected for a 20-minute period after 20 minutes of rest in the supine position and after a 5-minute acclimatization period under the ventilated hood. During this first experimental session, participants chose the foods they wanted for breakfast from a list of items on a validated food menu [30]. The generic name of the different food item was shown, with no other nutritional information. Each food item consumed during

Table 1: Energy and macronutrient composition of the experimental lunch.

	Energy (kcal/100 g)	Macronutrients (g/100 g)		
		Carbohydrate	Proteins	Lipids
Pasta plate	95.3	13.1	2.9	2.8
Vanilla yogurt	80.0	12.0	4.9	1.3
Oatmeal cookies	458.3	70.8	4.2	18.8

the first session was weighed and then used as a standardized breakfast for the next three experimental sessions. For the remaining 3 experimental sessions, participants were asked to arrive at 8:00 a.m. They were served exactly the same breakfast as that they had eaten during the first experimental session and had to consume everything. Although the amount and type of foods varied from one participant to the next, it is important to stress that each participant received exactly the same breakfast for all experimental sessions.

From 8:30 a.m. to 10:45 a.m., participants were allowed to do any sedentary activities of their choice in the laboratory. During 2 of the 4 experimental sessions, an exercise session (Ex) consisting of walking with an incline or running on a treadmill was performed (preceded by a proper warm-up of 5 minutes at 3.5 mph). The intensity was set at 70% of each participant's VO_{2peak}, as determined during the preliminary session. During this session, heart rate was monitored to determine the intensity of the Ex based on the linear relationship that exists between VO_2 and heart rate under the anaerobic threshold [31, 32]. Participants exercised until they had expended an estimated 300 kcal. The required duration of the Ex was calculated using the VO_2 that corresponded to 70% of the VO_{2peak} obtained during the preliminary session. The Weir equation was used to calculate the caloric equivalent of this VO_2 measure [33, 34] (mean duration of the Ex was 33 ± 5.4 minutes). During the resting sessions (Rest), participants were asked to stay seated in the laboratory and had to remain seated for the same duration as the Ex intervention (i.e., 33 ± 5.4 minutes). At 11:45 a.m., for all conditions, participants were required to take a 15-minute shower and were then offered the experimental lunch. Before leaving the laboratory, at 12:30, participants chose what they would like to eat for the remainder of the day as well as for the day that followed the experimental manipulations.

2.3. Anthropometric Measurements. Height was measured using a Tanita HR-200 height rod (Tanita Corporation of America, Inc., Arlington Heights, IL) and weight was assessed with a standard beam scale (HR-100, BWB-800AS, Tanita Corporation, Arlington Heights, IL). Body composition was determined using dual-X-ray absorptiometry (DXA) scanner (Lunar Prodigy, General Electric, Madison, WI). Body composition was only measured at baseline 2 hours into the postprandial period, whereas weight was assessed at the beginning of each experimental session, following a 12-hour overnight fast.

2.4. Energy Intake Assessment. Lunch was served at noon and included pasta with cream sauce, vanilla flavoured yogurt, and oatmeal cookies (see Table 1). The same meal was offered at each of the four experimental sessions and all three-food items were provided in ad libitum fashion. Because all women were tested during the follicular phase of the menstrual cycle, at least 1 month separated all experimental conditions. The characteristics of the meal were presented on a piece of paper and read to participants by the experimenter. On two occasions (Rest and Ex), the foods were described as "high in fat (HF)" using the following description: (1) pasta: pasta with creamy vegetable sauce made with 35% cream and a rich cheese, (2) yogurt: vanilla flavoured yogurt made with creamy whole milk, and (3) cookies: gourmet oatmeal cookies made with real butter and old-fashioned brown sugar. And on the two other occasions (Rest and Ex), this same meal was provided but presented as "low in fat (LF)" with the following labels: (1) pasta: whole-wheat pasta with fresh vegetables in a light sauce made with reduced fat cream and cheese, (2) yogurt: nonfat vanilla flavoured yogurt, and (3) cookies: cookies made with fibre rich whole-grain oatmeal. Participants were instructed to eat as much or as little as they wanted of each of these items over a 30-minute period. After lunch, participants received a standardized menu containing 61 food items [30] and were asked to select what they wanted to eat for the remainder of the day as well as for the following day. We opted to measure food intake over 48 hours because it has been shown that exercise and labelling have an influence on EI over a period lasting more than one meal [3, 35]. Participants were instructed not to eat food outside of those selected from the menu for the measurement period (the remainder of the day and the following day). The selected food items were prepared according to guidelines previously described by McNeil et al. [30]: that is, all foods were weighed and stored in coolers to allow participants to carry them home. They were also instructed to bring back all leftovers and packaging two days later. EI for the entire measurement period is available for 12 participants, as we were unable to obtain EI during the last 24 hours in two participants who moved to a new city just after the last experimental session and were unable to bring back the coolers. It is important to note that information for the meal that followed Ex was nonetheless available for these two participants.

2.5. Appetite and Food Perception Measurements. Before and after each meal, as well as before the Ex or the Rest sessions, participants were asked to complete 100 mm visual analogue scales (VAS) to assess their desire to eat, hunger, fullness, and prospective food consumption [36, 37]. Additionally, during lunch, participants were asked to rate their appreciation of each item presented during the lunch meal on how much they liked it using a visual analogue scale (anchored from "not at all" to "very much"). They were also asked to provide a score from 1 to 8 on the following questions: "how healthy does this plate look to you?" (1 = "very unhealthy"; 8 = "very healthy"), "If you were eating this plate regularly, how would it affect your weight?" (1 = "weight loss"; 8 = "weight gain"), and "Do you consider this plate as appropriate for a healthy menu?" (1 = "very inappropriate"; 8 = "very appropriate"). These questions were adapted from those used by Provencher et al. [12].

2.6. Statistical Analysis. Statistical analyses were performed using SPSS software (version 17; SPSS Inc., Chicago, IL). Normality of the distribution was first assessed using the Kolmogorov-Smirnov test. A two-way repeated measures analysis of variance (ANOVA) was used to determine the main effect of exercise (Ex/Rest) and meal labelling (HF/LF) on EI at lunch, as well as for the entire measurement period (standardized breakfast, experimental lunch, and ad libitum out-lab intake assessed with the standardized menu for the remainder of the day and the following day). The effect of exercise (Ex/Rest) and labelling (HF/LF) on the perceived healthiness (i.e., "healthiness," "effect on weight," and "appropriateness in a healthy menu" ratings) for each food item (pasta/yogurt/cookies) was assessed with a non-parametric Friedman's test as the scale used is an ordinal variable and the distribution was not normal. To adjust for multiple tests performed, we employed a Bonferroni correction and as a result the level of significance was set at $P \leq 0.005$. When nonparametric Friedman's test was found to be significant, Wilcoxon tests were used to find where significant differences existed. Paired T-tests were carried out to explore if Ex affected appetite (i.e., desire to eat, hunger, fullness, and prospective food consumption) before lunch. Two-way repeated measures ANOVA with exercise (Ex/Rest) and labelling (HF/LF) as within subject factors were used to assess the effects and interactions of these factors on appetite after the lunch. Finally, in order to describe variation in EI, Spearman's rank order correlations (ρ) were carried out to assess the relationships between perception ratings at lunch.

3. Results

3.1. Participant Characteristics. Participant characteristics are shown in Table 2. Body weight remained stable across experimental sessions ($P = 0.738$).

3.2. Energy Intake. The average EI for the standardized breakfast was 609.8 SD 163.6 kcal (24.8% of the energy intake of the day), and as mentioned in the methods each participant consumed the same breakfast at every experimental session. Energy and macronutrient intakes at lunch across sessions are shown in Table 3. There was no main effect of Ex ($P = 0.541$) or food labelling ($P = 0.984$) on EI at lunch. Moreover, contrary to our hypothesis, no significant interactions were noted between Ex and food labelling ($P = 0.248$). The effect size of this outcome was small (partial $\eta^2 = 0.101$; observed power: 20%) [38]. Fat-free mass, fat mass, and RMR

Table 2: Participants characteristics at baseline ($N = 14$).

	Mean (±SD)	Range
Age (years)	22.4 ± 2.7	19–28
Weight (kg)	68.9 ± 12.4	55.6–94.4
BMI (kg/m^2)	24.1 ± 3.6	18.2–31.9
Fat mass (kg)	22.2 ± 9.2	11.7–45.2
Fat-free mass (kg)	43.0 ± 4.4	34.6–51.2
Body fat (%)	33.0 ± 7.4	20.3–48.3
RMR (kcal/d)	1310.1 ± 124.3	1147.05–1585.9
VO_{2peak} (ml/kg·min)	40.8 ± 6.1	30.3–51.3
TFEQ score (/51)	22.1 ± 8.0	9–34

BMI, body mass index; RMR, resting metabolic rate; and TFEQ, Three-Factor Eating Questionnaire.

were included in the model as covariate because they are known to be important predictors of EI [39], but they did not demonstrate a significant cofounding effect and neither did participants' restraint, disinhibition, and hunger levels as assessed by the TFEQ. EI ($F(3, 39) = 0.203$ $P = 0.894$) and appreciation of the foods (degree to which participants liked the meal on a scale from "not at all" to "very much") were not significantly affected by the order of experimental sessions. Energy and macronutrient intakes over 48 hours were not different across sessions (Table 3).

3.3. Appetite Rating. There was no effect of Ex on prelunch appetite ratings. However, a significant main effect of Ex ($F(1, 7) = 7.252$ $P = 0.018$) and of food labelling ($F(1, 7) = 4.697$ $P = 0.049$) on prospective food consumption after lunch was observed. More specifically, participants reported being able to eat more food after Ex as well as after the LF meal sessions (Rest + LF: 8.7 SD 8.2 mm; Rest + HF: 6.3 SD 6.6 mm; Exercise + LF: 13.1 SD 8.4 mm; Exercise + HF: 10.4 SD 7.8 mm on a 100 mm scale), although they did not significantly eat more during the rest of the day.

3.4. Perceived Healthiness. There was no effect of Ex on healthiness rating ($P = 0.240$), on the perceived effects on weight ($P = 0.360$), or on the appropriateness in a healthy menu ($P = 0.173$). Food items labelled as LF were globally perceived as healthier ($P < 0.001$) and more appropriate in a healthy menu ($P < 0.001$) than food items labelled as HF. However, labels did not influence perceived effect on weight ($P = 0.180$). Table 4 presents perceived healthiness ratings for each item across experimental conditions. The Friedman test revealed that labelling did not affect perceived healthiness of cookies the same way as it did on the other food items. Indeed, no significant difference was observed in the perceived healthiness rating ($\chi^2(3) = 11.713$ $P = 0.006$) and the capacity to induce weight gain ($\chi^2(3) = 10.705$ $P = 0.01$) across conditions (using the 0.005 level of significance adjusted for multiple comparisons) suggesting that the perception of the cookies was not affected by label manipulations. The yogurt was globally perceived as healthier ($P < 0.001$), more appropriate in a healthy menu ($P < 0.001$),

TABLE 3: Lunch and total (48 hours) energy (kcal) and macronutrient (g) intake for all four experimental conditions.

	RL	RH	EL	EH	P^c		
					Exercise status	Labelling	Exercise status* labelling
Lunch energy intake (kcal)[a]	622.5 ± 186.1	660.0 ± 186.1	685.0 ± 190.2	648.3 ± 201.5	0.541	0.984	0.248
Carbohydrate (g)[a]	93.1 ± 28.7	94.9 ± 27.2	98.5 ± 28.0	93.1 ± 29,5	0.766	0.567	0.445
Lipids (g)[a]	19.1 ± 6.2	19.5 ± 5.9	20.4 ± 6.7	19.5 ± 6.2	0.676	0.744	0.544
Proteins (g)[a]	20.0 ± 6.4	21.0 ± 6.0	21.3 ± 4.7	19.7 ± 6.4	0.975	0.714	0.129
Total energy intake (kcal)[b]	4276.2 ± 1193.5	4215.1 ± 665.1	4377.9 ± 823.7	4671.4 ± 993.3	0.182	0.605	0.301
Carbohydrate (g)[b]	592.2 ± 204.3	551.5 ± 86.5	574.4 ± 121.6	631.2 ± 152.9	0.299	0.792	0.129
Lipids (g)[b]	155.5 ± 56.9	155.2 ± 54.7	167.2 ± 43.1	173.8 ± 38.6	0.188	0.692	0.541
Proteins (g)[b]	145.2 ± 45.1	143.7 ± 27.5	152.9 ± 42.4	157.3 ± 40.3	0.190	0.846	0.619

Means ± s.d.

[a] $N = 14$; [b] $N = 12$. ∗ indicates the interaction.

[c] P value for the main effects and interaction of the ANOVA.

Sessions: RL: Rest and low fat; RH: resting and high fat; EL: Exercise and low fat; EH: Exercise and high fat.

Total energy intake includes the self-selected standardized breakfast, the experiment lunch, and energy intake outside the laboratory (total of 48 hours).

Table 4: Perceived healthiness rating of the lunch for all four experimental conditions ($N = 14$).

	RL	RH	EL	EH	Between condition differences	Exact sig. (P) Labelling	Exact sig. (P) Exercise status	Pairs differences
Healthiness (/8(SD))								
Pasta	5.9 (1.2)	3.8 (1.4)	5.5 (1.3)	4.2 (1.5)	<0.001*	<0.001*	0.488	RL-RH RL-EH RH-EL EL-EH
Yogurt	6.4 (1.0)	4.8 (1.4)	6.4 (1.7)	4.7 (1.8)	0.001*	<0.001*	0.5	RL-RH RL-EH
Cookies	3.9 (1.5)	3.3 (1.9)	3.6 (1.3)	2.6 (1.3)	0.006	NA	NA	NA
Effect on weight (/8(SD))								
Pasta	4.7 (1.1)	6.4 (1.2)	5.0 (0.7)	6.1 (1.1)	<0.001*	<0.001*	0.478	RL-RH RL-EH RH-EL EL-EH
Yogurt	4.1 (0.9)	5.1 (1.1)	3.9 (0.9)	5.1 (1.2)	<0.001*	<0.001*	0.247	RL-RH RL-EH RH-EL EL-EH
Cookies	5.8 (1.3)	6.5 (1.3)	5.9 (1.2)	6.6 (1.1)	0.01	NA	NA	NA
Appropriateness in a healthy menu (/8(SD))								
Pasta	6.1 (1.1)	3.5 (1.7)	5.4 (1.3)	3.7 (1.8)	<0.001*	<0.001*	0.169	RL-RH RL-EH RH-EL EL-EH
Yogurt	6.7 (1.2)	4.9 (1.7)	6.5 (1.6)	4.6 (1.7)	0.003*	<0.001*	0.223	RL-RH RL-EH
Cookies	3.9 (1.6)	2.6 (1.2)	3.9 (1.6)	3.0 (2.0)	0.002*	0.001*	0.477	RL-RH

Between condition differences are tested with Friedman test.
Main effect and pairs differences are tested with Wilcoxon test only when Friedman test is found to be significant. * $P < 0.001$.
Bonferroni correction is used to correct for multiple analysis and as a result the level of significance is set at $P \leq 0.005$.

and less associated with weight gain ($P < 0.001$) when compared with pasta and cookies.

3.5. Association between Perceived Healthiness and Food Consumption. Correlation analyses demonstrated that a higher rating of perceived healthiness was associated with a reduced perceived capacity to affect weight ($\rho = -0.747$, $P < 0.001$) and higher ratings of the appropriateness in a healthy menu ($\rho = 0.831$, $P < 0.001$). A positive correlation was also observed between the perceived healthiness rating and the weight of food consumed (g) when all three-food items were pooled together ($\rho = 0.339$, $P < 0.001$), though no significant correlation was found between the perceived healthiness and EI (kcal). The appreciation rating was also positively associated with an increased consumption of pasta ($\rho = 0.472$, $P < 0.001$) and cookies ($\rho = 0.267$, $P = 0.047$).

4. Discussion

We set to investigate whether food labelling interacts with exercise to influence postexercise EI, the perceived healthiness of meals, and appetite in sedentary women. We also assessed whether variations in EI correlated with variations in health perception of the meals. To our knowledge, this is the first study to evaluate the effects of both exercise and food labelling on postexercise EI within the same study design. Contrary to our hypothesis, neither exercise nor labelling the lunch as HF or LF had an impact on EI acutely (lunch) or for the 48-hour testing period. However, as hypothesized, food items labelled as LF were perceived as healthier and associated with higher prospective food consumption after the meal. We also show that the food items with the highest score for perceived healthiness were consumed in larger amounts as shown by the positive correlation between perceived healthiness rating and the weight (g) of the different food item consumed.

A number of studies have shown that a bout of exercise does not acutely impact EI [6, 40], which is in accordance with the results presented in the current study. Indeed, no significant differences were observed for EI at lunch, after Ex or Rest, or for the total 48 hours, meaning that the participants did not compensate for the EE induced by the Ex. Ex only slightly influence appetite perception after lunch. Indeed, participants reported being able to eat a larger amount of food after Ex than after Rest, even if they did not.

Unlike Shide et al., Wooley [41], and Provencher et al. [12] who observed an increase in EI after the ingestion of a food labelled as LF or healthier, no differences in EI were observed between the different fat content labelling in the present study. In accordance with our results, Bowen et al. [42] did not observe any effects of labelling (HF versus LF) on milkshake consumption in a group of women, which is similar to the results reported by Gravel et al. [43] in a mixed population. The methodological diversity of the different study protocols complicates the comparison of study results as far as the impact of labelling on EI is concerned. It is important to mention that, contrary to most of the protocols currently published on the influence of labelling on food intake [8, 12], a complete meal was manipulated and used in our study to assess EI at lunch, compared to single item like milkshakes, yogurt, or cookies. Our results thus illustrated that even if label does influence healthiness perception of food, initial knowledge about nutritional characteristics of the items would exceed the impact of label. Also, those characteristics seem to be further highlighted when different items are presented side by side. As reported by Oakes and colleagues [7, 44], food items often carry the reputation of being good or bad for health and body weight control, and this preconception strongly influences perception and caloric estimations of the product. The lunch meal proposed to the participants in our protocol contained food items with good (yogurt), neutral (pasta), and bad (cookies) reputations to ensure a better representation of real life food variety. Food items were also different in terms of their energy density (0.8 kcal/g for the yogurt versus 4.58 kcal/g for the cookies; see Table 1). This distinction explains why we observed a significant correlation between the weight of food consumed (g) (but not EI (kcal)) and perceived healthiness. We found that the labelling affected the perceived healthiness of a product, but this rating varied substantially between the different food items, which reiterated the importance of testing complete meals and not just focusing on single food items.

As hypothesized, the items labelled LF were perceived as healthier, but this manipulation had more impact on the perception of the pasta and the yogurt than on that of the cookies, which were perceived as unhealthy no matter how they were labelled. Buckland et al. [45] demonstrated that a diet-congruent starter (e.g., a salad) was associated with a significant reduction in EI at lunch when compared with a hedonic starter (e.g., garlic bread) in dieters. The labelling manipulation thus likely had reduced impact on the cookies because they are not a diet-congruent food item. It is also in accordance with the conclusion of recent review from Provencher and Jacob [46] which states that labelling influences health perception but that the impact on energy intake is less consistent.

Limitations. Although the crossover protocol used for this project is robust and experimental conditions were rigorous and well controlled, limitations need to be mentioned. First, the sample size is relatively small and limited to young women, mostly university students, which limits the generalizability of the results. A posteriori power analysis revealed that a sample of 78 individuals would have been needed to obtain a power of 0.80 [47] and statistically different effects on the average difference between session, which were between 10 and 60 kcal pour EI at lunch. Although the study was indeed underpowered to detect a difference in EI of this magnitude, the clinical relevance of such a difference must also be put into perspective. There is always a possibility that the appreciation of the meal decreased across sessions, as the same meal was presented each time, but as the sessions were randomized with at least one month separating each session, the likelihood of this occurring is substantially reduced. In fact, no effect of the order of the sessions was noted on EI and appreciation at lunch as presented in the results. We also must stress the acute nature of the present study design. Caution is warranted before extrapolating short-term outcomes to long-term exposure, particularly when dealing with energy balance outcomes.

5. Conclusion

In summary, labelling a meal as HF or LF did not alter postexercise EI. However, we show for the first time that Ex did influence the effect of labelling on perception, even if actual EI was not significantly changed. Future study designs should assess the effects of the presentation of a wider range of food items on their perception and intake. It would also be important to assess whether EI is affected when manipulations of labelling are maintained over longer periods of time, where it may lead to variations in energy balance and, ultimately, energy stores.

Abbreviations

ANOVA: Analysis of variance
BMI: Body mass index
CSEP: Canadian Society of Exercise Physiology
RH: Resting and high fat session
RL: Resting and low fat session
Rest: Resting session
DXA: Dual X-ray absorptiometry
EE: Energy expenditure
e.g.: Example
EI: Energy intake
EH: Exercise and high fat session
EL: Exercise and low fat session
Ex: Exercise session
HF: High fat label
i.e.: In other words
Kcal: Kilocalorie
Kg: Kilogram
Min: Minute
Mph: Miles per hour
LF: Low fat label
P: Probability that observed data are consistent with the null hypothesis
RMR: Resting metabolic rate
s.d.: Standard deviation
VAS: Visual analogue scales
VO_{2peak}: Measured peak oxygen consumption.

Disclosure

This research received no specific grant from any funding agency and commercial or not-for-profit sectors.

Authors' Contributions

Jacynthe Lafrenière and Éric Doucet designed the research. Jacynthe Lafrenière and Jessica McNeil conducted the research. Jacynthe Lafrenière, Jessica McNeil, Véronique Provencher, and Éric Doucet conceptualized the analysis of the data. Jacynthe Lafrenière and Jessica McNeil analysed the data. Jacynthe Lafrenière, Éric Doucet, and Véronique Provencher wrote the manuscript. All authors critically appraised and approved the final version of the manuscript.

Acknowledgments

The authors would like to thank the participants for their devoted contribution in this project. The authors especially want to thank Dr. Gilles Lamothe for his expert advice on the statistical analysis.

References

[1] N. A. King, P. Caudwell, M. Hopkins et al., "Metabolic and behavioral compensatory responses to exercise interventions: barriers to weight loss," *Obesity*, vol. 15, no. 6, pp. 1373–1383, 2007.

[2] J. Mayer, P. Roy, and K. P. Mitra, "Relation between caloric intake, body weight, and physical work: studies in an industrial male population in West Bengal," *The American Journal of Clinical Nutrition*, vol. 4, no. 2, pp. 169–175, 1956.

[3] M. Pomerleau, P. Imbeault, T. Parker, and E. Doucet, "The Effects of exercise intensity on food intake and appetite in women," *The American Journal of Clinical Nutrition*, vol. 80, no. 5, pp. 1230–1236, 2004.

[4] R. J. Stubbs, A. Sepp, D. A. Hughes et al., "The effect of graded levels of exercise on energy intake and balance in free-living women," *International Journal of Obesity*, vol. 26, no. 6, pp. 866–869, 2002.

[5] E. Jokisch, A. Coletta, and H. A. Raynor, "Acute energy compensation and macronutrient intake following exercise in active and inactive males who are normal weight," *Appetite*, vol. 58, no. 2, pp. 722–729, 2012.

[6] J. A. King, L. K. Wasse, and D. J. Stensel, "Acute exercise increases feeding latency in healthy normal weight young males but does not alter energy intake," *Appetite*, vol. 61, no. 1, pp. 45–51, 2013.

[7] M. E. Oakes and C. S. Slotterback, "Judgements of food healthfulness: food name stereotypes in adults over age 25," *Appetite*, vol. 37, no. 1, pp. 1–8, 2001.

[8] D. J. Shide and B. J. Rolls, "Information about the fat content of preloads influences energy intake in healthy women," *Journal of the American Dietetic Association*, vol. 95, no. 9, pp. 993–998, 1995.

[9] M. E. Oakes, "Beauty or beast: does stereotypical thinking about foods contribute to overeating?" *Food Quality and Preference*, vol. 16, no. 5, pp. 447–454, 2005.

[10] M. E. Oakes and C. S. Slotterback, "Too good to be true: dose insensitivity and stereotypical thinking of foods' capacity to promote weight gain," *Food Quality and Preference*, vol. 16, no. 8, pp. 675–681, 2005.

[11] P. Chandon and B. Wansink, "The biasing health halos of fast-food restaurant health claims: lower calorie estimates and

higher side-dish consumption intentions," *Journal of Consumer Research*, vol. 34, no. 3, pp. 301–314, 2007.

[12] V. Provencher, J. Polivy, and C. P. Herman, "Perceived healthiness of food. If it's healthy you can eat more!," *Appetite*, vol. 52, no. 2, pp. 340–344, 2009.

[13] J. M. Brunstrom, N. G. Shakeshaft, and E. Alexander, "Familiarity changes expectations about fullness," *Appetite*, vol. 54, no. 3, pp. 587–590, 2010.

[14] S. M. Willbond, M. A. Laviolette, K. Duval, and É. Doucet, "Normal weight men and women overestimate exercise energy expenditure," *The Journal of Sports Medicine and Physical Fitness*, vol. 50, no. 4, pp. 377–384, 2010.

[15] M. Spence, M. Livingstone, L. E. Hollywood et al., "A qualitative study of psychological, social and behavioral barriers to appropriate food portion size control," *International Journal of Behavioral Nutrition and Physical Activity*, vol. 10, no. 1 article 92, 2013.

[16] J. M. Jakicic, "The role of physical activity in prevention and treatment of body weight gain in adults," *The Journal of Nutrition*, vol. 132, no. 12, pp. 3826S-3829S, 2002.

[17] S. J. Long, K. Hart, and L. M. Morgan, "The ability of habitual exercise to influence appetite and food intake in response to high- and low-energy preloads in man," *The British Journal of Nutrition*, vol. 87, no. 5, pp. 517–523, 2002.

[18] C. Martins, H. Truby, and L. M. Morgan, "Short-term appetite control in response to a 6-week exercise programme in sedentary volunteers," *The British Journal of Nutrition*, vol. 98, no. 4, pp. 834–842, 2007.

[19] G. Cowburn and L. Stockley, "Consumer understanding and use of nutrition labelling: a systematic review," *Public Health Nutrition*, vol. 8, no. 1, pp. 21–28, 2005.

[20] M. E. Oakes, "Differences in judgments of food healthfulness by young and elderly women," *Food Quality and Preference*, vol. 14, no. 3, pp. 227–236, 2003.

[21] M. S. Tremblay, D. E. R. Warburton, I. Janssen et al., "New Canadian physical activity guidelines," *Applied Physiology, Nutrition and Metabolism*, vol. 36, no. 1, pp. 36–46, 2011.

[22] A. M. Gorczyca, L. A. Sjaarda, E. M. Mitchell et al., "Changes in macronutrient, micronutrient, and food group intakes throughout the menstrual cycle in healthy, premenopausal women," *European Journal of Nutrition*, vol. 55, no. 3, pp. 1181–1188, 2015.

[23] J. McNeil, J. D. Cameron, G. Finlayson, J. E. Blundell, and É. Doucet, "Greater overall olfactory performance, explicit wanting for high fat foods and lipid intake during the mid-luteal phase of the menstrual cycle," *Physiology & Behavior*, vol. 112-113, pp. 84–89, 2013.

[24] D. P. Swain, B. C. Leutholtz, M. E. King, L. A. Haas, and J. David Branch, "Relationship between % heart rate reserve and % VO2 reserve in treadmill exercise," *Medicine and Science in Sports and Exercise*, vol. 30, no. 2, pp. 318–321, 1998.

[25] American College of Sport Medicine, *ACSM's Guidelines for Exercise Testing & Prescriptions*, Lippincott Williams & Wilkins, Philadelphia, Pa, USA, 7th edition, 2005.

[26] Canadian Society for Exercise Physiology, *Professional Fitness & Lifestyle Consultant Resource Manual*, Canadian Society for Exercise Physiology, Ottawa, Canada, 1996.

[27] G. A. V. Borg, "Psychophysical bases of perceived exertion," *Medicine and Science in Sports and Exercise*, vol. 14, no. 5, pp. 377–381, 1982.

[28] M. J. Chen, X. Fan, and S. T. Moe, "Criterion-related validity of the Borg ratings of perceived exertion scale in healthy individuals: a meta-analysis," *Journal of Sports Sciences*, vol. 20, no. 11, 2002.

[29] A. J. Stunkard and S. Messick, "The three-factor eating questionnaire to measure dietary restraint, disinhibition and hunger," *Journal of Psychosomatic Research*, vol. 29, no. 1, pp. 71–83, 1985.

[30] J. McNeil, M.-È. Riou, S. Razmjou, S. Cadieux, and É. Doucet, "Reproducibility of a food menu to measure energy and macronutrient intakes in a laboratory and under real-life conditions," *The British Journal of Nutrition*, vol. 108, no. 7, pp. 1316–1324, 2012.

[31] J. Achten and A. E. Jeukendrup, "Heart rate monitoring: applications and limitations," *Sports Medicine*, vol. 33, no. 7, pp. 517–538, 2003.

[32] B. R. Londeree and S. A. Ames, "Trend analysis of the % VO2 max-HR regression," *Medicine and Science in Sports and Exercise*, vol. 8, no. 2, pp. 123–125, 1976.

[33] P. I. Mansell and I. A. Macdonald, "Reappraisal of the Weir equation for calculation of metabolic rate," *The American Journal of Physiology*, vol. 258, no. 6 part 2, pp. R1347-R1354, 1990.

[34] J. B. Weir, "New methods for calculating metabolic rate with special reference to protein metabolism," *The Journal of Physiology*, vol. 109, no. 1-2, pp. 1–9, 1949.

[35] C. A. Roberto, P. D. Larsen, H. Agnew, J. Baik, and K. D. Brownell, "Evaluating the impact of menu labeling on food choices and intake," *American Journal of Public Health*, vol. 100, no. 2, pp. 312–318, 2010.

[36] A. Flint, A. Raben, J. E. Blundell, and A. Astrup, "Reproducibility, power and validity of visual analogue scales in assessment of appetite sensations in single test meal studies," *International Journal of Obesity*, vol. 24, no. 1, pp. 38–48, 2000.

[37] R. J. Stubbs, D. A. Hughes, A. M. Johnstone et al., "The use of visual analogue scales to assess motivation to eat in human subjects: a review of their reliability and validity with an evaluation of new hand-held computerized systems for temporal tracking of appetite ratings," *The British Journal of Nutrition*, vol. 84, no. 4, pp. 405–415, 2000.

[38] P. E. Morris and C. O. Fritz, "Effect sizes in memory research," *Memory*, vol. 21, no. 7, pp. 832–842, 2013.

[39] J. E. Blundell, G. Finlayson, C. Gibbons, P. Caudwell, and M. Hopkins, "The biology of appetite control: do resting metabolic rate and fat-free mass drive energy intake?" *Physiology & Behavior*, vol. 152, pp. 473–478, 2015.

[40] L. Balaguera-Cortes, K. E. Wallman, T. J. Fairchild, and K. J. Guelfi, "Energy intake and appetite-related hormones following acute aerobic and resistance exercise," *Applied Physiology, Nutrition and Metabolism*, vol. 36, no. 6, pp. 958–966, 2011.

[41] S. C. Wooley, "Physiologic versus cognitive factors in short term food regulation in the obese and nonobese," *Psychosomatic Medicine*, vol. 34, no. 1, pp. 62–68, 1972.

[42] D. Bowen, P. Green, N. Vizenor, C. Vu, P. Kreuter, and B. Rolls, "Effects of fat content on fat hedonics: cognition or taste?" *Physiology and Behavior*, vol. 78, no. 2, pp. 247–253, 2003.

[43] K. Gravel, É. Doucet, C. P. Herman et al., "'Healthy,' 'diet,' or 'hedonic'. How nutrition claims affect food-related perceptions and intake?" *Appetite*, vol. 59, no. 3, pp. 877–884, 2012.

[44] M. E. Oakes, "Stereotypical thinking about foods and perceived capacity to promote weight gain," *Appetite*, vol. 44, no. 3, pp. 317–324, 2005.

[45] N. J. Buckland, G. Finlayson, and M. M. Hetherington, "Slimming starters. Intake of a diet-congruent food reduces meal intake in active dieters," *Appetite*, vol. 71, pp. 430–437, 2013.

[46] V. Provencher and R. Jacob, "Impact of perceived healthiness of food on food choices and intake," *Current Obesity Reports*, vol. 5, no. 1, pp. 65–71, 2016.

[47] J. Cohen, "Statistical power analysis," *Current Directions in Psychological Science*, vol. 1, no. 3, pp. 98–101, 1992.

2

Limited Effects of Endurance or Interval Training on Visceral Adipose Tissue and Systemic Inflammation in Sedentary Middle-Aged Men

Joshua H. F. Cooper,[1] Blake E. G. Collins,[1] David R. Adams,[1] Robert A. Robergs,[2] and Cheyne E. Donges[1]

[1] *School of Exercise Science, Sport and Health, Charles Sturt University, Bathurst, NSW, Australia*
[2] *Queensland University of Technology, Brisbane, QLD, Australia*

Correspondence should be addressed to Cheyne E. Donges; cdonges@csu.edu.au

Academic Editor: Chris I. Ardern

Purpose. Limited data exists for the effects of sprint-interval training (SIT) and endurance training (ET) on total body composition, abdominal visceral adipose tissue, and plasma inflammation. Moreover, whether "active" or "passive" recovery in SIT provides a differential effect on these measures remains uncertain. *Methods.* Sedentary middle-aged men ($n = 62$; 49.5 ± 5.8 y; 29.7 ± 3.7 kg·m^2) underwent abdominal computed tomography, dual-energy X-ray absorptiometry, venepuncture, and exercise testing before and after the interventions, which included the following: 12 wks 3 d·wk^{-1} ET ($n = 15$; 50–60 min cycling; 80% HR_{max}), SIT ($4–10 \times 30$ s sprint efforts) with passive (P-SIT; $n = 15$) or active recovery (A-SIT; $n = 15$); or nonexercise control condition (CON; $n = 14$). Changes in cardiorespiratory fitness, whole-body and visceral fat mass, and plasma systemic inflammation were examined. *Results.* Compared to CON, significant increases in interpolated power output (P-SIT, $P < 0.001$; ET, $P = 0.012$; A-SIT, $P = 0.041$) and test duration (P-SIT, $P = 0.001$; ET, $P = 0.012$; A-SIT, $P = 0.046$) occurred after training. Final VO_2 consumption was increased after P-SIT only ($P < 0.001$). Despite >90% exercise compliance, there was no change in whole-body or visceral fat mass or plasma inflammation ($P > 0.05$). *Conclusion.* In sedentary middle-aged men, SIT was a time-effective alternative to ET in facilitating conditioning responses yet was ineffective in altering body composition and plasma inflammation, and compared to passive recovery, evidenced diminished conditioning responses when employing active recovery.

1. Introduction

Excessive abdominal visceral adipose tissue (VAT) quantity and associated inflammatory cytokine secretion are linked to the development of insulin resistance (IR) and type 2 diabetes (T2D) mellitus [1, 2]. In turn, IR and T2D are precursors to increased atherosclerotic disease progression and end-point cardiovascular disease [3, 4]. Prevalence of obesity, metabolic dysfunction, and consequent disease risk increases with age [5]. Ageing is also associated with sedentary lifestyle and physical inactivity, thus presenting a confluence of factors for the development of whole-body and central obesity in middle-aged populations [6]. A key perception cited for the development of sedentary lifestyle is lack of time to engage in (what is deemed to be) the appropriate volume of physical activity [7].

Recent research indicates that sprint-interval training (SIT) is a time-efficient modality that provides similar and/or comparable health benefits to conventional endurance training (ET) [8–11]. SIT has been shown to increase muscle oxidative capacity [8, 9], cardiorespiratory fitness [10], endurance performance [8–10], and importantly from a disease perspective, insulin sensitivity, and glucose metabolism [11]. It has been suggested that, as is historically observed following ET, SIT may also produce similarly commensurate reductions in whole-body fat mass (FM) and VAT. Further, SIT may prove to be a more time-effective alternative to ET given that most middle-aged individuals do not meet recommended physical

Table 1: Baseline subject characteristics.

Measure	ET	P-SIT	A-SIT	CON
Age (y)	51.1 ± 5.7	47.2 ± 5.1	49.1 ± 5.3	51.2 ± 7
Height (cm)	177.3 ± 4.4	177.9 ± 8.3	177.0 ± 8.9	176.5 ± 6.3
BMI (kg·m^2)	30.6 ± 3.4	29.7 ± 4.1	29.7 ± 4.0	28.7 ± 3.6
Waist (cm)	104 ± 9	102 ± 11	100 ± 12	96 ± 9
WHR	1.00 ± 0.06	0.96 ± 0.05	0.97 ± 0.06	0.96 ± 0.06
Total chol. (mmol·L^{-1})	5.6 ± 1.3	5.6 ± 0.8	5.2 ± 1.2	5.8 ± 1.0
LDL chol. (mmol·L^{-1})	3.7 ± 1.2	3.7 ± 0.7	3.6 ± 0.9	3.8 ± 1.0
HDL chol. (mmol·L^{-1})	1.1 ± 0.2	1.1 ± 0.4	1.1 ± 0.3	1.2 ± 0.3
CHR	5.5 ± 1.6	5.7 ± 1.8	4.9 ± 1.5	5.1 ± 1.5
Triglycerides (mmol·L^{-1})	1.9 ± 1.1	1.8 ± 0.8	1.2 ± 0.7	1.7 ± 1.0
Glucose (mmol·L^{-1})	5.8 ± 0.4	5.7 ± 0.5	5.8 ± 0.6	5.4 ± 0.5
SBP (mmHg)	135 ± 12	131 ± 12	136 ± 13	138 ± 15
DBP (mmHg)	86 ± 10	81 ± 9	87 ± 10	92 ± 14

Data are mean ± standard deviation. ET: endurance training condition (n = 15); P-SIT: passive sprint-interval training condition (n = 15); A-SIT: active sprint-interval training condition (n = 15); CON: nonexercising control condition (n = 14). BMI: body mass index; WHR: waist to hip ratio; chol: cholesterol; LDL: low-density lipoprotein; HDL: high-density lipoprotein; CHR: cholesterol hazard ratio; SBP: systolic blood pressure; DBP: diastolic blood pressure. One-way ANOVA comparisons showed no differences between conditions for baseline measures ($P > 0.05$).

activity guidelines [6, 12]; however, studies evidencing the safety and outcome efficacy of SIT in middle-aged men are emerging but remain limited.

While ET is largely a well-researched and accepted modality for the reduction of whole-body FM and abdominal VAT in multiple population groups [13, 14], limited evidence exists to date as to whether SIT can produce similar results to ET. There have been some recent studies which have investigated the effect of interval-type training on central obesity; however, the involved exercise was not maximal (i.e., sprint-type) [15, 16], or there was no inclusion of reference methods to assess abdominal VAT such as magnetic resonance imaging or computed tomography [10, 16, 17]. Despite these shortcomings, in the studies of SIT, there were decreases in measures of central obesity as well as whole-body fat mass [10, 17]. Accordingly, there may be beneficial effects of SIT on abdominal VAT reduction, yet, to the authors knowledge, there has been no study to use reference method VAT analysis of SIT, especially in comparison to conventional ET. Moreover, the current SIT-central obesity data are limited in application to middle-aged adults given that most data pertains to younger trained/recreationally active participants [10, 17]. In addition, some studies include only a SIT condition (i.e., no ET or variation of SIT as a comparison) [10] or a cosex design, thereby introducing potential sex-specific conflict in pooled-sex analysis [10, 17]. Thus, further research is needed in more appropriately examining the effects of SIT on whole-body fat and abdominal VAT.

Importantly, abdominal VAT is a reported site for the release of proinflammatory cytokines, which participate in insulin signal transduction abnormalities and atherosclerotic disease processes [1, 2, 5]. Of the previously studied modalities, ET evidences the greatest capacity for abdominal VAT reduction [13, 14]. That said, ET is the most extensively studied modality, with minimal evidence thus far for SIT. To date, ET appears to produce the most beneficial response in, respectively, decreasing proinflammatory (e.g., tumor necrosis factor-α [TNF-α], interleukin-6 [IL-6], and C-reactive protein [CRP]) and increasing anti-inflammatory cytokines (e.g., IL-4, and IL-10), collectively facilitating cytokine profile (i.e., balance) towards a more normoglycaemic/atheroprotective state [18–21]. Again, the effects of SIT remain relatively unstudied and poorly understood. A recent study concluded no effect of SIT on plasma systemic inflammation, despite only incorporating a 2 wk intervention period [22]. Regardless of the lack of research for SIT, it appears possible that if SIT elicits VAT reduction, decreases may also be observed in plasma markers of chronic systemic inflammation.

The purpose of this study was to compare 12 wks conventional ET to SIT for effects on whole-body FM, abdominal VAT, and systemic inflammation in sedentary middle-aged men. A further aim was to examine whether additional between-interval ET activity (i.e., passive versus active recovery) would confer a different magnitude (i.e., greater extent) of response on outcome data. We hypothesised that ET would decrease whole-body FM, abdominal VAT, and systemic inflammation to a greater extent than the SIT conditions, with active SIT being more effective than passive SIT.

2. Methods

2.1. Participants. Sixty-two middle-aged (40–60 y) men volunteered for this study (data in Table 1). Participants were sedentary at baseline, defined as no regular structured or incidental exercise or physical activity >2 d·wk^{-1} in the 12 months priorly. Participants were screened by a physician for preexisting diabetes, cardiovascular disease, renal or hepatic disorders, immunological irregularities, rheumatoid arthritis, periodontal disease, chronic obstructive pulmonary disease, and any other condition linked to systemic inflammatory responses. Volunteers who were tobacco smokers

(<1 y cessation), had orthopaedic limitations, or were taking lipid-lowering, antihypertensive, anti-inflammatory, or other potentially confounding medications were not involved in the study. Following recruitment, participants attended an information seminar and received written and verbal information of all study procedures. Participants provided verbal and written informed consent prior to becoming involved. The study was approved by the Institutional Ethics committee and conformed to standards for the use of human subjects in research as outlined in 5th revision of the Declaration of Helsinki.

2.2. Study Overview. After prescreening and recruitment, eligible participants attended an information seminar where all procedures were explained and discussed. In a fasted and rested state, participants attended the Institutional Laboratory between 0530 and 0830 h for baseline testing and sequentially completed computed tomography (CT), dual-energy X-ray absorptiometry (DXA), blood pressure assessment, anthropometry, venous blood collection, and a submaximal exercise stress test (GXT). Participants were then randomized into endurance (ET; $n = 15$), "active" recovery sprint-interval training (A-SIT; $n = 15$), "passive" recovery sprint-interval training (P-SIT; $n = 15$), or a nonexercising control condition (CON; $n = 14$). Participants in the exercise groups completed 12 wk, 3 d·wk^{-1} fully supervised, periodized, and progressive programs. After the 12 wk intervention period and in a standardized manner (same time of day, same equipment, same tester, etc.) according to pretesting, participants returned to the laboratories and repeated all baseline test procedures. Participants received no remuneration or incentives for their involvement in the study.

2.3. Diet and Physical Activity Control. At the preintervention information and familiarisation seminar and regularly throughout the interventions, all participants were briefed verbally and in writing of the importance of maintaining previous dietary and physical activity habits. Participants were asked to maintain regular food and beverage type, macronutrient content, cooking preparation, portion size, consumption time, and so forth as closely as possible to preintervention dietary patterns during the 12 wk study period. Although sedentary at study baseline, participants in the interventions were asked to maintain their prestudy incidental physical activity habits and to not engage in any additional planned or incidental physical activities during the 12 wk training period.

2.4. Graded Exercise Testing. Human ethics, Exercise and Sports Science, Australia, and the American College of Sports Medicine guidelines advocate the need for physician supervision during maximal exercise testing as well as SIT in the recruited cohort given age and risk-factor status. It was not logistically possible to have a physician in attendance at all exercise testing and training sessions. Thus, submaximal GXT and SIT procedures were consequently administered with 85% of estimated heart rate (85% HR_{max}) maximum serving as termination criteria in all study exercise procedures. Blood pressure and electrocardiographic analysis were conducted during the GXT for anomaly identification. Participants were assessed (supervised by RR) for pressure and trace anomalies associated with underlying disease (e.g., hypertensive responses, ST-segment abnormalities, ectopic activity, and bundle-branch blocks) likely to be exacerbated by exercise, as previously recommended [23]. One participant was identified as having concerning anomalies and was excluded; all others were randomized to a study condition.

An electronically braked cycle ergometer (CASE ECG Stress Test System, General Electric Medical Systems, Milwaukee, WI) was used to conduct the GXT. An initial power output of 50 W was followed by increments in power output of 25 W·min^{-1} until 85% of estimated heart rate maximum (HR_{max}) was achieved, as identified via a cohort-specific equation ($205.9 - 0.685 \times$ age) [24]. Expired gases and flow volumes were collected during the GXT and analysed by a calibrated metabolic cart (TrueOne 2400, ParvoMedics, Salt Lake City, Utah) to provide oxygen uptake measures. The GXT was terminated at the predetermined 85% HR_{max} value. Interpolated 85% workload (last completed workload + fraction of last attempted workload) and test duration (time to 85%) were recorded to provide intervention outcome data and assist the respective training intervention programs.

2.5. Exercise Training Interventions. As exercise session duration is a primary consideration in time cost: benefit for middle-aged cohorts, we opted to provide the advocated guidelines as an upper limit for the ET methods (e.g., 150–180 min) and appropriately progressive SIT programs that were matched to each other for session duration but considerably shorter in duration (50%) than the ET condition. All exercise sessions were directly administered and supervised by the research team (JC and BC), with participant attendance and compliance being documented and monitored throughout. Training was standardized for time of day for each participant and occurred within a climate-controlled laboratory at the Institution. Heart rate, rating of perceived exertion (RPE), cycling duration, pedalling resistance, interval repetitions, and recovery time periods were all monitored and controlled throughout the 12 wk intervention. All exercise group participants received verbal familiarisation with the exercise session structure, physiological demands, and equipment used prior to commencing training and received strong verbal encouragement throughout each session of the program.

2.5.1. Endurance Training (ET). The ET program consisted of cycle ergometry (828e, Monark AB, Varberg, Sweden) at a workload which elicited ~80–85% of age-predicted HR_{max} or (initially) ~90% of the final workload obtained in the GXT. Training commenced at 50 min·session^{-1} for Wks 1–6 and increased to 60 min·session for Wks 7–12. Mean session Watts, RPE, and heart rate were recorded in each session. As participants conditioning increased, the workload was increased so as to maintain an intensity of ~80–85% of HR_{max}.

2.5.2. Passive Recovery Sprint-Interval Training (P-SIT). The P-SIT training program involved cycle ergometry (828E, Monark Exercise AB, Varberg, Sweden) and included a 5 min

TABLE 2: Cardiorespiratory fitness measures.

Measure	ET	P-SIT	A-SIT	CON
Study compliance (%)	90.9 ± 7.3	91.2 ± 4.4	91.4 ± 7.6	—
Time GXT (s)				
Pre	373 ± 98	380 ± 90	393 ± 87	389 ± 98
Post	446 ± 109^	470 ± 98^	455 ± 89^	400 ± 96
Raw Δ	73 ± 54*	90 ± 41*	62 ± 57	10 ± 49
% Δ	21 ± 17	25 ± 14	18 ± 17	3 ± 15
Peak output GXT (W)				
Pre	180 ± 41	183 ± 38	189 ± 36	187 ± 41
Post	211 ± 46^	222 ± 38^	215 ± 36^	191 ± 40
Raw Δ	30 ± 23*	39 ± 18*	26 ± 24*	4 ± 20
% Δ	18 ± 14	23 ± 13	15 ± 14	3 ± 12
VO_2 GXT ($L\cdot min^{-1}$)				
Pre	2.26 ± 0.46	2.33 ± 0.54	2.61 ± 0.47	2.33 ± 0.49
Post	2.60 ± 0.50	2.82 ± 0.55^	2.91 ± 0.53	2.41 ± 0.40
Raw Δ	0.34 ± 0.28	0.49 ± 0.22*	0.30 ± 0.29	0.07 ± 0.26
% Δ	16 ± 15	22 ± 12	12 ± 12	5 ± 13
VO_2 GXT ($mL\cdot kg^{-1}\cdot min^{-1}$)				
Pre	23.6 ± 4.2	24.8 ± 4.8	28.2 ± 4.0	26.4 ± 6.0
Post	27.4 ± 5.2	29.9 ± 5.1^	31.3 ± 3.8	27.1 ± 4.9
Raw Δ	3.8 ± 3.3	5.1 ± 2.4*	3.1 ± 3.2	0.7 ± 3.3
% Δ	17 ± 16	22 ± 11	12 ± 12	4 ± 14

Data mean ± standard deviation. ET: endurance training condition (n = 15); P-SIT: passive sprint-interval training condition (n = 15); A-SIT: active sprint-interval training condition (n = 15); CON: nonexercising control condition (n = 14). *Significant within-group change from baseline ($P < 0.05$). ^Significant between-group change ($P < 0.05$). GXT: graded exercise test at 85% of age-predicted heart rate maximum (HR_{max}); VO_2: volume of oxygen uptake.

(limited) light-moderate warm-up/cool-down of either side of a SIT component. The SIT component is comprised of 1 : 6 work : rest cycles, via 30 s sprint efforts followed by 3 min of passive recovery. Training commenced with four interval efforts, increasing by one effort per fortnight, with 10 efforts being completed at program completion. Pilot testing in an analogous cohort revealed that a cadence of 120 $rev\cdot min^{-1}$ and 5-6% body mass resistance optimized the 30 s work stimulus (e.g., required a "maximal" effort). In the between-interval period, P-SIT participants either remained stationary on the bike or were allowed restricted movement (slow walking; limited in distance) around the training room (60 m^2).

2.5.3. Active Recovery Sprint-Interval Training (A-SIT). The A-SIT training program was identical in all program aspects as the P-SIT program (same ergometers, number of efforts, work cadence, progression, etc.); however, it consisted of 3 min (between-interval) periods involving continued cycling at 60 $rev\cdot min^{-1}$ at a lightened resistance (e.g., 1.0–1.5 kp, depending on the participant). Pilot testing confirmed that this combination of cadence and resistance permitted sufficient recovery so as to ensure that participants were to achieve 120 rpm for similar time duration as P-SIT participants during each ensuing interval effort.

2.6. Measures

2.6.1. Computed Tomography. At baseline testing, participants firstly arrived at a local radiology facility for computed tomography of the abdominal region. Upon arrival, participants voided the bladder and were positioned as central as possible in the gantry regarding vertex-pubis symphysis alignment. An anterior-posterior scanogram (scout radiograph) of the lower abdomen and pelvis was conducted using a 64-slice multidetector CT (Toshiba Aquilion, Toshiba Medical Systems, Tokyo, Japan). A volume acquisition compartment 77 mm in length was obtained (120 kv, 50 mA, and 0.5 s tube rotation) cephalically from the superior end-plate of L4 during suspended inspiration. After scanning, eleven 7.0 mm contiguous axial images were reconstructed in a maximal display field of view (500 mm) for volume calculation with an attenuation range of −180 to −30 Hounsfield units, and the total adipose tissue (TAT), VAT and subcutaneous adipose tissue (SAT) compartments were determined as described previously [25].

2.6.2. Dual-Energy X-Ray Absorptiometry, Anthropometry and Blood Pressure Assessment. A supine DXA scan was undertaken to estimate whole-body composition (Norland XR800, Cooper Surgical Company, Turnbull, CT, USA). Participants were positioned centrally on the bench of the DXA machine and a whole-body scan was completed with a resolution of 4.5 × 9.0 mm and scanning speed of 130 $mm\cdot sec^{-1}$. The scan was then analysed with customized software (Illuminatus DXA, version 4.2.0, Turnbull, CT, USA) for FM and fat free mass (FFM) which are reported in absolute (kg) and relative (%) terms. All pre- and postintervention scanning

TABLE 3: Body mass and composition data.

Measure	ET	P-SIT	A-SIT	CON
Body mass (kg)				
Pre	96.2 ± 11.4	94.8 ± 20.2	93.9 ± 18.9	89.4 ± 12.1
Post	95.7 ± 12.4	95.7 ± 21.2	94.1 ± 19.1	89.8 ± 12.2
Raw Δ	−0.5 ± 3.5	0.8 ± 1.6	0.2 ± 1.2	0.5 ± 1.2
% Δ	−0.6 ± 3.9	0.7 ± 1.6	0.2 ± 1.4	0.5 ± 1.4
FFM (kg)				
Pre	70.8 ± 7.5	71.4 ± 10.7	70.9 ± 11.6	67.7 ± 6.6
Post	71.2 ± 7.8	72.8 ± 11.2	71.9 ± 11.6	69.2 ± 6.7
Raw Δ	0.37 ± 1.5	1.5 ± 1.9	1.0 ± 1.6	1.4 ± 1.0
% Δ	0.5 ± 2.2	2.0 ± 2.4	1.4 ± 2.2	2.1 ± 1.3
FM (kg)				
Pre	27.2 ± 8.7	24.8 ± 10.9	24.4 ± 8.7	23.3 ± 7.6
Post	28.2 ± 9.6	25.2 ± 11.8	25.1 ± 9.4	23.5 ± 7.1
Raw Δ	1.0 ± 2.1	0.4 ± 2.0	0.7 ± 1.7	0.2 ± 1.3
% Δ	3.5 ± 9.1	1.3 ± 8.5	2.7 ± 6.5	1.8 ± 7.4
FM (%)				
Pre	27.3 ± 6.5	25.0 ± 5.8	25.0 ± 5.3	25.1 ± 5.4
Post	27.9 ± 7.0	24.8 ± 6.0	25.2 ± 5.4	24.9 ± 4.6
Raw Δ	0.6 ± 1.6	−0.2 ± 1.7	0.2 ± 1.4	−0.2 ± 1.2
% Δ	1.9 ± 6.5	−0.5 ± 7.8	1.0 ± 5.7	0.0 ± 6.4
SAT (cm^3)				
Pre	2396 ± 843	1952 ± 773	2153 ± 788	1852 ± 719
Post	2415 ± 918	1924 ± 746	2179 ± 873	1886 ± 660
Raw Δ	19 ± 163	−29 ± 113	26 ± 188	34 ± 161
% Δ	0.1 ± 7.5	−1.3 ± 6.3	0.7 ± 7.2	4.2 ± 12.2
VAT (cm^3)				
Pre	1474 ± 427	1540 ± 596	1353 ± 568	1225 ± 448
Post	1489 ± 447	1482 ± 588	1331 ± 705	1441 ± 569
Raw Δ	16 ± 338	−58 ± 302	−22 ± 367	216 ± 280
% Δ	3.2 ± 23.6	−3.0 ± 14.8	−1.3 ± 20.2	18.4 ± 22.5
TAT (cm^3)				
Pre	3870 ± 1031	3492 ± 1162	3506 ± 1253	3077 ± 1038
Post	3904 ± 1210	3405 ± 1246	3510 ± 1453	3327 ± 1095
Raw Δ	35 ± 427	−87 ± 238	4 ± 452	250 ± 294
% Δ	0.4 ± 11.8	−3.0 ± 5.8	−0.3 ± 9.7	8.8 ± 10.7
VAT (%)				
Pre	38.8 ± 8.5	44.0 ± 8.4	37.8 ± 7.9	40.3 ± 8.4
Post	38.8 ± 7.4	43.3 ± 6.4	37.0 ± 8.6	43.0 ± 7.6
Raw Δ	0.1 ± 4.8	−0.7 ± 4.8	−0.8 ± 4.5	2.7 ± 5.5
% Δ	1.7 ± 12.8	−0.4 ± 10.6	−1.8 ± 12.2	8.2 ± 13.7

Data are mean ± standard deviation. ET: endurance training exercise group, $n = 15$; P-SIT: passive sprint-interval training exercise group, $n = 15$; A-SIT: active sprint-interval training exercise group, $n = 15$; CON: control group, $n = 14$. FFM: total body fat free mass; FM: total body fat mass; SAT: subcutaneous adipose tissue; VAT: abdominal visceral adipose tissue; TAT: total abdominal adipose tissue. There were no significant pre-to-post or between-condition differences in body composition measures after the study interventions ($P > 0.05$).

procedures and analyses were standardized pre to post (e.g., fasted, rested, no alcohol in the prior 24 h, scan settings, and participant positioning).

TABLE 4: Measures of plasma systemic inflammation.

Measure	ET	P-SIT	A-SIT	CON
CRP ($mg{\cdot}L^{-1}$)				
Pre	2.8 ± 1.6	2.7 ± 1.3	2.1 ± 1.4	2.1 ± 1.5
Post	2.9 ± 1.6	2.1 ± 0.9	1.9 ± 1.2	2.1 ± 1.6
Raw Δ	0.2 ± 1.2	−0.6 ± 1.0	−0.2 ± 0.9	0.0 ± 0.9
% Δ	11.8 ± 40.9	−12.3 ± 50.7	−1.5 ± 34.6	24.3 ± 118.5
IL-6 ($pg{\cdot}L^{-1}$)				
Pre	3.16 ± 1.36	3.11 ± 1.04	3.29 ± 0.53	3.27 ± 0.64
Post	3.55 ± 0.75	3.18 ± 0.63	3.57 ± 0.38	3.65 ± 0.81
Raw Δ	0.40 ± 1.03	0.08 ± 1.01	0.28 ± 0.46	0.37 ± 0.77
% Δ	22.8 ± 30.6	10.9 ± 35.5	10.1 ± 14.0	12.9 ± 23.2
TNF-α ($pg{\cdot}L^{-1}$)				
Pre	6.1 ± 1.7	6.8 ± 1.5	6.6 ± 1.8	5.2 ± 1.4
Post	6.8 ± 2.1	6.6 ± 1.9	6.4 ± 1.9	5.7 ± 1.3
Raw Δ	0.7 ± 1.6	−0.2 ± 2.2	−0.2 ± 1.3	0.5 ± 1.5
% Δ	13.7 ± 28.8	1.3 ± 31.9	−1.6 ± 23.1	16.0 ± 33.5
MCP-1 ($pg{\cdot}L^{-1}$)				
Pre	121 ± 43	137 ± 43	145 ± 46	111 ± 86
Post	121 ± 38	129 ± 33	141 ± 43.02	109 ± 84
Raw Δ	−0.2 ± 33.0	−7.5 ± 43.3	−4.1 ± 34.1	−1.8 ± 61.6
% Δ	7.7 ± 37.9	4.0 ± 41.0	3.1 ± 28.8	25.8 ± 92.2
IL-10 ($pg{\cdot}L^{-1}$)				
Pre	3.72 ± 2.78	3.77 ± 3.03	3.32 ± 2.32	4.98 ± 2.40
Post	5.31 ± 5.25	5.77 ± 4.59	2.93 ± 1.47	5.35 ± 3.17
Raw Δ	1.59 ± 3.72	2.00 ± 4.08	−0.39 ± 2.00	0.38 ± 1.97
% Δ	53.2 ± 85.2	118.0 ± 218.3	16.7 ± 84.5	8.8 ± 42.6

Data are mean ± standard deviation. ET: endurance training exercise group, $n = 15$; P-SIT: passive sprint-interval training exercise group, $n = 15$; A-SIT: active sprint-interval training exercise group, $n = 15$; CON: control group, $n = 14$. CRP: C-reactive protein; IL-6: interleukin 6; TNFα: tumor necrosis factor α; MCP-1: monocyte chemoattractant protein 1; IL-10: interleukin 10. There were no significant pre-to-post or between-condition differences in plasma CRP and cytokine measures after the study interventions ($P > 0.05$).

Following DXA, measurements of body mass and waist and hip circumference were obtained for each participant. Body mass was taken wearing minimal clothing and standardized before and after intervention. Waist and hip circumference measurements were collected as described previously [26] and by the same tester before/after intervention (CD). Blood pressure was measured via auscultation after ~10 min of rest. Systolic and diastolic pressures were recorded three times with a 1 min rest period between measurements. The lowest paired systolic and diastolic values were recorded.

2.6.3. Venous Blood Collection and Analysis. Participants then underwent venepuncture procedures in which a cannula was inserted into a medial antecubital vein and blood was manually drawn by syringe and gently ejected into prechilled (on ice) tubes treated with ethylenediaminetetraacetic acid and serine protease inhibitor (Pefabloc SC, Sigma-Aldrich, Sydney, Australia) to prevent cytokine degradation. Drawn blood was also ejected into serum separator tubes and left to clot within ~20–30 min. The prechilled and clotted serum tubes were centrifuged (refrigerated) for 10 min at 4°C, and plasma and serum specimens were stored at −80°C until analysis (<2 wks after collection).

Serum was analysed for total cholesterol, high-density lipoprotein cholesterol, triglycerides, glucose, and CRP on a high-throughput automated blood analyser according to the manufacturer and respective kit instructions (Dimension EXL, Siemens Healthcare Diagnostics, Sydney, Australia). The Friedewald equation was used to estimate low-density lipoprotein cholesterol as described previously [26]. Intra- and interassay coefficient of variation (CV) were less than 6.1% for all measured analytes. Commercially available enzyme-linked immunosorbent assays (Jomar Life Research, Melbourne) were used to analyse plasma for IL-6, IL-10, TNF-α, and MCP-1. Each participant pre- and postsample was loaded sequentially on the same plate, and all standard curves were $R \geq 0.99$. Intra- and interassay CV were reported (manufacturer) <10% for all analytes.

2.7. Statistical Analysis. A sample size of ≥10 participants per condition was required in order to acquire an effect size of 0.25 at $\alpha = 0.05$ according to *a priori* analysis [27] (G*Power v.3). However, >14 participants were involved to help avoid type II error. The subject sample size used in this study is similar to recent studies which have reported significant intervention effects of ET and SIT on measures of body composition [10, 16, 17]. Repeated-measures analysis of covariance (ANCOVA) was used to assess condition × time interactions with baseline data (for each respective variable) used as the covariate. If a main effect was observed in the ANCOVA, one-way ANOVA with Bonferroni's multiple comparison *post hoc* tests applied to determine significant differences. Effect size (ES) data for pre-to-post change and between-group differences were determined using unbiased Hedges Cohen's *d* calculation (trivial: <0.20; small: 0.20–0.49; moderate: 0.50–0.79; or large: >0.80). Statistical significance for the ANCOVA and one-way ANOVA was accepted when $P < 0.05$. ES data was only reported if deemed to have an upper moderate or large effect ($d > 0.70$). All data are presented as mean ± standard deviation (SD).

3. Results

3.1. Exercise Training Compliance. All subjects attended >30 of the 36 organised exercise training sessions (~91%), with mean session attendance being 32 of the 36 sessions (see Table 2). One-way ANOVA revealed that there was no significant difference in training compliance between groups ($P > 0.05$). While there were no adverse events arising from the exercise training interventions, 3 participants, one from each of the P-SIT, A-SIT, and CON groups, respectively, did not complete the 12 wk interventions ($1n$ = orthopaedic limitations; $2n$ = time constraints) and were excluded from analysis, resulting in final numbers: ET ($n = 15$), P-SIT ($n = 15$), A-SIT ($n = 15$), and CON ($n = 14$).

3.2. Cardiorespiratory Fitness Measures. A significant main effect was identified for increases in VO_2 uptake, power output, and GXT time duration at 85% HR_{max} ($P < 0.05$). One-way ANOVA identified increases for peak output (P-SIT, $P < 0.001$; ET, $P = 0.009$; A-SIT, $P = 0.05$), time duration (P-SIT, $P = 0.001$; ET, $P = 0.01$), and VO_2 at 85% HR_{max} ($L{\cdot}min^{-1}$) (P-SIT, $P = 0.001$) (Table 2). In comparison to CON, at 85% HR_{max}, there was a significant pre-to-post difference by the exercise interventions for increases in power output (P-SIT, $P < 0.001$; ET, $P = 0.012$; A-SIT, $P = 0.041$), time duration (P-SIT, $P = 0.001$; ET, $P = 0.012$; A-SIT, $P = 0.046$), and VO_2 ($L{\cdot}min^{-1}$) (P-SIT, $P < 0.001$) (Table 2). Although no significant differences in change of VO_2 at 85% HR_{max} ($L{\cdot}min^{-1}$) were observed between the CON and ET ($P = 0.063$) or CON and A-SIT ($P = 0.055$), between-group ES data showed a trend for difference (ET versus CON, $d = 0.97$; A-SIT versus CON, $d = 0.81$).

3.3. Body Composition, Abdominal CT, and Anthropometry. There was no significant difference in anthropometry measures after the interventions ($P > 0.05$) and only trivial to moderate ES data for pre-to-post and between-condition comparisons (all $d < 0.60$). Further, there were no significant changes in FM, FFM, or abdominal CT measures pre-to-post or between conditions ($P > 0.05$) (see Table 3). The ES data indicated only trivial to small (all $d < 0.22$) ES data for changes in FM and FFM. Although a large effect between CON-ET groups presented for FFM increase ($d = 1.36$), ES data for pre-to-post change in abdominal CT were small to trivial (all $d < 0.41$). However, for VAT (cm^3), a large and moderate ES, respectively, presented between P-SIT and CON ($d = 0.91$) and A-SIT and CON ($d = 0.70$). For VAT (%), a moderate ES presented between A-SIT and CON ($d = 0.78$) and P-SIT and CON ($d = 0.78$).

3.4. Biochemistry, Plasma CRP, and Cytokines. There were no significant pre-to-post or between-condition differences of fasting glucose, cholesterol, LDL, HDL or triglycerides ($P > 0.05$). Aside from moderate ES data for a pre-to-post difference in glucose between CON and A-SIT ($d = 0.77$), all pre-to-post (all $d < 0.57$) and between-group (all $d < 0.58$) biochemistry ES data were trivial to moderate. There were no significant pre-to-post or between-condition differences for plasma CRP or studied cytokines ($P > 0.05$; see Table 4). The ES data showed a moderate ES for CRP reduction between P-SIT and ET ($d = 0.70$) and for IL-10 moderate ES for increase between P-SIT and A-SIT ($d = 0.71$). Otherwise, only trivial to moderate ES data were detected for pre-to-post (all $d < 0.59$) and between-group (all $d < 0.65$) changes of CRP and the studied cytokines.

4. Discussion

This study compared conventional ET to age/health-status appropriate SIT for respective effects on whole-body composition, abdominal VAT, and pro- and anti-inflammatory cytokine concentrations in a sedentary overweight middle-aged male population. This study also examined whether a passive (P-SIT) or active (A-SIT) recovery period (between-intervals efforts) would facilitate a differential magnitude of response in outcome measures. Specifically, in addition to completing the P-SIT program, the A-SIT group completed further 27–81 mins (range from Wks 1–12) of moderate intensity exercise per week. We incorporated this study design to ascertain whether the coupling of ET with P-SIT (in recovery) offered additive effects to outcome measures. After intervention, we observed significant improvements in fitness measures across all exercise conditions, yet, surprisingly, increases observed in P-SIT appeared more robust in comparison to A-SIT, despite matching of the 30 s interval efforts. Accordingly, while requiring further elucidation, in the studied population, there may be evidence of an inhibitory effect of combining ET with SIT, exacerbated via the absence of sufficient between-effort "recovery" periods. Previously, ET and SIT have both been reported to significantly reduce body fat [10, 16, 17]; however, to date, of ET and SIT, only evidence exists for a positive effect of ET on abdominal VAT [13]. In the studied cohort, our 12 wk intervention did not result in a reduction of FM or abdominal VAT following either of the SIT interventions. In addition, we observed no changes in inflammatory measures following all exercise interventions. Such a response raises further questions regarding the efficacy of exercise training without caloric restriction to facilitate favourable changes in body composition, abdominal VAT, and chronic systemic inflammation.

Accumulating evidence supports that SIT is a time-efficient alternative to conventional ET for the facilitation of musculoskeletal adaptations associated with oxidative metabolism [8–11]. In this study, all three exercise conditions improved measures of cardiorespiratory fitness; however, P-SIT appeared to elicit the greatest relative changes and difference to the CON across each cardiorespiratory fitness measure. These data further support the work of these previous studies and further highlight the role of exercise intensity (compared with duration) in eliciting rapid exercise-induced conditioning-based adaptations. However, the blunted cardiorespiratory fitness improvements observed in A-SIT (when compared to P-SIT) indicate that an inhibitory effect may be present in the A-SIT data. Nader [28] has previously outlined the concurrent training "effect," wherein the combination of strength and endurance exercise results in potential molecular interference in phenotype-specific adaptive signalling and diminished adaptation in comparison to single-mode completion (e.g., strength or endurance alone). The A-SIT sessions here could be viewed as inducing short-duration high-intensity periods of maximal force with similar duration to 8–10 RM strength-training set, yet combined with continuous moderate intensity endurance exercise in the recovery period. Thus, the A-SIT condition essentially parallels aspects of "Fartlek-"style training, which is ingrained in training programs of many well-conditioned/prepared athletes [29, 30]. Nevertheless, in the studied population group, there may have been a detrimental effect given their lack of condition to accommodate the intense training stimulus. As reported previously, potential inhibitory mechanisms observed as a result of a concurrent training effect include diminished neural activation rapidity, impaired glycogen regulation, muscle fiber-type transformation, ADP-ATP ratio, and associated effect on molecular signalling processes orchestrating muscle protein turnover [28]. Further research may be warranted in investigating these mechanisms in response to A-SIT (compared to P-SIT) in deconditioned middle-aged populations.

Contrary to the findings in this study, SIT and ET have previously been shown to decrease body mass and whole-body FM, thereby positively influencing relative whole-body composition [10, 16, 17]. Accumulating data indicates that 150 $min{\cdot}wk^{-1}$ of moderate intensity exercise may be insufficient to reduce body mass and may only serve to maintain or ameliorate gain in weight [12, 31]. In our study, the ET group commenced at 150 and progressed to 180 $min{\cdot}wk^{-1}$ and cycled at a moderate-to-vigorous intensity. The data shows lack of change in whole-body FM and raises questions as to whether middle-aged populations should be increasing session and thus total weekly duration or focusing on optimization of intensity. Accordingly, we sought to appraise an appropriate SIT intervention as an alternative to ET, and, like ET, we observed a limited effect of SIT on whole-body FM. Keating et al. [16] recently reported that moderate intensity cycling ~108–144 $min{\cdot}wk^{-1}$ over a 12 wk intervention elicited significant reductions in whole-body FM; however, a SIT condition in this study did not alter whole-body or trunk FM. In contrast, prior research has demonstrated that SIT can be effective in reducing whole-body FM [10, 17]. These reductions observed generally appear to be comparable to reductions after ET, yet, in some studies, SIT is reportedly more effective than ET in decreasing whole-body FM [10, 17]. As evidence, Macpherson et al. observed that a SIT protocol of 4–6 repetitions of 30 s maximal running efforts 3 $sessions{\cdot}wk^{-1}$ for 6 weeks elicited a 12.4% decrease in FM opposed to a 5.8% decrease in a ET group (program range: 90–180 $min{\cdot}wk^{-1}$). However, this study investigated recreationally active men and women (24 y mean age) and thus whether these age-based and sex-pooled findings apply to overweight middle-aged men remains uncertain. Although data support suggests that SIT may be as effective as ET as a regular exercise alternative [8–11], no current physical guidelines for SIT have been implemented and its effect on health-related outcomes such as whole-body FM are thus far inconsistent and require further elucidation.

Mounting evidence substantiates that the extent (quantity) and dysfunctional regulation (atherogenicity) of abdominal VAT are associated with the extent and progression of metabolic and cardiovascular disease [5, 25]. These findings support why the reduction of VAT currently occupies a central focus in the prevention of these diseases [32]. In this study, there were no differences observed in abdominal VAT in response to the ET or SIT exercise interventions. Historically, ET appears to be the most effective exercise modality for the reduction of abdominal VAT, as shown by a recent meta-analysis and systematic review [13]. Currently, data for the effect of SIT on VAT remain sparse, especially in combination with whole-body FM data. However, similar to our study, others have also reported no effect of SIT on trunk fat (via DXA) [17]. While data are lacking for the effects of SIT on abdominal VAT (CT/MRI-derived) and/or trunk fat (DXA-derived), some interval-type exercise research has reported decreases in measures of central obesity [33, 34]. Hottenrott et al. [33] observed that a high-intensity running-based SIT program (4 × 30 min sessions with 30–120 s intervals) resulted in significant decreases in abdominal VAT; however, these authors used bioelectrical impedance for assessment of abdominal VAT rather than CT or MRI. Furthermore, although theoretically matched for training duration to an ET condition, the SIT condition included greater training frequency and a substantial incorporation of ET, thus raising questions as to whether it was the isolated effect of SIT *per se*. In using similar exercise methodology to our study, Trapp et al. [34] observed a significant reduction in trunk fat mass following a 20 min 3 d·wk^{-1} high-intensity intermittent sprint condition (cycles of 8 s sprint: 12 s recovery). While our interventions found no pre-to-post differences for abdominal VAT, the CON group marginally increased visceral FM. As such, it appears that ET and SIT may have potentially offset gain in VAT across the intervention period, siding with prior research that exercise may serve as a preventative tool against increases in VAT [35].

Equivocal and inconsistent evidence precludes current understanding of the capacity for exercise to decrease markers of chronic systemic inflammation. Some studies report no change in CRP or inflammatory cytokines following exercise intervention [20, 21, 26, 36, 37], while other studies report significant reductions [18–21, 38, 39]. Despite conflicting data to date, in studies where plasma concentrations of CRP and cytokine concentrations reductions are observed, ET appears the more effective modality [18, 19, 21, 39, 40]. The effects of SIT on positively influencing cytokine profile (reducing proinflammatory; increasing anti-inflammatory) are still uncertain. Leggate et al. [22] examined the effect of a 2 wk SIT intervention on inflammation and reported no change in TNF-α, IL-6, MCP-1, or IL-10, suggesting that SIT may be relatively ineffective in changing cytokine profile. The limited duration of their intervention would likely have promoted limited/no change in VAT and (theoretically) associated inflammation, which appears to be a consistent finding in other studies [1, 2, 5]. We opted to investigate a longer duration SIT intervention period in order to increase the likelihood of a reduction in VAT and thus associated proinflammatory cytokines (TNF-α, IL-6, CRP, and MCP-1). The lack of change in these measures may be explained by the lack of change in abdominal VAT. Further research is needed to verify whether exercise-induced reduction of VAT is essential for reduction of these markers, as our data are inconclusive to show such an effect.

In addition, we examined whether SIT (or ET) may have imparted an anti-inflammatory effect, as would be indicated via increased IL-10 concentrations after training [18, 20, 21, 40]. Despite no significant change denoted in IL-10 for this study, both P-SIT and ET exercise groups evidenced a trend for an increase. However, a large SD, due to large interindividual response variance may have precluded significance. Despite power analyses indicating n of 15 per group sufficient to yield statistical significance, and that recent studies have incorporated a similar [16] or smaller [10] sample sizes as this study, a larger sample size in our study may have further substantiated a limited effect of the exercise interventions. In addition, there is existing evidence that 12 wks may induce adaptations which are associated with enhanced metabolic and/or immune regulatory function, yet subsequent effects of these adaptations are not observed until ensuing periods (i.e., at 6 or 12 months). Thus, a limitation of the current study may also be that a longer time frame is required to impart a significant effect on body composition and related plasma inflammatory measures. An additional limitation to our study is that it cannot be ruled out that changes in habitual diet and physical activity may have influenced the study data. In this view, while we strongly emphasised the maintenance of diet and planned/incidental physical activity across the 12 wk period, it is possible that that there may have been some alteration in satiety (in response to the exercise) and/or a decrease in incidental activity given potential training-induced weariness/fatigue from the conducted exercise training sessions.

In undertaking SIT, participants are required to complete supramaximal sprint efforts which are metabolically anaerobic in nature and physically demanding given the involved intensity. Even though, SIT was well-tolerated in this study by all participants, with optimal study compliance and very low study attrition. Accordingly, this method of exercise may be favourable for adoption in the general public, obviously after thorough preexercise medical health screening. Nevertheless, further research is needed to identify a more appropriate means of monitoring the interplay between exercise intensity and cardiovascular work given that, in SIT exercise, participants are undertaking exercise with maximal exertion, yet with delay in the heart rate response. Accordingly, relative submaximal HR_{max} criteria arguably appear redundant given our observation that most participants did not breach 85% HR_{max} until the conclusion of or immediately after interval.

In conclusion, 12 wks of ET, P-SIT, or A-SIT in an overweight middle-aged male population appeared ineffective in altering whole-body FM, abdominal VAT, or plasma markers underlying chronic systemic inflammation. The lack of change in body composition and abdominal VAT may underline the lack of change in the inflammatory markers. Aligning with previous research, this study has shown P-SIT to promote comparable cardiorespiratory fitness improvements to that of ET. However, it is worth emphasising that the present fitness improvements were based on the use of participant's baseline data with VO_{2peak} as the covariate. However, given that the A-SIT condition presented evidence of a diminished conditioning response in comparison to P-SIT, questions are raised regarding the use of "active" recovery periods in SIT programs involving deconditioned cohorts. Further research may be warranted in examining whether inhibitory mechanisms may be involved in A-SIT versus P-SIT in initially sedentary or deconditioned adults.

Competing Interests

There are no competing interests associated with this manuscript.

Acknowledgments

This study was funded solely by an Internal Charles Sturt University Research Grant. The research team would like to thank the participants for volunteering their time for this study. They would also like to acknowledge the Institutional Staff for their technical assistance.

References

[1] L. Fontana, J. C. Eagon, M. E. Trujillo, P. E. Scherer, and S. Klein, "Visceral fat adipokine secretion is associated with systemic inflammation in obese humans," *Diabetes*, vol. 56, no. 4, pp. 1010–1013, 2007.

[2] G. S. Hotamisligil, N. S. Shargill, and B. M. Spiegelman, "Adipose expression of tumor necrosis factor-α: direct role in obesity-linked insulin resistance," *Science*, vol. 259, no. 5091, pp. 87–91, 1993.

[3] S. A. Lear, K. H. Humphries, S. Kohli, A. Chockalingam, J. J. Frohlich, and C. L. Birmingham, "Visceral adipose tissue accumulation differs according to ethnic background: results of the Multicultural Community Health Assessment Trial (M-CHAT)," *The American Journal of Clinical Nutrition*, vol. 86, no. 2, pp. 353–359, 2007.

[4] H. C. McGill Jr., C. A. McMahan, E. E. Herderick et al., "Obesity accelerates the progression of coronary atherosclerosis in young men," *Circulation*, vol. 105, no. 23, pp. 2712–2718, 2002.

[5] J.-P. Després and I. Lemieux, "Abdominal obesity and metabolic syndrome," *Nature*, vol. 444, no. 7121, pp. 881–887, 2006.

[6] W. L. Haskell, I.-M. Lee, R. R. Pate et al., "Physical activity and public health: updated recommendation for adults from the American College of Sports Medicine and the American Heart Association," *Circulation*, vol. 116, no. 9, pp. 1081–1093, 2007.

[7] M. J. Gibala and S. L. McGee, "Metabolic adaptations to short-term high-intensity interval training: a little pain for a lot of gain?" *Exercise and Sport Sciences Reviews*, vol. 36, no. 2, pp. 58–63, 2008.

[8] K. A. Burgomaster, K. R. Howarth, S. M. Phillips et al., "Similar metabolic adaptations during exercise after low volume sprint interval and traditional endurance training in humans," *Journal of Physiology*, vol. 586, no. 1, pp. 151–160, 2008.

[9] M. J. Gibala, J. P. Little, M. van Essen et al., "Short-term sprint interval versus traditional endurance training: similar initial adaptations in human skeletal muscle and exercise performance," *Journal of Physiology*, vol. 575, no. 3, pp. 901–911, 2006.

[10] R. E. K. Macpherson, T. J. Hazell, T. D. Olver, D. H. Paterson, and P. W. R. Lemon, "Run sprint interval training improves aerobic performance but not maximal cardiac output," *Medicine and Science in Sports and Exercise*, vol. 43, no. 1, pp. 115–122, 2011.

[11] J. A. Babraj, N. B. J. Vollaard, C. Keast, F. M. Guppy, G. Cottrell, and J. A. Timmons, "Extremely short duration high intensity interval training substantially improves insulin action in young healthy males," *BMC Endocrine Disorders*, vol. 9, article 3, 2009.

[12] J. E. Donnelly, S. N. Blair, J. M. Jakicic, M. M. Manore, J. W. Rankin, and B. K. Smith, "Appropriate physical activity intervention strategies for weight loss and prevention of weight regain for adults," *Medicine & Science in Sports & Exercise*, vol. 41, no. 2, pp. 459–471, 2009.

[13] I. Ismail, S. E. Keating, M. K. Baker, and N. A. Johnson, "A systematic review and meta-analysis of the effect of aerobic vs. resistance exercise training on visceral fat," *Obesity Reviews*, vol. 13, no. 1, pp. 68–91, 2012.

[14] R. J. Verheggen, M. F. Maessen, D. J. Green, A. R. Hermus, M. T. Hopman, and D. H. Thijssen, "A systematic review and meta-analysis on the effects of exercise training versus hypocaloric diet: distinct effects on body weight and visceral adipose tissue," *Obesity Reviews*, vol. 17, no. 8, pp. 664–690, 2016.

[15] H. Zhang, T. K. Tong, W. Qiu, J. Wang, J. Nie, and Y. He, "Effect of high-intensity interval training protocol on abdominal fat reduction in overweight Chinese women: a randomized controlled trial," *Kineziologija*, vol. 47, no. 1, pp. 57–66, 2015.

[16] S. E. Keating, E. A. Machan, H. T. O'Connor et al., "Continuous exercise but not high intensity interval training improves fat distribution in overweight adults," *Journal of Obesity*, vol. 2014, Article ID 834865, 12 pages, 2014.

[17] B. J. Sawyer, *Effects of eight weeks of high-intensity interval training on blood glucose regulation, endothelial function, and visceral fat in obese adults [thesis]*, Arizona State University, Tempe, Ariz, USA, 2013.

[18] E. Goldhammer, A. Tanchilevitch, I. Maor, Y. Beniamini, U. Rosenschein, and M. Sagiv, "Exercise training modulates cytokines activity in coronary heart disease patients," *International Journal of Cardiology*, vol. 100, no. 1, pp. 93–99, 2005.

[19] M. L. Kohut, D. A. McCann, D. W. Russell et al., "Aerobic exercise, but not flexibility/resistance exercise, reduces serum IL-18, CRP, and IL-6 independent of β-blockers, BMI, and psychosocial factors in older adults," *Brain, Behavior, and Immunity*, vol. 20, no. 3, pp. 201–209, 2006.

[20] S. Balducci, S. Zanuso, A. Nicolucci et al., "Anti-inflammatory effect of exercise training in subjects with type 2 diabetes and the metabolic syndrome is dependent on exercise modalities and independent of weight loss," *Nutrition, Metabolism and Cardiovascular Diseases*, vol. 20, no. 8, pp. 608–617, 2010.

[21] K. M. Beavers, T. E. Brinkley, and B. J. Nicklas, "Effect of exercise training on chronic inflammation," *Clinica Chimica Acta*, vol. 411, no. 11-12, pp. 785–793, 2010.

[22] M. Leggate, W. G. Carter, M. J. C. Evans, R. A. Vennard, S. Sribala-Sundaram, and M. A. Nimmo, "Determination of inflammatory and prominent proteomic changes in plasma and adipose tissue after high-intensity intermittent training in overweight and obese males," *Journal of Applied Physiology*, vol. 112, no. 8, pp. 1353–1360, 2012.

[23] R. J. Gibbons, G. J. Balady, J. T. Bricker et al., "ACC/AHA 2002 guideline update for exercise testing: summary article: a report of the American College of Cardiology/American Heart Association Task Force on Practice Guidelines (committee to update the 1997 exercise testing guidelines)," *Journal of the American College of Cardiology*, vol. 40, no. 8, pp. 1531–1540, 2002.

[24] O. Inbar, A. Oren, M. Scheinowitz, A. Rotstein, R. Dlin, and R. Casaburi, "Normal cardiopulmonary responses during incremental exercise in 20-to 70-yr-old men," *Medicine & Science in Sports & Exercise*, vol. 26, no. 5, pp. 538–546, 1994.

[25] C. Couillard, N. Bergeron, D. Prud'homme et al., "Gender difference in postprandial lipemia: Importance of visceral adipose tissue accumulation," *Arteriosclerosis, Thrombosis, and Vascular Biology*, vol. 19, no. 10, pp. 2448–2455, 1999.

[26] C. E. Donges, R. Duffield, and E. J. Drinkwater, "Effects of resistance or aerobic exercise training on interleukin-6, C-reactive protein, and body composition," *Medicine and Science in Sports and Exercise*, vol. 42, no. 2, pp. 304–313, 2010.

[27] F. Faul, E. Erdfelder, A.-G. Lang, and A. Buchner, "G* Power 3: a flexible statistical power analysis program for the social, behavioral, and biomedical sciences," *Behavior Research Methods*, vol. 39, no. 2, pp. 175–191, 2007.

[28] G. A. Nader, "Concurrent strength and endurance training: from molecules to man," *Medicine and Science in Sports and Exercise*, vol. 38, no. 11, pp. 1965–1970, 2006.

[29] J. Helgerud, K. Hoydal, E. Wang et al., "Aerobic high-intensity intervals improve $V^{\bullet}O_{2max}$ more than moderate training," *Medicine & Science in Sports & Exercise*, vol. 39, no. 4, pp. 665–671, 2007.

[30] L. V. Billat, "Interval training for performance: a scientific and empirical practice," *Sports Medicine*, vol. 31, no. 1, pp. 13–31, 2001.

[31] D. MacAuley, A. Bauman, and P. Frémont, "Exercise: not a miracle cure, just good medicine," *The British Medical Journal*, vol. 350, no. 416, pp. 1107–1108, 2015.

[32] K. G. M. Alberti, P. Zimmet, J. Shaw, and IDF Epidemiology Task Force Consensus Group, "The metabolic syndrome—a new worldwide definition," *The Lancet*, vol. 366, no. 9491, pp. 1059–1062, 2005.

[33] K. Hottenrott, S. Ludyga, and S. Schulze, "Effects of high intensity training and continuous endurance training on aerobic capacity and body composition in recreationally active runners," *Journal of Sports Science and Medicine*, vol. 11, no. 3, pp. 483–488, 2012.

[34] E. G. Trapp, D. J. Chisholm, J. Freund, and S. H. Boutcher, "The effects of high-intensity intermittent exercise training on fat loss and fasting insulin levels of young women," *International Journal of Obesity*, vol. 32, no. 4, pp. 684–691, 2008.

[35] G. R. Hunter, D. W. Brock, N. M. Byrne, P. C. Chandler-Laney, P. Del Corral, and B. A. Gower, "Exercise training prevents regain of visceral fat for 1 year following weight loss," *Obesity*, vol. 18, no. 4, pp. 690–695, 2010.

[36] T. Christiansen, S. K. Paulsen, J. M. Bruun, S. B. Pedersen, and B. Richelsen, "Exercise training versus diet-induced weight-loss on metabolic risk factors and inflammatory markers in obese subjects: a 12-week randomized intervention study," *American Journal of Physiology—Endocrinology and Metabolism*, vol. 298, no. 4, pp. E824–E831, 2010.

[37] S. R. Gray, G. Baker, A. Wright, C. F. Fitzsimons, N. Mutrie, and M. A. Nimmo, "The effect of a 12 week walking intervention on markers of insulin resistance and systemic inflammation," *Preventive Medicine*, vol. 48, no. 1, pp. 39–44, 2009.

[38] C. E. Donges, R. Duffield, K. J. Guelfi, G. C. Smith, D. R. Adams, and J. A. Edge, "Comparative effects of single-mode vs. duration-matched concurrent exercise training on body composition, low-grade inflammation, and glucose regulation in sedentary, overweight, middle-aged men," *Applied Physiology, Nutrition and Metabolism*, vol. 38, no. 7, pp. 779–788, 2013.

[39] S. M. Abd El-Kader, "Aerobic versus resistance exercise training in modulation of insulin resistance, adipocytokines and inflammatory cytokine levels in obese type 2 diabetic patients," *Journal of Advanced Research*, vol. 2, no. 2, pp. 179–183, 2011.

[40] N. P. E. Kadoglou, F. Iliadis, N. Angelopoulou et al., "The anti-inflammatory effects of exercise training in patients with type 2 diabetes mellitus," *European Journal of Cardiovascular Prevention and Rehabilitation*, vol. 14, no. 6, pp. 837–843, 2007.

3

Obesity Might Be a Predictor of Weight Reduction after Smoking Cessation

Charlotta Pisinger,[1] Helle Øster Nielsen,[2] Caroline Kuhlmann,[2] and Susanne Rosthøj[3]

[1] *Research Centre for Prevention and Health, Glostrup Hospital, Building 84/85, 2600 Glostrup, Denmark*
[2] *Faculty of Health and Medical Sciences, University of Copenhagen, 1123 Copenhagen K, Denmark*
[3] *Section of Biostatistics, Institute of Public Health, University of Copenhagen, 1014 Copenhagen, Denmark*

Correspondence should be addressed to Caroline Kuhlmann; carolinekuhlmann@live.dk

Academic Editor: Chris I. Ardern

Background and Objectives. Approximately one in five ex-smokers reduces or maintains weight after smoking cessation but little is known about who succeeds to avoid weight gain. The purpose of this study was to identify predictors of weight reduction after long-term smoking cessation in a general population. *Methods.* Data was obtained from two Danish population-based cohorts (the Inter99 and the Helbred2006 study). Anthropometric measurements were performed by trained research staff. Out of 3.577 daily smokers at baseline 317 participants had quit smoking at the five-year follow-up for at least one year. Multiple logistic regression analysis was performed to determine predictors of weight reduction. *Results.* Thirteen percent reduced weight by at least 1 kg and 4% maintained their weight. Quitters with obesity had more than seven times higher odds than normal weight quitters to lose weight (OR 7.13 (95% CI 2.76–19.71)), and they had the largest median weight loss of 4.45 kg. The only other significant predictor of weight reduction was low tobacco consumption at baseline. *Conclusions.* Predictors of weight reduction after smoking cessation were high body mass index and low tobacco consumption at baseline. This study might motivate smokers with obesity to quit smoking and health professionals to give them support.

1. Introduction

Tobacco kills nearly six million people each year worldwide and unless action is taken, the annual death toll could increase to more than eight million by 2030 [1]. The benefits of smoking cessation are huge both when it comes to reduction of risk of specific diseases and to a substantial life extension [2]. Smoking cessation is one of the most cost-effective methods to prevent disease in a population [3] and it is estimated that smokers require $ 1,046 each year in additional health care expenses compared to nonsmokers [4]. Even though about three out of four smokers wish to quit [5] many smokers experience barriers when it comes to serious quit attempts. A fear of weight gain is one of the concerns reported by many smokers and weight gain is also a frequent reason given by those who relapse [6, 7].

Smokers gain weight after they quit smoking mainly because of the removal of nicotine's effects on the central nervous system [8]. Adult smokers weigh, on average, approx. 4 kg less than nonsmokers and ex-smokers gain on average the "missing" 4-5 kg after smoking cessation [9]. The mechanisms of weight gain after smoking cessation are complex and include increased appetite and energy intake, increased intake of sugar, decreased resting metabolic rate, and increased lipoprotein lipase activity [10], but the molecular mechanisms are not fully understood. Animal studies have shown that nicotine significantly decreased body weight and food intake via a decrease in meal size and a longer intermeal interval [11]. Nicotine increases energy expenditure both by direct effects on peripheral tissues, largely mediated by catecholamines, and by effects on central nervous system neuroendocrine circuits. The effect of nicotine on the brain also leads to suppression of appetite, and smoking per se (hand to mouth behaviour) can serve as an alternative to eating [12].

Limited information has been reported in relation to maintenance or reduction of weight after smoking cessation, even though up to one out of five ex-smokers actually reduce or maintain weight after smoking cessation [13]. Many studies have investigated predictors of weight gain but to our knowledge only one study has identified predictors for weight loss after smoking cessation [14]. The unilateral focus on weight gain might have contributed to the misunderstanding in the general population that weight gain is an inevitable consequence of smoking cessation.

Two more recent Danish population-based studies followed smokers over a period of five years, giving us the opportunity to explore the topic of weight reduction after smoking cessation.

The aim of this study was to identify predictors for weight reduction after long-term smoking cessation. Furthermore, we wanted to determine the proportion of ex-smokers with weight reduction or maintenance after smoking cessation and the median weight reduction over a five-year period.

2. Materials and Methods

2.1. Study Design and Participants. The study population is based on data from two population-based cohorts, the Inter99 study and the Helbred2006 study. The two studies included persons living in the south-western area of Copenhagen randomly selected from the Danish Civil Registration System and took place at Research Centre for Prevention and Health, Rigshospitalet-Glostrup. A written consent form was obtained from all participants. Both studies were approved by the Ethical Committee of Copenhagen County. The Helbred2006 study was approved by the Danish Data Protection Agency and the Inter99 study was approved by the Danish Health and Medicines Authority.

The Inter99 study is the largest randomized lifestyle intervention study in Denmark (1999–2006) including 61,301 persons aged 30–60 years. The aim of the Inter99 study was to assess the effect of a preventive strategy including individualized risk assessment; multifactorial nonpharmacological intervention based on tailored information, motivation, and support; and a programme for maintenance [15]. The subjects were prerandomized into control group (n = 48,285; no data on smoking or weight available) or intervention group (n = 13,016). Eighty-two persons had died, disappeared, or emigrated, leaving 12,934 for invitation in the intervention group. Out of these, 6,784 participants were included (inclusion = day of first examination). Participation rate (= attended the baseline visit) was 52.5%; 2,804 were daily smokers at baseline. Participation rate at 5-year follow-up visit (2004–2006) was 69.2%. The Inter99 study is described in detail elsewhere by Jorgensen et al. [15].

The aim of the Helbred2006 study (2006–2008) including 7,931 persons aged 18–69 years was to investigate prevalence and predictors of lifestyle-related chronic diseases such as coronary heart disease, diabetes, musculoskeletal disorders, asthma, allergy, chronic lung diseases, and mental disorders. Out of the almost eight thousand invited, 3,471 persons attended the baseline visit; participation rate was 44.7% (same definition as above); 773 were daily smokers at baseline. Participation rate at 5-year follow-up visit (2011) was 66.5%. Further details about the Helbred2006 cohort are described by Thuesen et al. [16].

All participants in both studies completed a questionnaire about health, lifestyle, and sociodemographic factors at inclusion. Anthropometric measurements (e.g., weight and height) performed by trained research staff were obtained.

A total of 3,577 (2,804 + 773) daily smokers were included in both studies at baseline. This paper is based on the 262 daily smokers in the Inter99 study and the 55 in the Helbred2006 study (total n = 317) who reported that they had quit smoking for at least 12 months at the five-year follow-up, independently of smoking status at other follow-up visits (minimal length of smoking abstinence being 12 months and maximal up to five years).

2.2. Variables. Weight reduction was defined as ≥1 kg lower weight at five-year follow-up than at baseline. Weight maintenance was defined as having the same or <1 kg lower weight at five-year follow-up than at baseline.

Weight gain was defined as increased weight at the five-year-follow-up compared to baseline.

Tobacco consumption was measured in grams of tobacco in the following way: one cigarette/gram of pipe tobacco = 1 gram, one cheroot/cigarillo = 3 grams, and one cigar = 5 grams. Light smokers were defined as smoking ≤15 cigarettes daily and heavy smokers >15 cigarettes daily, a common cut-point in tobacco related studies.

Height was measured without shoes to the nearest cm. Weight was measured without shoes and overcoat to the nearest kg and body mass index (BMI) was calculated (kg/m^2). BMI was divided into three categories: normal weight (<24.9), overweight (25–29.9), and obese (>30 kg/m^2).

Sociodemographic variables were self-reported: socioeconomic status (SES) defined by the length of completed vocational training/academic education (low: <2 years/medium: 2–4 years/high: >4 years).

Lifestyle variables were self-reported at baseline. Dietary quality score, a three-classed variable, was generated for each of the four food-groups (fish, vegetable, fruit, and fat) from a 52-item food frequency questionnaire. Summation of the four variables resulted in a score ranging from zero to eight. Subsequently participants were categorized into three classes: healthy dietary habits (score 7–9), average dietary habits score 4–6), and unhealthy dietary habits (score 1–3). The dietary quality score has previously been validated (see also the discussion section) [17]. Physical activity at baseline was based on leisure time physical activity: "During leisure time, which statement best describes your physical activity?" (read, watch TV, or be engaged in other sedentary activity/go for a walk, use your bike, or perform light physical activity for at least 4 hours a week/active athlete or performing heavy gardening, housework, etc., at least 3 times a week/vigorous training or participation in competitive sports several times a week), categorized into two groups (insufficiently active and active (light activity, moderate activity, and vigorous activity))

[18]. Alcohol consumption at baseline was calculated by adding the mean weekly intake of units of beer, strong beer, liquor, wine, and spirits in the last 12 months. Consumption was categorized to three groups (≤7, 8–14, and >14 units alcohol per week).

2.3. Statistical Analysis. Proportions or medians were used to describe the characteristics of the study population. Proportions were compared across subgroups using the Pearson chi-square or the Fisher exact test and the Kruskal-Wallis test was used to compare quantitative variables.

Multiple logistic regression analysis was performed to determine the associations between weight reduction and the explanatory variables. The analyses included BMI, tobacco consumption, lifestyle variables (diet, physical activity, and alcohol), sociodemographic variables (SES, sex, and age), and cohort. Possible interactions between cohort and the remaining explanatory variables were investigated, but no such interactions were found in any of the models.

To identify a set of predictive explanatory variables, a reduced model was defined using the Allen-Cady modified backwards selection procedure [19]. The explanatory variables were ranked by importance and in each step, the risk factor with the lowest rank was excluded from the model if the corresponding p value was below 0.05. The procedure ends when the explanatory variable with the lowest rank cannot be eliminated from the model. In this procedure the explanatory variables were ranked in the following order: BMI, tobacco consumption, lifestyle variables (diet, physical activity, and alcohol), sociodemographic variables (SES, sex, and age), and cohort.

To evaluate the discriminatory power of the models, the area (AUC) under the receiver operating characteristic curve (ROC) was determined for the logistic regression models.

To assess the robustness of the results, the analysis based on the reduced regression model was repeated using the outcome variable "no weight gain" (maintained or reduced weight).

Statistical analyses were performed using SAS version 9.2 (SAS Institute, Cary, NC, USA). The level of significance was set to 5%.

3. Results

Of those who were daily smokers at baseline 8.9 percent had been abstinent from smoking for at least 12 months at the five-year follow-up (317 out of 3,577). A total of 262 (82.6%) of the ex-smokers had gained weight at five-year follow-up, 41 (13%) had reduced weight by ≥1 kg, and 14 (4%) had maintained their weight.

The 41 ex-smokers who had reduced weight had a significantly higher BMI and lighter intensity of smoking at baseline than those who did not reduce weight. There were no significant differences regarding age, sex, SES, cohort, or lifestyle (Table 1). The median weight change in all ex-smokers was an increase of 5.0 kg (IQR 1.6–8.9). The median weight reduction was 3.5 kg (IQR 2.1–5.5) in those who had a weight reduction of at least 1 kg at five-year follow-up. Only tobacco consumption and cohort were associated with the size of the weight reduction, whereas BMI was borderline associated with the size of the weight reduction ($p = 0.06$) (Table 2).

In the reduced multiple logistic regression model, BMI and tobacco consumption were the only predictors of the outcome (Table 3). The effects of these two predictors were similar in the full and the reduced model.

The ROC curve analysis showed the predictive value (AUC) of the reduced model to be 0.72 (CI 95% 0.63–0.80), corresponding to a "fair" predictive value. The odds of reducing weight for heavy ex-smokers were reduced with two-thirds compared to light ex-smokers. Ex-smokers with obesity had more than seven times higher odds and overweight ex-smokers almost three times higher odds of weight reduction than those with normal weights (Table 3).

The robustness of the results analysis of the reduced logistic regression model considering "no weight gain" (weight reduction/maintenance) as outcome thereby increasing the number of cases from 41 to 55 showed attenuated effect of obesity (OR 5.03 (CI 95% 1.90–13.32)) but not of overweight (OR 2.27 (CI 95% 1.02–5.00)). Heavy smokers at baseline had less than half the chance of weight reduction/maintenance compared to heavy smokers (OR 0.42 (CI 95% 0.20–0.89)).

4. Discussion

This population-based study found that almost one in six persons who had quit smoking for at least one year had lost or maintained their weight. A predictor of weight reduction was a high BMI at baseline, even when adjusted for lifestyle factors and socioeconomic status. Quitters with obesity had more than seven times higher odds than normal weight quitters to lose weight. Of those of the quitters who lost weight after smoking cessation, persons with obesity at baseline had the largest median weight loss of 4.45 kg (Table 1). The only other predictor of weight reduction was low tobacco consumption at baseline, whereas baseline lifestyle factors, sex, age, and socioeconomic status, and cohort were not found to be associated with weight reduction.

A meta-analysis based on 62 studies found that 16 to 21% of ex-smokers had lost or maintained their weight [13] and a Cochrane review from 2012 found that 13% had lost weight [9]. This corresponds very well with the 13% who lost weight by ≥1 kg, and the 4% who maintained their weight in our study. The smoke-free follow-up period was 12 months in both reviews, whereas it was minimum one and up to five years in our study, so we had a longer follow-up and cessation period. For comparison, 31.4% of the whole Inter99 study population (6.784 smokers, ex-smokers, and never-smokers at baseline) had lost weight by ≥1 kg at 5-year follow-up. It is well-known that most smokers gain weight when they quit.

Predictors of weight *gain* found in previous studies have been female sex, younger age, lower socioeconomic status, and being African-American descent [8, 13, 20–22]. These factors were not significantly associated with weight loss in our study but the tendency was pointing in the same direction (ethnicity was not tested due to low number of persons with other ethnicity than Danish). Neither were cohorts, diet, or

Table 1: Baseline characteristic of ex-smokers with long-term abstinence at five-year follow-up ($N = 317$).

Baseline variables	Weight reduction min. 1 kg No (%) 276 (87)	Weight reduction min. 1 kg Yes (%) 41 (13)	*p* value
Body mass index kg/m^2			**<0.01**
Obese BMI ≥ 30	31 (11.2)	12 (29)	
Overweight BMI 25–29.9	107 (38.8)	20 (49)	
Normal weight BMI 18,5–24.9	138 (50.0)	9 (22)	
Tobacco consumption			**0.02**
Light smoker < 15 g tobacco/day	139 (50.6)	29 (70.7)	
Heavy smoker ≥ 15 g tobacco/day	136 (49.5)	12 (29.3)	
	Missing n = 1		
Cohort			*0.17
Inter1999	228 (82.6)	34 (82.9)	
Health2006	48 (17.4)	7 (17.1)	
Socioeconomic status (length of education)			0.41
High (>4 years)	27 (10.9)	7 (17.9)	
Middle (2–4 years)	180 (72.6)	25 (65.1)	
Low (<2 years)	41 (16.5)	7 (17.9)	
	Missing n = 30		
Sex			0.68
Male	151 (54.7)	21 (51.2)	
Female	125 (45.3)	20 (48.8)	
Age groups			0.85
18–39 years	40 (14.5)	5 (12.2)	
40–49 years	120 (43.5)	17 (41.5)	
50–69 years	116 (42)	19 (46.3)	
Diet score			0.53
Healthy (7–9)	26 (9.5)	6 (16.6)	
Average (4–6)	201 (74.2)	30 (73.1)	
Unhealthy (1–3)	44 (16.2)	5 (12.2)	
	Missing n = 5		
Physical activity (leisure time)			0.84
Active	211 (77)	31 (75.6)	
Insufficiently active	63 (23)	10 (24.4)	
	Missing n = 2		
Alcohol units per week			0.42
>14	82 (33.3)	10 (26.3)	
8–14	56 (22.7)	7 (18.4)	
≤7	105 (42.7)	20 (52.6)	
	Missing n = 33		

*Fischer's exact test.

physical activity at baseline significant predictors of weight loss.

Several studies have reported a high prequit tobacco consumption or high nicotine addiction to be positively associated with weight gain [8, 23]. This supports our finding of more than 60% increased odds of weight loss in persons with low tobacco consumption.

To our knowledge, only one previous study has investigated predictors of weight *reduction* after smoking cessation [14]. This study from 1980 followed over 1700 adult males over five years and found, exactly like we did, that postcessation weight loss was associated with lighter smoking and "stoutness of build." Strong conclusions cannot be drawn, based on two studies only, but it is interesting that a study performed more than 30 years ago concluded the same.

As previous studies have found that persons with obesity experience the largest weight gain [24, 25] it was surprising that we found that persons with obesity had the highest odds of weight reduction and the highest mean weight loss in our study. However, the findings are not irreconcilable. First of

Table 2: Baseline characteristics of ex-smokers at five year follow-up with a weight reduction of minimum 1 kg ($N = 41$).

Baseline variables	N	Weight loss (%)		Weight reduction (kg)		p-value
		Median (upper-lower quartile)	Mean	Median (upper-lower quartile)	Mean	
Body Mass Index kg/m^2						0.06
Obese BMI ≥ 30	12	4.98 (2.8–10.9)	8.04	4.45 (2.6–10.9)	7.37	
Overweight BMI 25–29.9	20	5.37 (2.7–6.9)	6.08	4.15 (2.1–5.7)	4.93	
Normal weight BMI 18,5–24.9	9	3.25 (2.4–4.9)	3.61	2.30 (1.6–2.9)	2.37	
Tobacco consumption						**<0.01**
Light ≤ 15 g tobacco/day	29	3.25 (2.6–5.9)	4.59	2.50 (1.9–4.4)	3.50	
Heavy > 15 g tobacco/day	12	6.18 (4.8–14.6)	9.79	5.10 (3.7–15.4)	8.92	
Cohort						**0.04**
Inter99	34	4.96 (2.8–7.2)	6.69	3.65 (2.2–5.9)	5.61	
Health2006	7	2.92 (1.4–5.7)	3.29	1.90 (1.2–4.3)	2.53	
Socioeconomic Status (length of education)						0.24
High (>4 years)	7	7.16 (2.7–13.7)	7.49	4.70 (2.1–13.8)	7.16	
Middle (2–4 years)	25	3.59 (2.6–5.7)	5.21	3.00 (1.9–4.4)	3.99	
Low (<2 years)	7	5.73 (4.0–7.8)	7.73	4.20 (3.6–6.1)	6.69	
	Missing $n = 2$					
Sex						0.28
Male	21	4.55 (2.8–7.8)	6.44	3.70 (2.2–6.1)	5.92	
Female	20	4.76 (2.6–6.4)	5.76	2.95 (1.9–4.6)	4.21	
Age groups						0.54
18–39 years	5	4.91 (2.0–6.6)	4.72	2.50 (1.6–5.5)	3.80	
40–49 years	17	4.61 (3.5–6.6)	6.40	3.60 (3.0–5.9)	5.49	
50–69 years	19	3.25 (2.6–6.2)	6.22	2.30 (1.9–4.7)	5.06	
Diet score						0.30
Healthy (7–9)	6	3.61 (2.0–5.7)	3.73	2.40 (1.4–4.2)	2.67	
Average (4–6)	30	4.25 (2.8–6.6)	6.24	3.55 (2.1–5.8)	5.33	
Unhealthy (1–3)	5	5.00 (4.9–8.1)	8.18	4.10 (2.5–8.1)	6.54	
Physical activity (leisure time)						0.72
Active	31	3.95 (2.6–6.6)	5.85	5.20 (1.9–5.5)	4.89	
Insufficiently active	10	4.96 (3.1–8.1)	6.92	3.40 (2.3–8.1)	5.69	
Alcohol units per week						0.29
>14	10	2.90 (2.0–5.7)	4.77	2.15 (1.6–4.3)	3.65	
8–14	7	7.16 (2.7–13.7)	7.53	4.70 (2.1–13.8)	7.17	
≤7	21	4.76 (2.8–6.0)	6.38	3.50 (2.2–4.4)	5.12	
	Missing $n = 3$					
Ex-smokers with weight reduction	41	4.61 (2.6–6.6)	6.11	3.50 (2.1–5.5)	5.09	

all, the studies (including ours) have used BMI (or weight) as proxy for obesity which does not distinguish between fat and musculature. The above-mentioned "stoutness of build" [14] might reflect that persons with postcessation weight loss were more muscular than fat. Second, even though most persons with obesity will gain weight some persons with obesity might be very determined not to put on additional weight after quitting smoking whereas most normal/low-weight smokers have been able to eat more or less what they desired as long as they smoked and therefore did not reduce intake of fattening food items or calories after they have quit. Also, regression towards the mean might be an attributing factor.

Unfortunately, several smoking cessation programs focusing on weight have resulted in lower quit rates [26, 27] so introducing weight-control in a smoking cessation program might actually undermine the effect of it. A Cochrane

TABLE 3: Predictors of ex-smokers' weight reduction after five years. Model 1 including all tested predictors. Model 4 including final predictors.

Baseline variables	Model 1 incl. all explanatory variables ($N = 257$) Estimate OR	CI 95%	p value	Overall test	Model 4 ($N = 316$) Estimate OR	CI 95%	p value	Overall test
Heavy smoker	0.37	(0.16–0.86)	**0.02**	**0.02**	0.34	(0.16–0.72)	**<0.01**	**<0.01**
Light smoker (ref.)	1.00				1.00			
Obese	7.13	(2.46–20.69)	**<0.01**	**0.00**	7.38	(2.76–19.71)	**<0.01**	**<0.01**
Overweight	2.72	(1.10–6.73)	**0.03**		3.10	(1.34–7.16)	**0.01**	
Normal weight (ref.)	1.00				1.00			
Inter99	1.25	(0.43–3.65)	0.68	0.68	—	—	—	
Health2006 (ref.)	1.00							
High socioeconomic status	0.85	(0.23–3.23)	0.81	0.59	—	—	—	
Middle socioeconomic status	0.60	(0.21–1.77)	0.36		—	—	—	
Low socioeconomic status (ref.)	1.00				—	—	—	
Male	1.37	(0.59–3.18)	0.47	0.47	—	—	—	
Female (ref.)	1.00				—	—	—	
Age (years)	1.02	(0.98–1.08)	0.34	0.34	—	—	—	
Healthy diet	1.36	(0.30–6.23)	0.70	0.82	—	—	—	
Average diet	0.94	(0.28–3.22)	0.93		—	—	—	
Unhealthy diet (ref.)	1.00				—	—	—	
Active (physical activity)	0.65	(0.25–1.67)	0.37	0.38	—	—	—	
Insufficiently active (ref.)	1.00				—	—	—	
>14 alcohol units/week	0.68	(0.27–1.67)	0.40	0.47	—	—	—	
8–14 alcohol units/week	0.56	(0.29–1.59)	0.28		—	—	—	
≤7 alcohol units/week (ref.)	1.00				—	—	—	
ROC	AUC	CI 95%			AUC	CI 95%		
Predictive value	0.72	(0.63–0.80)			0.75	(0.67–0.83)		

Area under the ROC-curve (AUC).

review identified exercise interventions (median −2.1 kg) and personalized weight management support (median −2.6 kg) as the only two effective treatments to prevent postcessation weight gain after one year, without undermining long-term quit rates. However, the review concluded that there are too few data to be sure [9]. It is important to have in mind that most trials aimed at preventing weight gain typically enrolled weight concerned women, which reduces their generalisability. Weight management education only, very low calorie intake, cognitive behavioural therapy to allay concern about weight gain, and pharmacotherapy for smoking cessation were not associated with long-term weight gain [9].

For many smokers, the anticipation of weight gain can hinder smoking cessation [28]. Unfortunately, we still experience overweight smokers report that health professionals have warned them not to quit, for example, after a myocardial infarction. Many health professionals have the misperception that obesity is a larger danger to health than smoking. The benefits of quitting smoking will however mostly outweight the risks of increased weight. It has been calculated that a postcessation weight gain of almost 16 BMI units (kg/m^2) is required for to offset the detrimental effect of continued smoking on coronary heart disease mortality. This corresponds to a weight gain of 42 kg (93 lb) for a woman 163 cm (64 in.) tall [29]. Health professionals should very early after smoking cessation detect people gaining excessive weight and intervene to prevent this by referring to exercise interventions and personalized weight management support. Results from this study need to be replicated but might hopefully motivate smokers with obesity and overweight to quit and health professionals to give them full support.

4.1. Weaknesses. The major weakness of this study is that out of many thousands of citizens included in two large population-based studies there were only few individuals/baseline-smokers who succeeded to quit smoking on long term and to lose weight. Results based on 41 persons must be interpreted with caution and analyses should be repeated in larger populations. Also, only a minority of persons with obesity are affected by these results.

A large weight gain might lead to smoking relapse, which would mean that those who put on large amounts of weight early in their quit attempt and relapsed were not represented by our data. People with obesity could be those with the lowest tolerance of weight gain and have high relapse rates early in the smoking cessation process, so only those who did not put on weight/lost weight are abstinent at long term. This selection-bias would highly influence our conclusions. However, no clear association between weight gain and the risk of relapse has been found [30]. We used point prevalence data in our analyses instead of continuous abstinence, but this should not affect the weight change estimates [13]. Waist circumference is found to be independently associated with cardiovascular disease, diabetes, and total mortality [31] and might have been a good alternative to BMI. Abstinence from smoking was self-reported (validation of abstinence was performed in the Inter99 study, but not the Helbred2006 study), which could lead to information-bias. This would be reflected in a lower weight gain in general but should not necessary influence our conclusions on predictors. By including only those who claimed long-term abstinence, we hope to have reduced this bias. It might be a weakness that we do not have the same length of abstinence for all participants; we measured long-term abstinence in order to look at long-term weight changes. Use of categories instead of quantitative variables imposes the risk of misclassification and reduces the power. Definition of BMI < 25 as normal weight misclassifies those who are underweight. Use of self-reported lifestyle variables might lead to underreporting of unhealthy lifestyle, especially in persons with obesity, thereby underestimating the influence of lifestyle. The dietary quality score has been shown to be associated with higher dietary quality in general, including a low intake of fat, especially saturated fat, a high intake of fiber, various vitamins and minerals, fruit, fish, vegetables, and whole-grain products and to be significantly negatively associated with total cholesterol, triglyceride, low-density lipoprotein-cholesterol, and the absolute risk of ischemic heart disease (in adjusted analyses). However, the score does not include information on sweets, sweetened beverages, or specific food as processed meet. There is a risk of underestimation of calorie intake. Physical activity at baseline was unfortunately based on leisure time physical activity only, thus underestimating energy consumption. Use of baseline lifestyle variables can be criticized as lifestyle might have changed during the long follow-up time, especially after quitting. Measuring socioeconomic status is very complex and each measurement has different strengths and weaknesses. There is no single best indicator of socioeconomic status but education has many strengths. We expected that participants in the Inter99 study, where all smokers were offered assistance to quit and all participants with obesity were offered group-based counselling to lose weight, had a higher probability of losing weight after smoking cessation. However, we did not find an association between cohort and weight reduction, which is in concordance with previous studies showing no difference in weight gain between trials that aimed to prevent weight gain after cessation and the treatment trials without this aim [5]. Defining weight loss we required a loss of 1 kg or more, to minimize measurement bias. There is no evidence for choosing this cut-off; mostly studies have only investigated if weight was higher/lower than before quitting smoking. As very few smokers had quit smoking for at least one year too few persons would have been included if the cut-off had been weight loss of, for example, 5% of body weight or more, which would be clinically more relevant. It is well-known that weight is not as stable as, for example, height, and weight cycling is rather common, especially among overweight persons, which also is a weakness in this study. The analysis of the reduced logistic regression model considering "no weight gain" (weight reduction/maintenance) as outcome thereby increasing the number of cases to 55 showed attenuated effect of obesity but not of overweight. The possibility of residual confounding due to unknown or unmeasured confounders always exists.

4.2. Strengths. Both cohorts were population-based and results therefore have a higher generalizability than results from randomized controlled trials on smoking cessation. We included a population of daily smokers to begin with to find the 371 persons with long-term abstinence from smoking, and compared to the existing literature we followed the cohorts for a long time. Information on weight and height was objectively measured by experienced health professionals. Analyses were consistent with or without inclusion of lifestyle- and sociodemographic factors and the cohort variable.

5. Conclusion

In two large Danish population-based cohorts we found that 13% had lost weight and 4% had maintained their weight after smoking cessation. A predictor of weight reduction was a high BMI, even when adjusted for lifestyle factors and socioeconomic status. Quitters with obesity had more than seven times higher odds than normal weight quitters to lose weight, and they had the largest median weight loss of 4.45 kg. The only other predictor of weight reduction was low tobacco consumption at baseline, whereas baseline lifestyle factors, sex, age, socioeconomic status, and cohort were not found to be associated with weight reduction. For many smokers, the anticipation of weight gain can hinder smoking cessation and many lay people and health professionals have the misperception that obesity is a larger danger to health than smoking. The benefits of quitting smoking will however mostly out-weight the risks of increased weight; almost 16 kg/m^2 BMI units is required for to offset the detrimental effect of smoking. Results from this study might hopefully motivate smokers with obesity and overweight to quit and health professionals to give them full support.

Disclosure

The researchers are independent of the founders who had no influence on study design, conduct, analyses, or interpretation of results. This manuscript is based on Helle Øster Nielsen's master thesis.

Authors' Contributions

Charlotta Pisinger was involved in the design of the Inter99 study and development of the intervention. Helle Øster

Nielsen, Susanne Rosthøj, and Charlotta Pisinger were all involved in design of the actual study. Helle Øster Nielsen analyzed data, assisted by Susanne Rosthøj. All discussed data analyses and interpretation and contributed to first version of the manuscript. Caroline Kuhlmann contributed to update of literature and revision of later versions of the manuscript. All critically revised the manuscript and approved the final version of the manuscript.

Acknowledgments

The authors thank the whole staff of the Inter99 study and the Helbred2006 study and all persons participating in these studies. The Inter99 study was initiated by Professor Torben Jorgensen, D.M.S. (principal investigator), Knut Borch-Johnsen, D.M.S. (principal investigator on the diabetes part), Troels Thomsen, Ph.D., and Hans Ibsen, D.M.S. The present steering committee of the Inter99 study are Professor Torben Jorgensen, D.M.S. (principal investigator), and Charlotta Pisinger, Ph.D. and M.P.H. The Helbred2006 study was initiated by Professor Torben Jorgensen, D.M.S. (principal investigator), Allan Linneberg. The Danish Health Foundation funded CP's work with this paper.

References

[1] WHO. Tobacco No. 339; 2016.

[2] R. Doll and R. Peto, "The causes of cancer: quantitative estimates of avoidable risks of cancer in the United States today," *Journal of the National Cancer Institute*, vol. 66, no. 6, pp. 1191–1308, 1981.

[3] R. Kahn, R. M. Robertson, R. Smith, and D. Eddy, "The impact of prevention on reducing the burden of cardiovascular disease," *Diabetes Care*, vol. 31, no. 8, pp. 1686–1696, 2008.

[4] T. Bush, J. C. Lovejoy, M. Deprey, and K. M. Carpenter, "The effect of tobacco cessation on weight gain, obesity, and diabetes risk," *Obesity (Silver Spring)*, vol. 24, no. 9, pp. 1834–1841, 2016.

[5] (DK) N. B. o. H. Danskernes Sundhed. Den Nationale Sundhedsprofil 2013, Copenhagen: National Board of Health; 2014.

[6] R. C. Klesges, A. W. Meyers, L. M. Klesges, and M. E. La Vasque, "Smoking, body weight, and their effects on smoking behavior: a comprehensive review of the literature," *Psychological Bulletin*, vol. 106, no. 2, pp. 204–230, 1989.

[7] R. C. Klesges and S. A. Shumaker, "Understanding the relations between smoking and body weight and their importance to smoking cessation and relapse," *Health Psychology*, vol. 11, supplement 1-3, 1992.

[8] M. Komiyama, H. Wada, S. Ura et al., "Analysis of factors that determine weight gain during smoking cessation therapy," *PLoS ONE*, vol. 8, no. 8, Article ID e72010, 2013.

[9] A. C. Farley, P. Hajek, D. Lycett, and P. Aveyard, "Interventions for preventing weight gain after smoking cessation," *Cochrane database of systematic reviews (Online)*, vol. 1, Article ID CD006219, 2012.

[10] C. Filozof, M. C. Fernandez Pinilla, and A. Fernandez-Cruz, "Smoking cessation and weight gain," *Obesity Reviews*, vol. 5, no. 2, pp. 95–103, 2005.

[11] G. Miyata, M. M. Meguid, M. Varma, S. O. Fetissov, and H. J. Kim, "Nicotine alters the usual reciprocity between meal size and meal number in female rat," *Physiology and Behavior*, vol. 74, no. 1-2, pp. 169–176, 2001.

[12] J. Audrain-Mcgovern and N. L. Benowitz, "Cigarette smoking, nicotine, and body weight," *Clinical Pharmacology and Therapeutics*, vol. 90, no. 1, pp. 164–168, 2011.

[13] H.-J. Aubin, A. Farley, D. Lycett, P. Lahmek, and P. Aveyard, "Weight gain in smokers after quitting cigarettes: meta-analysis," *BMJ (Online)*, vol. 345, Article ID e4439, 2012.

[14] R. Bosse, A. J. Garvey, and P. T. Costa Jr., "Predictors of weight change following smoking cessation," *International Journal of the Addictions*, vol. 15, no. 7, pp. 969–991, 1980.

[15] T. Jorgensen, K. Borch-Johnsen, T. F. Thomsen, H. Ibsen, C. Glumer, and C. Pisinger, "A randomized non-pharmacological intervention study for prevention of ischaemic heart disease: baseline results Inter99," *European Journal of Cardiovascular Prevention and Rehabilitation*, vol. 10, no. 5, pp. 377–386, 2003.

[16] B. H. Thuesen, C. Cerqueira, M. Aadahl et al., "Cohort profile: the health2006 cohort, research centre for prevention and health," *International Journal of Epidemiology*, vol. 43, no. 2, Article ID dyt009, pp. 568–575, 2014.

[17] U. Toft, L. H. Kristoffersen, C. Lau, K. Borch-Johnsen, and T. Jorgensen, "The dietary quality score: validation and association with cardiovascular risk factors: the inter99 study," *European Journal of Clinical Nutrition*, vol. 61, no. 2, pp. 270–278, 2007.

[18] B. Saltin and G. Grimby, "Physiological analysis of middle-aged and old former athletes. Comparison with still active athletes of the same ages," *Circulation*, vol. 38, no. 6, pp. 1104–1115, 1968.

[19] E. G. D. Vittinghoff, S. C. Shiboski, and C. E. McCulloch, *Regression Methods in Biostatistics: Linear, Logistic, Survival, and Repeated Measures Models*, Springer, Heidelberg, 2005.

[20] L. C. Dale, D. R. Schroeder, T. D. Wolter, I. T. Croghan, R. D. Hurt, and K. P. Offord, "Weight change after smoking cessation using variable doses of transdermal nicotine replacement," *Journal of General Internal Medicine*, vol. 13, no. 1, pp. 9–15, 1998.

[21] P. O'Hara, J. E. Connett, W. W. Lee, M. Nides, R. Murray, and R. Wise, "Early and late weight gain following smoking cessation in the lung health study," *American Journal of Epidemiology*, vol. 148, no. 9, pp. 821–830, 1998.

[22] G. E. Swan and D. Carmelli, "Characteristics associated with excessive weight gain after smoking cessation in men," *American Journal of Public Health*, vol. 85, no. 1, pp. 73–77, 1995.

[23] D. F. Williamson, J. Madans, R. F. Anda, J. C. Kleinman, G. A. Giovino, and T. Byers, "Smoking cessation and severity of weight gain in a national cohort," *The New England Journal of Medicine*, vol. 324, no. 11, pp. 739–745, 1991.

[24] S. Veldheer, J. Yingst, J. Zhu, and J. Foulds, "Ten-year weight gain in smokers who quit, smokers who continued smoking and never smokers in the United States, NHANES 2003-2012," *International Journal of Obesity*, vol. 39, no. 12, pp. 1727–1732, 2015.

[25] D. Lycett, M. Munafo, E. Johnstone, M. Murphy, and P. Aveyard, "Associations between weight change over 8 years and baseline body mass index in a cohort of continuing and quitting smokers," *Addiction*, vol. 106, no. 1, pp. 188–196, 2011.

[26] A. L. Copeland, P. D. Martin, P. J. Geiselman, C. J. Rash, and D. E. Kendzor, "Smoking cessation for weight-concerned women: Group vs. individually tailored, dietary, and weight-control follow-up sessions," *Addictive Behaviors*, vol. 31, no. 1, pp. 115–127, 2006.

[27] S. M. Hall, C. D. Tunstall, K. L. Vila, and J. Duffy, "Weight gain prevention and smoking cessation: Cautionary findings,"

American Journal of Public Health, vol. 82, no. 6, pp. 799–803, 1992.

[28] A. W. Meyers, R. C. Klesges, S. E. Winders, K. D. Ward, B. A. Peterson, and L. H. Eck, "Are weight concerns predictive of smoking cessation? A prospective analysis," *Journal of Consulting and Clinical Psychology*, vol. 65, no. 3, pp. 448–452, 1997.

[29] D. L. McGee Sr., "Smoking, body weight, and CHD mortality in diverse populations," *Preventive Medicine*, vol. 38, no. 6, pp. 834–840, 2004.

[30] S. M. Hall, D. Ginsberg, and R. T. Jones, "Smoking cessation and weight gain," *Journal of Consulting and Clinical Psychology*, vol. 54, no. 3, pp. 342–346, 1986.

[31] T. L. S. Visscher, J. C. Seidell, A. Molarius, D. van der Kuip, A. Hofman, and J. C. A. Witteman, "A comparison of body mass index, waist-hip ratio and waist circumference as predictors of all-cause mortality among the elderly: the rotterdam study," *International Journal of Obesity*, vol. 25, no. 11, pp. 1730–1735, 2001.

4

Establishing Waist-to-Height Ratio Standards from Criterion-Referenced BMI Using ROC Curves in Low-Income Children

Ryan D. Burns,[1] Timothy A. Brusseau,[1] Yi Fang,[1] You Fu,[2] and James C. Hannon[3]

[1] *Department of Health, Kinesiology, and Recreation, University of Utah, 250 S. 1850 E., HPER North, RM 241, Salt Lake City, UT 84112, USA*
[2] *School of Community Health Sciences, University of Nevada, Reno, 1664 North Virginia Street, Reno, NV 89557, USA*
[3] *College of Physical Activity and Sport Sciences, West Virginia University, P.O. Box 6116, 375 Birch St., Morgantown, WV 26505-6116, USA*

Correspondence should be addressed to Ryan D. Burns; ryan.d.burns@utah.edu

Academic Editor: Li Ming Wen

The purpose of this study was to establish health-related waist-to-height ratio (WHtR) cut-points associating with FITNESSGRAM's body mass index (BMI) criterion-referenced standards in low-income children. A secondary aim was to examine the classification agreement between the derived WHtR cut-points and various cardiometabolic blood markers using current recommendations. Participants were 219 children from low-income schools (mean age = 10.5 ± 0.6 years). Waist circumference, height, weight, and cardiometabolic blood markers were collected in a fasting state before school hours. Receiver operating characteristic (ROC) curves were used to determine WHtR cut-points that associated with a child meeting FITNESSGRAM's age- and sex-specific criterion-referenced standards for BMI. The derived WHtR cut-point was 0.50 (AUC = 0.89, $p < 0.001$; sensitivity = 0.86, specificity = 0.82, and accuracy = 84.3%). Classification agreement using the derived WHtR cut-point with various blood marker standards was statistically significant but considered weak to fair (kappa 0.14–0.34, agreement = 59%–67%, and $p < 0.01$). The WHtR cut-point of 0.50 can be used with strong accuracy to distinguish low-income children who met FITNESSGRAM's criterion-referenced standards for body composition; however, the evidence was weaker for its use in distinguishing low-income children meeting specific cardiometabolic blood marker recommendations.

1. Introduction

Optimizing health-related fitness (HRF) is an effective strategy for attenuating cardiometabolic disease health risk in the pediatric population [1, 2]. HRF consists of five components including body composition, cardiorespiratory endurance, muscular strength and endurance, and flexibility [3]. Of these five components, body composition and cardiorespiratory endurance have the strongest links to health outcomes in children and adolescents [4, 5]. Therefore, optimizing body composition and cardiorespiratory endurance may decrease the incidence of cardiometabolic disease risk factors [6]. This may especially be important in low-income children where the prevalence of obesity and unfavorable obesity-related cardiometabolic disease risk factors is significantly greater compared to higher socioeconomic status pediatric populations [7, 8].

Currently in the USA, HRF is assessed using the FITNESSGRAM, the national fitness test battery (http://www.fitnessgram.net). For body composition, FITNESSGRAM recommends the use of percent of body fat or body mass index (BMI) [9–11]. Because of the logistic limitations of acquiring estimated percent of body fat from sum of skinfolds assessment in physical education settings, BMI is often used because of its ease of administration and calculation. The BMI standards are currently age- and sex-specific when employing the FITNESSGRAM [3]. Instead of providing a child with an absolute BMI score, children are classified into Healthy Fitness Zones, which gives the child personalized messages based on their current estimated body composition [12].

The two primary Healthy Fitness Zones include the Healthy Fitness Zone (HFZ), a zone where a child is given a message stating that he or she is at a level of good health, and the Needs Improvement (NI), a zone that gives the message that a child should strive to improve their BMI to attenuate health risk. The current version of FITNESSGRAM (v.10) states that the cut-points for BMI are adjusted to align with the age- and sex-specific Centers for Disease Control and Prevention BMI percentiles, using the 83rd and 92nd percentiles for boys and the 80th and 90th percentiles for girls. These cut-points have been validated using a metabolic syndrome criterion in a large sample of adolescents aged 12–19 years from the National Health and Nutrition Examination Survey [13].

Despite the benefits of BMI in field settings, specifically in physical education, the index contains inherent limitations. The original development for BMI was for population surveillance, to monitor body composition within large groups of people [14]. However, it is currently widely used for individual body composition assessment [15]. Its use at the individual level has been under scrutiny because of its inability to distinguish between fat mass and fat-free mass [16]. BMI also does not specify where fat is distributed on a person's body, as visceral adipose deposits have been shown to pose more of a health risk compared to subcutaneous deposits [17].

An increasingly popular alternative to BMI is waist-to-height ratio (WHtR) [18]. WHtR is simply an individual waist circumference divided by their height. Some studies have shown that this index is better at distinguishing children and adolescents with unfavorable cardiometabolic risk factors than BMI [19]. However, the discordance in BMI and WHtR estimations of individual body composition may be more evident after the commencement of puberty in both girls and boys, when hormonal changes elicit different fat and fat-free mass distributions and deposit rates on the body [20]. Despite this, the use of WHtR in younger children still may have utility, especially to monitor central adiposity. Indeed, in the low-income pediatric population, central (or visceral) adiposity has been shown to be more prevalent compared to children of a higher socioeconomic status [20, 21].

No study to date has developed WHtR cut-points associating current FITNESSGRAM standards for body composition. Also, examining the agreement of the derived WHtR cut-point with cardiometabolic blood marker recommendations will give evidence for the strength of its utility in clinical settings for identifying low-income children at risk for early onset cardiometabolic disease. Therefore, the purpose of this study was to derive a WHtR cut-point associating with meeting FITNESSGRAM's age- and sex-specific criterion-referenced standards for BMI in low-income children from the USA. A secondary aim was to examine the classification agreement between children meeting the derived WHtR cut-point with meeting standards for various cardiometabolic blood markers using recommendations from the National, Heart, Lung, and Blood Institute.

2. Material and Methods

2.1. Participants. Participants were a nonprobability convenience sample of 219 children from five low-income schools from the Mountain West region of the US (mean age = 10.5 ± 0.6 years; 126 girls and 93 boys). Children were recruited from the fourth through the sixth grades and were primarily of a Hispanic ethnic background (210/219, 95.8%). Approximately 91%–96% of the children at each school were from low-income families. Written assent was obtained from each child and written consent was obtained from each child's parent or guardian prior to data collection. There were no exclusion criteria given for recruitment of the children and all children were in good physical condition for physical assessment. The University Institutional Review Board approved the protocols employed in this study.

2.2. Measures

2.2.1. Body Mass Index and Waist-to-Height Ratio. Height was measured to the nearest 0.5 centimeter using a portable stadiometer (SECA 213; Hanover, MD, USA). With shoes off, weight was measured to the nearest 0.1 kg using a portable medical scale (BD-590; Tokyo, Japan). BMI was calculated taking each child's weight (in kg) divided by square of height (in meters). Waist circumference was measured in a private screening area where three abdominal circumference measurements were taken at the level of the superior border of the iliac crest on the participant's right side using a standard measuring tape. All measurements were estimated to the nearest 0.5-centimeter with the average of the three measurements used for data analysis. WHtR was calculated taking the child's waist circumference in centimeters divided by their height in centimeters. The anthropometric measures (i.e., BMI and waist circumference) were collected by a trained graduate research assistant to maintain testing consistency and were collected in accordance with the American College of Sports Medicine guidelines.

2.2.2. Cardiometabolic Blood Markers. Each child's cardiometabolic biomarkers were collected using the Cholestech LDX system (Alere Inc., Waltham, MA, USA). Individual blood markers included total cholesterol, LDL cholesterol, HDL cholesterol, triglycerides, and blood glucose. A capillary blood sample was collected between the hours of 6 am and 8 am before the start of the school day. All blood samples were collected in a fasting state, verbally verified by both the child and the child's parent or guardian. Blood samples were collected using a finger stick on each child's right index finger using a 40 μL capillary tube and injected into a Lipid Profile-Glucose Cassette (Alere Inc., Waltham, MA, USA) to be subsequently analyzed. The puncture site was cleaned and bandaged and all materials were properly disposed of in a biohazard container.

Blood pressure was measured using an electronic blood pressure device (CONTEC08A, Contec Medical Systems Co., Qinhuangdao, China). Systolic blood pressure and diastolic blood pressure measurements were taken on each child's right arm with the right arm rested and elevated at heart level and both feet flat on the ground. Blood pressure measurements were collected while the children were seated, immediately following a seated five-minute relaxation period.

2.3. Procedures. Anthropometric measurements (i.e., BMI and WHtR), blood markers, and blood pressure measurements were collected on the same testing day. Anthropometric measurements were collected first, blood markers collected second, and blood pressure measurements collected third for all students. Students not reporting to the data collection site in a fasting state were rescheduled.

2.4. Data Processing. Each child's BMI was stratified into FITNESSGRAM's HFZ or NI [22]. Only two of the three FITNESSGRAM fitness zones were used for classification in order to create a binary predictor variable for BMI. The cardiometabolic blood marker continuous variable scores were also stratified into a binary classification scheme based on US National Heart, Lung, and Blood Institute recommendations [23]. Unfavorable cardiometabolic measurements were defined as having total cholesterol ≥ 170 mg/dL, LDL cholesterol ≥ 110 mg/dL, HDL cholesterol ≤ 45 mg/dL, triglycerides ≥ 90 mg/dL, blood glucose ≥ 100 mg/dL, and systolic and diastolic blood pressure measurements ≥ 95th percentile as determined by age and sex. The aforementioned binary variables were coded as 0 = not meeting recommendations and 1 = meeting recommendations for WHtR and blood markers and 0 = NI and 1 = HFZ for BMI.

2.5. Statistical Analysis. For descriptive purposes, differences between sex groups on all continuous measures were examined using independent *t*-tests. The primary analysis involved using a Receiver Operating Characteristic (ROC) curve to determine the optimal WHtR cut-point needed to accurately discriminate children who did and who did not achieve FITNESSGRAM's age- and sex-specific recommendations for BMI. Overall diagnostic power was determined using the area-under-the-curve (AUC). AUC scores of ≥0.90 were considered excellent; 0.80–0.89, good; 0.70–0.79, fair; and <0.70, poor [21]. The optimal WHtR cut-point was determined using maximum Youden's J statistic (J_{max}), which was calculated using STATA's "senspec" command. Youden's J is the point on the ROC curve that maximizes the sum of sensitivity and specificity (J_{max} = max((sensitivity + specificity) − 1)). Sensitivity was the probability that a child achieved a WHtR cut-point (T^+) given that he or she met the FITNESSGRAM standard for BMI (D^+), or $P(T^+ \mid D^+)$. Sensitivity is synonymous with the probability of achieving a true positive. Specificity was the probability that a child did not meet a WHtR cut-point (T^-) given that he or she did not meet the FITNESSGRAM standard for BMI, $P(T^- \mid D^-)$, or a true negative [24]. Maximizing sensitivity and specificity associates with the datum closest to (0, 1) on the ROC curve and is a WHtR cut-point that is likely to yield strong classification accuracy.

Classification agreement between children meeting the WHtR cut-point and children meeting each cardiometabolic blood marker standard was examined using kappa statistics and percentage of agreement. The kappa statistics were interpreted as weak if <0.20, fair if 0.20–0.39, moderate if 0.40–0.59, good if 0.60–0.79, and very good if ≥0.80 [25]. Alpha level was set at $p \leq 0.05$ and all analyses were carried out using STATA v14.0 statistical software package (College Station, TX, USA).

3. Results

The descriptive statistics for all continuous variables are presented in Table 1 for the total sample and within sex groups. Comparing sex groups, girls displayed higher triglycerides than boys (mean difference = 12.4 mg/dL, $p < 0.01$) and boys displayed higher diastolic blood pressure than girls (mean difference = 3.6 mmHg, $p < 0.01$). There were no other statistically significant differences between sexes for any other measure. Table 2 presents the distribution of children meeting cardiometabolic blood marker recommendations from the National Heart, Lung, and Blood Institute. The range for meeting the various recommendations was 51.5% for triglycerides to 91.7% for blood glucose.

Figure 1 is the ROC curve showing the range of sensitivity and 1 − specificity for various WHtR cut-points associating with a child meeting FITNESSGRAM's age- and sex-specific criterion-referenced standards for BMI. Results from the ROC curve analysis yielded an optimal WHtR cut-point of 0.50 (J_{max} = 0.68, AUC = 0.89, and $p < 0.001$; sensitivity = 0.86, specificity = 0.82, and accuracy = 84.3%). The AUC was considered good. Using the derived cut-point, approximately 55% of the sample displayed a WHtR ≤ 0.50 (120/219). Table 3 presents the agreement statistics between children meeting the derived WHtR cut-point with children meeting the recommendations for each cardiometabolic blood marker. All kappa statistics were statistically significant except for LDL cholesterol. Statistically significant kappa statistics were considered weak to fair and ranged from kappa = 0.14 for total cholesterol to kappa = 0.34 for systolic blood pressure. The percentage agreement thus ranged from 58.6% for total cholesterol to 66.8% for systolic blood pressure.

4. Discussion

The purpose of this study was to establish a WHtR cut-point that associated with FITNESSGRAM's age- and sex-specific criterion-reference standards for BMI. A secondary aim was to use the cut-point to analyze classification agreement with various cardiometabolic blood markers using recommendations from the National Heart, Lung, and Blood Institute. The primary finding from this study was that the derived WHtR cut-point of 0.50 strongly agreed with BMI criterion-referenced standards used in the FITNESSGRAM battery. Approximately 84% of children were correctly classified using the 0.50 cut-point and only 16% of children were misclassified. The 0.50 WHtR cut-point has been recommended in other works within the child and adolescent populations [24, 26, 27].

The simple recommendation of keeping a waist circumference less than one-half of height holds merit in the low-income pediatric population as well when distinguishing children who achieved FITNESSGRAM's body composition standards. In other work, this cut-point has been shown to relate moderately well to cardiometabolic risk factors in

TABLE 1: Descriptive data for the total sample and within sex groups (means and standard deviations).

	Total sample (N = 219)	Girls (n = 126)	Boys (n = 93)
BMI[a] (kg/m^2)	19.1 (4.3)	18.9 (4.6)	19.3 (3.8)
WHtR[b]	0.49 (0.08)	0.48 (0.08)	0.50 (0.07)
Total cholesterol (mg/dL)	153.1 (27.7)	153.1 (26.4)	153.2 (29.4)
LDL cholesterol (mg/dL)	87.1 (26.7)	85.3 (24.4)	90.0 (29.9)
HDL cholesterol (mg/dL)	44.6 (13.2)	44.5 (12.1)	44.7 (14.6)
Triglycerides (mg/dL)	112.6 (82.8)	**112.0† (94.1)**	99.6 (62.2)
Glucose (mg/dL)	86.1 (9.6)	86.1 (10.0)	86.1 (9.0)
Systolic blood pressure (mmHg)	112.9 (14.6)	113.0 (14.4)	112.9 (15.0)
Diastolic blood pressure (mmHg)	67.1 (10.9)	65.6 (10.5)	**69.2† (11.2)**

Note. [a]BMI stands for body mass index; [b]WHtR stands for waist-to-height ratio; bold indicates statistical differences compared to the opposite sex, $^\dagger p < 0.01$.

TABLE 2: Number of children meeting standards/recommendations for each measure (expressed as counts and percentages).

	Meeting	% meeting	Not meeting
BMI	118	53.8%	101
Total cholesterol	172	78.5%	47
LDL cholesterol	193	88.1%	26
HDL cholesterol	98	44.7%	121
Triglycerides	113	51.5%	106
Glucose	201	91.7%	18
Systolic blood pressure	107	48.8%	112
Diastolic blood pressure	138	63.0%	81

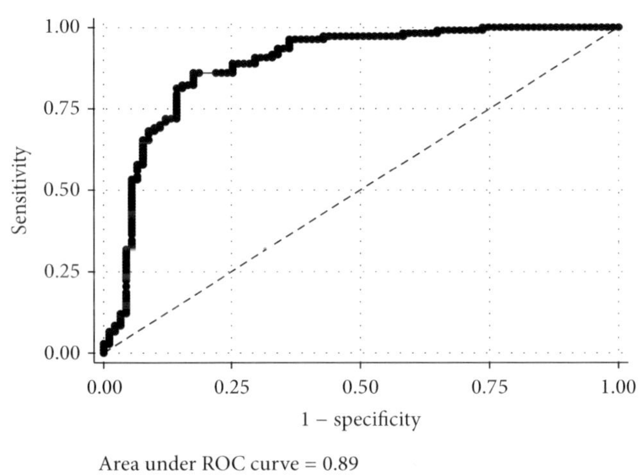

FIGURE 1: Receiver operating characteristic curve displaying the sensitivity and 1 − specificity scores for waist-to-height ratio cut-points associating with children meeting FITNESSGRAM's body composition criterion-referenced standards.

children, adolescents, and adults [28, 29]. The established WHtR cut-point has the benefit of being developed from FITNESSGRAM's criterion-referenced standards for BMI. FITNESSGRAM's criterion-referenced standards for BMI were developed from percent of body fat estimated from skinfold thickness, which was linked to the metabolic syndrome using a large sample of children and adolescents from the US National Health and Nutrition Examination Survey [11]. The BMI standards are currently used as part of a comprehensive fitness test battery in physical activity or physical education settings. Other researches have found WHtR cut-points ranging between 0.60 in obese Mexican adolescents [30], 0.47 in young Brazilian children [31], 0.465 in female and 0.455 in male South African children [32], and 0.475 in female and 0.485 in male Chinese children [18]. The discordance in developed WHtR cut-points may be the result of the referent variable used for comparison (e.g., metabolic syndrome, percent of body fat, and BMI), genetics, diet, age, sex, and the procedures and instrumentation used to collect anthropometric and health measurements [33]. Despite this, the cut-points derived from various studies approximate the 0.5 cut-point found in this study, which is in exact accordance with the weighted mean boundary found from a recent meta-analysis [33].

In addition to its relative ease of interpretation, WHtR also has the benefit of capturing visceral adipose deposition, which has been shown to increase low-grade systemic inflammation in the body, a possible genesis for early incident cardiometabolic disease risk factors [34]. One limitation of WHtR is that some administered training may be needed to yield a reliable and valid waist circumference measurement, whereas, with BMI, no training is needed. However, WHtR in many studies has been shown to classify individuals of all ages with greater accuracy than BMI because of its ability to isolate central adiposity [35]. Height and bone structure confounding is partially controlled for when dividing the waist measurement by height; therefore its validity as a body composition index is robust regardless of stature.

Although WHtR strongly agreed with BMI standards, its ability to distinguish children who did or did not meet individual cardiometabolic blood markers was classified as weak to fair. Most studies show an association between WHtR and individual and clustered cardiometabolic biomarkers [36]. WHtR has also been found to be associated with certain health behaviors in children such as TV viewing, sedentary behavior, and irregular breakfast [37]. In this study the accuracy in distinguishing children with unfavorable cardiometabolic biomarkers has been found to be similar compared to previous research [31, 32]. The relative lower accuracy of WHtR in children compared to older cohorts may

TABLE 3: Classification agreement using the derived WHtR cut-point and cardiometabolic blood marker recommendations.

	Kappa (95% CI)	p value	% of agreement
Total cholesterol	**0.14 (0.01, 0.26)**	0.015	58.6%
LDL cholesterol	0.04 (−0.07, 0.16)	0.215	53.1%
HDL cholesterol	**0.33 (0.20, 0.46)**	<0.001	66.5%
Triglycerides	**0.22 (0.08, 0.36)**	0.001	61.5%
Glucose	**0.13 (0.04, 0.21)**	0.002	59.1%
Systolic blood pressure	**0.34 (0.21, 0.48)**	<0.001	66.8%
Diastolic blood pressure	**0.26 (0.13, 0.39)**	<0.001	64.0%

be because of the greater difficulty to detect unfavorable risk factors because these traits may take several years to develop. Indeed, the prevalence for unfavorable biomarkers was less than 50% for most measures, except for HDL cholesterol and diastolic blood pressure, and quite low for total cholesterol, LDL cholesterol, and fasting glucose. Another reason for the weak accuracy in WHtR classifying children may have been because of the use of a capillary blood sample to collect the biomarkers. Capillary blood sampling, although convenient, may overestimate certain biomarkers compared to venous blood sampling [38]. Future research should use venous blood sampling to possibly yield more valid results.

This is the first study to establish a WHtR cut-point associating with FITNESSGRAM's criterion-references standards for BMI in low-income children. This is also the first study to associate WHtR with standards developed from FITNESSGRAM. Practically, the results from this study yield certain implications. WHtR can be used as an alternative to BMI in field settings, specifically in physical education settings for body composition assessment. As stated previously, WHtR has the benefit of capturing central adipose deposits that pose more of a health threat compared to subcutaneous deposits on a child's body [30]. Screening for central adiposity at an early age may help attenuate the risk of developing visceral adipose deposits later in life and thus attenuate incidence of unfavorable cardiometabolic disease risk factors. Although the accuracy of distinguishing low-income children with unfavorable cardiometabolic disease risk was weak to fair, statistically significant agreement was still found; therefore there is still utility for WHtR's use as a cardiometabolic screening tool. However, future research needs to explore these associations further using larger sample sizes, venous blood sampling, and more ethnically diverse samples.

There are limitations to this study that must be considered before generalizations can be made. First, the sample consisted of low-income children, primarily Hispanic, from schools located within the Mountain West region of the USA. Therefore, the external validity of the results is questionable if the results are to be generalized to higher socioeconomic status children or to samples comprising different ethnic representation. Second, a capillary blood sample was obtained to analyze the cardiometabolic blood markers, which may overestimate levels within 5% compared to venous blood samples. Third, the acquired sample size of 219 children is relatively low for cross-sectional descriptive studies employing ROC curves analysis; therefore future research should address the research question using larger sample sizes to improve statistical power and the internal validity of the results. Finally, diet was not accounted for in the analysis, which may influence cardiometabolic health markers. Future research should account for the potential confounding of diet when examining the relationship between WHtR and cardiometabolic health.

5. Conclusion

In conclusion, the derived WHtR cut-point of 0.50 strongly agreed with FITNESSGRAM's criterion-referenced standards for BMI. The WHtR = 0.50 cut-point has also been indicated in prior research within the adolescent and adult populations and may provide a valid alternative to BMI as a body composition assessment metric in low-income children. Despite the strong agreement with BMI, its ability to distinguish low-income children who achieved individual blood marker recommendations was weak to fair. This may have been because of the low prevalence of certain risk factors or the use of capillary blood sampling. This study was the first to establish a WHtR cut-point that associated with criterion-referenced BMI using a sample of low-income children from the USA. The WHtR = 0.50 cut-point can be used with strong accuracy in field settings to distinguish children who would meet standards using FITNESSGRAM's BMI, but its use for screening for a child's cardiometabolic disease risk needs further exploration.

Competing Interests

The authors declare that there is no conflict of interests regarding the publication of this paper.

Acknowledgments

The authors would like to thank the US Department of Education for funding this study (Grant no. S215F140118). They would also like to thank the students who participated in this study.

References

[1] R. G. McMurray and L. B. Andersen, "The influence of exercise on metabolic syndrome in youth: a review," *American Journal of Lifestyle Medicine*, vol. 4, no. 2, pp. 176–186, 2010.

[2] F. B. Ortega, J. R. Ruiz, M. J. Castillo, and M. Sjöström, "Physical fitness in childhood and adolescence: a powerful marker of health," *International Journal of Obesity*, vol. 32, no. 1, pp. 1–11, 2008.

[3] G. J. Welk, S. B. Going, J. R. Morrow Jr., and M. D. Meredith, "Development of new criterion-referenced fitness standards in the FITNESSGRAM program: rationale and conceptual overview," *American Journal of Preventive Medicine*, vol. 41, no. 4, pp. S63–S67, 2011.

[4] J. R. Ruiz, F. B. Ortega, N. S. Rizzo et al., "High cardiovascular fitness is associated with low metabolic risk score in children: the European Youth Heart Study," *Pediatric Research*, vol. 61, no. 3, pp. 350–355, 2007.

[5] K. Sasayama, E. Ochi, and M. Adachi, "Importance of both fatness and aerobic fitness on metabolic syndrome risk in Japanese children," *PLoS ONE*, vol. 10, no. 5, Article ID e0127400, 2015.

[6] J. C. Eisenmann, G. J. Welk, M. Ihmels, and J. Dollman, "Fatness, fitness, and cardiovascular disease risk factors in children and adolescents," *Medicine and Science in Sports and Exercise*, vol. 39, no. 8, pp. 1251–1256, 2007.

[7] C. L. Ogden, M. M. Lamb, M. D. Carroll, and K. M. Flegal, "Obesity and socioeconomic status in children: United States 1988–1994 and 2005–2008," in *NCHS Data Brief no 51*, National Center for Health Statistics, Hyattsville, Md, USA, 2010.

[8] Y. Wang and Q. Zhang, "Are American children and adolescents of low socioeconomic status at increased risk of obesity? Changes in the association between overweight and family income between 1971 and 2002," *American Journal of Clinical Nutrition*, vol. 84, no. 4, pp. 707–716, 2006.

[9] K. R. Laurson, J. C. Eisenmann, and G. J. Welk, "Development of youth percent body fat standards using receiver operating characteristic curves," *American Journal of Preventive Medicine*, vol. 41, no. 4, supplement 2, pp. S93–S99, 2011.

[10] K. R. Laurson, J. C. Eisenmann, and G. J. Welk, "Body fat percentile curves for U.S. children and adolescents," *American Journal of Preventive Medicine*, vol. 41, no. 4, supplement 2, pp. S87–S92, 2011.

[11] K. R. Laurson, J. C. Eisenmann, and G. J. Welk, "Body mass index standards based on agreement with health-related body fat," *American Journal of Preventive Medicine*, vol. 41, no. 4, supplement 2, pp. S100–S105, 2011.

[12] W. Zhu, M. T. Mahar, G. J. Welk, S. B. Going, and K. J. Cureton, "Approaches for development of criterion-referenced standards in health-related youth fitness tests," *American Journal of Preventive Medicine*, vol. 41, no. 4, pp. S68–S76, 2011.

[13] K. R. Laurson, G. J. Welk, and J. C. Eisenmann, "Diagnostic performance of BMI percentiles to identify adolescents with metabolic syndrome," *Pediatrics*, vol. 133, no. 2, pp. e330–e338, 2014.

[14] G. Eknoyan, "Adolphe Quetelet (1796–1874)—the average man and indices of obesity," *Nephrology Dialysis Transplantation*, vol. 23, no. 1, pp. 47–51, 2008.

[15] A. M. Prentice and S. A. Jebb, "Beyond body mass index," *Obesity Reviews*, vol. 2, no. 3, pp. 141–147, 2001.

[16] A. M. Nevill, A. D. Stewart, T. Olds, and R. Holder, "Relationship between adiposity and body size reveals limitations of BMI," *American Journal of Physical Anthropology*, vol. 129, no. 1, pp. 151–156, 2006.

[17] M. L. Cruz, R. N. Bergman, and M. I. Goran, "Unique effect of visceral fat on insulin sensitivity in obese Hispanic children with a family history of type 2 diabetes," *Diabetes Care*, vol. 25, no. 9, pp. 1631–1636, 2002.

[18] W. Yan, H. Bingxian, Y. Hua et al., "Waist-to-height ratio is an accurate and easier index for evaluating obesity in children and adolescents," *Obesity*, vol. 15, no. 3, pp. 748–752, 2007.

[19] P. Brambilla, G. Bedogni, M. Heo, and A. Pietrobelli, "Waist circumference-to-height ratio predicts adiposity better than body mass index in children and adolescents," *International Journal of Obesity*, vol. 37, no. 7, pp. 943–946, 2013.

[20] J. C. Dekkers, R. H. Podolsky, F. A. Treiber, P. Barbeau, B. Gutin, and H. Snieder, "Development of general and central obesity from childhood into early adulthood in African American and European American males and females with a family history of cardiovascular disease," *The American Journal of Clinical Nutrition*, vol. 79, no. 4, pp. 661–668, 2004.

[21] D. E. Kendzor, M. O. Caughy, and M. T. Owen, "Family income trajectory during childhood is associated with adiposity in adolescence: a latent class growth analysis," *BMC Public Health*, vol. 12, no. 1, article 611, 2012.

[22] S. A. Plowman and M. D. Meredith, *Fitnessgram/Activitygram Reference Guide*, The Cooper Institute, Dallas, Tex, USA, 4th edition, 2013.

[23] National Heart, Lung, and Blood Institute, "Expert panel on integrated guidelines for cardiovascular health and risk reduction in children and adolescents: summary report," *Pediatrics*, vol. 128, supplement 5, pp. S213–S256, 2011.

[24] M. Ashwell and S. D. Hsieh, "Six reasons why the waist-to-height ratio is a rapid and effective global indicator for health risks of obesity and how its use could simplify the international public health message on obesity," *International Journal of Food Sciences and Nutrition*, vol. 56, no. 5, pp. 303–307, 2005.

[25] D. G. Altman, *Practical Statistics for Medical Research*, Chapman and Hall/CRC, London, UK, 1st edition, 1990.

[26] I. de Padua Cintra, M. A. Zanetti Passos, L. C. Dos Santos, H. da Costa Machado, and M. Fisberg, "Waist-to-height ratio percentiles and cutoffs for obesity: a cross-sectional study in Brazilian adolescents," *Journal of Health, Population, and Nutrition*, vol. 32, no. 3, pp. 411–419, 2014.

[27] R. W. Taylor, S. M. Williams, A. M. Grant, B. J. Taylor, and A. Goulding, "Predictive ability of waist-to-height in relation to adiposity in children is not improved with age and sex-specific values," *Obesity*, vol. 19, no. 5, pp. 1062–1068, 2011.

[28] J. S. Mokha, S. R. Srinivasan, P. DasMahapatra et al., "Utility of waist-to-height ratio in assessing the status of central obesity and related cardiometabolic risk profile among normal weight and overweight/obese children: the Bogalusa Heart Study," *BMC Pediatrics*, vol. 10, article 73, 2010.

[29] S. C. Savva, D. Lamnisos, and A. G. Kafatos, "Predicting cardiometabolic risk: waist-to-height ratio or BMI. A meta-analysis," *Diabetes, Metabolic Syndrome and Obesity: Targets and Therapy*, vol. 6, pp. 403–419, 2013.

[30] E. R. Rodea-Montero, M. L. Evia-Viscarra, and E. Apolinar-Jiménez, "Waist-to-height ratio is a better anthropometric index than waist circumference and BMI in predicting metabolic syndrome among obese Mexican adolescents," *International Journal of Endocrinology*, vol. 2014, Article ID 195407, 9 pages, 2014.

[31] V. M. Kuba, C. Leone, and D. Damiani, "Is waist-to-height ratio a useful indicator of cardio-metabolic risk in 6-10-year-old children?" *BMC Pediatrics*, vol. 13, no. 1, article 91, 2013.

[32] T. E. Matsha, A.-P. Kengne, Y. Y. Yako, G. M. Hon, M. S. Hassan, and R. T. Erasmus, "Optimal waist-to-height ratio values for cardiometabolic risk screening in an ethnically diverse sample

of South African urban and rural school boys and girls," *PLoS ONE*, vol. 8, no. 8, article e71133, 2013.

[33] L. M. Browning, S. D. Hsieh, and M. Ashwell, "A systematic review of waist-to-height ratio as a screening tool for the prediction of cardiovascular disease and diabetes: 0.5 could be a suitable global boundary value," *Nutrition Research Reviews*, vol. 23, no. 2, pp. 247–269, 2010.

[34] C. S. Tam, L. K. Heilbronn, C. Henegar et al., "An early inflammatory gene profile in visceral adipose tissue in children," *International Journal of Pediatric Obesity*, vol. 6, no. 2, pp. e360–e363, 2011.

[35] M. Ashwell, L. Mayhew, J. Richardson, and B. Rickayzen, "Waist-to-height ratio is more predictive of years of life lost than body mass index," *PLoS ONE*, vol. 9, no. 9, Article ID e103483, 2014.

[36] R. Jayawardana, P. Ranasinghe, M. H. R. Sheriff, D. R. Matthews, and P. Katulanda, "Waist to height ratio: a better anthropometric marker of diabetes and cardio-metabolic risks in South Asian adults," *Diabetes Research and Clinical Practice*, vol. 99, no. 3, pp. 292–299, 2013.

[37] R. Lehto, C. Ray, M. Lahti-Koski, and E. Roos, "Health behaviors, waist circumference and waist-to-height ratio in children," *European Journal of Clinical Nutrition*, vol. 65, no. 7, pp. 841–848, 2011.

[38] J. H. Stein, C. M. Carlsson, K. Papcke-Benson, J. A. Einerson, P. E. McBride, and D. A. Wiebe, "Inaccuracy of lipid measurements with the portable Cholestech L·D·X analyzer in patients with hypercholesterolemia," *Clinical Chemistry*, vol. 48, no. 2, pp. 284–290, 2002.

5

FTO rs9939609 Does Not Interact with Physical Exercise but Influences Basal Insulin Metabolism in Brazilian Overweight and Obese Adolescents

Gabrielle Araujo do Nascimento,[1] Neiva Leite,[2] Lupe Furtado-Alle,[1] Mayza Dalcin Teixeira,[1] Ricardo Lehtonen Rodrigues de Souza,[1] Gerusa Eisfeld Milano,[2] Larissa Rosa da Silva,[2] Juliana Pizzi,[2] Wendell Arthur Lopes,[3] Maria de Fátima Aguiar Lopes,[2] Ana Cláudia Kapp Titski,[2] and Luciane Viater Tureck[1,4]

[1]*Department of Genetics, Centro Politécnico, Setor de Ciências Biológicas, Federal University of Paraná, Francisco H. dos Santos, 210 Jardim das Américas, 81531-970 Curitiba, PR, Brazil*
[2]*Department of Physical Education, Federal University of Paraná, Coração de Maria, 92 Jardim Botânico, 80215-370 Curitiba, PR, Brazil*
[3]*Department of Physical Education, State University of Maringa, Av. Colombo 5790, 87020-900 Maringa, PR, Brazil*
[4]*Academic Department of Education, Federal University of Technology–Paraná, Av. Monteiro Lobato Km 04, 84016-210 Ponta Grossa, PR, Brazil*

Correspondence should be addressed to Luciane Viater Tureck; luviater@gmail.com

Academic Editor: Moonseong Heo

Purpose. The rs9939609 SNP (T > A) in *FTO* gene is associated with obesity and type 2 diabetes. The present study aimed at verifying whether this SNP influenced biochemical outcomes of children and adolescents who are overweight/obese submitted to a program of physical exercise and also if there was influence on basal levels of these biochemical variables. *Methods.* The sample was composed by 432 children and adolescents grouped in three ways (obese, overweight, and normal weight); of these, 135 children and adoloescents who are obese and overweight were submitted to a physical exercise program for 12 weeks. All were genotyped by TaqMan SNP genotyping assay. *Results.* The children and adolescents who are overweight/obese and carriers of AA genotype had higher levels of insulin ($p = 0.03$) and HOMA ($p = 0.007$) and lower levels of glucose ($p = 0.003$), but the SNP did not modulate the response to physical exercise. *Conclusions.* In our study, the rs9939609 AA genotype was associated with parameters related to insulin metabolism but did not interact with physical exercise.

1. Introduction

Obesity is a multifactorial disease influenced by several genetic factors, including the fat mass and obesity-associated (*FTO*) gene [1, 2], which is expressed in the whole organism, mainly in hypothalamus, and thus associated with energy balance regulation [3]. *FTO* gene product is a 2-oxoglutarate dependent nucleic acid demethylase [4] which can have several target genes, including genes related to metabolism.

One of its most studied SNPs is the rs9939609 SNP (T > A), associated with obesity, type 2 diabetes, and other metabolic complications [1, 5, 6]. The body weight increase associated with rs9939609 A-allele could be related to an increase in *FTO* expression, since *FTO* transcripts are more abundant in risk allele carriers [7].

Many studies have shown association between A-allele and increased food intake and reduced satiety [8–11]; however, the interaction of the rs9939609 SNP with energy expenditure has not yet been clarified, since some studies found interaction and others did not [12].

Besides the effect induced by rs9939609 A-allele in several basal metabolic parameters [13–16], it can also interfere in the response promoted by physical and/or dietary interventions. Some studies have found a reduction in levels of cholesterol, low-density lipoprotein cholesterol (LDL-C), insulin, and HOMA-IR in A-allele carries in response to diet [17, 18]. Regarding the physical exercise, any study that analyzed the interaction of the rs9939609 A-allele on biochemical outcomes was not found.

Efforts have been adopted to understand the interactions between genetic and environmental factors underlying the complex pathologies. In this sense, the identification of modifiable factors that may contribute to decrease the genetic predisposition on metabolic disorders is important for prevention and treatment. Considering the potential influence of rs9939609 on biochemical variables that predict essential metabolic functions, and the lack of studies with *FTO* and physical exercise interaction, the present study investigated the rs9939609 SNP ($T > A$) effect on biochemical outcomes induced by physical exercise in children and adolescents who are overweight/obese.

2. Materials and Methods

2.1. Subjects. The study was composed by 432 children and adolescents (290 boys and 142 girls), of which 169 had normal weight and 263 had overweight or were obese (80 overweight and 183 obese), according to parameters defined by WHO [19]. The mean overall age was 13.51 ± 0.09 years old (aged 8–17 y), and the mean BMI *Z*-score in the overweight/obese group was 2.69 before the exercise and 2.73 after the exercise. In the normal weight group, the mean BMI *Z*-score was −0.22. This study was limited to analysis of the biochemical variables in these individuals. Some of them were analyzed in a previous study that was limited to anthropometric variables analysis [20].

The recruitment of children and adolescents was carried out in public schools of the state of Paraná, Southern Brazil, with the following inclusion criteria: children and adolescents who have medical liberation for physical exercise and do not use drugs that could interfere on weight control and/or lipid levels. An invitation to participate in the research was made to those individuals who met the criteria and those who accepted signed the free and informed consent term, along with the legal responsible consent [20]. The study was approved by the ethics committee of the Federal University of Paraná (UFPR) (protocol number 765.184/2003-11) [20].

Weight and height were measured with an accuracy of 0.1 kg and 0.1 cm, respectively. BMI was calculated as weight in kilograms divided by the square of height in meters and then converted into BMI *Z*-score according to WHO [19]. The children and adolescents were considered overweight when their BMI *Z*-score was between +1 and +2 and obese when their BMI *Z*-score was more than +3 [19].

2.2. Biochemical Variables. The blood samples were collected, and total cholesterol (TC), HDL-C, and TG were measured by standard procedures in private partner laboratories and in the clinical analyzes laboratory of UFPR. Blood glucose levels were determined by the enzymatic method, and insulin was measured by the chemiluminescence immunoassay technique by automated equipment. LDL-C levels were calculated using the Friedewald equation [21], homeostatic model assessment for insulin resistance (HOMA-IR) was calculated using the formula fasting blood glucose (μU/ml) × insulin (mMol/l)/22.5 [22], and the quantitative insulin sensitivity check index (QUICKI) was calculated using the formula 1/(log (fasting insulin) (mU/ml) × log (fasting blood glucose) (mMol/l)) [23]. These variables were measured before and after the exercise program.

2.3. Physical Exercise Intervention Program. Of the 263 children and adolescents who are overweight or obese and who participated in the study, 135 were submitted to an after-school exercise program. This research is part of a larger project the objective of which was to analyze the response of the children and adolescents who are overweight or obese to different physical exercises [24–27].

The exercise intervention programs were carried out in a special session offered in the school gym (land-based aerobic exercise, high-intensity interval training (HIIT), and combined training) or in the university setting (water walking).

Each student participated in one of the four different physical exercise programs: land-based aerobic exercise, HIIT, combined training, or water walking. Each physical exercise program consisted of 3 sessions per week for 12 weeks. They were instructed in the FITT principles (frequency, intensity, time, and type of exercise) by physical education teachers in the school or in the university setting. The minimal adherence accepted was 70% of attendance.

The details of exercise programs are described below and also in previously published works [20,24–27].

The land-based aerobic exercise ($n = 53$) was performed in a total of 110 minutes, divided into 45 minutes of walking, 45 minutes of indoor cycling, and 20 minutes of stretching. The reserve heart rate (RHR) was accessed, with 35% to 55% in the first to fourth week, 45% to 65% in the fifth to eight week, and 55% to 75% in the last weeks [24].

HIIT ($n = 27$) was performed in 45 minutes in each session, and the students did warming-up exercises, running for 30 seconds at 100% speed peak effort, walking for 60 seconds at 50% peak velocity (active recovery period), and relaxing. The exercise was composed by two sets, and there were four minutes of rest between sets. The training progressed as the weeks passed: in the first week, the set was composed by 4 × 30 s/60 s; in the week 2, it was composed by 5 × 30 s/60 s; in the week 3, it was 6 × 30 s/60 s; in the weeks 4 and 5, it was 7 × 30 s/60 s; in the weeks 6 to 9, the recovery period was reduced to 45 s (8 × 30 s/45 s); and in the last two weeks, it was 8 × 30 s/30 s [25].

The combined training ($n = 29$) was a combination of resistance and aerobic training, and each session lasted 60 minutes. In the resistance training, the students realized six exercises: leg press, leg extension, leg curl, bench press, lateral pull down, and arm curl. It was composed by three sets of 6–10 repetitions at 60–70% 1 RM (maximum repetition), and

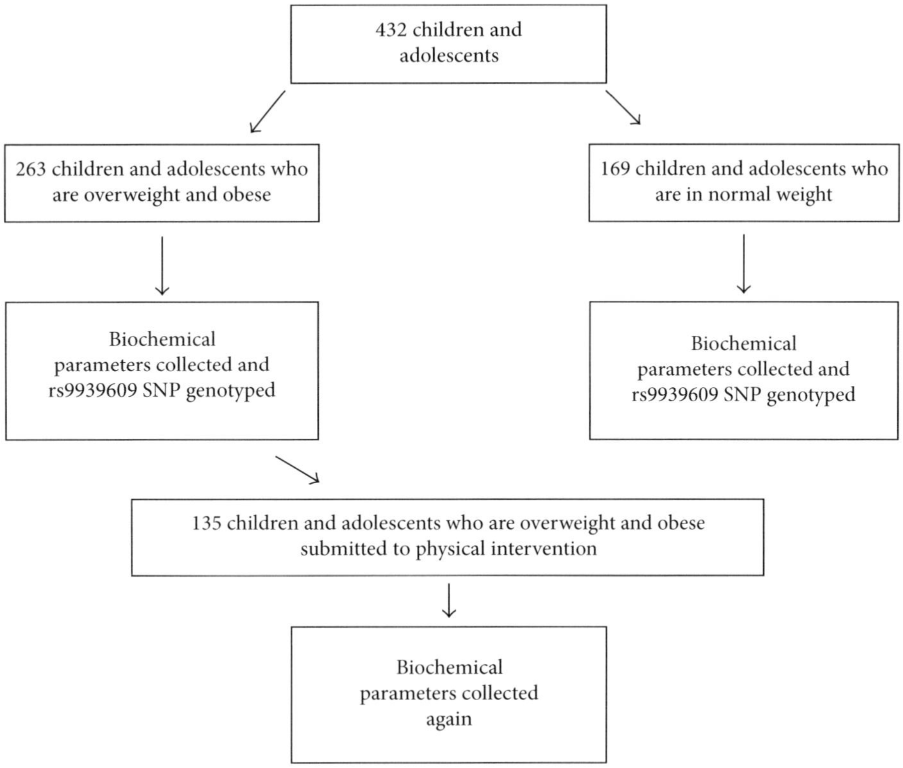

Figure 1: Study design.

the load was adjusted weekly. In the aerobic training, the students walked/ran in an athletic track for 30 minutes, and the intensity was 50–80% of VO_{2peak} [26].

The water-walking exercise ($n = 26$) was realized with the support of a float vest attached to the waist, and it is a simulation of walking on land without the contact of the feet with the bottom of the pool. The students realized five minutes of warming up, 45 minutes of walking, and 10 minutes of recovering, totalizing 60 minutes in a session. The exercise intensity was 40% to 60% of the RHR and increased in the fifth and ninth weeks [27].

In the statistical analyzes, these groups were analyzed together due to the small number of participants in each one; however, in some analyzes, the type of exercise was added as a correction factor. The analysis of some variables was realized with a smaller number of individuals, since it was not possible to obtain data on all variables from all individuals who completed the program ($n = 135$).

The experimental procedure applied is demonstrated in Figure 1.

2.4. DNA Extraction and Genotyping. DNA were extracted from peripheral blood according to a salting-out technique [28] and then diluted to 20 ng/μl. *FTO* rs9939609 SNP was genotyped with a TaqMan SNP genotyping assay (Applied Biosystems). The reactions were done using the following conditions: 60°C for 30 s, 95°C for 10 min, 50 cycles of 95°C for 15 s and 60°C for 1 min, and 60°C for 30 s. In each reaction, three previously sequenced control samples were included, representative of each of the possible genotypes.

2.5. Statistical Analysis. The frequencies of genotypes and alleles were obtained by direct counting and compared between the group of overweight/obese and normal weight by chi-square test, which was also used to check the Hardy–Weinberg equilibrium. The continuous variables were tested for normality using the Kolmogorov–Smirnov test with the Lilliefors correction. The recessive, dominant, and lack of dominance models of allelic interaction were tested. The recessive model was adopted for analysis that involved the sample stratification by rs9939609 SNP genotype. For each variable, the means were compared between genotypes by parametric or no parametric tests (*t* test or Mann–Whitney, resp.). The comparisons between initial and final means (before and after physical exercise) were conducted by the Wilcoxon test or *t* test for dependent samples.

A two-way mixed ANOVA with repeated measures was used to verify the genotype influence on the response to physical exercise, and the nonparametric variables were normalized by logarithmic transformation. Multiple regression analysis was also applied. Statistical significance adopted for the tests was 0.05 (5%).

3. Results

The risk allele (A) was not associated with obesity in our study (overweight/obese and normal weight group with similar allelic frequency $p = 0.71$). In the overweight and obese group ($n = 263$), 38.02% were TT carriers, 48.67% AT, and 13.31% AA. The genotype frequencies in the normal weight group ($n = 169$) were 37.28% (TT), 52.66% (AT),

TABLE 1: Initial and final averages of biochemical variables stratified by rs9939609 *FTO* SNP genotype and effect of exercise (p value training), genotype (p value genotype), and training × genotype interaction (p value T × G).

Variables	TT + AT (mean ± SD)				AA (mean ± SD)				p value		
	n	Before	After	%Δ	n	Before	After	%Δ	Training	Genotype	T × G
TC (mg/dl)	118	163 ± 35.81	157 ± 32.79	−3.68	17	161 ± 31.75	148 ± 29.26	−8.07	**0.002**	0.55	0.20
HDL-C (mg/dl)	117	48 ± 10.9	46 ± 11.81	−4.17	17	52 ± 11.95	46 ± 9.91	−11.54	**0.005**	0.43	0.05
LDL-C (mg/dl)	118	94 ± 29.5	90 ± 27.42	−4.26	17	92 ± 24.27	83 ± 30.94	−9.78	**0.02**	0.44	0.34
TG (mg/dl)	117	104.44 ± 53.98	102.71 ± 52.84	−1.66	17	85.85 ± 30.35	98.06 ± 68.54	14.22	0.4	0.34	0.26
Glucose (mg/dl)	117	87 ± 9.39	86 ± 8.06	−1.15	18	82 ± 9.6	80 ± 5.76	−2.44	0.07	**0.003**	0.77
Insulin (uIU/ml)	94	15.54 ± 10.93	12.68 ± 7.81	−18.40	15	20 ± 14.06	17.58 ± 9.8	−12.10	**0.02**	0.07	0.84
HOMA-IR	48	1.86 ± 1.18	1.4 ± 0.88	−24.73	8	2.86 ± 1.73	2.53 ± 1.43	−11.54	0.06	**0.007**	0.74
QUICKI	43	0.34 ± 0.04	0.36 ± 0.04	5.88	7	0.32 ± 0.03	0.33 ± 0.03	3.13	**0.03**	0.07	0.70

TC: total cholesterol; HDL-C: high-density lipoprotein cholesterol; LDL-C: low-density lipoprotein cholesterol; TG: triglycerides; HOMA-IR: homeostatic model assessment for insulin resistance; QUICKI: quantitative insulin sensitivity check index; SD: standard deviation; %Δ: percentage variation; T × G: training × genotype interaction; the test applied was two-way mixed ANOVA.

and 10.06% (AA). Both groups are in Hardy–Weinberg equilibrium.

A mixed two-way ANOVA test was performed to investigate possible effects of physical intervention (within subject factor: before and after training); genotype (between subject factor: AA × AT + TT); and training × genotype interaction on the biochemical variables (Table 1). It was possible to observe that the physical intervention and genotype independently influenced the biochemical variables of the children and adolescents who were overweight and obese.

The physical exercise, independently of the *FTO* rs9939609 genotype, improved the metabolic profile: TC, LDL-C, and insulin levels decreased after the intervention ($p = 0.002$, $p = 0.02$, and $p = 0.02$, resp.), and QUICKI increased ($p = 0.03$), indicating insulin sensitivity improvement of the children who are overweight and obese (Table 1).

The *FTO* genotype influenced the glucose levels ($p = 0.03$) and HOMA-IR index ($p = 0.007$) (Table 1). Higher HOMA-IR was associated with AA carriers before and after the physical exercise ($p = 0.006$ and $p = 0.01$, resp.). The same genotype was associated with lower glucose levels only after the intervention ($p = 0.002$) (Supplementary Table 1). According to the ANOVA analysis, the AA carriers trend toward higher levels of insulin ($p = 0.07$) after the physical exercise and lower values of QUICKI ($p = 0.07$) before and after the physical exercise, compared to TT + AT carriers (Table 1 and Supplementary Table 1), suggesting that AA genotype could be associated with less favorable insulin profiles. There was no genotype × training interaction, since the changes in variables after the intervention were not different among genotypes (Table 1).

To investigate the observed trends in ANOVA and identify other factors that contributed to the insulinic profile of children who are overweight and obese, we conducted multiple regression analysis with the initial measures (before), final measures (after), and also with the differences between final and initial values (difference). All the multiple regression analyses were corrected for age, sex, and BMI Z-score. Regression analysis with the final and differences values was corrected for the type of exercise practiced (land-based aerobic exercise, high-intensity interval training (HIIT), combined training, or water walking) (Table 2).

The effect of the *FTO* rs9939609 genotype on the biochemical variables of children and adolescents with normal weight was also evaluated. The comparisons of mean levels of the variables between carriers and noncarriers of AA genotype did not present significant results (Supplementary Table 2), as well as multiple regression analyses (corrected for age, sex, and BMI Z-score) (Table 2).

The regression analysis results confirmed the rs9939609 AA genotype effect in children who are overweight and obese, even after the applied corrections. The initial and final insulin levels were influenced by *FTO* SNP ($p = 0.04$ and $p = 0.03$, resp.), as well as the initial HOMA-IR ($p = 0.01$), and final glucose levels ($p = 0.003$). The differences in biochemical variables levels (initial levels – final levels) were not influenced by *FTO* SNP, which corroborates the absence of the *FTO* SNP × training interaction, observed in ANOVA.

4. Discussion

Our study was designed to investigate the interaction between *FTO* rs9939609 SNP and a program of physical exercise on biochemical outcomes of the children and adolescents who were overweight and obese. In this sense, the interaction between the *FTO* rs9939609 SNP and physical exercise did not affect the biochemical outcomes; however, the *FTO* rs9939609 SNP was associated with insulin, HOMA-IR, and glucose levels of the children and adolescents who were overweight and obese.

Our study identified an important relationship between AA genotype and less favorable insulin profiles: the mean values of insulin in AA individuals were higher than those recommended by some authors [29]. There are at least two possible ways that would explain this relationship, both involving the *FTO* overexpression related to rs9939609 A-allele [7].

The most direct relationship between rs9939609 and insulin resistance is suggested by Tschritter and colleagues [30]. They found association between the *FTO* rs8050136 SNP and cerebrocortical insulin resistance in humans [30], but this polymorphism is in linkage disequilibrium with rs9939609 (rs9939609, $D' = 0.9998$ [31]); so we cannot rule out a causal effect of the rs9939609 SNP. Tschritter and colleagues observed a reduction of the insulin effect in cortical activity, which

TABLE 2: Models of multiple regression analysis before and after the physical exercise, with difference values in children and adolescents who are overweight/obese and normal weight.

Dependent variable	Independent variables considered	Overweight and obese Before (n = 263)		After (n = 135)		Difference (n = 135)	
		$\beta \pm$ SD	p	$\beta \pm$ SD	p	$\beta \pm$ SD	p
Glucose (mg/dl)	Genotype	0.06 ± 0.06	0.36	0.26 ± 0.09	**0.003**	−0.03 ± 0.09	0.76
	Age	0.07 ± 0.06	0.28	−0.03 ± 0.09	0.74	0.08 ± 0.09	0.35
	Sex	−0.06 ± 0.06	0.36	0.16 ± 0.09	0.07	−0.07 ± 0.09	0.42
	BMI Z-score (kg/m^2)	0.08 ± 0.06	0.20	0.11 ± 0.09	0.23	−0.23 ± 0.09	**0.01**
	Type of physical exercise	—	—	−0.08 ± 0.09	0.38	−0.17 ± 0.09	0.07
Insulin (uIU/ml)	Genotype	−0.13 ± 0.06	**0.04**	−0.19 ± 0.09	**0.03**	−0.004 ± 0.10	0.97
	Age	0.16 ± 0.07	**0.01**	0.24 ± 0.09	**0.01**	−0.03 ± 0.10	0.79
	Sex	0.17 ± 0.06	**0.009**	0.11 ± 0.09	0.24	0.13 ± 0.10	0.20
	BMI Z-score (kg/m^2)	0.35 ± 0.07	**10^{-4}**	0.36 ± 0.09	**0.0002**	−0.0008 ± 0.10	0.99
	Type of physical exercise	—	—	0.32 ± 0.09	**0.0005**	0.05 ± 0.10	0.60
HOMA-IR	Genotype	−0.24 ± 0.09	**0.01**				
	Age	0.14 ± 0.10	0.14				
	Sex	0.16 ± 0.09	0.09	*		*	
	BMI Z-score (kg/m^2)	0.27 ± 0.10	**0.006**				
	Type of physical exercise	—	—				
QUICKI	Genotype	0.12 ± 0.09	0.20				
	Age	0.05 ± 0.1	0.59				
	Sex	−0.27 ± 0.09	**0.004**	*		*	
	BMI Z-score (kg/m^2)	−0.38 ± 0.10	**0.0002**				
	Type of physical exercise	—	—				

Dependent variable	Independent variables considered	Normal weight (n = 169) $\beta \pm$ SD	p
Glucose (mg/dl)	Genotype	−0.07 ± 0.08	0.37
	Age	−0.04 ± 0.08	0.58
	Sex	−0.24 ± 0.08	**0.002**
	BMI Z-score (kg/m^2)	0.02 ± 0.08	0.82
Insulin (uIU/ml)	Genotype	−0.06 ± 0.07	0.39
	Age	−0.03 ± 0.07	0.73
	Sex	0.39 ± 0.07	**10^{-4}**
	BMI Z-score (kg/m^2)	0.10 ± 0.07	0.18
HOMA-IR	Genotype	−0.12 ± 0.09	0.17
	Age	0.17 ± 0.09	0.06
	Sex	0.20 ± 0.09	**0.02**
	BMI Z-score (kg/m^2)	0.02 ± 0.09	0.79
QUICKI	Genotype	0.09 ± 0.11	0.42
	Age	0.19 ± 0.11	0.09
	Sex	−0.14 ± 0.11	0.21
	BMI Z-score (kg/m^2)	−0.04 ± 0.11	0.70

HOMA-IR: homeostatic model assessment for insulin resistance; QUICKI: quantitative insulin sensitivity check index; β: regression coefficient; SD: standard deviation; Genotype: TT + AT and AA (recessive model). *HOMA-IR and QUICKI after physical exercise and differences values have no sufficient variance for the regression analysis; therefore, no results are displayed.

decreases the cerebrocortical response to insulin [30]. Therefore, AA genotype carriers may have reduced insulin effect in the brain, which has led to increased insulin production, resulting in higher insulin values and HOMA index compared to AA genotype noncarriers.

After training, the insulin levels remained higher, and the glucose levels in these individuals were significantly lower compared to AA genotype noncarriers. The practice of physical exercise promotes a reduction in glucose levels, since the muscle contractions generate an increase in glucose uptake through an enhancement in glucose transporter type four (GLUT4) production [32, 33]. However, more studies are necessary to understand the interaction between the rs993960AA genotype, exercise, and glucose outcome.

A less direct relationship between rs9939609 and insulin levels may involve the demethylase function of the FTO [4]. Merkestein and colleagues [34] found that male mice with *FTO* overexpression have lower adiponectin levels after 20 weeks, which agrees with the reduction in adiponectin levels found in humans who are obese [35]. Adiponectin is a hormone produced mainly in white adipose tissue and has a negative correlation with obesity. All the adiponectin functions are not known exactly, but it is probably involved in glucose, TG, and fatty acids decrease. Low levels of this hormone increase the susceptibility to insulin resistance and type 2 diabetes [36]. By binding to its receptors (AdipoR1 and AdipoR2), adiponectin activates the AMP-activated protein kinase (AMPK), which stimulates glucose utilization and fatty-acid combustion. Therefore, the reduction in adiponectin levels would impair the glucose metabolism and insulin sensitivity [37, 38]. Thus, the *FTO* rs9939609 SNP can contribute to the adiponectin modulation, and consequently, for the glucose metabolism.

Another possible target of FTO is the *ghrelin* gene. Karra and colleagues [39] found that cells with *FTO* overexpression have increased expression of ghrelin mRNA [39]. Ghrelin is a hormone synthesized by the stomach that promotes increased appetite and food intake and decreased insulin sensitivity, among other functions [40]. Therefore, the effects in glucose metabolism observed in the present study can also be explained by ghrelin overexpression.

Additionally, similar to our findings, other studies also observed association of AA genotype with insulin levels and insulin resistance index [15, 41, 42]. Considering that the *FTO* target genes are not fully known, there is a wide variety of possible genes related to metabolism that may had their expression altered in function of *FTO* rs9939609 genotype.

We did not find any effect of the rs9939609 AA genotype on biochemical outcomes in response to training physical program. The studies regarding interactions between *FTO* and physical exercise have controversial results, since some works found interaction [43, 44] and some did not [3,10,45–47]. Those discrepant results could be attributed to the different samples and different ways to analyze the physical activity. Regarding the samples, some studies included children and adolescents [3, 48] while others involved adults [43–46]. Kilpeläinen and colleagues [49] showed that the age is an important factor that modulates the *FTO* and physical exercise interaction, since they observed the interaction between rs9939609 SNP and physical activity only in adults, and not in children and adolescents [49]. Probably other factors also contribute to the heterogeneity in study results, such as gender, ethnicity, and metabolic status.

Moreover, the method of measuring physical activity can also contribute to the heterogeneity, which requires caution in comparisons. Some authors used questionnaires [44, 45, 48], which also differ between them; and other studies analyzed the maximal oxygen uptake (VO_2max), resting energy expenditure, and basal metabolic rate [3, 10, 41]. Our study is one of the few that evaluated the rs9939609 effect on biochemical outcomes of the children and adolescents who were overweight and obese submitted to a physical intervention program, which promoted benefits, improving homeostasis regarding CT, LDL-C, insulin, and QUICKI levels.

4.1. Limitations. Our work has some limitations, as the sample size, which did not make possible to separate children and adolescents by gender, age, or type of physical exercise. However, the type of physical exercise was included in the multiple regression analysis, adjusting our results to this variable.

4.2. Conclusions. In conclusion, we found that the rs9939609 AA genotype influenced parameters related to insulin metabolism and did not interact with physical exercise. Studies that seek to identify the effect of the genetic polymorphisms in metabolic markers are important because they can help with prevention alternatives and more individualized treatments, according to the genetic background of each patient. Additionally, these studies may identify different metabolic pathways in which of these genes participate, and, possibly, indicate new insights into pharmaceutical researches.

Acknowledgments

This work was supported by Fundação Araucária de Apoio ao Desenvolvimento Científico e Tecnológico do Estado do Paraná, Coordenação de Aperfeiçoamento de Pessoal de Nível Superior (CAPES), and Conselho Nacional de Desenvolvimento Científico e Tecnológico (CNPq). The authors would also like to thank the members of "Núcleo de Qualidadede Vida" (Department of Physical Education, Federal University of Paraná) for the data collection.

References

[1] T. M. Frayling, N. J. Timpson, M. N. Weedon et al., "A common variant in the *FTO* gene is associated with body mass index and predisposes to childhood and adult obesity," *Science*, vol. 316, no. 5826, pp. 889–893, 2007.

[2] J. E. Cecil, R. Tavendale, P. Watt, M. M. Hetherington, and C. N. A. Palmer, "An obesity-associated *FTO* gene variant and increased energy intake in children," *New England Journal of Medicine*, vol. 359, no. 24, pp. 2558–2566, 2008.

[3] K. A. Fawcett and I. Barroso, "The genetics of obesity: *FTO* leads the way," *Trends in Genetics*, vol. 26, no. 6, pp. 266–274, 2010.

[4] T. Gerken, C. A. Girard, Y.-C. L. Tung et al., "The obesity-associated *FTO* gene encodes a 2-oxoglutarate-dependent nucleic acid demethylase," *Science*, vol. 318, no. 5855, pp. 1469–1472, 2007.

[5] J. K. Hertel, S. Johansson, E. Sonestedt et al., "*FTO*, type 2 diabetes, and weight gain throughout adult life: a meta-analysis of 41,504 subjects from the scandinavian HUNT, MDC, and MPP studies," *Diabetes*, vol. 60, no. 5, pp. 1637–1644, 2011.

[6] R. Liguori, G. Labruna, A. Alfieri et al., "The *FTO* gene polymorphism (rs9939609) is associated with metabolic syndrome in morbidly obese subjects from southern Italy," *Molecular and Cellular Probes*, vol. 28, no. 4, pp. 195–199, 2014.

[7] T. Berulava and B. Horsthemke, "The obesity-associated SNPs in intron 1 of the *FTO* gene affect primary transcript levels," *European Journal of Human Genetics*, vol. 18, no. 9, pp. 1054–1056, 2010.

[8] J. Wardle, C. Llewellyn, S. Sanderson, and R. Plomin, "The *FTO* gene and measured food intake in children," *International Journal of Obesity*, vol. 33, no. 1, pp. 42–45, 2009.

[9] J. R. Speakman, K. A. Rance, and A. M. Johnstone, "Polymorphisms of the *FTO* gene are associated with variation in energy intake, but not energy expenditure," *Obesity*, vol. 16, no. 8, pp. 1961–1965, 2008.

[10] N. J. Timpson, P. M. Emmett, T. M. Frayling et al., "The fat mass–and obesity-associated locus and dietary intake in children," *American Journal of Clinical Nutrition*, vol. 88, no. 4, pp. 971–978, 2008.

[11] H.-J. Lee, I. K. Kim, J. H. Kang et al., "Effects of common *FTO* gene variants associated with BMI on dietary intake and physical activity in Koreans," *Clinica Chimica Acta*, vol. 411, no. 21-22, pp. 1716–1722, 2010.

[12] J. R. Speakman, "The "Fat Mass and Obesity Related" (*FTO*) gene: mechanisms of impact on obesity and energy balance," *Current Obesity Reports*, vol. 4, no. 1, pp. 73–91, 2015.

[13] R. M. Freathy, N. J. Timpson, D. A. Lawlor et al., "Common variation in the *FTO* gene alters diabetes-related metabolic traits to the extent expected given its effect on BMI," *Diabetes*, vol. 57, no. 5, pp. 1419–1426, 2008.

[14] D. A. De Luis, R. Aller, O. Izaola, D. Primo, and E. Romero, "Association of the rs9939609 gene variant in *FTO* with insulin resistance, cardiovascular risk factor and serum adipokine levels in obese patients," *Nutrición Hospitalaria*, vol. 33, no. 5, pp. 1108–1115, 2016.

[15] C. Muñoz-Yáñez, R. Pérez-Morales, H. Moreno-Macías et al., "Polymorphisms *FTO* rs9939609, *PPARG* rs1801282 and *ADIPOQ* rs4632532 and rs182052 but not lifestyle are associated with obesity related-traits in Mexican children," *Genetics and Molecular Biology*, vol. 39, no. 4, pp. 547–553, 2016.

[16] J. Prakash, B. Mittal, A. Srivastava, S. Awasthi, and N. Srivastava, "Association of *FTO* rs9939609 SNP with obesity and obesity-associated phenotypes in a North Indian population," *Oman Medical Journal*, vol. 31, no. 2, pp. 99–106, 2016.

[17] D. A. Luis, R. Aller, O. Izaola, and D. Pacheco, "Role of rs9939609 *FTO* gene variant in weight loss, insulin resistance and metabolic parameters after a high monounsaturated vs. a high polyunsaturated fat hypocaloric diets," *Nutrición Hospitalaria*, vol. 32, no. 1, pp. 175–181, 2015.

[18] D. A. de Luis, R. Aller, O. Izaola et al., "Evaluation of weight loss and adipocytokines levels after two hypocaloric diets with different macronutrient distribution in obese subjects with rs9939609 gene variant," *Diabetes/Metabolism Research and Reviews*, vol. 28, no. 8, pp. 663–668, 2012.

[19] World Health Organization, *Health Topics: Obesity*, September 2016, http://www.who.int/topics/obesity/en/.

[20] G. A. do Nascimento, M. Dalcin Teixeira, L. Furtado-Alle et al., "*FTO* rs9939609 A allele influences anthropometric outcome in response to dietary intervention, but not in response to physical exercise program," *European Journal of Nutrition*, pp. 1–10, 2017.

[21] W. T. Friedewald, R. I. Levy, and D. S. Fredrickson, "Estimation of the concentration of low-density lipoprotein cholesterol in plasma, without use of the preparative ultracentrifuge," *Clinical Chemistry*, vol. 18, no. 6, pp. 499–502, 1972.

[22] D. R. Matthews, J. P. Hosker, A. S. Rudenski, B. A. Naylor, D. F. Treacher, and R. C. Turner, "Homeostasis model assessment: IR and beta-cell function from fasting plasma glucose and insulin concentration in man," *Diabetologia*, vol. 28, no. 7, pp. 412–419, 1985.

[23] A. Katz, S. S. Nambi, K. Mather et al., "Quantitative insulin sensitivity check index: a simple, accurate method for assessing insulin sensitivity in humans," *Journal of Clinical Endocrinology & Metabolism*, vol. 85, no. 7, pp. 2402–2410, 2000.

[24] G. E. Milano, N. Leite, T. J. Chaves, G. E. Milano, R. L. R. de Souza, and L. F. Alle, "Atividade da butirilcolinesterase e fatores de risco cardiovascular em adolescentes obesos submetidos a um programa de exercícios físicos," *Arquivos Brasileiros de Endocrinologia & Metabologia*, vol. 57, no. 7, pp. 533–537, 2013.

[25] J. Pizzi, L. Furtado-Alle, D. Schiavoni et al., "Reduction in butyrylcholinesterase activity and cardiovascular risk factors in obese adolescents after 12-weeks of high-intensity interval training," *Journal of Exercise Physiology Online*, vol. 20, no. 3, pp. 110–121, 2017.

[26] W. A. Lopes, N. Leite, L. R. da Silva et al., "Effects of 12 weeks of combined training without caloric restriction on inflammatory markers in overweight girls," *Journal of Sports Sciences*, vol. 34, no. 20, pp. 1902–1912, 2016.

[27] M. F. A. Lopes et al., "The effects of water walking on the anthropometrics and metabolic aspects in young obese," *Revista Brasileira de Cineantropometria & Desempenho Humano*, vol. 17, no. 2, pp. 146–155, 2015.

[28] D. K. Lahiri and J. I. Numberger, "A rapid non-enzymatic method for the preparation of HMW DNA from blood for RFLP studies," *Nucleic Acids Research*, vol. 19, p. 5444, 1991.

[29] S. Ten and N. Maclaren, "Insulin resistance syndrome in children," *Journal of Clinical Endocrinology & Metabolism*, vol. 89, no. 6, pp. 2526–2539, 2004.

[30] O. Tschritter, H. Preissl, Y. Yokoyama, F. Machicao, H.-U. Häring, and A. Fritsche, "Variation in the *FTO* gene locus is associated with cerebrocortical insulin resistance in humans," *Diabetologia*, vol. 50, no. 12, pp. 2602-2603, 2007.

[31] W. Chuenta, B. Phonrat, A. Tungtrongchitr et al., "Common variations in the *FTO* gene and obesity in Thais: a family-based study," *Gene*, vol. 558, no. 1, pp. 75–81, 2015.

[32] S. Mann, C. Beedie, S. Balducci et al., "Changes in insulin sensitivity in response to different modalities of exercise: a review of the evidence," *Diabetes/Metabolism Research and Reviews*, vol. 30, no. 4, pp. 257–268, 2014.

[33] A. García-Hermoso, J. M. Saavedra, Y. Escalante, M. Sanchez-Lopez, and V. Martinez-Vizcaino, "Endocrinology and adolescence: aerobic exercise reduces insulin resistance markers in obese youth: a meta-analysis of randomized controlled trials," *European Journal of Endocrinology*, vol. 171, no. 4, pp. R163–R171, 2014.

[34] M. Merkestein, J. S. McTaggart, S. Lee et al., "Changes in gene expression associated with *FTO* overexpression in mice," *PLoS One*, vol. 9, no. 5, article e97162, 2014.

[35] Y. Arita, S. Kihara, N. Ouchi et al., "Paradoxical decrease of an adipose-specific protein, adiponectin, in obesity," *Biochemical and Biophysical Research Communications*, vol. 257, no. 1, pp. 79–83, 1999.

[36] A. Shehzad, W. Iqbal, O. Shehzad, and Y. S. Lee, "Adiponectin: regulation of its production and its role in human diseases," *Hormones*, vol. 11, no. 1, pp. 8–20, 2012.

[37] T. Kadowaki, T. Yamauchi, N. Kubota, K. Hara, K. Ueki, and K. Tobe, "Adiponectin and adiponectin receptors in insulin resistance, diabetes, and the metabolic syndrome," *Journal of Clinical Investigation*, vol. 116, no. 7, pp. 1784–1792, 2006.

[38] N. Kubota, Y. Terauchi, T. Yamauchi et al., "Disruption of adiponectin causes insulin resistance and neointimal

formation," *Journal of Biological Chemistry*, vol. 227, no. 29, pp. 25863–25867, 2002.

[39] E. Karra, O. G. O'Daly, A. I. Choudhury et al., "A link between *FTO*, ghrelin, and impaired brain food-cue responsivity excellence cluster on cellular stress responses in aging-associated diseases," *Journal of Clinical Investigation*, vol. 123, no. 8, pp. 3539–3551, 2013.

[40] L. Mihalache, A. Gherasim, O. Niţă et al., "Effects of ghrelin in energy balance and body weight homeostasis," *Hormones*, vol. 15, no. 2, pp. 186–196, 2016.

[41] S. I. I. Kring, C. Holst, E. Zimmermann et al., "*FTO* gene associated fatness in relation to body fat distribution and metabolic traits throughout a broad range of fatness," *PLoS One*, vol. 3, no. 8, article e2958, 2008.

[42] S. Tan, A. Scherag, O. E. Janssen et al., "Large effects on body mass index and insulin resistance of fat mass and obesity associated gene (*FTO*) variants in patients with polycystic ovary syndrome (PCOS)," *BMC Medical Genetics*, vol. 11, no. 1, p. 12, 2010.

[43] M. Muc, C. Padez, and L. Manco, "Influence of physical activity on the association between the *FTO* variant rs9939609 and adiposity in young adults," *American Journal of Human Biology*, vol. 27, no. 5, pp. 734–738, 2015.

[44] J. Petkeviciene, A. Smalinskiene, J. Klumbiene, V. Petkevicius, V. Kriaucioniene, and V. Lesauskaite, "Physical activity, but not dietary intake, attenuates the effect of the *FTO* rs9939609 polymorphism on obesity and metabolic syndrome in Lithuanian adult population," *Public Health*, vol. 135, pp. 23–29, 2016.

[45] A. Jonsson, F. Renström, V. Lyssenko et al., "Assessing the effect of interaction between an *FTO* variant (rs9939609) and physical activity on obesity in 15,925 Swedish and 2,511 Finnish adults," *Diabetologia*, vol. 52, no. 7, pp. 1334–1338, 2009.

[46] T. Berentzen, S. I. I. Kring, C. Holst et al., "Lack of association of fatness-related *FTO* gene variants with energy expenditure or physical activity," *Journal of Clinical Endocrinology & Metabolism*, vol. 93, no. 7, pp. 2904–2908, 2008.

[47] A. Leońska-duniec, Z. Jastrzębski, A. Zarębska, A. Maciejewska, K. Ficek, and P. Cięszczyk, "Assessing effect of interaction between the *FTO* A/T polymorphism (rs9939609) and physical activity on obesity-related traits," *Journal of Sport and Health Science*, vol. 352, 2016.

[48] E. T. Liem, J. M. Vonk, P. J. Sauer et al., "Influence of common variants near *INSIG2*, in *FTO*, and near *MC4R* genes on overweight and the metabolic profile in adolescence: The TRAILS (TRacking Adolescents' Individual Lives Survey) Study," *American Journal of Clinical Nutrition*, vol. 91, no. 2, pp. 321–328, 2010.

[49] T. O. Kilpeläinen, L. Qi, S. Brage et al., "Physical activity attenuates the influence of *FTO* variants on obesity risk: a meta-analysis of 218,166 adults and 19,268 children," *PLoS Medicine*, vol. 8, no. 11, p. e1001116, 2011.

6

FTO Gene Associates and Interacts with Obesity Risk, Physical Activity, Energy Intake, and Time Spent Sitting

Bolaji Fatai Oyeyemi,[1,2] Charles Ayorinde Ologunde,[2] Ayonposi Bukola Olaoye,[2,3] and Nanfizat Abiket Alamukii[4]

[1] *Integrative Biology Unit, Transcriptional Regulation Group, International Centre for Genetic Engineering and Biotechnology, New Delhi, India*
[2] *Department of Science Technology, The Federal Polytechnic Ado-Ekiti, Ado-Ekiti, Nigeria*
[3] *Institute of Biological, Environmental and Rural Sciences, Aberystwyth University, Aberystwyth, UK*
[4] *Cell Biology and Genetics Unit, Department of Zoology, University of Ibadan, Ibadan, Nigeria*

Correspondence should be addressed to Bolaji Fatai Oyeyemi; bolaji@icgeb.res.in

Academic Editor: Aron Weller

Fat mass and obesity-associated (FTO) gene influences obesity but studies have shown that environmental/lifestyle variables like physical activity (PA), time spent sitting (TSS), and energy intake might mediate the effect. However, this is poorly understood in Nigeria due to scarce studies. We demystified association and interaction between FTO rs9939609, obesity, PA, TSS, and energy intake in Nigeria. FTO gene variant was genotyped by restriction fragment length polymorphism and gene sequencing analysis in 103 people with obesity and 98 controls. Anthropometrics and environmental variables were measured using standard procedures. Significant associations were found between FTO rs9939609 with obesity and environmental/lifestyle variables before and after adjusting for age. Carriers of allele A have significantly higher odds of being overweight/obese using BMI [0.191 (0.102–0.361), $p < 0.001$] but this was attenuated by PA ($p_{[\text{interaction}]} = 0.029$); odds of being overweight reduced from 0.625 (0.181–2.159) to 0.082 (0.009–0.736) for low and high PA, respectively. Mediation analysis of total indirect effect also confirmed this by showing a simultaneous mediating role of total PA, energy intake, and TSS in the relationship between FTO and BMI (unstandardized coefficient = 1.60, 95% CI. 1.26–2.22). This study shows a relationship between FTO and obesity phenotype and environmental/lifestyle factors might be an important modulator/mediator in the association.

1. Introduction

Increasing number of overweight/obese people has contributed immensely to public health challenge throughout the world. Studies in Nigeria had reported a higher rate of obesity and cardiovascular risk factors [1]. Thus Nigeria is not exempted from the scourge. Therefore, there is the need for greater attention and proactive step to stem the tide. The interactions between environmental and individual factors, including genetic makeup, explain the variability in body size between individuals in a given population [2–5], implying that gene-environment interaction might be germane in the development/progression of overweight/obesity [6].

One of the most known genetic factors predisposing humans to nonmonogenic obesity is a polymorphism in the fat mass and obesity-associated (FTO) gene [7, 8] especially first intron rs9939609 (A/T variant) [9–12]. Individuals carrying this risk allele have been reported to have about 1.09 kg, 0.54 kg/m^2, and 1.07 cm more weight, BMI, and waist circumference (WC), respectively [10]. However, there are still many unknown attributes regarding the biology of this locus [5, 6].

Human carriers of the susceptible single nucleotide polymorphisms (SNPs) in *FTO* (rs9939609 A/T variant) have also been shown to have a strong relationship with satiety and nutrient preference; this suggests that FTO variant is germane in the dietary macronutrient composition of an individual [5]. To lend credence to this, a recent study suggested that there was FTO (rs9939609 A/T variant) genotype-specific enhancement of neural sensitivity to food stimuli. Thus it seems to be predisposing individual to addiction-supportive food perception [13, 14]. However, Gustavsson et al. [15] reported no evidence of interactions between FTO genotype and macronutrient intake on cardiovascular heart disease risk or BMI. This might be a result of the difference in genetic and environmental variables of their study population; it thus shows that genetic and environmental factors are germane in demystifying obesity.

A high ratio of second to fourth digit finger length (2D : 4D) is widely associated with increased BMI, body size, and coronary heart disease [16–18]. Thus it might be related to the FTO rs9939609 gene variant. Several studies have elucidated the effects of environment and FTO variant on obesity, evident in the well-studied time spent sitting (TSS), physical activity (PA), and dietary correlates of obesity [9, 10, 12, 19]. The first study on FTO gene polymorphism in a well-characterized African (Gambians living in traditional lifestyle) reported that FTO gene variant seems not to influence BMI [20]. But this is slowly being understood in Nigerian context due to limited reports. Studies have shown that some anthropometric variables (ratio of second to the fourth finger (2D : 4D), WC, neck circumference (NC), waist to height ratio (WHtR), and waist to hip ratio (WHR)) might be a surrogate marker for overweight/obesity [21–23]. This study explored those anthropometric traits relationship with FTO rs9939609 variant and the modulating roles of environmental variables (PA, TSS, and energy intake) among young adults. This study combined gene sequencing and restriction fragment length polymorphism (RFLP) to unravel FTO polymorphism in Nigeria population.

2. Materials and Methods

This case-control pilot study was conducted among randomly selected unrelated young adults with the mean age of 22.6 (103 people with obesity [BMI $\geq$ 25.0 Kg/m^2] and 98 controls) at the Federal Polytechnic Ado-Ekiti (FPA), Nigeria. The study (including informed consent forms and the proposed participant recruitment strategy) was approved by the Research Ethics Committee of the Ekiti State Teaching Hospital Ethical Committee and the FPA Ethical Committee (approval number: FPA/ETH/13-028). We conducted this study in accordance with the Declaration of Helsinki, and all participants gave written informed consent.

Digit length was measured as previously described by Manning et al. [24]. Briefly, subjects kept their hands supine on a flat surface with the palm facing up and the digits straight in the same plane and fingers wide opened in a posture of ease (not kept together tight under artificial pressure).

Body weight, height, WC, HC, and NC were measured with standard procedure while BMI, WHtR, and WHR were calculated as weight (kg) divided by height (m) squared, WC divided by height, and WC divided by HC, respectively.

PA and TSS were measured with self-reported International Physical Activity Questionnaire-Short (IPAQ-SF) form which had been adapted to one of the Nigeria major languages by [25]. Total physical activity was computed and categorized as described by http://www.ipaq.ki.se. Briefly, each category of physical activity was multiplied by their estimated intensity (MET) and reported day(s); the sum of all categories was the total physical activity of the individual. MET intensity includes vigorous (8 METs), moderate (4 METs), and walking (3.3 METs). One MET is the energy dissipated in an inactive state which is 3.5 mL/kg/min of VO_2 [26].

We used semiquantified food frequency questionnaire (FFQ) to collect information about the dietary habits of our participants as described by [27].

Genomic DNA was isolated from EDTA-anticoagulated whole blood samples using Quick-gDNAMiniPrep kits (ZymoResearch, USA) according to the manufacturer's protocol and stored at −20°C. Genotyping of SNP in rs9939609 was done with PCR-RFLP assay as described by [28]. Briefly, genomic DNA (20 ng) was incubated in a 10 μL solution containing 1 NH4 buffer, 2.5 mmol/liter magnesium, 200 μmol/liter each dNTP, 20 pmol forward (5′-AACTGGCTCTTGAATGAAATAGGATTCAGA-3′) and reverse (5′-AGAGTAACAGAGACTATCCAAGTGCAGTAC-3′) oligonucleotide primers, and 0.5 U Taq DNA polymerase (Inqaba West Africa). The PCR mix was incubated using a touchdown programme at 94°C for 2 minutes followed by 35 cycles of 93°C for 15 seconds, 65°C–56°C for 20 seconds (dropping 0.5°C per cycle), 72°C for 30 seconds, 72°C for 5 minutes, and 10°C ∞. This was then incubated at 37°C for 3 hours with 2 U ScaI (Inqaba, West Africa). Genotype success rate was 98%.

To confirm results from PCR-RFLP, we proceeded to sequence analysis of the FTO rs9939609 gene: sequencing reactions were performed using the ABI Big Dye Terminator Cycle Sequencing kit version 3.1 (Applied Biosystems Inc., Foster City, CA). Cycling conditions include 94°C/1 minute; 25 cycles of 96°C/10 seconds, and 60°C/4 minutes. Reactions were carried out in a total volume of 20 μL, which included 1–3 ng/μL purified PCR product, 3.2 pmol primer, and 8 μL ABI Prism Big Dye Terminator mix, v3.1 (Applied Biosystems). The sequencing products were cleaned using the ZR-96 DNA Sequencing Clean-up kitTM (Zymo Research Corporation©, Irvine, CA, 2005-2006). Products were analyzed on the Applied Biosystems/Hitachi 3130 9-1-Genetic Analyser. The FTO rs9939609 gene was sequenced bidirectionally in every participant to confirm the observed variants.

2.1. Statistical Analysis. Statistical analysis was performed using IBM SPSS 22 and GraphPad Prism 7 for Mac while sample size was computed using G*Power (version 3.1; Heinrich Heine University, Düsseldorf, Germany) [29] and method described by Viechtbauer et al. [30] for a pilot study. Power, significance, and minor or risk allele frequencies (MAF) for cases and controls were 95%, 5%, 40%, and 27%, respectively; thus our sample size appears to be sufficient for pilot study.

Data are expressed as frequencies and percentage or as means (standard deviation) unless otherwise stated. Allelic

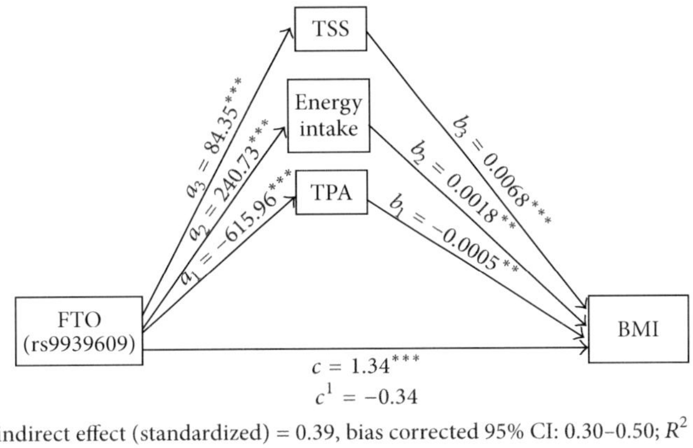

FIGURE 1: Multiple mediation models of the relationship between FTO rs9939609, TPA, energy intake, TSS, and BMI. (TPA, energy intake, and TSS are mediators). Standardized coefficients are presented and tested for significance with 95% confidence intervals calculated using the bias-corrected bootstrap method (5000 samples). a = standardized IV to Med coefficient, b = standardized Med to DV coefficient, c = standardized total effect (IV to DV), and c^1 = specific indirect effect (indirect path). $^{**}p < 0.01$; $^{***}p < 0.001$. BMI: body mass index, TPA: total physical activity, TSS: time spent sitting, IV: independent variable, DV: dependent variable, and Med: mediator.

and genotypic frequencies were determined by counting the genotypes and distribution of genotypes in different groups was compared by Chi-square or Fisher exact test. Robust logistic regression was used to evaluate the associations between the FTO rs9939609 genotype (genotype coded as 0 for TT, 1 for AT, and 2 for AA), obesity measures, 2D : 4D, and energy intake (controlled for sex and age). Models were also created for the categorical outcome (overweight/obesity versus control) by robust logistic regression where FTO rs9939609 was included. Analyses were adjusted for sex and age, and odds ratios (OR) with 95% confidence intervals (CI) were calculated to estimate the association between genotypes and measurements. Differences were checked by T-test and ANOVA (Significant ANOVA results were further examined using the Bonferroni post hoc test). Differences in data that did not follow a normal distribution (physical activity) were analyzed with nonparametric Kruskal–Wallis and Mann–Whitney tests.

A statistical method which is known as tests of mediation, which examines the effect of a presumed mediator(s) on the outcome of a predictor on the response variable, is used to investigate possible mediating effects of PA, TSS, and energy intake on the association between our distal variable (FTO rs9939606 genotype) and outcome (BMI). In recent times, studies have employed this method for mediating analysis of mediator(s) on obesity risk allele and BMI [9, 31]. We followed approaches developed by [32] for the multiple mediation analysis on our mediators on the relationship between FTO rs9939609 and BMI. Briefly, we named path coefficient linking the predictor with mediators and path coefficient of a mediator to the outcome as paths a and b, respectively. Paths c and c' refer to the total and indirect effect of FTO rs9939609on BMI in the absence and presence of the mediators, respectively (Figure 1). Bootstrapping was used to create 95% confidence intervals around the "true" value of this cross-product (referred to as the indirect effect). If zero is not within this confidence interval, then the indirect (i.e., mediating) effect is significant. The SPSS "indirect" macro developed to accompany the paper by [32] was used to test the significance. We also checked the mediating effect of each mediator separately and of BMI on the association of FTO rs9939609 on TSS using the same method described above.

A p value < 0.05 was considered to have statistical significance.

3. Results

We arrived at the sample size with G*Power (version 3.1; Heinrich Heine University, Düsseldorf, Germany) [29] and method described by Viechtbauer et al. [30] for a pilot study. Power, significance, and MAF for cases and controls were 95%, 5%, 40%, and 27%, respectively. Thus our sample size appears to be sufficient for this pilot study.

The demographics of the two hundred and one unrelated participants (age range from 17 to 39 years) stratified by sex are presented in Table 1; 51.20%, 32.3%, 53.2%, and 54.7% of individuals were people with obesity using BMI, WC, WHR, and WHtR benchmarks. Cutoff values include BMI ≥ 25.0 kg/m^2, WC ≥ 80.0 cm for female and ≥94.0 cm for male, and WHR ≥ 0.45 for female and ≥0.5 for male while values ≥0.5 were used for WHtR in both sexes. There was a statistical difference in total physical activity in female and male but not time spent sitting. The ratio of second and fourth digits of both hands was also different (2D : 4D) (Table 1).

All participants were genotyped for FTO SNP rs9939609; thirty-six (17.9%) were homozygous for the obesity risk allele (AA), 90 (44.8%) were heterozygous (AT), and 75 (37.3%) were wild type (TT). The frequency of allele A in this study is 0.40, while it is 0.53 and 0.27 for overweight/obesity and healthy control, respectively. None of these allelic frequencies differs from Hardy-Weinberg equilibrium ($p > 0.05$).

We reported significantly high obesity risk factors in AA, followed by AT and TT, respectively, while the opposite was reported in physical activity pattern (Table 2, Supplementary Table 1, and Supplementary Figures 1–4 in Supplementary material available online at https://doi.org/10.1155/2017/3245270). As shown in Table 3 and Supplementary Figures 1

Table 1: Characteristics of the study population.

Characteristics	Overall (n = 201)	Female (n = 102)	Male (n = 99)	p
Age (years)	22.64 (3.61)	23.05 (3.69)	22.22 (3.50)	0.105
Anthropometric				
Body weight (kg)	66.98 (9.54)	62.54 (7.80)	71.56 (9.03)	<0.001
BMI (kg/m^2)	25.96 (3.06)	25.52 (3.15)	26.41 (2.91)	0.044
Normal (n; %)[a]	98; 48.80	45; 22.40	53; 26.40	0.182
Overweight/obesity (n; %)[b]	103; 51.20	57; 28.40	46; 22.90	0.322
NC (cm)	31.24 (4.00)	30.78 (5.06)	31.25 (4.34)	0.121
WC (cm)	81.67 (8.02)	80.91 (7.50)	82.47 (8.48)	0.169
Central obesity (n; %)[c]	65; 32.30	56; 27.90	9; 4.50	<0.001
WHR	0.881 (0.081)	0.862 (0.070)	0.899 (0.088)	0.001
Central obesity (n; %)[d]	107; 53.20	57; 28.40	50; 24.90	0.445
WHtR	0.507 (0.055)	0.514 (0.053)	0.499 (0.056)	0.038
Visceral obesity (n; %)[e]	110; 54.70	62; 30.80	48; 23.90	0.08
R2D : 4D	0.9711 (0.027)	0.9819 (0.027)	0.9600 (0.022)	<0.001
L2D : 4D	0.9684 (0.024)	0.9791 (0.023)	0.9573 (0.021)	<0.001
Energy intake (kcal/day)[f]	1848.76 (431.17)	1763.73 (397.96)	1936.36 (448.23)	0.004
Time spent siting (minutes/week)	411.19 (183.12)	400.98 (173.53)	421.72 (192.82)	0.424
Physical activity (PA)				
Total PA (MET-minutes/week)**	678 (4177–40)	643.5 (3405–40)	1335 (4177–188.5)	<0.001
Light PA (MET-minutes/week)**	396 (1782–0)	280.5 (1782–0)	495 (1782–33)	<0.001
Moderate PA (MET-minutes/week)**	180 (1800–0)	120 (1800–0)	320 (1680–0)	<0.001
Vigorous PA (MET-minutes/week)**	80 (1800–0)	0 (1800–0)	80 (1800–0)	0.072

Data are presented as means (standard deviation (SD) values shown in parenthesis) except stated otherwise. The difference was evaluated using Student's T-test and Chi-square test for continuous and categorical variables, respectively; BMI: body mass index, NC: neck circumference, WC: waist circumference, WHR: waist to hip ratio, WHtR: waist to height ratio, R2D : 4D: ratio of right hand second to fourth digit, and L2D : 4D: ratio of left hand second to the fourth digit; n = number of samples; % = percentage; [a]normal BMI < 25 kg/m^2 while [b]overweight/obesity BMI ≥ 25 kg/m^2; [c]central obesity was defined as WC > 80 cm for female and > 94 cm for male; [d]central obesity was defined as WHR > 0.85 for female and >0.90 for male; [e]visceral obesity was defined as WHtR > 0.5; [f]total energy intake per day from carbohydrate sources; **data expressed by median (range); Mann–Whitney U test.

and 2, presence of at least one copy of the risk allele (A) was associated with some units higher (β) obesity risk factors as categorized by body weight (β: 3.11 kg per risk allele, 95% CI: 0.39–5.83, $p < 0.001$), BMI (β: 1.74 kg/m^2 per risk allele, 95% CI: 0.89–2.58, $p < 0.001$), WC (β: 5.73 cm per risk allele, 95% CI: 3.58–7.88, $p < 0.001$), and NC (β: 2.55 cm per risk allele, 95% CI: 1.45–3.65, $p < 0.001$). We also observed that 2D : 4D in both hands showed marked increased in individuals with the risk allele (β: 0.018 per risk allele, 95% CI: 0.011–0.025, $p < 0.001$ and β: 0.016 per risk allele, 95% CI: 0.010–0.022, $p < 0.001$) for right and left hand, respectively (Table 3 and Supplementary Figure 3). A similar trend was observed for energy intake (354.4 Kcal/day more per risk allele) and TSS (190.5 minutes more per risk allele) (Tables 2 and 3 and Supplementary Figure 4).

Participants with FTO risk allele (A) had significantly higher odds of being overweight/obese (OR: 0.19 (0.10–0.36), $p < 0.001$), central obesity (OR: 0.33 (0.15–0.71), $p = 0.005$), and visceral obesity (OR: 0.12 (0.06–0.23), $p < 0.001$) than individuals with the T allele only (Table 3). But the odds were attenuated with increased physical activity levels as shown in Table 4. The odds of overweight/obesity reduced from 0.63 (95% CI: 0.18–2.16) per copy of the risk allele in participants with lower levels of PA to 0.08 (95% CI: 0.009–0.736) in participants with high PA ($p_{(\text{interaction})} = 0.029$) (Table 4). Similar odds trends were found in WHR central obesity (low PA: 0.517 versus high PA: 0.057 per copy of the risk allele, $p_{(\text{interaction})} = 0.007$) and WHtR visceral obesity (low PA: 0.356 versus high PA: 0.142 per copy of the risk allele, $p_{(\text{interaction})} = 0.010$). This was further confirmed in Figures 2–4 where the least square mean of obesity traits in FTO genotypes is different in low and high PA. There was also gene-PA interaction effect on energy intake and time spent sitting with significant $p_{(\text{FTO}*\text{PA})}$ interaction values of 0.008 and 0.027 was reported, respectively (Figure 4). From the preceding, we might predict that there are mediating effects of PA, TSS, and energy intake on BMI, thus mediation analysis.

Multiple regression analyses were conducted to assess effects of mediator(s) on the relationship between FTO rs9939609 and BMI using mediation model. First, it was found that FTO rs9939609 variant was associated with BMI ($B = 1.34$, $t(199) = 4.68$, and $p < 0.001$) (path c). It was also found that FTO rs9939609 variant was significantly related to all mediator TPA ($B = -615.96$, $t(199) = -5.69$, and

TABLE 2: Anthropometric traits of overweight and control subjects stratified by FTO rs6639609 variants.

Characteristics	Overall (n = 201) TT (n = 75)	TA (n = 90)	AA (n = 36)	p
Body weight (kg)	65.03 (8.04)[a]	66.67 (10.49)[a]	71.82 (8.47)	0.007[a]
BMI (kg/m^2)	24.95 (2.50)[a]	26.10 (3.24)[a]	27.70 (2.88)	0.006[a]
NC (cm)	29.72 (2.63)[a]	30.91 (3.78)[a]	35.20 (4.39)	<0.001[a]
WC (cm)	78.20 (7.14)	82.70 (7.46)	86.33 (8.21)	0.026
WHtR	0.481 (0.05)	0.519 (0.05)[a]	0.532 (0.06)[a]	0.006[a]
WHR	0.840 (0.07)	0.883 (0.07)	0.957 (0.08)	0.002
R2D : 4D	0.9586 (0.02)	0.9742 (0.02)	0.9894 (0.04)	0.0026
L2D : 4D	0.9570 (0.02)	0.9726 (0.02)	0.9816 (0.03)	0.013
Energy intake (kcal/day)	1662.00 (377.76)	1891.67 (370.25)	2273.89 (537.91)	0.008
TSS (minutes/week)	300.13 (129.75)	465.22 (151.73)	541.94 (160.62)	0.003
TPA**	1668.00 (4177–99)	625.25 (4120–40)	645.00 (2826–89.5)	<0.001
VPA**	792.00 (1782–0)	297.00 (1782–0)	231.00 (1386–33)	<0.001
MPA**	480.00 (1800–0)	170.00 (1760–0)	120.00 (1440–0)	<0.001
LPA**	96.00 (1800–0)	0 (1680–0)	0 (1800–0)	0.066

Data are expressed as mean (SD values presented in parenthesis) except stated otherwise; ANOVA test (Bonferroni multiple comparability test) was used to compare means across genotype while Kruskal–Wallis test was used to test the difference in physical activity; BMI: body mass index, NC: neck circumference, WC: waist circumference, WHR: waist to hip ratio, WHtR: waist to height ratio, R2D : 4D: ratio of right hand second to fourth digit, and L2D : 4D: ratio of left hand second to fourth digit; TSS: time spent sitting, TPA: total physical activity, VPA: vigorous physical activity, MPA: moderate physical activity, and LPA: low physical activity; [a]data expressed with the same superscript in the same row are not statistically different at $p < 0.05$; **data are expressed by median (range); Kruskal–Wallis test (comparability test Dunns).

TABLE 3: Association of FTO rs9939609 genotype with obesity-related traits.

Variables Anthropometrics	Estimated change per unit A allele (95% CI)	p
Body weight (kg)	3.109 (0.392–5.827)	0.025
BMI (kg/m^2)	1.735 (0.89–2.579)	<0.001
WC (cm)	5.73 (3.58–7.88)	<0.001
WHR	0.068 (0.047–0.089)	<0.001
WHtR	0.041 (0.026–0.055)	<0.001
NC (cm)	2.55 (1.45–3.65)	<0.001
Overweight or obesity[a]	0.191 (0.102–0.361)	<0.001
Central obesity[b]	0.328 (0.151–0.714)	0.005
Central obesity[c]	0.131 (0.068–0.253)	<0.001
Visceral obesity[d]	0.12 (0.062–0.232)	<0.001
Energy intake (kcal/day)	354.40 (231.71–477.10)	<0.001
TSS (minutes/week)	190.52 (147.8–233.23)	<0.001
R2D : 4D	0.018 (0.011–0.025)	<0.001
L2D : 4D	0.016 (0.01–0.022)	<0.001

Data presented as beta coefficient (for continuous outcome) or odd ratio (OR) (for binary outcome) with corresponding 95% confidence interval (CI). Models were adjusted for age and sex; BMI: body mass index, NC: neck circumference, WC: waist circumference, WHR: waist to hip ratio, WHtR: waist to height ratio, R2D : 4D: ratio of the right hand second digit to the fourth, and L2D : 4D: ratio of the left hand second digit to the fourth; [a]overweight or obesity was defined as BMI ≥ 25.0 kg/m^2; [b]central obesity was defined as WC > 80 cm for female and >94 cm for male; [c]central obesity was defined as WHR > 0.85 for female and >0.90 for male; [d]visceral obesity was defined as WHtR > 0.5.

$p < 0.001$) (path a_1), energy intake ($B = 240.73$, $t(198) = 5.71$, and $p < 0.001$) (path a_2), and TSS ($B = 84.35$, $t(197) = 5.44$, and $p < 0.001$) (path a_3). Lastly, results indicated that all mediator, TPA, energy intake, and TSS were associated with BMI ($B = -0.0005$, $t(196) = -2.79$, and $p < 0.01$ (path b_1); $B = 0.0018$, $t(196) = 3.99$, and $p < 0.01$ (path b_2); and $B = 0.0068$, $t(198) = 5.33$, and $p < 0.001$ (path b_3)), respectively. Because all a and b paths were significant, multiple mediation analyses were tested using the bootstrapping method with bias-corrected confidence estimates and 95% confidence interval of the indirect effects was obtained with 5000 bootstrap resamples [32].

Table 4: Association between FTO rs9939609 genotype and obesity measures by category of PA.

Variable	Low PA ($n = 77$) OR (95% CI)	p	Moderate PA ($n = 75$) OR (95% CI)	p	High PA ($n = 49$) OR (95% CI)	p	$p_{(FTO*PA)}$
Overweight[a]	0.625 (0.181–2.159)	0.46	0.113 (0.033–0.387)	0.001	0.082 (0.009–0.736)	0.026	0.029
Central obesity[b]	0.78 (0.212–2.872)	0.71	0.273 (0.065–1.151)	0.077	0.187 (0.037–0.952)	0.043	0.345
Central obesity[c]	0.517 (0.174–1.539)	0.24	0.047 (0.011–0.194)	<0.001	0.057 (0.01–0.323)	0.001	0.007
Visceral obesity[d]	0.356 (0.116–1.089)	0.07	0.039 (0.01–0.16)	<0.001	0.142 (0.032–0.636)	0.011	0.010

Data presented as the odd ratio (OR) with corresponding 95% confidence interval (CI). Models were adjusted for age and sex; BMI: body mass index, WC: waist circumference, WHR: waist to hip ratio, and WHtR: waist to height ratio; [a]overweight or obesity was defined as BMI $\geq 25.0\,kg/m^2$; [b]central obesity was defined as WC > 80 cm for female and >94 cm for male; [c]central obesity was defined as WHR > 0.85 for female and >0.90 for male; [d]visceral obesity was defined as WHtR > 0.5.

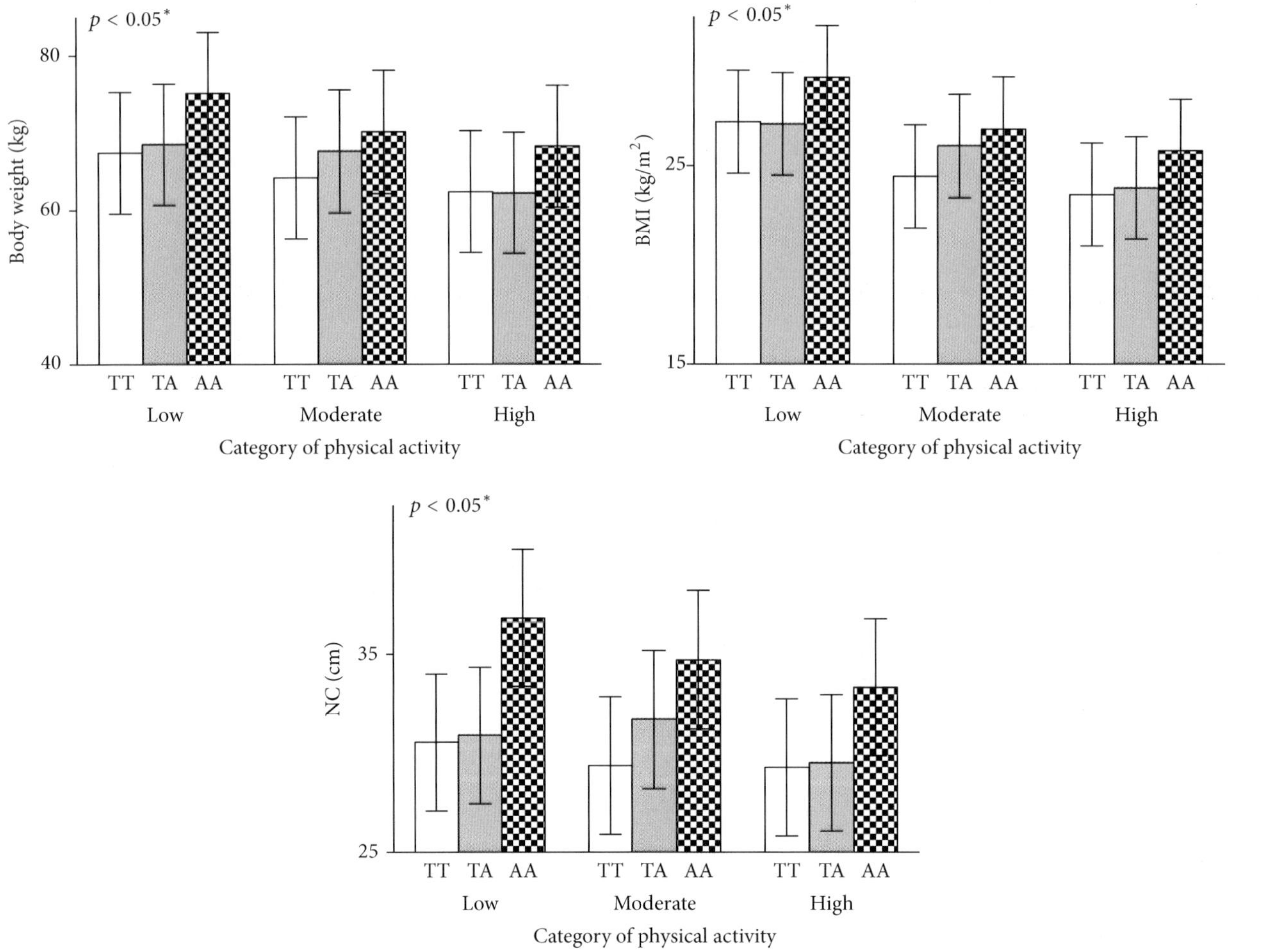

Figure 2: Effect of the FTO rs9939609 genotype on adiposity measures (body weight, BMI, and NC) stratified by category of PA. p values are for the interaction between the FTO variant and PA category; least-squares means of different genotypes across all PA groups were calculated using Robust Linear Regression analysis, after adjusting for age and sex. Allele frequency by PA category was low: 20/43/14; moderate: 28/34/13; high: 27/13/9 for TT, TA, and AA genotypes, respectively. BMI: body mass index; NC: neck circumference. *Mean of each variable with genotype for high PA is different from mean of each genotype for low PA at $p < 0.05$ but not in NC TA and TT genotype.

Results of the mediation analysis of total indirect effect confirmed the simultaneous mediating role of TPA, energy intake, and TSS in the relation between FTO gene variant and BMI (the *total indirect effect* was statistically significant while unstandardized-coefficient = 1.68; 95% CI: 1.26–2.22). Also, results indicated that the direct effect of FTO gene variant on BMI was reduced drastically though significant ($B = -0.34$, $t(196) = -1.13$, and $p > 0.05$) (path c^1) when controlling for mediators, thus suggesting full mediation (Figure 1). Each mediator (TPA, energy intake, and TSS) was tested separately, and they all showed full mediating ability on the interaction between FTO rs9939609 and BMI (Supplementary Figures 5–7). Mediation model was created for the effect of BMI on the association of FTO rs9939609

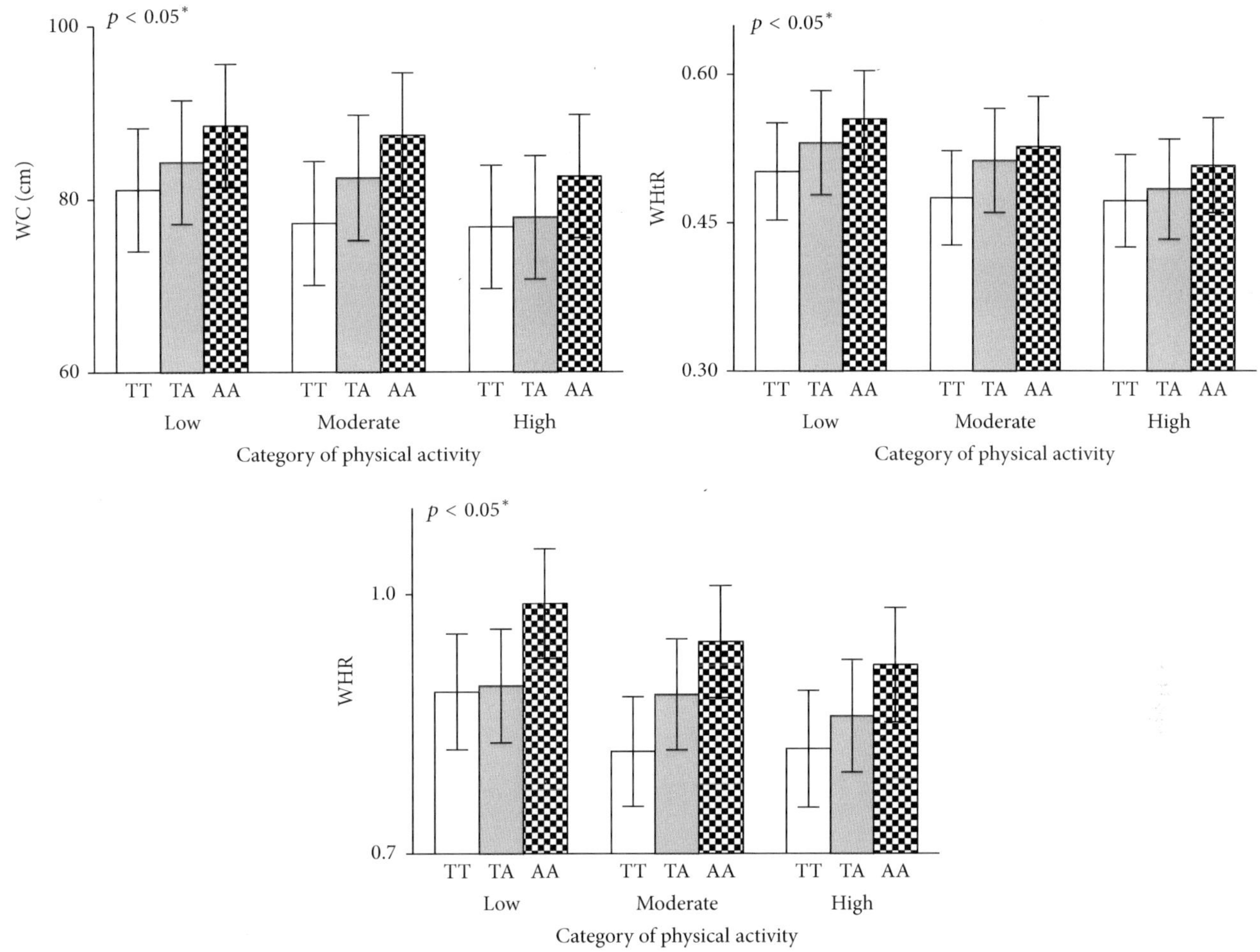

FIGURE 3: Effect of the FTO rs9939609 genotype on adiposity measures (WC, WHtR, and WHR) stratified by category of PA. p values are for the interaction between the FTO variant and PA category; least-squares means of different genotypes across all PA groups were calculated using Robust Linear Regression analysis, with adjustment for age and sex. Allele frequency by PA category was low: 20/43/14; moderate: 28/34/13; high: 27/13/9 for TT, TA, and AA genotypes, respectively. WC: waist circumference, WHtR: waist to height ratio, and WHR; waist to hip ratio. *Mean of each variable with genotype for high PA is different from the mean of each genotype for low PA at $p < 0.05$ but not in WC AA genotype and WHR TA genotype.

with TSS and TPA, and it showed that BMI exerts full mediation in both cases (Supplementary Figures 8-9).

4. Discussion

In this pilot study, we analyzed SNP rs9939609 of the FTO gene in a group of people with obesity and control in Nigeria. Individuals with the FTO risk allele (A) and low PA level had significantly high obesity risk factors (BMI, WC, NC, WHR, WHtR, body weight, 2D : 4D, energy intake, and TSS). Furthermore, PA, energy intake, and TSS play a mediating role in the effect of the FTO gene variant to BMI. These relationships indicate that the genetic variant and some environmental variables (PA, TSS, and energy intake) might be playing a relevant role in obesity. This study thus elucidated the relationships between FTO genotype, PA, anthropometrics, energy intake, and 2D : 4D in a population residing in Nigeria. But further studies are required to confirm or to refute these observations.

The AA genotype proportion of the FTO rs9939609 reported in this study was significantly higher in people with obesity when compared with control (25.2% to 10.2%); this is in agreement with earlier studies [8, 11, 33]. Our results are in tandem with previous studies as carriers of risk alleles showed higher obesity-related traits [8–11], thus confirming the relationship between FTO rs9939609 and obesity.

This study reported a 1.74 (95% CI 0.47 to 1.10) kg/m^2 increase in BMI per A allele. This is higher than 1.66, 1.55, 0.79, and 0.54 reported in France, Roma/Gypsy population, and China and across seven European countries [10, 34–36] but lower than 2.8 (95% CI 1.3–6.0) reported in Pakistan female [37]. This shows that our result is comparable to what was reported from other parts of the world. More so, our result is not in agreement with Li et al. [38] that reported no relationship between FTO rs9939609 and BMI in Chinese Han population; this discrepancy might be due to difference in environmental variables, obesity categorization, ethnic

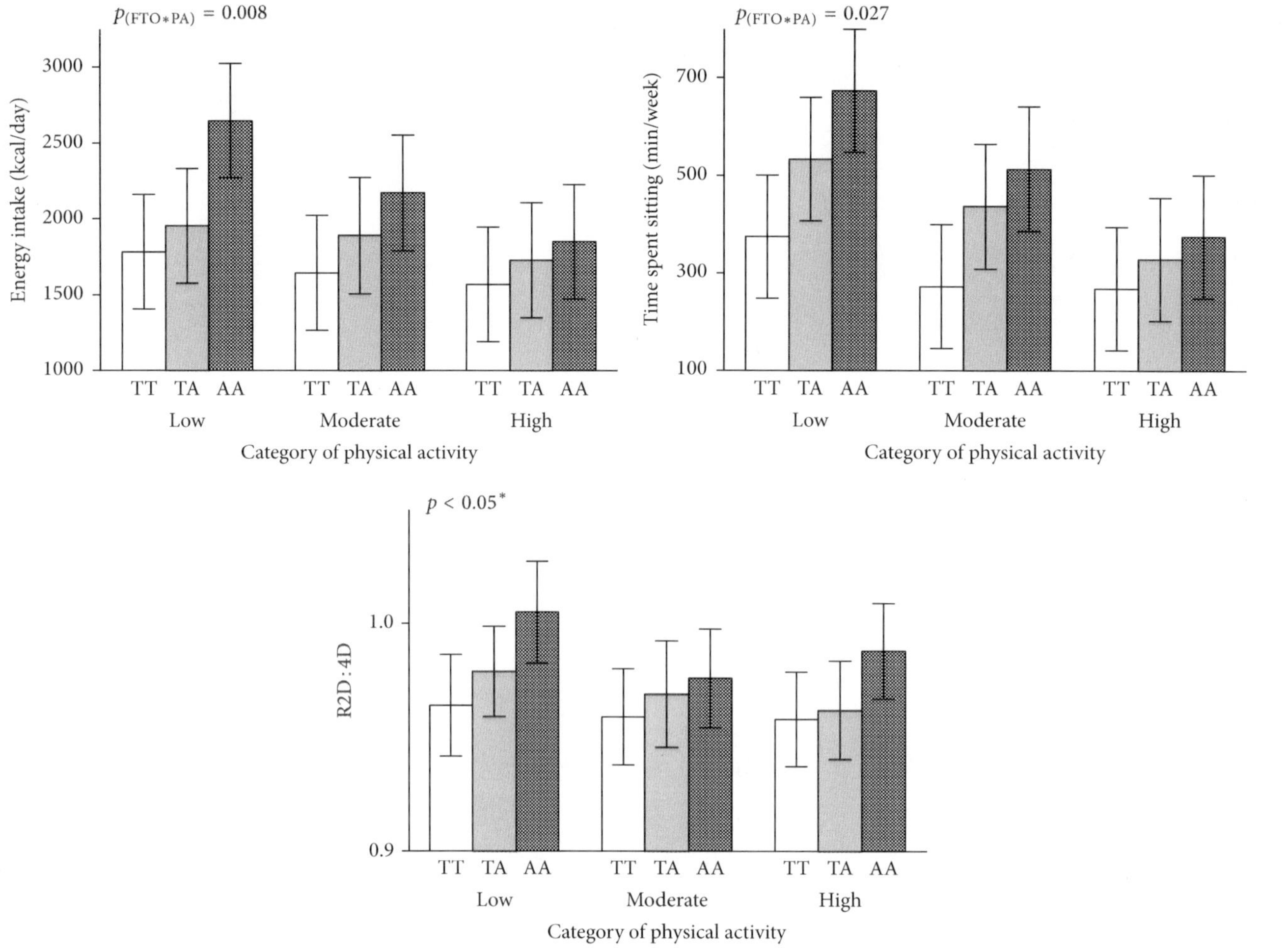

FIGURE 4: Effect of the FTO rs9939609 genotype on energy intake, TSS, and R2D : 4D stratified by category of PA. p values are for the interaction between the FTO variant and PA category; least-squares means of different genotypes across all PA groups were calculated by using Robust Linear Regression analysis, with adjustment for age and sex. Allele frequency by PA category was low: 20/43/14; moderate: 28/34/13; high: 27/13/9 for TT, TA, and AA genotypes, respectively. TSS: time spent sitting. R2D : 4D; ratio of the left hand second digit to the fourth, and TSS; time spent sitting. *Mean of each variable with genotype for high PA is different from mean of each genotype for low PA at $p < 0.05$ but not in R2D : 4D TT and AA genotype.

difference, and their low MAF, thereby making it having little power to affect obesity in that region. In this study, we reported MAF of 40%, slightly similar to 35.54 reported in Gambia by Hennig et al. [20], higher than (12.1%) reported in China by [36, 38], and lower than (~45%) reported among European population [8].

Similarly, this study shows that FTO rs9939609 A allele carriers had an increased risk (odds) of overweight/obesity [OR = 0.19 (95% CI: 0.10, 0.36); $p < 0.001$], central obesity [OR = 0.33 (95% CI: 0.15, 0.71); $p < 0.001$], and visceral obesity [OR = 0.12 (95% CI: 0.06, 0.23); $p < 0.001$] compared with the TT homozygotes. This is less than the results from other studies across seven European countries [10] and France [34]. The reason might be due to the difference in sample size power, environmental variables, central obesity categorization, and variants in data collection procedure and to different linkage disequilibrium patterns across FTO intron 1 between the various ethnic groups, particularly in populations of African ancestry [4, 5]. Subsequently, our study suggests that the odds of being overweight/obesity was substantially attenuated by active lifestyle (PA). This is similar to other studies that showed that PA might mitigate the effects of gene variant FTO rs9939609 on obesity [10, 19, 36, 39]. But contrary to what was reported in Finland, they reported leisure-time PA [40]. We also reported A allele-dependent increase in energy intake and TSS; this is in line with some recent works [9, 14].

From the foregoing, we might infer that environmental variables (PA, energy intake, and TSS) might have a mediating role in the interaction between FTO rs9939609 and BMI, mediation analysis. Results from multiple mediation analysis showed that all our environmental variables have a full mediating effect on the interaction between FTO rs9939609 and BMI; this is incongruent with other studies by [9, 14, 31].

Studies have shown the importance of both FTO rs9939609 and 2D : 4D as a surrogate marker for obesity and coronary heart disease [8–11, 16–18] but none have studied the relationship between them. We reported an association between FTO gene variant and 2D : 4D with individual carrying FTO risk allele having increased 2D : 4D; thus 2D : 4D might be used to predict individual FTO rs9939609 genotype in future, but further studies are required to buttress and refute this.

Full role of FTO first intron rs9939609 on obesity etiology and their role in energy expenditure need more to be done. Speakman [6] reported that there is inconclusive evidence (like epistatic or gene-environment interaction) in the relationship between FTO, PA, and energy expenditure. Thus, we can explore gene-environment interaction to demystify biology of FTO.

This study presents evidence about the role of genetic variant and gene-environment interaction concerning obesity in a Nigerian youth population which is based case-control study with good response rate and low selection bias. Also, our study had the power to detect the association of rs9939609 with obesity in Nigerian youth. However, several limitations should also be noted. First, this study was carried out in a Polytechnic campus which might affect response to some parameters like PA because the layout of the school seems to encourage PA. Second, we need an objective measure of environmental variables like accelerometer for PA to be sure of the PA level. Lastly, only one SNP of *FTO* was measured in this study, so it is unclear whether the identified association is due to this particular sequence variant or another variant in tight linkage disequilibrium with rs9939609 [40].

Power value (95%) and Bonferroni correction for multiple testing used in this study reduce both the risk of false positive and false negative results; thus we might draw some conclusion from our results. Nigeria relies on results from other parts of the world on the interaction of genetic and environmental impact on obesity; this might not be good because studies have shown variations from the different ethnic population [2–5]. Thus this study made an indigenous genetic study of obesity available, thus paving the way for proper management of obesity because PA, TSS, and energy intake showed modulating/mediating effect on the interaction between FTO and obesity. Lastly, such evidence of gene-environmental/lifestyle interaction will be of great importance because environment/lifestyle can be modified easily unlike gene that is inherent in the particular population.

5. Conclusions

Our study suggests that environmental/lifestyle factors like PA, TSS, and energy intake might be substantial modulator and/or mediator in the association between FTO rs9939609 and BMI in Nigeria because they mediate the influence of FTO variant on BMI, offering new insight into the interrelationship between FTO genetic variants, TPA, energy intake, and TSS in Nigeria. Our data attest the previously reported association regarding the genetic variability in intron 1 of FTO gene and obesity risk. This might propose a mechanism of understanding of FTO-linked weight gain and obesity in the Nigerian context, but further study with larger sample size and objective measures of environmental variable is warranted.

Disclosure

The founding sponsors had no role in the design of the study; in the collection, analyses, or interpretation of data; in the writing of the manuscript; and in the decision to publish the results.

Authors' Contributions

Bolaji Fatai Oyeyemi, Charles Ayorinde Ologunde, and Ayonposi Bukola Olaoye conceived and designed the experiments; Bolaji Fatai Oyeyemi and Nanfizat Abiket Alamukii performed the experiments; Bolaji Fatai Oyeyemi, Charles Ayorinde Ologunde, and Ayonposi Bukola Olaoye analyzed the data; Bolaji Fatai Oyeyemi, Charles Ayorinde Ologunde, and Ayonposi Bukola Olaoye contributed reagents/materials/analysis tools; Bolaji Fatai Oyeyemi wrote the paper; all authors read and approved the final manuscript.

Acknowledgments

This study was funded by Tertiary Education Trust Fund (TETFund). The authors thank Ajimola Odunayo, Olomeye Olubunmi, Sholatan Kehinde, Egbeyemi Ita, and Kolawole Omoseebi for assistance with collection of anthropometric measurements and blood samples and Professor Ademowo O. G. and staff of Molecular Biology Laboratory, Institute for Advanced Medical Research and Training (IMRAT), University College Hospital, Ibadan, for allowing them to use their laboratory for part of the work. They also appreciate the staff of Bioscience Unit and Inqaba West Africa, International Institute for Tropical Agriculture (IITA), Ibadan, for allowing them to use their laboratory for genetic analysis and sequencing and their effort in seeing the success of this work. Lastly, they thank Dr Neel S. Bhavesh of ICGEB for the support in providing a conducive intellectual space that allows for the draft and writing of the manuscript.

References

[1] S. N. Akarolo-Anthony, W. C. Willett, D. Spiegelman, and C. A. Adebamowo, "Obesity epidemic has emerged among Nigerians," *BMC Public Health*, vol. 14, no. 1, article 455, 2014.

[2] M. R. Wing, J. M. Ziegler, C. D. Langefeld et al., "Analysis of FTO gene variants with obesity and glucose homeostasis measures in the multiethnic Insulin Resistance Atherosclerosis Study cohort," *International Journal of Obesity*, vol. 35, no. 9, pp. 1173–1182, 2011.

[3] B. A. Swinburn, G. Sacks, K. D. Hall et al., "The global obesity pandemic: shaped by global drivers and local environments," *The Lancet*, vol. 378, no. 9793, pp. 804–814, 2011.

[4] K. L. Monda, G. K. Chen, K. C. Taylor et al. et al., "A meta-analysis identifies new loci associated with body mass index in individuals of African ancestry," *Nature Genetics*, vol. 45, no. 6, pp. 690–696, 2013.

[5] R. J. F. Loos and G. S. H. Yeo, "The bigger picture of FTO: the first GWAS-identified obesity gene," *Nature Reviews Endocrinology*, vol. 10, no. 1, pp. 51–61, 2014.

[6] J. R. Speakman, "The 'fat mass and obesity related' (FTO) gene: mechanisms of impact on obesity and energy balance," *Current Obesity Reports*, vol. 4, no. 1, pp. 73–91, 2015.

[7] C. Dina, D. Meyre, S. Gallina et al., "Variation in FTO contributes to childhood obesity and severe adult obesity," *Nature Genetics*, vol. 39, no. 6, pp. 724–726, 2007.

[8] T. M. Frayling, N. J. Timpson, M. N. Weedon et al., "A common variant in the FTO gene is associated with body mass index and predisposes to childhood and adult obesity," *Science*, vol. 316, no. 5826, pp. 889–894, 2007.

[9] Y. C. Klimentidis, A. Arora, A. Chougule, J. Zhou, and D. A. Raichlen, "FTO association and interaction with time spent sitting," *International Journal of Obesity*, vol. 40, no. 3, pp. 411–416, 2016.

[10] C. Celis-Morales, C. F. M. Marsaux, K. M. Livingstone et al., "Physical activity attenuates the effect of the FTO genotype on obesity traits in European adults: the Food4Me study," *Obesity*, vol. 24, no. 4, pp. 962–969, 2016.

[11] C. Duicu, C. O. MǍrginean, S. VoidǍzan, F. Tripon, and C. BǍnescu, "FTO rs 9939609 SNP is associated with adiponectin and leptin levels and the risk of obesity in a cohort of romanian children population," *Medicine (United States)*, vol. 95, no. 20, Article ID e3709, 2016.

[12] K. M. Livingstone, C. Celis-Morales, S. Navas-Carretero et al., "Fat mass-and obesity-associated genotype, dietary intakes and anthropometric measures in European adults the Food4Me study," *British Journal of Nutrition*, vol. 115, no. 3, pp. 440–448, 2015.

[13] A. B. Kühn, D.-L. Feis, L. Schilbach et al., "FTO gene variant modulates the neural correlates of visual food perception," *NeuroImage*, vol. 128, pp. 21–31, 2016.

[14] Q. Qi, M. K. Downer, T. O. Kilpelainen et al., "Dietary Intake, FTO genetic variants, and adiposity: a combined analysis of over 16,000 children and adolescents," *Diabetes*, vol. 64, no. 7, pp. 2467–2476, 2015.

[15] J. Gustavsson, K. Mehlig, K. Leander et al., "FTO gene variation, macronutrient intake and coronary heart disease risk: a gene–diet interaction analysis," *European Journal of Nutrition*, vol. 55, no. 1, pp. 247–255, 2016.

[16] B. F. Oyeyemi, O. A. Iyiola, A. W. Oyeyemi, K. A. Oricha, A. T. Anifowoshe, and N. A. Alamukii, "Sexual dimorphism in ratio of second and fourth digits and its relationship with metabolic syndrome indices and cardiovascular risk factors," *Journal of Research in Medical Sciences*, vol. 19, no. 3, pp. 234–239, 2014.

[17] B. Fink, J. T. Manning, and N. Neave, "The 2nd–4th digit ratio (2D : 4D) and neck circumference: implications for risk factors in coronary heart disease," *International Journal of Obesity*, vol. 30, no. 4, pp. 711–714, 2006.

[18] J. T. Manning and P. E. Bundred, "The ratio of 2nd to 4th digit length and age at first myocardial infarction in men: a link with testosterone?" *British Journal of Cardiology*, vol. 8, no. 12, 2001.

[19] T. O. Kilpelainen, L. Qi, S. Brage et al., "Physical activity attenuates the influence of FTO variants on obesity risk: a meta-analysis of 218,166 adults and 19,268 children," *PLOS Medicine*, vol. 8, no. 11, Article ID e1001116, 2011.

[20] B. J. Hennig, A. J. Fulford, G. Sirugo et al., "FTO gene variation and measures of body mass in an African population," *BMC Medical Genetics*, vol. 10, no. 1, article 21, 2009.

[21] K. G. M. M. Alberti, P. Zimmet, and J. Shaw, "The metabolic syndrome—a new worldwide definition," *The Lancet*, vol. 366, no. 9491, pp. 1059–1062, 2005.

[22] World Health Organization, *Waist Circumference and Waist-Hip Ratio: Report of A WHO Expert Consultation, Geneva, 8–11 December 2008*, World Health Organization, Geneva, Switzerland, 2011.

[23] M. Ashwell, P. Gunn, and S. Gibson, "Waist-to-height ratio is a better screening tool than waist circumference and BMI for adult cardiometabolic risk factors: systematic review and meta-analysis," *Obesity Reviews*, vol. 13, no. 3, pp. 275–286, 2012.

[24] J. T. Manning, D. Scutt, J. Wilson, and D. I. Lewis-Jones, "The ratio of 2nd to 4th digit length: a predictor of sperm numbers and concentrations of testosterone, luteinizing hormone and oestrogen," *Human Reproduction*, vol. 13, no. 11, pp. 3000–3004, 1998.

[25] A. L. Oyeyemi, A. Y. Oyeyemi, B. O. Adegoke et al., "The short international physical activity questionnaire: cross-cultural adaptation, validation and reliability of the Hausa language version in Nigeria," *BMC Medical Research Methodology*, vol. 11, article 156, 2011.

[26] C. E. Garber, B. Blissmer, M. R. Deschenes et al., "Quantity and quality of exercise for developing and maintaining cardiorespiratory, musculoskeletal, and neuromotor fitness in apparently healthy adults: guidance for prescribing exercise," *Medicine and Science in Sports and Exercise*, vol. 43, no. 7, pp. 1334–1359, 2011.

[27] S. N. Akarolo-Anthony, F. O. Odubore, S. Yilme et al., "Pattern of dietary carbohydrate intake among urbanized adult Nigerians," *International Journal of Food Sciences and Nutrition*, vol. 64, no. 3, pp. 292–299, 2013.

[28] A. López-Bermejo, C. J. Petry, M. Díaz et al., "The association between the FTO gene and fat mass in humans develops by the postnatal age of two weeks," *Journal of Clinical Endocrinology and Metabolism*, vol. 93, no. 4, pp. 1501–1505, 2008.

[29] F. Faul, E. Erdfelder, A. Buchner, and A.-G. Lang, "Statistical power analyses using G*Power 3.1: tests for correlation and regression analyses," *Behavior Research Methods*, vol. 41, no. 4, pp. 1149–1160, 2009.

[30] W. Viechtbauer, L. Smits, D. Kotz et al., "A simple formula for the calculation of sample size in pilot studies," *Journal of Clinical Epidemiology*, vol. 68, no. 11, pp. 1375–1379, 2015.

[31] Z. Yilmaz, C. Davis, N. J. Loxton et al., "Association between MC4R rs17782313 polymorphism and overeating behaviors," *International Journal of Obesity*, vol. 39, no. 1, pp. 114–120, 2015.

[32] K. J. Preacher and A. F. Hayes, "Asymptotic and resampling strategies for assessing and comparing indirect effects in multiple mediator models," *Behavior Research Methods*, vol. 40, no. 3, pp. 879–891, 2008.

[33] H. Mangge, W. Renner, G. Almer, D. Weghuber, R. Möller, and R. Horejsi, "Rs9939609 variant of the fat mass and obesity-associated gene and trunk obesity in adolescents," *Journal of Obesity*, vol. 2011, Article ID 186368, 4 pages, 2011.

[34] C. M. Phillips, E. Kesse-Guyot, R. Mcmanus et al., "High dietary saturated fat intake accentuates obesity risk associated with the fat mass and obesity-associated gene in adults," *Journal of Nutrition*, vol. 142, no. 5, pp. 824–831, 2012.

[35] S. Macekova, I. Bernasovsky, D. Gabrikova et al., "Association of the FTO rs9939609 polymorphism with obesity

in ROMA/GYPSY population," *American Journal of Physical Anthropology*, vol. 147, no. 1, pp. 30–34, 2012.

[36] B. Xi, Y. Shen, M. Zhang et al., "The common rs9939609 variant of the fat mass and obesity-associated gene is associated with obesity risk in children and adolescents of Beijing, China," *BMC Medical Genetics*, vol. 11, no. 1, article 107, 2010.

[37] A. Shahid, S. Rana, S. Saeed, M. Imran, N. Afzal, and S. Mahmood, "Common variant of FTO Gene, rs9939609, and obesity in Pakistani females," *BioMed Research International*, vol. 2013, Article ID 324093, 7 pages, 2013.

[38] H. Li, Y. Wu, R. J. F. Loos et al., "Variants in the fat mass- and obesity-associated (FTO) gene are not associated with obesity in a Chinese Han population," *Diabetes*, vol. 57, no. 1, pp. 264–268, 2008.

[39] S. Karasawa, M. Daimon, S. Sasaki et al., "Association of the common fat mass and obesity associated (FTO) gene polymorphism with obesity in a Japanese population," *Endocrine Journal*, vol. 57, no. 4, pp. 293–301, 2010.

[40] M. Hakanen, O. T. Raitakari, T. Lehtimäki et al., "FTO genotype is associated with body mass index after the age of seven years but not with energy intake or leisure-time physical activity," *Journal of Clinical Endocrinology and Metabolism*, vol. 94, no. 4, pp. 1281–1287, 2009.

7

Prospective Associations of the Short Form Health Survey Vitality Scale and Changes in Body Mass Index and Obesity Status

Cathrine Lawaetz Wimmelmann,[1,2] Emilie Rune Hegelund,[1] Anna Paldam Folker,[3] Emilie Just-Østergaard,[1,2] Merete Osler,[4,5,6,7,8] Erik Lykke Mortensen,[1,2] and Trine Flensborg-Madsen[1,2]

[1]*Section of Environmental Health, Department of Public Health, University of Copenhagen, Øster Farimagsgade 5A, 1353 Copenhagen K, Denmark*
[2]*Center for Healthy Aging, Faculty of Health and Medical Sciences, University of Copenhagen, Copenhagen, Denmark*
[3]*National Institute of Public Health, University of Southern Denmark, Øster Farimagsgade 5A, 1353 Copenhagen K, Denmark*
[4]*Research Center for Prevention and Health, Glostrup Hospital, Glostrup, Denmark*
[5]*Danish Aging Research Center, University of Aarhus, Aarhus, Denmark*
[6]*Danish Aging Research Center, University of Southern Denmark, Odense, Denmark*
[7]*Danish Aging Research Center, University of Copenhagen, Copenhagen, Denmark*
[8]*Section of Social Medicine, Department of Public Health, University of Copenhagen, Øster Farimagsgade 5A, 1353 Copenhagen K, Denmark*

Correspondence should be addressed to Cathrine Lawaetz Wimmelmann; calw@sund.ku.dk

Academic Editor: Michele D. Levine

Objectives. The objectives of the current study were to prospectively investigate the predictive value of the vitality scale of the Short Form Health Survey for changes in body mass index and development of obesity. *Methods.* The study population comprised 2864 (81.5%) men and 648 (18.5%) women from the Metropolit Project and the Danish Longitudinal Study on Work, Unemployment and Health, who participated in a follow-up examination in 2009–2011 corresponding to a follow-up period of 3–7 years. Associations of vitality with body mass index and obesity were investigated separately for men and women in linear and logistic regression models adjusting for age, baseline body mass index, education, physical activity, smoking, and obesity-related diseases. *Results.* Vitality was significantly associated with change in body mass index among men ($p < 0.001$) and women ($p < 0.05$) gaining weight after adjusting for age, baseline body mass index, education, physical activity, smoking, and obesity-related diseases. No significant associations of vitality with BMI change were observed among individuals maintaining or losing weight during the follow-up period. Furthermore, vitality significantly predicted development of obesity among women. *Conclusion.* The study indicates that vitality is of predictive value for increases in BMI over time among individuals gaining weight and may further predict the development of obesity among women. This identification of poor vitality as a potential risk indicator for weight gain and development of obesity may be beneficial in clinical practice.

1. Introduction

Obesity, defined as a body mass index (BMI) $\geq 30\,kg/m^2$, is a major public health problem [1] and is associated with various medical comorbidities such as type 2 diabetes, cardiovascular disease, and stroke [2]. In addition to the medical comorbidities, a growing body of research has investigated the psychological and social correlates of obesity. Especially, health-related quality of life (HRQOL) has received attention [3–5]. HRQOL has been defined as a multidimensional construct comprising physical, emotional, and social well-being, which reflects an individual's subjective evaluation and reaction to health or illness [4]. The Short Form Health Survey (SF-36) [6] is a widely used generic measure of HRQOL comprising eight subscales that can be divided into a physical and a mental HRQOL component. By applying generic measures of HRQOL such as the SF-36 [6], cross-sectional studies have shown that HRQOL varies with BMI [7, 8]. Most consistently, individuals with obesity seem to have lower HRQOL [9, 10]. Furthermore, cohort studies have shown decreases in HRQOL over time in overweight individuals and in individuals with obesity with the largest reductions observed in the physical domains of HRQOL [11, 12]. Finally, weight loss has been associated with increases in several HRQOL domains especially vitality, general health perception, and physical role functioning [13, 14].

However, BMI and obesity may not merely predict decreases in HRQOL but may also be a consequence of HRQOL. Thus, HRQOL may be a predictor of BMI and obesity, but until now, only one study has investigated whether HRQOL predicts weight changes over time. This study [11] indicated a bidirectional relationship between HRQOL and obesity. Interestingly, individuals in the lowest tertile of the HRQOL domains related to the mental component gained significantly more weight over the five-year follow-up period than individuals in the highest tertile. That is, where previous research has emphasized the impact of obesity on the physical aspects of HRQOL [10, 12], this study suggested that mental aspects of HRQOL is of importance for weight changes over time.

The SF-36 vitality scale is a subscale included in the mental component of the SF-36 and assesses different aspects of fatigue. This scale has been suggested as the best of the eight SF-36 subscales at discriminating between levels of health [6, 15], and it has previously been associated with several medical conditions, including cardiovascular disease and mortality risk [15, 16], suggesting that somatic aspects of health is also captured by the SF-36 vitality scale.

As knowledge about the possible effects of HRQOL on weight status is extremely scarce, the aim of the current study was to investigate the predictive value of the SF-36 vitality scale for both changes in BMI and development of obesity. We set out to examine this question in a longitudinal study design using two large Danish cohorts that were examined in 2004 and 2006, respectively, and included a follow-up study of these cohorts 3 to 7 years later. As sociodemographic factors, lifestyle, and health factors consistently have been associated with both HRQOL [17, 18] and weight status [19, 20], the effects of such factors on the associations between SF-36 vitality and BMI and obesity will be included in the analyses of this relation.

2. Methods

2.1. Study Cohorts and Baseline Data

2.1.1. The Metropolit 1953 Danish Male Birth Cohort (MP). The Metropolit 1953 Danish Male Birth Cohort [21] comprises 11532 men born in 1953 in the metropolitan area of Copenhagen who were alive and living in Denmark in 1968. In 2004, a questionnaire was sent to all members of the cohort who had a postal address in Denmark, assessing different aspects of health, social position, and health behavior. A total of 6292 men aged 51 years completed the questionnaire which included the SF-36 vitality scale and information on self-reported height and weight.

2.1.2. The Danish Longitudinal Study on Work, Unemployment and Health (DALWUH). The Danish Longitudinal Study on Work, Unemployment and Health (DALWUH) [22] is a random sample of 10% of the Danish population born in 1949 and 1959. Questionnaire data concerning health, social relations, psychosocial factors, and work environment were collected in 2000 and again in 2006. A total of 6151 men and women aged 47 and 57 years participated in the 2006 follow-up, which included the SF-36 vitality scale and information on self-reported height and weight.

2.1.3. The Copenhagen Aging and Midlife Biobank (CAMB). In 2009–2011, members from the MP and the DALWUH were invited to participate in the Copenhagen Aging and Midlife Biobank (CAMB) [23]. Participants in the CAMB completed a questionnaire assessing health, lifestyle behaviors, social position, and social relations. In addition, they participated in a clinical examination including an assessment of BMI and a blood draw. Written consent was obtained from all participants prior to examination. Complete information on the SF-36 vitality scale at baseline and BMI at baseline and follow-up were available for 2378 men from the MP and 1142 men and women from the DALWUH. To avoid outliers with regard to BMI, eight men were eliminated from the analyses due to an extreme BMI change from baseline to the CAMB examination. Thus, the final study sample for the current study comprised 3512 participants with a mean age of 51.6 years (SD: 3.0 years) (Figure 1).

The study protocols of the described studies were approved by local institutional review committees prior to study initiation of the studies.

3. Measures/Variables

3.1. Outcomes

3.1.1. Body Mass Index and Obesity. BMI was calculated as weight (kg)/height $(m)^2$. At follow-up, height and weight were measured at a clinical examination [23], while BMI at baseline was based on self-reported height and weight. BMI change was estimated as "follow-up BMI−baseline BMI" and used as a continuous outcome variable in linear regression analyses.

Obesity was constructed as a binary variable defining participants with a BMI $\geq 30\,kg/m^2$ as having obesity and participants with a BMI $<30\,kg/m^2$ as not having obesity.

3.2. Predictor

3.2.1. SF-36 Vitality. Vitality was assessed using the vitality scale of the Short Form Health Survey (SF-36) [6], which

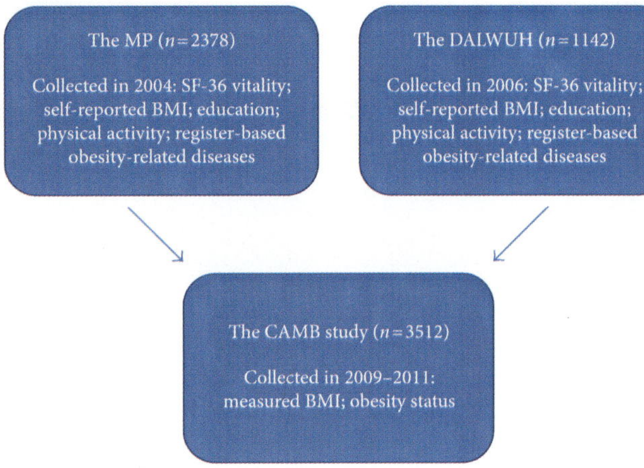

Figure 1: Baseline cohorts and follow-up sample. MP, Metropolit cohort; DALWUH, the Danish Longitudinal Study on Work, Unemployment and Health; CAMB, Copenhagen Aging and Midlife Biobank.

consists of four items evaluating the vitality domain of HRQOL by questions on tiredness and energy level. For instance, one question was "*How much time during the past 4 weeks did you feel full of pep?*" Answers ranged from 1 ("All of the time") to 6 ("None of the time"). Raw scores from the SF-36 vitality scale were transformed to scores ranging from 0 to 100 with 100 indicating the highest level of vitality. Based on the tertiles of the SF-36 vitality scale scores, a categorical variable with three categories corresponding to high, medium, and low vitality was constructed and used in the main analyses.

3.3. Covariates. Variables that have previously been shown to affect both HRQOL and weight status were considered as covariates.

3.3.1. Educational Level. Educational level provides information about the length and the level of the participants' vocational training at baseline assessed on six categories ranging from 1 ("No vocational training") to 6 ("Higher level education >4 years"). Based on this information, three categories were derived corresponding to low, medium, and high level of education.

3.3.2. Leisure Time Physical Activity. "Leisure time physical activity" was self-reported at baseline. Participants in the MP were asked which of the following four statements best described their general level of leisure time physical activity: hard exercise at elite level several times a week; exercise or heavy domestic work at least 4 hours a week; easy physical activity such as walking and cycling at least 4 hours a week; or sedentary activity such as reading and television watching. Participants in the DALWUH were asked to report the average number of hours per week they were physically active. Answers ranged from 1 ("0 hours") to 6 (">7 hours"). Information about physical activity level in the two cohorts was combined in a categorical variable. Based on the distribution of answers on the cohort-specific physical activity items, three categories were constructed corresponding to low, medium, and high physical activity level.

3.3.3. Smoking. A question about current smoking status was administered to participants in the two cohorts. All participants were asked whether they were currently smoking on a daily basis; currently smoking but not on a daily basis; had stopped smoking; or never had smoked. Based on this information, a binary variable was constructed with participants who reported that they were currently smoking either daily or regularly categorized as "smokers" and participants who reported to have stopped smoking or never had smoked categorized as "nonsmokers."

3.3.4. Obesity-Related Disorders. The Danish National Patient Registry was used to identify participants who had received one or more of the following obesity-related diagnoses prior to the baseline assessments in 2004 (the MP) and 2006 (the DALWUH): type 2 diabetes mellitus (ICD-8 code: 250; ICD-10 code: E11), essential hypertension (ICD-8 codes: 400, 401; ICD-10 code: I10), ischemic heart disease (ICD-8 codes: 410–413; ICD-10 codes: I20, I21, I24, I25), or other hypothyroidism (ICD-8 code: 242; ICD-10 code: E03). These conditions were selected as they are frequent among elderly persons and have been included in prior studies of HRQOL and BMI [11]. Four variables corresponding to the four conditions were constructed and scored such that 0 reflected "no diagnosis" and 1 reflected "diagnosis."

3.3.5. Statistical Analysis. Descriptive statistics were used to analyze participant characteristics. Differences between the two cohorts and between men and women were examined using chi-square tests or independent *t*-tests depending on the nature of the dependent variable. Also, to analyze the distribution of BMI change in relation to the three SF-36 vitality categories, the tertiles of BMI change were calculated and used as a categorical variable in chi-square tests.

Preliminary analyses showed sex differences in several key variables including BMI and SF-36 vitality, and a significant interaction of sex and SF-36 vitality on the risk of developing obesity was observed ($p = 0.049$). In line with previous studies, the main analyses were therefore stratified by sex. Also, cohort differences were found on all characteristics. Accordingly, cohort status was adjusted for in all the conducted analyses.

Changes in BMI from baseline to follow-up assessment were analyzed in four models: Model 1 adjusted for cohort, age, and baseline BMI; Model 2 adjusted for cohort, age, baseline BMI, and level of education; Model 3 adjusted for cohort, age, baseline BMI, smoking, and level of physical activity; Model 4 adjusted for cohort, age, baseline BMI, and obesity-related diseases including type 2 diabetes, hypertension, ischemic heart disease, and other hypothyroidism. Analyses of BMI were conducted using linear regression analyses and are shown for three different populations. First, associations of SF-36 vitality with BMI change were investigated in the full sample. Secondly, as previous research has suggested that prospective associations of BMI and HRQOL differ between individuals gaining and losing weight [11], the associations were investigated separately for participants gaining weight and participants either maintaining or losing weight over the follow-up period.

The risk of becoming obese was analyzed in four models with the same covariates as described above. Participants with BMI ≥30 kg/m^2 at baseline were excluded from these analyses, and logistic regression was applied to investigate associations of SF-36 vitality with obesity as outcome. Because preliminary analyses showed that no women in the high SF-36 vitality category were obese at follow-up, a binary SF-36 vitality variable was used in all analyses of obesity with the high and the medium categories merged.

4. Results

Table 1 presents participant characteristics including sex, age, BMI, obesity status, follow-up BMI, obesity status at follow-up, level of education, level of physical activity, smoking, prevalence of obesity-related diseases, and the distribution of the SF-36 vitality categories separately for the two baseline cohorts. By design, the two cohorts included in the study differ on sex as the MP consists of men only, while the DALWUH includes both men and women. The total sample of the present study, therefore, consists of 2864 (81.5%) men and 648 (18.5%) women with a mean age of 52 years. The mean baseline BMI was 26.0 kg/m^2 and 24.6 kg/m^2 for men and women, respectively, and 326 (11.4%) men and 62 (9.6%) women were categorized as obese at baseline. Of the total 3512 participants in the current study, almost 40% reported to have high educational level and 30% reported a high physical activity level. However, only 19.4% of the participants were categorized as high on SF-36 vitality and 37.5% fell in the low SF-36 vitality category.

Table 1: Characteristics of participants in the Metropolit 1953 Danish Male Birth Cohort, the Danish Longitudinal Study on Work, Unemployment and Health, and the total study sample.

	MP	DALWUH	p value[1]
N	2371	1141	—
Sex (%)			*0.000* (by design)
Men	100.0	42.7	
Women	0	57.3	
Age, M (SD)	51.0 (0.2)	52.8 (5.0)	*0.000* (by design)
Level of education (%)			0.070
High	39.4	41.0	
Medium	47.3	48.5	
Low	13.3	10.5	
BMI at baseline, M (SD)	25.9 (3.8)	25.4 (4.2)	*0.000*
Obesity baseline (%)			0.304
Yes	10.7	11.8	
No	89.3	88.2	
BMI at follow-up, M (SD)	26.3 (3.8)	25.9 (4.4)	*0.000*
Obesity follow-up (%)			0.166
Yes	15.8	14.0	
No	85.2	86.0	
Physical activity (%)			*0.000*
High	27.3	34.6	
Medium	58.5	56.5	
Low	14.2	8.9	
Smoking (%)			*0.000*
Yes	34.0	25.0	
No	66.0	75.0	
Obesity-related diseases (%)			
Type 2 diabetes	1.6	2.1	*0.039*
Hypertension	3.5	3.7	0.100
Ischemic heart disease	3.9	3.2	0.829
Hypothyroidism	0.2	0.7	*0.002*
SF-36 vitality, M (SD)	68.0 (18.9)	62.0 (19.7)	*0.000*
SF-36 vitality (%)			*0.000*
High	21.8	14.5	
Medium	45.2	38.4	
Low	32.0	47.1	

[1] p value of the chi-square test or independent t-test of differences between the means—categorical and continuous outcomes, respectively. SD, standard deviation; M, mean; MP, the Metropolit 1953 Danish Male Birth Cohort; DALWUH, the Danish Longitudinal Study on Work, Unemployment and Health.

The tertiles of BMI change and the chi-square tests of SF-36 vitality with the tertiles of BMI change are shown for men and women in Table 2. Among both men and women, those scoring high on SF-36 vitality were most likely to have a small weight gain corresponding to the second tertile of BMI change. However, these associations were only significant among women ($p = 0.002$).

Associations of SF-36 vitality with BMI are shown in Table 3 for the full sample and for the weight gain group and the weight loss group, respectively. For the *full sample*, SF-36 vitality was significantly associated with BMI change among men independently of cohort, age, baseline BMI, level of education, and obesity-related diseases. A trend was observed when adjusting for level of physical activity and smoking in addition to cohort, age, and baseline BMI. Men scoring low on SF-36 vitality had a 0.05–0.07 ($p < 0.05$) standard deviation larger BMI increase than high-scoring men depending on the investigated model. SF-36 vitality did not predict BMI change in any of the investigated models among women.

Of the total sample, 2377 participants gained weight over the follow-up period while 1135 maintained or lost weight with a mean BMI increase of 1.4 (SD: 1.3) and a mean BMI decrease of 1.1 (SD: 1.1) in the two groups, respectively. In the *weight gain group*, significant associations of SF-36 vitality were found for both men and women. Among men, the low SF-36 vitality group had a significantly higher BMI increase over the follow-up period compared with the high SF-36 vitality group ($p < 0.001$ in all models). BMI increases were 0.09–0.13 standard deviations larger among men with low baseline SF-36 vitality compared with men in the high vitality category. Men in the medium SF-36 vitality category did not differ significantly from their high-scoring counterparts with regards to BMI changes from baseline to follow-up. Among women, SF-36 vitality also predicted BMI

Table 2: Tertiles of change in BMI for men and women by SF-36 vitality category. p values for chi-square tests are presented.

	Change in BMI (tertiles)		
Men			
SF-36 vitality	−9.4–0 BMI units	0.1–1.1 BMI units	1.2–11.0 BMI units
High (%)	35	35	30
Medium (%)	34	35	31
Low (%)	33	32	35
p value[1]			0.126
Women			
SF-36 vitality	−13.7–0.3 BMI units	0.4–1.1 BMI units	1.2–8.5 BMI units
High (%)	26	43	31
Medium (%)	42	32	26
Low (%)	37	26	37
p value[1]			**0.002**

[1]p value for the chi-square test of association between SF-36 category and the tertiles of change in BMI.

Table 3: Linear regression (standardized beta) of SF-36 vitality on BMI change among men and women. Full sample and separate for men and women gaining and maintaining/losing weight.

	Model 1[a]		Model 2[b]		Model 3[c]		Model 4[d]		Model 1[a]		Model 2[b]		Model 3[c]		Model 4[d]	
	β	p[1]	β	p[1]	β	p[1]	β	p[1]	β	p[1]	β	p[1]	β	p[1]	β	p[1]
Full sample			Men (N = 2864)								Women (N = 648)					
SF-36 vitality		**0.011**		**0.036**		0.062		**0.022**		0.159		0.182		0.241		0.112
High	—		—		—		—		—		—		—		—	
Medium	0.02		0.02		0.01		0.02		−0.08		−0.08		−0.07		−0.08	
Low	0.07*		0.06*		0.05*		0.06*		0.01		0.0		0.01		0.02	
Weight gain			Men (N = 1920)								Women (N = 457)					
SF-36 vitality		**<0.001**		**<0.001**		**0.001**		**<0.001**		**<0.001**		**0.001**		**0.002**		**<0.001**
High	—		—		—		—		—		—		—		—	
Medium	0.03		0.02		0.02		0.03		−0.02		−0.03		−0.04		−0.03	
Low	0.13**		0.12**		0.09*		0.13**		0.12		0.11		0.11		0.13	
Weight loss			Men (N = 944)								Women (N = 191)					
SF-36 vitality		0.139		0.143		0.294		0.114		0.523		0.613		0.661		0.523
High	—		—		—		—		—		—		—		—	
Medium	−0.03		−0.03		−0.03		−0.03		0.00		0.00		0.03		0.03	
Low	−0.08		−0.07		−0.06		−0.08		−0.03		−0.01		0.01		0.00	

[a]Adjusted for cohort, age, and baseline BMI. [b]Adjusted for cohort, age, baseline BMI, and education. [c]Adjusted for cohort, age, baseline BMI, physical activity, and smoking. [d]Adjusted for cohort, age, baseline BMI, and obesity-related diseases. [1]p value of the F-test. *Significantly different from reference value at $p < 0.05$. **Significantly different from reference value at $p < 0.001$.

increases in all models. However, women in the medium and low SF-36 vitality category did not differ significantly from the high-scoring women possibly reflecting the relatively small number of women in the current study.

In the *weight maintenance/weight loss group*, SF-36 vitality at baseline was not associated with BMI change among men or women in any of the investigated models.

Table 4 presents associations of baseline SF-36 vitality with obesity status at follow-up in men and women. SF-36 vitality did not predict obesity at follow-up among men. In contrast, among women, SF-36 vitality predicted obesity at follow-up in all the investigated models with women in the low SF-36 vitality category having 6.3 (p = 0.006) times higher odds of becoming obese at follow-up than women in the high SF-36 vitality group. Furthermore, this association remained significant when adjusting for level of education, level of physical activity, smoking, and obesity-related diseases in addition to cohort, age, and baseline BMI (odds ratios ranging from 5.8–7.1; $p < 0.05$). The previously described significant interaction of sex and SF-36 vitality on the risk of becoming obese (p = 0.049) indicates that the different results for men and women were statistically significant.

5. Discussion

To our knowledge, this is one of the first studies to investigate the effect of SF-36 vitality on BMI changes and the development of obesity. Results indicated that SF-36 vitality was of predictive value for changes in BMI among men and women gaining weight over the five-year follow-up period with larger increases in BMI observed in individuals with low SF-36 vitality at baseline compared with individuals reporting high baseline SF-36 vitality. In contrast, SF-36 vitality was not related to changes in BMI among men and women losing weight. Furthermore, SF-36 vitality was significantly associated with development of obesity among women.

TABLE 4: Logistic regression of associations between SF-36 vitality (high/low) and obesity (BMI ≥30 kg/m^2) among men and women.

	Men (N = 2543)								Women (N = 586)							
	Model 1[a]		Model 2[b]		Model 3[c]		Model 4[d]		Model 1[a]		Model 2[b]		Model 3[c]		Model 4[d]	
	OR (95% CI)	p^1	OR (95% CI)	p^1	OR (95% CI)	p^1	OR (95% CI)	p^1	OR (95% CI)	p^1	OR (95% CI)	p^1	OR (95% CI)	p^1	OR (95% CI)	p^1
SF-36 vitality		0.253		0.255		0.560		0.271		**0.006**		**0.010**		**0.005**		**0.008**
High	—		—		—		—		—		—		—		—	
Low	1.2 (0.9; 1.8)		1.2 (0.9; 1.8)		1.1 (0.8; 1.6)		1.2 (0.9; 1.8)		6.3 (1.7; 23.8)*		5.8 (1.5; 21.9)*		7.1 (1.8; 28.2)*		6.0 (1.6; 22.4)*	

[a]Adjusted for cohort, age, and baseline BMI. [b]Adjusted for cohort, age, baseline BMI, and education. [c]Adjusted for cohort, age, baseline BMI, physical activity, and smoking. [d]Adjusted for cohort, age, baseline BMI, and obesity-related diseases. [1]p value of the F-test. *Significantly different from reference value at $p < 0.05$. **Significantly different from reference value at $p < 0.001$. CI, confidence interval.

The average BMI change of men and women in the current study was modest (0.62 (SD: 1.7) BMI units for men and 0.64 (SD: 1.8) for women). The results in Table 2 revealed that most women in the high SF-36 vitality group fell in the second tertile corresponding to a minor BMI increase of 0.4–1.1 BMI units. This is in line with previous research showing that people in developed countries typically gain weight until they are about 60 years old [24]. Furthermore, there is consistent evidence that excess weight does not constitute the same health risk among middle-aged and elderly individuals as it does among younger individuals, but may in fact be protective of age-related health problems [25]. Thus, studies emphasize a distinction between smaller weight gains that may be expected in certain age groups and greater weight gains, which may reflect underlying pathological causes, resulting in obesity.

5.1. Associations of SF-36 Vitality with BMI Change and Obesity. There is convincing evidence that HRQOL varies with BMI, and further that HRQOL is substantially reduced among obese individuals [10, 26]. However, while longitudinal studies have recognized the predictive value of BMI and obesity on HRQOL, research that prospectively has investigated the reverse association, the influence of HRQOL on BMI and/or obesity, is extremely scarce. In the current study, we found that SF-36 vitality is not merely a consequence of weight gain or obesity but may also be regarded as a predictor of weight status over time. Interestingly, SF-36 vitality was only of predictive value for BMI changes among individuals with increasing BMI during the follow-up period. These results are in line with the only previous study prospectively investigating the effect of HRQOL on obesity [11]. In their study, Cameron et al. [11] followed 5985 Australian men and women with a mean age of 51.3 years over a five-year follow-up period and found that the mental components of HRQOL including the SF-36 vitality scale predicted weight gain over the follow-up period. More specifically, individuals in the lowest baseline SF-36 vitality tertile gained more BMI units than individuals in the medium and high SF-36 vitality tertiles though the exact estimates were not reported. However, findings from both the current study and the Cameron et al. [11] study indicate that there is no clear dose-dependent relationship between SF-36 vitality and increases in BMI as only individuals with the lowest baseline vitality had significantly greater increases in BMI.

5.2. Possible Underlying Mechanisms. The SF-36 vitality scale is included in the mental component of the SF-36. However, studies have consistently reported moderate to strong correlations between the physical and mental components of HRQOL [27, 28], emphasizing the complex relation between physical and mental factors in HRQOL. Previous research has suggested that weight gain and obesity mainly are predictors of the physical components of HRQOL [12]. However, in line with the Cameron et al. [11] study who emphasized the effect of the mental component on weight gain, the current findings suggested that SF-36 vitality is of importance for increases in BMI and development of obesity. Thus, results of the current study further add to the evidence that different components of HRQOL are relevant for associations of HRQOL and weight status depending on the direction of this relation.

Several plausible mechanisms may link SF-36 vitality and weight gain. Reduced vitality may lead to increases in BMI through a lack of motivation, energy, and/or capacity to engage in physical activity. In fact, previous research has suggested that individuals with poor SF-36 vitality report significantly more sedentary activity compared with individuals with high SF-36 vitality [29]. However, in the current study, adjusting for level of physical activity did not influence the association between SF-36 vitality and changes in BMI or obesity substantially. Thus, our results are not supportive of this hypothesis. Furthermore, the correlation between SF-36 vitality at baseline and level of physical activity at follow-up was weak ($r = 0.16$), indicating that level of physical activity from baseline to follow-up does not influence the reported associations between SF-36 vitality and weight gain.

Possible biological explanations for the observed associations between SF-36 vitality and BMI change and development of obesity were not investigated in the present study. For instance, reduced SF-36 vitality may contribute to weight gain and obesity through stress-related systems including the hypothalamic-pituitary-adrenal axis [30]. Such biological pathways have been suggested to contribute to the relation between depression and increased BMI and obesity [31, 32], and it is possible that similar mechanisms are responsible for the associations between mental components of HRQOL and obesity found in prior research [11] and more specifically, between SF-36 vitality and weight status observed in the current study. Future studies examining the relation between HRQOL and weight status should include potential underlying biological mechanisms.

Lastly, psychological pathways related to eating behavior and body dissatisfaction may underlie associations of SF-36 vitality and obesity. Interestingly, in the current study, low SF-36 vitality predicted development of obesity among women in all the tested models with ORs ranging from 5.8 to 7.1 ($p < 0.05$) while this association was not significant among men. Thus, results of the current study indicate that sex differences may exist in the relation between SF-36 vitality and obesity. Research has consistently linked emotionally induced eating [33, 34] and body dissatisfaction with obesity [35] especially among women. Thus, the observed sex differences in the relation between SF-36 vitality and obesity may indicate that psychological mechanisms play a greater role in the development of obesity among women than among men. We did not observe substantial sex differences in the relation between SF-36 and BMI change, and it may be hypothesized that psychological mechanisms constitute a more important factor for the development of obesity than for variations within the nonobese BMI range.

5.3. Strengths and Limitations. This study has several strengths including a prospective study design, a large community-based sample, objectively measured weight and height at follow-up, detailed information about socio-demographic factors and physical activity, and register-based information about obesity-related medical diseases. Yet, some limitations should be mentioned.

The average BMI increase among weight gainers was 1.5 BMI points (SD: 1.3) for men and 1.4 (SD: 1.2) for women during the follow-up period, which must be considered moderate changes. However, the follow-up period of the current study was 3–7 years, and it may be that BMI changes become clinically relevant when they are considered over the years of a lifetime.

Also, baseline BMI was based on self-reported height and weight, while BMI at follow-up was physically measured at an examination. Considering the consistently found tendency to underreport weight [36], BMI changes in the current study may have been overestimated. However, the mean measured and self-reported BMI at follow-up did not differ (26.33 kg/m^2 versus 26.33 kg/m^2), indicating that participants in the current study are not prone to underreport their weight.

The availability of extensive data from two large community cohorts is an advantage of the current study. However, by design, there is very little age variation within the cohorts. Age has previously been found to be one of the most consistent predictors of overweight and obesity with middle-aged and older individuals at higher risk of being obese than their younger counterparts [37, 38]. Members of the included cohorts were all either 47, 51, or 57 years of age at baseline, and thus results of the present study are only relevant for middle-aged individuals. Furthermore, cultural differences may affect public and individual perspectives on obesity [39], and it is therefore uncertain whether the current results can be generalized beyond the Danish population. Furthermore, the CAMB had a relatively modest response rate of 30%, which should be considered when interpreting the results. For instance, it is likely that participants and nonparticipants in the CAMB study differ on individual characteristics such as level of education and general health [23] with only the more resourceful individuals participating in the follow-up study. That is, the effect of SF-36 vitality on weight status may possibly have been underestimated in the current study.

Lastly, as discussed earlier, we did not investigate the effect of biological mechanisms on the SF-36 vitality-BMI change/obesity relation. Likewise, the current study focused on the vitality scale, which is encompassed in the mental component of the SF-36. However, it would have been interesting to also examine the predictive value of other SF-36 scales, especially to include subscales from the physical SF-36 component. Unfortunately, this information was not available in the current study.

6. Conclusion

The study findings indicate that the SF-36 vitality scale is of predictive value for increases in BMI over time among individuals gaining weight, but not among individuals maintaining or losing weight. Furthermore, SF-36 vitality seems to be of importance for the development of obesity among women. Thus, it seems that some sex differences exist in the relation between SF-36 vitality and obesity possibly related to previously reported sex differences in the psychological correlates of obesity. It is plausible that different mechanisms underlie variations within the nonobese BMI range and variations in obesity emphasizing the importance of distinguishing between smaller weight changes and larger increases leading to obesity. Nevertheless, the identification of poor SF-36 vitality as a potential risk indicator for weight gain and development of obesity may be beneficial in clinical practice.

Acknowledgments

The authors thank IMK Almene Fond who funded the current study through a grant to Trine Flensborg-Madsen. They acknowledge the crucial role of the initiators and steering committees of the Metropolit Cohort and the Danish Longitudinal Study on Work Unemployment and Health, and they thank for their permission to conduct this study. Furthermore, the authors thank Kirsten Avlund, Helle Bruunsgaard, Nils- Erik Fiehn, Åse Marie Hansen, Poul Holm-Pedersen, Rikke Lund, Erik Lykke Mortensen, and Merete Osler who initiated and established the Copenhagen Aging and Midlife Biobank from 2009 to 2011. They also thank the staff at the Institute of Public Health and the National Research Center for the Working Environment who undertook the CAMB data collection.

References

[1] World Health Organization (WHO), "Global status report on noncommunicable diseases," in *Target7-Halt the Rise in Diabetes and Obesity*, pp. 79–94, World Health Organization, Geneva, Switzerland, 2014.

[2] S. S. Lim, T. Vos, A. D. Flaxman et al., "A comparative risk assessment of burden of disease and injury attributable to 67 risk factors and risk factor clusters in 21 regions, 1990–2010: a systematic analysis for the Global Burden of Disease Study 2010," *The Lancet*, vol. 380, no. 9859, pp. 2224–2260, 2013.

[3] F. Corica, A. Corsonello, G. Apolone, M. Lucchetti, N. Melchionda, and G. Marchesini, "Construct validity of the short form-36 health survey and its relationship with BMI in obese outpatients," *Obesity*, vol. 14, no. 8, pp. 1429–1437, 2006.

[4] K. R. Fontaine and I. Barofsky, "Obesity and health-related quality of life," *Obesity Reviews*, vol. 2, no. 3, pp. 173–182, 2001.

[5] R. L. Kolotkin, K. Meter, and G. R. Williams, "Quality of life and obesity," *Obesity Reviews*, vol. 2, no. 4, pp. 219–229, 2001.

[6] J. B. Bjørner, K. Thunedborg, T. S. Kristensen, J. Modvig, and P. Bech, "The Danish SF-36 health survey: translation and preliminary validity studies," *Journal of Clinical Epidemiology*, vol. 51, no. 11, pp. 991–999, 1998.

[7] Z Ul-Haq, D. F. Mackay, E. Fenwick, and J. P. Pell, "Meta-analysis of the association between body mass index and health-related quality of life among adults, assessed by the SF-36," *Obesity*, vol. 21, no. 3, pp. E322–E327, 2013.
[8] E. S. Ford, D. G. Moriarty, M. M. Zack, A. H. Mokdad, and D. P. Chapman, "Self-reported body mass index and health-related quality of life: findings from the behavioral risk factor surveillance system," *Obesity Research*, vol. 9, no. 1, pp. 21–31, 2001.
[9] D. B. Sarwer, M. Lavery, and J. C. Spitzer, "A review of the relationships between extreme obesity, quality of life, and sexual function," *Obesity Surgery*, vol. 22, no. 4, pp. 668–676, 2012.
[10] C. L. Wimmelmann, E. Smith, M. T. Lund, M. Hansen, F. Dela, and E. L. Mortensen, "The psychological profile of bariatric patients with and without type 2 diabetes: baseline results of the longitudinal GASMITO-PSYC study," *Surgery for Obesity and Related Diseases*, vol. 11, no. 2, pp. 412–418, 2015.
[11] A. J. Cameron, D. J. Magliano, D. W. Dunstan et al., "A bi-directional relationship between obesity and health-related quality of life: evidence from the longitudinal AusDiab study," *International Journal of Obesity*, vol. 36, no. 2, pp. 295–303, 2012.
[12] M. L. Daviglus, K. Liu, L. L. Yan et al., "Body mass index in middle age and health-related quality of life in older age: the Chicago Heart Association detection project in industry study," *Archives of Internal Medicine*, vol. 163, no. 20, pp. 2448–2455, 2003.
[13] K. R. Fontaine, I. Barofsky, R. E. Andersen et al., "Impact of weight loss on health-related quality of life," *Quality of Life Research*, vol. 8, no. 3, pp. 275–277, 1999.
[14] C. L. Wimmelmann, M. T. Lund, M. Hansen, F. Dela, and E. L. Mortensen, "The effect of preoperative type 2 diabetes and physical fitness on mental health and health-related quality of life after Roux-en-Y Gastric bypass," *Journal of Obesity*, vol. 2016, Article ID 3474816, 9 pages, 2016.
[15] S. Maynard, G. Keijzers, Å. M. Hansen et al., "Associations of subjective vitality with DNA damage, cardiovascular risk factors and physical performance," *Acta Physiologica*, vol. 213, no. 1, pp. 156–170, 2015.
[16] J. B. Bjorner, G. V. Wallenstein, M. C. Martin et al., "Interpreting score differences in the SF-36 vitality scale: using clinical conditions and functional outcomes to define the minimally important difference," *Current Medical Research and Opinion*, vol. 23, no. 4, pp. 731–739, 2007.
[17] E. Pappa, N. Kontodimopoulos, A. A. Papadopoulos, and D. Niakas, "Assessing the socio-economic and demographic impact on health-related quality of life: evidence from Greece," *International Journal of Public Health*, vol. 54, no. 4, pp. 241–249, 2009.
[18] F. J. Penedo and J. R. Dahn, "Exercise and well-being: a review of mental and physical health benefits associated with physical activity," *Current Opinion in Psychiatry*, vol. 18, no. 2, pp. 189–193, 2005.
[19] J. Sundquist and S. E. Johansson, "The influence of socio-economic status, ethnicity and lifestyle on body mass index in a longitudinal study," *International Journal of Epidemiology*, vol. 27, no. 1, pp. 57–63, 1998.
[20] P. Clarke, P. M. O'Malley, L. D. Johnston, and J. E. Schulenberg, "Social disparities in BMI trajectories across adulthood by gender, race/ethnicity and lifetime socio-economic position: 1986–2004," *International Journal of Epidemiology*, vol. 38, no. 2, pp. 499–509, 2008.
[21] M. Osler, R. Lund, M. Kriegbaum, U. Christensen, and A-M. Nybo Andersen, "Cohort profile: the metropolit 1953 Danish male birth cohort," *International Journal of Epidemiology*, vol. 35, no. 3, pp. 541–545, 2005.
[22] U. Christensen, R. Lund, M. T. Damsgaard et al., "Cynical hostility, socioeconomic position, health behaviors, and symptom load: a cross-sectional analysis in a Danish population-based study," *Psychosomatic Medicine*, vol. 66, no. 4, pp. 572–577, 2004.
[23] K. Avlund, M. Osler, E. L. Mortensen et al., "Copenhagen aging and midlife biobank (CAMB) an introduction," *Journal of Aging and Health*, vol. 26, no. 1, pp. 5–20, 2014.
[24] D. T. Villareal, C. M. Apovian, R. F. Kushner, and S. Klein, "Obesity in older adults: technical review and position statement of the American Society for Nutrition and NAASO, the obesity society," *American Journal of Clinical Nutrition*, vol. 82, no. 5, pp. 923–934, 2005.
[25] S. L. Miller and R. R. Wolfe, "The danger of weight loss in the elderly," *Journal of Nutrition Health and Aging*, vol. 12, no. 7, pp. 487–491, 2008.
[26] A. Renzaho, M. Wooden, and B. Houng, "Associations between body mass index and health-related quality of life among Australian adults," *Quality of life research*, vol. 19, no. 4, pp. 515–520, 2010.
[27] C. A. McHorney, J. E. Ware Jr., and A. E. Raczek, "The MOS 36-item short-form health survey (SF-36): II. psychometric and clinical tests of validity in measuring physical and mental health constructs," *Medical Care*, vol. 31, no. 3, pp. 247–263, 1993.
[28] S. S. Farivar, W. E. Cunningham, and R. D. Hays, "Correlated physical and mental health summary scores for the SF-36 and SF-12 Health Survey, V.1," *Health and Quality of Life Outcomes*, vol. 5, no. 1, p. 54, 2007.
[29] T. Balboa-Castillo, L. M. León-Muñoz, A. Graciani, F. Rodríguez-Artalejo, and P. Guallar-Castillón, "Longitudinal association of physical activity and sedentary behavior during leisure time with health-related quality of life in community-dwelling older adults," *Health and Quality of Life Outcomes*, vol. 9, no. 1, p. 47, 2011.
[30] S. I. Lindeberg, F. Eek, E. Lindbladh, P.-O. Östergren, Å. M. Hansen, and B. Karlson, "Exhaustion measured by the SF-36 vitality scale is associated with a flattened diurnal cortisol profile," *Psychoneuroendocrinology*, vol. 33, no. 4, pp. 471–477, 2008.
[31] F. S. Luppino, L. M. de Wit, P. F. Bouvy et al., "Overweight, obesity, and depression: a systematic review and meta-analysis of longitudinal studies," *Archives of General Psychiatry*, vol. 67, no. 3, pp. 220–229, 2010.
[32] P. Björntorp, "Do stress reactions cause abdominal obesity and comorbidities?," *Obesity Reviews*, vol. 2, no. 2, pp. 73–86, 2001.
[33] D. B. Allison and S. Heshka, "Social desirability and response bias in self-reports of "emotional eating"," *Eating Disorders*, vol. 1, no. 1, pp. 31–38, 1993.
[34] N. P. Hays, G. P. Bathalon, M. A. McCrory, R. Roubenoff, R. Lipman, and S. B. Roberts, "Eating behavior correlates of adult weight gain and obesity in healthy women aged 55–65 y," *American Journal of Clinical Nutrition*, vol. 75, no. 3, pp. 476–483, 2002.
[35] D. B. Sarwer, T. A. Wadden, and G. D. Foster, "Assessment of body image dissatisfaction in obese women: specificity, severity, and clinical significance," *Journal of Consulting and Clinical Psychology*, vol. 66, no. 4, pp. 651–654, 1998.
[36] H. Nawaz, W. Chan, M. Abdulrahman, D. Larson, and D. L. Katz, "Self-reported weight and height: implications for

obesity research," *American Journal of Preventive Medicine*, vol. 20, no. 4, pp. 294–298, 2001.

[37] C. L. Ogden, C. L. Johnson, M. D. Carroll, L. R. Curtin, and K. M. Flegal, "Prevalence of overweight and obesity among US children, adolescents, and adults, 1999-2002," *JAMA*, vol. 291, no. 23, pp. 2847–2850, 2004.

[38] C. L. Ogden, M. D. Carroll, L. R. Curtin, M. A. McDowell, C. J. Tabak, and K. M. Flegal, "Prevalence of overweight and obesity in the United States, 1999-2004," *JAMA*, vol. 295, no. 13, pp. 1549–1555, 2006.

[39] K. E. Friedman, S. K. Reichmann, P. R. Costanzo, A. Zelli, J. A. Ashmore, and G. J. Musante, "Weight stigmatization and ideological beliefs: relation to psychological functioning in obese adults," *Obesity Research*, vol. 13, no. 5, pp. 907–916, 2005.

8

School Engagement in Relation to Body Mass Index and School Achievement in a High-School Age Sample

Kristin E. Finn[1] **Myles S. Faith**[2] **and Young S. Seo**[2]

[1]*School of Education and Human Services, Canisius College, 2001 Main Street, Buffalo, NY 14208, USA*
[2]*Department of Counseling, School, and Educational Psychology, University at Buffalo–State University of New York, 420 Baldy Hall, Buffalo, NY 14260-1000, USA*

Correspondence should be addressed to Kristin E. Finn; finnk@canisius.edu

Academic Editor: Michele D. Levine

Purpose. Research has documented an inverse relationship between body mass index (BMI) and school achievement but has failed to empirically explain it. We tested whether this association among adolescents can be explained in part by student engagement. *Methods.* A self-report survey about health and school behaviors was completed by 196 high school students; BMI and achievement data were obtained from school records. Three forms of engagement were assessed: behavioral, presenteeism, and affective. Associations of engagement with BMI and achievement were examined, and mediation analyses were conducted. *Results.* The simple relationship between BMI and achievement was confirmed and demonstrated that BMI was negatively related to academic achievement. Higher BMI was also significantly correlated with lower classroom participation. Mediation tests showed the significant relationship between BMI and achievement was reduced after accounting for behavioral engagement but not affective engagement. *Conclusions.* These novel findings shed light on why heavier students often experience lower academic achievement. Intervention studies targeting barriers to classroom engagement among overweight and obese youth are needed so that their academic potential is not compromised.

1. Introduction

Childhood obesity is a major public health problem in the US and around the world. A well-established literature suggested childhood obesity is associated with numerous medical complications and comorbidities [1], psychosocial complications [2], poorer body image [3], and reduced health-related quality of life [4]. In addition to these health complications, emerging interest has focused on the link between obesity and academic achievement. A slowly growing but consistent body of evidence demonstrates that obesity is negatively related to academic performance. A review by Taras and Potts-Datema [5] suggests poorer school performance for children who are overweight or obese for all 10 studies in their review. Indicators of poor performance included lower math and reading scores, IQ scores, grade point average (GPA), educational persistence, absenteeism, grade retention, and placement in special education and remedial classes. Since their review, more recent investigations also consistently demonstrate worse academic outcomes for students with obesity [6, 7]. As educational attainment predicts long-term health outcomes and reduced longevity [8], poorer academic achievement is a concerning comorbidity of childhood obesity.

Despite the prior findings, there is a lack of understanding about the mechanisms underlying the relationship between obesity and achievement [5, 9]. To date, few if any empirical studies have tested the multiple pathways by which obesity affects achievement. A comprehensive review by Caird et al. [10] reported that the association between obesity and educational attainment weakens after controlling for confounding variables such as socioeconomic status. Truong and Sturm [7] conjecture that medical conditions, stigma, and depression may serve as pathways through which obesity affects achievement. Although each factor is plausible, they argue that none of them are sufficient explanations and that most of the association between obesity and education is likely due to other pathways. New data are needed to formally test underlying pathways and mechanisms.

In the present study, we propose that the relationship between obesity and achievement may be mediated, at least in part, by student engagement, a central component of achievement. In the field of education research, "student engagement" is widely regarded as essential for school success. Engagement research and theory has shown tremendous growth over the past two decades [11], with abundant evidence that engagement is a strong predictor of student achievement, motivation, learning, and retention [12, 13]. Engagement is a complex construct and has been conceptualized more fully in the past decade to include affective, behavioral, and cognitive dimensions [14, 15]. In a seminal model of student disengagement, Finn [16] outlined the process of dropping out of school as beginning with a lack of behavioral engagement in school activities (attendance, homework completion, and classroom participation) which then leads to poor school performance and subsequently to a lack of emotional engagement in school (valuing school outcomes and sense of belonging in school). School success (and failure) is the result of a cycle of engagement experiences. This rich literature offers a novel framework for studying the link between childhood obesity and academic performance.

Childhood obesity may in fact have a significant impact on engagement and subsequent academic success. In school settings, students with obesity encounter lower expectations for school success [17, 18]. A recent qualitative review of adolescents in the UK summarized the negative experience of obesity as severe, unrelenting, abusive, and isolating [19]. There is extensive evidence for biases against youth who are obese in schools [20], including from teachers [20] and principals [21] in addition to peers [22]. This may result in disengagement and "presenteeism," which in the workplace is defined as being present at work, but less productive or not fully functioning due to a health problem [23]. In one study of manufacturing employees, moderately or extremely obese workers experienced greater health-related loss in productivity than those with lower BMIs [24]. Studies of costs associated with lost productivity show that workers who are obese miss more work days due to illness, injury, or disability [25]. Similarly, students who are obese compared to healthy weight may be "showing up for work" (i.e., school attendance) but with diminished engagement on academic tasks. Empirical tests of the relationship between obesity and engagement are beginning to emerge. For example, in a recent study using the National Survey of Children's Health, adolescents with obesity were significantly more likely to be absent from school and less engaged [26].

While it is theoretically reasonable, to our knowledge, no studies have directly assessed the pathway between obesity, engagement, and achievement. Further, there is a lack of consistency in the way that educational experiences such as engagement and achievement have been operationalized. For instance, engagement has been measured as failing grades and unexplained absences [27] as well as parent's reports of their child caring about doing well in school and completing required work [26]. In this study, engagement is conceptualized as proschool attitudes and behaviors that contribute to success in school; it is operationalized as having both external (behavioral) and internal (affective) factors. The purpose of this investigation was to test whether the relationship between child BMI and academic achievement is mediated by behavioral and affective indicators of school engagement.

2. Method

2.1. Participants. A sample of 196 students from a large suburban high school in the northeast were included in the present study. Once the study gained approval from the Internal Review Board from Canisius College, participants completed surveys during three separate periods of a health class during the school day. Most (95%) of the participants were in grade 9 (average age 14.65). The sample was evenly split between males (47%) and females (53%). About 70% of the respondents reported race as white, 15% as African American, 6% Hispanic, and 9% other.

2.2. Measures. Three forms of school engagement were assessed: behavioral, presenteeism, and affective. These measures represent engagement ranging from more specific, external classroom behaviors and actions (behavioral) to internal attitudes and values about school and education (affective).

2.2.1. Behavioral Engagement/Participation. Behavioral engagement in school was assessed with 6 items that measured the extent to which students participate in the classroom. Example items include "I pay attention in class," "I participate in class discussions," and "I come to class on time." The items were adapted from Finn's school participation questionnaire (see [28]). Each item used a 4-point Likert scale ranging from "strongly disagree" to "strongly agree." The internal reliability coefficient for the scale was 0.82 in this sample.

2.2.2. Presenteeism. Presenteeism was assessed with a 7-item scale adapted from the World Health Organization's Health and Work Performance Questionnaire [29]. The scale assessed the extent to which students reported limited performance at school during the past month (e.g., not working carefully, lower work quality, and performance limited by health problems). This form of engagement was generally external, but less specific and classroom-related than the participation engagement measure. Each item was assessed on a 4-point scale that ranged from "none of the time" to "most of the time." The internal reliability estimate for the scale was 0.78 in this sample.

2.2.3. Affective Engagement/Identification. Affective engagement was assessed with the 10-item identification with school questionnaire [30]. The measure indicates the degree

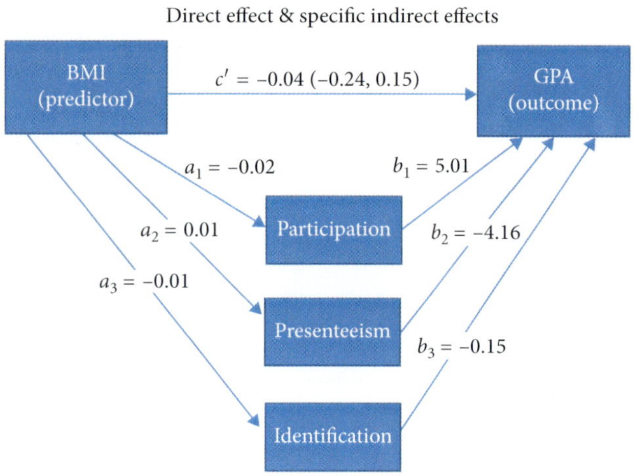

FIGURE 1: Parallel multiple mediation model tested through a set of paths controlling for gender and race. Note: direct effect (c') = −0.04 (−0.24, 0.15); specific indirect effect of participation (a_1b_1) = −0.09 (−0.18, −0.01); specific indirect effect of presenteeism (a_2b_2) = −0.05 (−0.14, 0.04); specific indirect effect of identification (a_3b_3) = 0.00 (−0.02, 0.03); total effect (c) = $c' + (a_1b_1 + a_2b_2 + a_3b_3)$.

to which students value both school and school-related outcomes and have a sense of belongingness in their school. Identification with school represents an internal form of engagement. Each item was assessed on a 4-point scale that ranged from "strongly disagree" to "strongly agree." Example items included "I feel proud of being part of my school," "I am treated with as much respect as other students in my class," and "School is one of the most important things in my life." The scale has good psychometric properties with an internal reliability coefficient of 0.79 in this sample.

2.2.4. GPA. Academic achievement was provided by school records indicating the student's current overall grades (GPAs) for their current year in school. Scores ranged from 61.58 to 99.56, with average GPA of 86.46 (standard deviation 9.03).

2.2.5. Body Mass Index. BMI (kg/m^2) for each student was obtained from school records. BMI was derived from children's weights and heights which were collected by New York State-certified physical education teachers during fitness testing which was part of the normal fitness unit curriculum at the beginning of the school year. A balance scale was used to measure weight, and a wall tape measure was used to record height. Body mass index for students, as reported by the school, ranged from 14.7 to 48.7 with an average BMI of 22.84 (standard deviation 5.5).

2.3. Data Analysis. Because obesity and school achievement are often associated with demographic characteristics, mediation analyses controlled for gender and race [7, 32]. The purpose of the present study was to examine whether engagement in school can be used to explain the link between obesity and achievement among adolescents. Specifically, regression analysis was used to test whether this relationship was mediated by three different indicators of school engagement.

Mediation analyses were conducted using SPSS PROCESS v.3 macro [33] to examine whether the relationship between student BMI and academic achievement was mediated through student participation, presenteeism, and identification with school. Specifically, a parallel multiple mediator model was employed by putting all three potential mediators simultaneously, thus allowing us to examine multiple mechanisms at the same time and to compare the magnitude of the indirect effects of student BMI through them. Compared with the traditional mediation approach suggested by Baron and Kenny [32], the total effect of the predictor on the outcome (here student BMI on GPA) may be obtained by summing the direct effect and specific indirect effects.

In Hayes' approach [33], both the direct and the indirect effects are obtained by estimating the coefficients from the three paths simultaneously as follows (Figure 1). First, student GPAs are regressed on student BMI while holding all three mediators, student gender, and race (white vs. nonwhite) constant (direct effect (c')). Second, student BMI predicts student participation at school (a_1), which in turn predicts student GPA (b_1) (specific indirect effect 1 (a_1b_1)). Third, student BMI predicts student presenteeism at school (a_2), which in turn predicts student GPA (b_2) (specific indirect effect 2 (a_2b_2)). Fourth, student BMI predicts student identification with school (a_3), which in turn predicts student GPA (b_3) (specific indirect effect 3 (a_3b_3)). Eventually, the total effect (not shown here) can be computed by adding direct effect (c') to the sum of specific indirect effects ($a_1b_1 + a_2b_2 + a_3b_3$). In order to check the robustness of the indirect effects, the bias-corrected bootstrap confidence intervals were computed which were derived by taking a random sample with 100,000 replacements.

3. Results

3.1. Descriptives. Descriptive statistics and correlation coefficients for the sample are given in Table 1. Gender was not significantly correlated with any of the other variables. Race was significantly correlated with both BMI and GPA; lower BMI and higher GPA were more typically associated with white students. Greater classroom participation and less presenteeism were also more likely among white students. Race was unrelated to level of school identification. Average student BMI for the sample was 22.84. The average BMI breakdown by gender and race was 22.7 for males, 22.9 for females, 22.1 for white, and 24.3 for nonwhite.

As expected, the inverse correlation between BMI and GPA was statistically significant ($r = -0.17$, $p = 0.019$) for the entire sample. The correlations further reveal important relationships for the three engagement measures. All three forms of engagement were interrelated with correlations ranging from 0.42 to 0.66. All forms of engagement measures were also significantly related to GPA, demonstrating the importance of engagement for academic success. Greater achievement was found for students with higher levels of

Table 1: Correlations among all variables.

	Gender	Race	BMI	GPA	Participation	Presenteeism	Identification
Gender	1.00	0.12	0.02	0.06	−0.05	0.03	−0.08
Race		1.00	0.18*	−0.29**	−0.24**	0.17*	−0.02
BMI			1.00	−0.17*	−0.21**	0.13	−0.06
GPA				1.00	0.53**	−0.51**	0.28**
Participation					1.00	−0.66**	0.57**
Presenteeism						1.00	−0.42**
Identification							1.00
Mean			22.84	86.46	3.15	2.00	3.03
Standard deviation			5.49	9.03	0.54	0.62	0.47

Note. Gender: 0 = male and 1 = female; race: 0 = white and 1 = nonwhite. $^{*}p < 0.05$; $^{**}p < 0.01$.

Table 2: Regression analyses predicting GPA from BMI, participation, presenteeism, and identification.

	Consequent															
Antecedent		M_1 (participation)				M_2 (presenteeism)				M_3 (identification)				Y (GPA)		
		b	SE	p		b	SE	p		b	SE	p		b	SE	p
X (BMI)	a_1	−0.02	0.01	0.012	a_2	0.01	0.01	0.142	a_3	−0.01	0.01	0.405	c'	−0.04	0.10	0.661
M_1 (participation)		—	—	—		—	—	—		—	—	—	b_1	5.01	1.49	0.001
M_2 (presenteeism)		—	—	—		—	—	—		—	—	—	b_2	−4.16	1.14	<0.001
M_3 (identification)		—	—	—		—	—	—		—	—	—	b_3	−0.15	1.40	0.916
Covariate: female		−0.04	0.08	0.598		0.02	0.09	0.862		−0.08	0.07	0.263		1.79	1.07	0.096
Covariate: nonwhite		−0.25	0.08	0.004		0.20	0.10	0.043		−0.00	0.08	0.973		−3.47	1.21	<0.01
Constant	i_{M_1}	3.64	0.16	<0.001	i_{M_2}	1.66	0.19	0.001	i_{M_3}	3.19	0.15	<0.001	i_Y	80.56	7.01	0.001
		$R^2 = 0.092$				$R^2 = 0.040$				$R^2 = 0.011$				$R^2 = 0.362$		
		$F(3,189) = 6.40$, $p < 0.001$				$F(3,189) = 2.62$, $p = 0.052$				$F(3,189) = 0.69$, $p = 0.557$				$F(6,186) = 17.58$, $p < 0.001$		

Note. Control variables included student gender and race.

classroom participation (0.53) and school identification (0.28) and lower levels of presenteeism (−0.51). In terms of BMI, the only engagement predictor to be significant was classroom participation (i.e., behavioral engagement) such that higher levels of BMI were associated with lower classroom participation ($r = -0.21$).

3.2. Partitions of Direct Effect and Indirect Effects. The direct effect of BMI, $c' = -0.04$, is the estimated differences in GPAs between students having the same school engagement (participation, presenteeism, and identification), gender, and race but differ by one unit in their BMI. As shown in Table 2, student GPAs did not differ as a function of student BMI when controlling for participation, presenteeism, identification, student gender, and race ($c' = -0.04$, $t(186) = -0.44$, $p = 0.66$, CI (−0.24, 0.15)). Thus, the association between BMI and GPA is nonsignificant after accounting for engagement mediators and control variables.

The indirect effects show the relationships between BMI and GPA as mediated by the effect of participation, presenteeism, and identification. The results of mediation analyses in Table 2 indicated that student BMI was inversely related to student participation at school ($a_1 = -0.02$, SE = 0.01, $p < 0.05$), which in turn was associated with a decline in student GPAs ($b_1 = 5.01$, SE = 1.49, $p = 0.001$). The indirect effect of student BMI on GPAs as modeled through student behavioral engagement (participation at school) was estimated as $a_1 b_1 = -0.02(5.01) = -0.09$. Students with a one unit higher BMI exhibited lower behavioral engagement (by 0.09 units), which in turn was associated with a decrease in their GPAs (bias-corrected bootstrap CI (−0.18, −0.01)). Thus, the relationship between BMI and GPA was significantly mediated by participation.

Indirect effects involving the other two engagement predictors showed that BMI was not significantly related to either presenteeism ($a_2 = 0.01$, SE = 0.001, $p > 0.05$) or identification ($a_3 = -0.01$, SE = 0.01, $p > 0.05$). The relationship between presenteeism and GPA was significant ($b_2 = -4.16$, SE = 1.14, $p < 0.001$) such that lower achievement was found for students who reported lower work quality at school. There was no significant relationship between identification with school and GPA ($b_3 = -0.15$, SE = 1.40, $p > 0.05$). Despite the relationship between presenteeism and GPA, there was no evidence of an indirect effect of presenteeism on the link between BMI and GPA. Similarly, no evidence was found to suggest that identification with school was a mediator of this relationship. Thus, the association between BMI and achievement was not influenced by student presenteeism at school ($a_2 b_2 = -0.05$, bias-corrected bootstrap CI (−0.14, 0.04)) and/or identification with school ($a_3 b_3 = -0.00$, bias-corrected bootstrap CI (−0.02, 0.03)).

4. Discussion

As discussed previously, there is ample evidence to show that being overweight or obese is related to poorer educational outcomes. In particular, research consistently finds an inverse relationship between BMI and academic achievement. What is unclear, however, is the causal explanation for this relationship. Given the widespread evidence that school engagement is necessary for academic success, we hypothesized that students who are overweight or obese may be less engaged in school which, in turn, explains why these students have worse academic outcomes. This hypothesis was tested with several forms of engagement among students.

Overall, our results confirmed that BMI was related to GPA and that student engagement was a significant mediator of this relationship. These are important findings since research so far has failed to clarify this relationship. Despite that all three forms of engagement were associated with achievement, our mediation hypotheses were only supported for the most behavioral form of engagement (i.e., classroom participation). Presenteeism in school and the affective form of engagement did not help to explain the effect of BMI on GPA. This suggests that specific, observable student behaviors in school such as participating in class discussions, handing in assignments, and putting forth effort are more important than internal attitudes about the value of school and feeling a sense of belonging. This is consistent with engagement research that shows that while attitudes about school are important predictors of school achievement, attitudes and perceptions are not sufficient alone and are most effective when coupled with academic behaviors [16]. Shernoff [34] argues that participation in schooling is essential for educational success and goes so far as to say "take away participation, and there can be no benefit of schooling" (p.10). Since all of our measures of engagement were intercorrelated and related to achievement, future research should examine the overlapping and unique effects of different types of engagement. A serial multiple mediator model could highlight potentially complex relationships among the mediators. It may be useful to establish how one engagement mediator affects another. For instance, does participation lead to identification or vice versa?

There are several possible reasons for why students with obesity may be less engaged in school. For instance, it is possible that weight bias may prevent or discourage students who are obese from being fully engaged in school. Obese compared to healthy weight children are more likely to be bullied in school. Such stigma and bullying among adolescents who are obese may result in diminished social, psychological, and physical health [35]. Students who feel ashamed and embarrassed may be reluctant to participate in class discussion or may avoid classes such as physical education. Students who are teased, bullied, or rejected may withdraw from others or avoid coming to school altogether. One study reported that the odds of skipping school because of weight-based teasing increased 5% per teasing incident for students who experience weight-based victimization [36]. In a study of 84 children enrolling in a family-based obesity treatment study, child-reported teasing/social rejection was associated with poorer child general academic ability as reported by teachers [37].

In addition, poor health may also contribute to lack of engagement. Daniels [38] review of the impact of obesity on school outcomes points to several health-related reasons for poor performance. Obesity-related problems such as poor nutrition, sedentary lifestyle, asthma, orthopedic problems, and sleep apnea may affect a student's ability to pay attention and stay focused in class, may impair cognitive functioning, contribute to mood disruptions, and increase tardiness and absenteeism. Students who have obesity-related health problems may miss school days because they do not feel well or have medical appointments. Sleep difficulties may make it difficult to arrive at school on time or pay attention in class. One study found that children referred by physicians to a special clinic for severely obese students missed a median of one day from school in the preceding month [39]. Additionally, Pan et al. [40] found that adolescents with obesity missed 37% more sick days due to health than adolescents with normal weight. A recent review of health and achievement shows that students with poor physical fitness and who do not maintain a healthy weight are at risk for poor school performance [9]. While not assessed in this study, it may be worthwhile to explore weight bias and health-related quality of life as impediments to school engagement in future investigations.

Limitations of this study include the inability to make causal connections with correlational data. For example, any causal effect of BMI on school achievement may be due in part to weight bias exposure. Mediation analyses shed light on the probable connection between obesity, engagement, and achievement; however, experimental or longitudinal designs would provide more definitive explanations. Also, the use of self-report data may result in biased estimates of behavioral engagement and work habits should be corroborated with teacher observations when possible. On the other hand, judgments of effort and concentration may be best assessed through self-report, and predictor and outcome variables were both obtained through school records. It should also be mentioned that students completed the survey during health classes which may have influenced some responses. Although most engagement items pertained to general school attitudes and behaviors, a small number of items on the presenteeism scale addressed limitations due to health issues which may have been more threatening for students who were overweight.

Our findings reveal an opportunity for novel intervention studies targeting barriers to school engagement among youth who are overweight or obese, such that academic potential is realized and not compromised. We are unaware of any such research, which could occur at a schoolwide level or target individual youth. There have been "universal" antibullying campaigns that have some successes in improving school climate [41]. School-based campaigns combating weight bias (e.g., discrimination among teachers and/or students) have not been studied to our knowledge but could be investigated. Alternatively, interventions might target specific youth who are weight teased, emotionally distressed from these experiences, and consequently disengaged in the classroom. Coping skills interventions for weight teasing have received only preliminary investigation [42] and could be studied in schools, especially if academic performance is compromised. Greater collaborations among education and obesity researchers could help cultivate new intervention research.

In summary, this study offers novel insight into an important and unresolved issue. To our knowledge, this is the first study to successfully test and identify engagement as an explanation for why achievement is threatened for students with obesity. Both status (e.g., race/ethnicity) and academic (e.g., grade retention) factors have been identified that place students at risk for educational failure and dropping out. Resilient students are those individuals who can overcome these barriers and succeed despite their level of risk. A large, influential study found impressive differences between resilient and nonresilient students on several measures of school engagement [12]. Thus, school engagement may be regarded as a protective factor in terms of educational risk [28]. Students who attend class, pay attention to the teacher, persist on difficult tasks, and complete assignments increase their likelihood of school success. Perhaps it is time to better recognize obesity as a risk factor for poorer achievement, and target students who are obese and less engaged in school and start to develop interventions that encourage engagement behaviors that foster daily learning.

Acknowledgments

This research was supported by a research support grant from the School of Education and Human Services at Canisius College to Kristin E. Finn. The authors are grateful to Joleen Reinholz and Peter J Heffley for assistance with data collection.

References

[1] W. H Dietz, "Health consequences of obesity in youth: childhood predictors of adult disease," *Pediatrics*, vol. 101, pp. 518–525, 1998.

[2] R. M. Puhl and J. D. Latner, "Stigma, obesity, and the health of the nation's children," *Psychological Bulletin*, vol. 133, no. 4, pp. 557–580, 2007.

[3] M. B. Schwartz and K. D. Brownell, "Obesity and body image," *Body Image*, vol. 1, no. 1, pp. 43–56, 2004.

[4] M. D. Tsiros, T. Olds, J. D. Buckley et al., "Health-related quality of life in obese children and adolescents," *International Journal of Obesity*, vol. 33, no. 4, pp. 387–400, 2009.

[5] H. Taras and W. Potts-Datema, "Obesity and student performance at school," *Journal of School Health*, vol. 75, no. 8, pp. 291–295, 2005.

[6] J. N. Booth, P. D. Tomporowski, J. M. Boyle et al., "Obesity impairs academic attainment in adolescence: findings from ALSPAC, a UK cohort," *International Journal of Obesity*, vol. 38, no. 10, pp. 1335–1342, 2014.

[7] K. Truong and R. Sturm, *Schooling and Human Capital*, Oxford University Press, New York, NY, USA, 2011.

[8] R. M. Kaplan, V. J. Howard, M. M. Safford, and G. Howard, "Educational attainment and longevity: results from the REGARDS U.S. national cohort study of blacks and whites," *Annals of Epidemiology*, vol. 25, no. 5, pp. 323–328, 2015.

[9] S. R. Shaw, P. Gomes, A. Polotskaia, and A. M. Jankowska, "The relationship between student health and academic performance: Implications for school psychologists," *School Psychology International*, vol. 36, no. 2, pp. 115–134, 2015.

[10] J. Caird, J. Kavanagh, K. Oliver et al., *Childhood Obesity and Educational Attainment*, Report No. CPPI-Center Report No 1901, EPPI-Centre, Social Science Research Unit, Institute of Education, University of London, London, UK, 2011.

[11] S. L. Christenson, A. L Reschly, and C. Wylie, *Handbook of Research on Student Engagement*, Springer, New York, NY, USA, 2012.

[12] J. D. Finn and D. A. Rock, "Academic success among students at risk for school failure," *Journal of Applied Psychology*, vol. 82, no. 2, pp. 221–234, 1997.

[13] F. M. Newmann, G. G. Wehlage, and S. D. Lamborn, "The significance and sources of student engagement," in *Student Engagement and Achievement in American Secondary Schools*, F. M. Newmann, Ed., pp. 11–39, Teachers College Press, New York, NY, USA, 1992.

[14] J. J. Appleton, S. L. Christenson, and M. J. Furlong, "Student engagement with school: Critical conceptual and methodological issues of the construct," *Psychology in the Schools*, vol. 45, no. 5, pp. 369–386, 2008.

[15] J. A. Fredricks, P. C. Blumenfeld, and A. H. Paris, "School engagement: potential of the concept, state of the evidence," *Review of Educational Research*, vol. 74, no. 1, pp. 59–109, 2004.

[16] J. D. Finn, "Withdrawing from school," *Review of Educational Research*, vol. 59, no. 2, pp. 117–142, 1989.

[17] J. L. Peterson, R. M. Puhl, and J. Leudicke, "An experimental assessment of physical educators' expections and attitudes: the importance of student weight and gender," *Journal of School Health*, vol. 82, no. 9, pp. 432–440, 2012.

[18] D. Neumark-Sztainer, M. Story, and T. Harris, "Beliefs and attitudes about obesity among teachers and school health care providers working with adolescents," *Journal of Nutritional Education*, vol. 31, no. 1, pp. 3–9, 1999.

[19] R. W. Rees, J. Caird, K. Dickson, C. Vigurs, and J. Thomas, "'It's on your conscience all the time': a systematic review of qualitative studies examining views on obesity among young people aged 12-18 years in the UK," *BMJ Open*, vol. 4, no. 4, article e004404, 2014.

[20] R. Puhl and K. D. Brownell, "Bias, discrimination, and obesity," *Obesity Research*, vol. 9, no. 12, pp. 788–805, 2001.

[21] J. H. Price, S. M. Desmond, and C. M. Stelzer, "Elementary school principals' perceptions of childhood obesity," *Journal of School Health*, vol. 57, no. 9, pp. 367–370, 1987.

[22] J. D. Latner and A. J. Stunkard, "Getting worse: the stigmatization of obese children," *Obesity Research*, vol. 11, no. 3, pp. 452–456, 2003.

[23] R. Z. Goetzel, S. R. Long, R. J. Ozminkowski, K. Hawkins, S. Wang, and W. Lynch, "Health, absence, disability, and presenteeism cost estimates of certain physical and mental health conditions affecting U.S. employers," *Journal of Occupational and Environmental Medicine*, vol. 46, no. 4, pp. 398–412, 2004.

[24] D. M. Gates, P. Succop, B. J. Brehm, G. L. Gillespie, and B. D. Sommers, "Obesity and presenteeism: the impact of body mass index on workplace productivity," *Journal of Occupational and Environmental Medicine*, vol. 50, no. 1, pp. 39–45, 2008.

[25] J. G. Trogdon, E. A. Finkelstein, T. Hylands, P. S. Dellea, and S. J. Kamal-Bahl, "Indirect costs of obesity: a review of the current literature," *Obesity Reviews*, vol. 9, no. 5, pp. 489–500, 2008.

[26] F. R. Carey, G. K. Singh, H. S. Brown III, and A. V. Wilkinson, "Educational outcomes associated with childhood obesity in the United States: cross-sectional results from the 2011-2012 National Survey of Children's Health," *International Journal of Behavioral Nutrition and Physical Activity*, vol. 12, no. S1, p. S3, 2015.

[27] R. Crosnoe, "Gender, obesity, and education," *Sociology of Education*, vol. 80, no. 3, pp. 241–260, 2007.

[28] J. D. Finn and K. S. Zimmer, "What is it? Why does it matter?," in *Handbook of Research on Student Engagement*, S. L. Christenson, A. L. Reschly, and C. Wylie, Eds., pp. 97–131, Springer, New York, NY, USA, 2012.

[29] R. C. Kessler, C. Barber, A. L. Beck et al., "The world health organization health and work performance questionnaire (HPQ)," *Journal of Occupational and Environmental Medicine*, vol. 45, no. 2, pp. 156–174, 2003.

[30] K. E. Voelkl, "Measuring students' identification with school," *Education and Psychological Measurement*, vol. 56, no. 5, pp. 760–770, 1996.

[31] R. M. Baron and D. A. Kenny, "The moderator-mediator variable distinction in social psychological research: conceptual, strategic, and statistical considerations," *Journal of Personality and Social Psychology*, vol. 51, no. 6, pp. 1173–1182, 1986.

[32] G. E. Bingham and L. Okagaki, "Ethnicity and student engagement," in *Handbook of Research on Student Engagement*, S. L. Christenson, A. L. Reschly, and C. Wylie, Eds., pp. 69–95, Springer, New York, NY, USA, 2012.

[33] A. F. Hayes, *Introduction to Mediation, Moderation, and Conditional Process Analysis: A Regression-Based Approach*, Guilford Press, New York, NY, USA, 2013.

[34] D. Shernoff, *Optimal Learning Environments to Promote Student Engagement*, Springer, New York, NY, USA, 2014.

[35] R. M. Puhl and K. M. King, "Weight discrimination and bullying," *Best Practices in Research on Clinical Endocrinology and Metabolism*, vol. 27, no. 2, pp. 117–127, 2013.

[36] R. M. Puhl and J. Leudicke, "Weight-based victimization among adolescents in the school setting: Emotional reactions and coping behaviors," *Journal of Youth and Adolescence*, vol. 41, no. 1, pp. 27–40, 2012.

[37] T. Gunnarsdottir, U. Njardvik, A. S. Olafsdottir, L. W. Craighead, and R. Bjarnason, "Teasing and social rejection among obese children enrolling in family-based behavioural treatment: effects on psychological adjustment and academic competencies," *International Journal of Obesity*, vol. 36, no. 1, pp. 35–44, 2012.

[38] D. Y. Daniels, "Examining attendance, academic performance, and behavior in obese adolescents," *Journal of School Nursing*, vol. 24, no. 6, pp. 379–387, 2008.

[39] J. B. Schwimmer, T. M. Burwinkle, and J. W. Varni, "Health-related quality of life of severely obese children and adolescents," *JAMA*, vol. 289, no. 14, pp. 1813–1819, 2003.

[40] L. Pan, B. Sherry, S. Park, and H. M. Blanck, "The association of obesity and school absenteeism attributed to illness or injury among adolescents in the United States, 2009," *The Journal of Adolescent Health*, vol. 52, no. 1, pp. 64–69, 2013.

[41] E. Cantone, A. P. Piras, M. Vellante et al., "Interventions on bullying and cyberbullying in schools: a systematic review," *Clinical Practice & Epidemiology in Mental Health*, vol. 11, no. 1, pp. 58–76, 2015.

[42] B. M. Panzer and S. Dhuper, "Designing a group therapy program for coping with childhood weight bias," *Social Work*, vol. 59, no. 2, pp. 141–147, 2014.

9

Positioning of Weight Bias: Moving towards Social Justice

Sarah Nutter,[1] Shelly Russell-Mayhew,[1] Angela S. Alberga,[2] Nancy Arthur,[1] Anusha Kassan,[1] Darren E. Lund,[3] Monica Sesma-Vazquez,[1] and Emily Williams[1]

[1] *Counselling Psychology, Werklund School of Education, University of Calgary, Calgary, AB, Canada*
[2] *Werklund School of Education, University of Calgary, Calgary, AB, Canada*
[3] *Curriculum and Learning, Werklund School of Education, University of Calgary, Calgary, AB, Canada*

Correspondence should be addressed to Sarah Nutter; snutter@ucalgary.ca

Academic Editor: Michele D. Levine

Weight bias is a form of stigma with detrimental effects on the health and wellness of individuals with large bodies. Researchers from various disciplines have recognized weight bias as an important topic for public health and for professional practice. To date, researchers from various areas have approached weight bias from independent perspectives and from differing theoretical orientations. In this paper, we examined the similarities and differences between three perspectives (i.e., weight-centric, non-weight-centric (health-centric), and health at every size) used to understand weight bias and approach weight bias research with regard to (a) language about people with large bodies, (b) theoretical position, (c) identified consequences of weight bias, and (d) identified influences on weight-based social inequity. We suggest that, despite differences, each perspective acknowledges the negative influences that position weight as being within individual control and the negative consequences of weight bias. We call for recognition and discussion of weight bias as a social justice issue in order to change the discourse and professional practices extended towards individuals with large bodies. We advocate for an emphasis on social justice as a uniting framework for interdisciplinary research on weight bias.

1. Introduction

Weight bias, or the stigma towards and negative stereotypes about individuals who have large bodies, has been described as "overt, expressible, and widely held" [1, p. 891]. Researchers have found weight bias to be the fourth most frequently reported form of discrimination and determined a 66% increase in its occurrence between 1995 and 2006 [2]. Individuals who live in large bodies are stereotypically characterized as being lazy, sloppy, weak-willed, physically and sexually unattractive, and gluttonous [3]. Research has documented weight bias in the attitudes of health care professionals [4], success in education [5], hiring practices in the workforce [6], interpersonal relationships of individuals with large bodies [7], and the influence of the media on weight bias [8]. Research has also documented numerous physical and psychological health consequences of weight bias, including, but not limited to, increased stress [9], decreased motivation to engage in physical activity [10], increased binge-eating behaviour [11], and depression [12].

Research areas such as fat studies, health care, and psychology have recognized weight bias as an important issue for research and professional practice [13]. However, despite the common interest in weight bias, each area remains relatively segregated to the point where each perspective may be associated with specific journals as the common outlets for research and review articles, with little overlap. Activists and researchers have been described as being "fundamentally engaged in framing contests over the nature and consequences of excess body weight" [14, p. 869]. Saguy and Riley [14] posited that, when such framing contests represent opposing positions, it may undercut the integration of the insights achieved by the conflicting perspectives. Consequently, few attempts have been made to name common interests for moving forward with interdisciplinary research.

Previous researchers have noted that body weight is often framed in one of two opposing ways: through the lens of body diversity or through the lens of excess weight as a preventable health risk [14, 15]. Each way of framing body weight constructs a different social problem and entails a different solution [14]. Each of the various perspectives engaged in weight bias research takes a unique position in understanding and explaining the origins and consequences of weight bias. Further, research areas also have different approaches to language, with some more frequently using the word *fat* to refer to individuals who have large bodies and others more frequently using the words *overweight* or *obese*. Differences are also present with respect to preference for person-first (e.g., *person with obesity*) or identity-first (e.g., *fat person*) language. In recent years, person-first language has become increasingly popular, as researchers have proposed that person-first language promotes openness and aids in the reduction of stigma and prejudice [16, 17]. This discussion has continued, however, as scholars in the area of disability studies have also argued for the continued use of identity-first language together with person-first language as a way to claim identity and to promote pride [17]. Proponents of using both person-first and identity-first terms flexibly have stated that it may acknowledge the roles and perspectives of different groups and that it will also allow for the opportunity to ask about preferred terms [17]. In relation to the field of weight bias, this may resemble openness to using *both* person-first (e.g., *person with obesity*) and identity-first (e.g., *fat person*) language, depending on the context as well as individual preference.

The purpose of this paper was to conduct a literature review of selected disciplines that contribute to weight bias research in order to overview the common, potentially competing, and emerging perspectives on this topic. Weight bias research was selected from multiple research disciplines, including fat studies, feminist literature, health at every size (HAES), health care, psychology, and sociology. The review targeted papers that provided a current conceptual and theoretical overview of different perspectives of weight bias. The similarities among, and differences between, each of these perspectives were examined with regard to five research questions: (a) what is the language used to refer to weight and individuals with large bodies? (b) through what general lens is discussion of weight bias approached? (c) what theoretical positions are used to discuss the source or causes of weight bias? (d) what consequences of weight bias are identified? and (e) how are these consequences discussed with regard to influence on weight-based inequity? In the following discussion, we introduce three perspectives of weight bias with regard to these five questions: the weight-centric perspective, the non-weight-centric perspective, and health at every size perspective. In addition to these perspectives, we also provide a brief overview of literature pertaining to the social determinants of health, as it supports our discussion of weight-based inequity identified among the three perspectives. Finally, we introduce a focus on social justice as a uniting perspective that offers a foundation for advancing interdisciplinary research on weight bias.

2. Differing Perspectives of Weight Bias

Saguy and Riley [14] described disagreements that surface when obesity is framed from different perspectives. For example, groups that understand obesity through a body diversity framework, versus a preventable risk framework, would have varying opinions about "if or why higher weights have adverse health consequences, what an ideal weight is or whether a universal ideal weight even exists, why people gain weight, why some weigh more than others, and whether weight loss improves health" (p. 874).

These body diversity and preventable risk frameworks have been commonly identified in the literature using the terms *weight-centric* and *non-weight-centric or health-centric* [18–20]. Researchers have also referred to these frameworks as *weight-normative* and *weight-inclusive* [21]. For the purposes of this paper, these terms will also be used to frame our discussion, with clarification. The term weight-centric has been previously defined as having the six following tenants: (a) the belief that weight is under individual control, (b) the belief that weight gain is caused by an imbalance in caloric intake and energy usage, (c) the belief that health status can be predicted by weight, (d) the belief that excess body weight causes disease and early death, (e) the belief that methods for successful long-term weight loss involve the modification of eating and exercise patterns, and (f) the belief that losing weight will result in better health [20]. However, for the purposes of this paper, the term weight-centric will be used to refer to research that typically discusses weight bias through a consideration of body weight and increasing rates of overweight and obesity, without the assumption of the six tenants described by O'Hara and Gregg [20]. Finally, it is also important to note that the perspectives described below are not mutually exclusive but may be regarded as emerging distinctions within the field of weight bias.

The literature represented in this paper provides a brief overview of each perspective and is not intended to be a comprehensive literature review. Articles for this paper were identified through two large multidisciplinary databases (i.e., Academic Search Complete and Web of Science), with a focus on identifying articles that presented a broad theoretical overview of one or more perspectives in addition to more focused experimental and correlational study-based articles. Multiple keyword search terms were used to aid in the collection of a broad range of articles representing each perspective. Various combinations of the following keyword search terms were used: anti-fat bias, body diversity, body size, body weight, epidemiology, fat acceptance, fat bias, fat oppression, fat shaming, fat stigma, fat studies feminism, health at every size, inequality, obesity, obesity stigma, weight bias, and weightism. This resulted in 173 articles that were reviewed for examination and comparison of the differing perspectives of weight bias that informed the current discussion. Articles were then scanned for the language used to refer to weight and individuals with large bodies as well as the theoretical orientation of the article in order to determine the perspective that the article best represented.

2.1. The "Weight-Centric" Perspective. The weight-centric perspective is characterized by the investigation of weight bias through the lens of increased prejudice and discrimination based on body weight, influenced in part by increasing rates of obesity [4, 22]. This perspective often includes researchers from fields such as health care and psychology, who identify weight bias as a prevalent social issue in need of further understanding [23]. Much of the research from this perspective has focused on documenting the prevalence of weight bias and discrimination within life domains (e.g., employment) [6] and among health care professionals and preprofessionals [4, 24]. Researchers have also examined the association of weight bias with other attitudes, such as racism and physical appearance concerns, as well as fundamental beliefs that serve as the basis for a political, economic, or social system [1, 25].

When referring to weight, researchers from the weight-centric perspective tend to use the terms *overweight* and *obesity*. When referring to individuals with large bodies, researchers tend to use both person-first (i.e., *person with obesity*) [26, 27] and identity-first (i.e., *obese person*) [8, 28] language. Professional associations such as the American Psychological Association encourage the use of person-first language [16] and person-first language has become increasingly popular within the medical community [29].

It is important to note that the current weight-centric perspective on weight bias has grown from a strong history of research documenting weight bias, especially among health professionals [4] and that this perspective has been, and continues to be, critiqued due to the "medicalization" of body weight. Weight has been used as an easily measurable proxy for health and, as such, individuals' weight and health have often been confounded. More specifically, researchers have critiqued obesity research as contributing to the belief that weight is within individual control, that it is as simple as calories in versus calories out, that weight and health are inextricably related, that excess weight causes disease and death and losing weight will result in health, and that methods for long-term weight loss are known and effective [15, 20, 30, 31].

2.1.1. Attribution Theory. Although there is no consensus within this perspective, researchers tend to utilize attribution theory to understand the origins of weight bias [4]. Attribution theory proposes that individuals are motivated to seek out causal explanations for outcomes or conditions and that negative bias towards individuals with large bodies arises from the tendency for weight to be regarded as under personal control [1, 22]. Research in attribution theory has suggested that when conditions are regarded as uncontrollable, individuals are likely to display increased liking and pity but that when conditions, such as obesity, are perceived as controllable, individuals are likely to display dislike, anger, and negative judgments [32]. Such reactions, specifically feelings of disgust, have been linked to weight bias and the treatment of individuals with large bodies [33]. Many researchers have regarded weight bias as occurring due to the view of obesity as a behavioural disorder that ignores the complexity of its causation and positions it as something to be treated or eradicated through behavioural change [3, 27, 34]. Researchers have asserted that complex biological processes are often overlooked in favour of common misconceptions, such as obesity being the result of low physical activity or an unhealthy diet and that anyone with willpower can lose weight [34]. Further, the success of behaviour modification obesity interventions is often measured through how much weight a person loses [35]; however, weight is not a behaviour. It would seem that the focus on the outcome of weight loss is measured without the consideration of the complex biological and contextual influences and that individual willpower and behaviour are commonly regarded as the cause of obesity. Research documenting the media effects of such "controllability" messages [8] as well as experimental investigations [36] has provided support for attribution theory.

2.1.2. Thin-Ideal Internalization. More recently, researchers from the weight-centric perspective have also proposed that weight bias reflects the degree to which an individual has bought into social standards of attractiveness [10]. Over the last several decades, ideal body standards have shifted, with the ideal body for women being prescribed as thin, with large breasts and toned muscles, and the ideal body for men being prescribed as lean and muscular, with wide shoulders and a narrow waist [37–39]. Recent research has provided support for the relationship between the internalization of thin-ideal body standards and weight bias [40]. For example, the physical appearance concerns related to the internalization of the thin-ideal may serve to increase disgust reactions towards individuals with large bodies, thus increasing weight bias [41].

2.1.3. Social Comparison Theory. Researchers have also suggested that weight bias is influenced by the tendency to make comparisons based on body weight [42]. Social comparison theory asserts that individuals are motivated to compare and evaluate their own opinions and abilities with the opinions and abilities of others, which instills a sense of validation [43]. Previous researchers have suggested that weight bias is a form of downward social comparison that serves to increase the self-esteem of the individual making the comparison [42]. For example, a social comparison perspective of weight bias asserts that individuals may compare their bodies to people who have larger bodies in order to feel better about their own body size, thus perpetuating weight bias.

2.1.4. Consequences of Weight Bias. Researchers operating from the weight-centric perspective have also identified significant negative consequences of weight bias. Among these, researchers have identified depression [12], increased binge-eating behaviour [11], anxiety [44], and stress [9], as well as decreased motivation to engage in physical activity [10]. Although researchers from this perspective have focused less on how weight bias influences social inequity, researchers have suggested that negative beliefs and judgments tend to be greater for girls and women with large bodies compared to men [45, 46]. Research has also suggested that weight bias can impact patient quality of care as well as equality of patient care, as health care professionals may spend less time with patients with large bodies and provide fewer treatment options [47]. Finally, it is important to note that researchers have stated that the consequences of experiencing weight bias may be more harmful than simply having a large body and that perhaps the health consequences attributed to obesity may be better explained by weight bias [48].

2.2. The "Non-Weight-Centric" or "Health-Centric" Perspective. The non-weight-centric perspective is characterized by the tendency to approach discussion of weight and weight bias by taking a critical stance to the popular obesity discourses [49, 50]. This perspective often includes researchers from interdisciplinary fields such as fat studies and feminist studies, as well as sociology, who identify that weight has become an indicator for social status whereby large bodies are regarded as less successful and less attractive [30]. Researchers from this perspective seek to understand discourses beyond the medicalization of obesity and to build a body-accepting and embodied culture [30, 49, 50], where the focus is on health, not weight. In other words, from this perspective, body size is conceptualized as existing on a continuum of natural body diversity and is not something that is to be corrected.

Researchers from the health-centric perspective examine the broader social forces that aid in shifting attention and concentration "away from the fat body itself and more towards positioning and contingent systems and structures" [49, p. 1020-1021]. More specifically, researchers in this area have examined weight bias in relation to a broad array of topics including body shame and sexual health [51, 52], media influence [53–55], the fashion industry [56], education [57–59], public health [60, 61], and health care [62]. In addition, feminist researchers have also been critical of the lack of attention paid to weight bias in relation to the attention paid to other weight-related topics, such as eating disorders [63]. Vincent Roehling [64] proposed that weight bias may be an issue more congruent with the second wave of feminism, in that it tends to impact White middle-class women the most, and may be incompatible with mainstream feminist thought that has emphasized the influences of gender, race, socioeconomic status, sexual orientation, and their intersections. Shaw and Lee [65] described current feminist thought as being inclusive and affirming of all women, as well as seeking to promote equality and justice for all women. Not only is an increased focus on weight within feminist thought important with regard to weight bias, but also it might highlight the similar barriers and systemic issues that create the social conditions for the occurrence of both eating disorders *and* weight bias.

When referring to weight, researchers from the health-centric perspective tend to use terms such as *fat*, *fatness*, or *fat bodies* as well as identity-first (i.e., *fat person*) [15, 30] language when referring to individuals with large bodies. Many researchers and activists from this perspective use the word *fat* intentionally as a way to reclaim power, to remove shame and stigma, and to position fat as one of many possible identity descriptors [15, 49]. In addition to being critical of the language used to describe weight and individuals with large bodies, researchers from the fat perspective examine weight bias through numerous theoretical approaches, including critical analysis of obesity discourses [30], critical fat studies [15, 66], feminist poststructuralism [62], and intersectionality [67]. Each of these theoretical approaches will be discussed below.

2.2.1. Critical Analysis of Obesity Discourse. Researchers who have approached weight bias through a critical examination of obesity discourses have identified two competing frames. The first frame is considered the dominant weight and beauty discourse, which recognizes the "slender" body as attractive and successful and large bodies as unhealthy, diseased, and representing failure, which results in body size being regarded as an individual responsibility [15, 30, 31]. Alternatively, the second frame recognizes this discourse as originating in Western patriarchal culture and that these widespread messages serve to devalue female body size and shape with serious consequences [30, 31]. Despite these two competing discourses, researchers have recognized that "obesity epidemic" discourse tends to dominate public discussion [30, 31]. This discourse is problematic, as the ongoing discussion of large bodies as an "epidemic," "infection," or a "plague" leaves no room for the acceptance of natural body diversity. By being complicit with this discourse of the "obesity epidemic," researchers have asserted that large bodies will continue to be excluded, marginalized, and regarded as immoral [15, 31].

2.2.2. Critical Fat Studies. Similar to the critical analysis of obesity discourses, critical fat studies have been described as a position that disputes weight bias in two ways [61]. First, by placing emphasis on the complex nature of body weight, critical fat studies challenges the dominant framing of obesity as an unbalanced relationship between calories in and calories out and as a personal choice [44, 61]. Rather, critical fat studies reframes body weight as a natural form of body diversity [14]. Second, critical fat studies seeks to challenge the assumption that large bodies are a serious threat to individual health as well as other "universal scientific 'truths'" often presented in research consistent with the dominant obesity discourse [15, p. 100, 66]. More specifically, researchers from this perspective challenge incorrect and biased assumptions about weight and body size that occur in research, policy, entertainment media, news media, and public health campaigns [15].

2.2.3. Feminist Poststructuralism. Many researchers within the non-weight-centric/health-centric perspective who operate within feminist studies approach the discussion of weight bias using poststructuralism, which emphasizes the examination of how the body and identity are shaped through social relations as well as cultural and institutional beliefs [30, 62]. This framework allows for the consideration of diverse perspectives like race, ethnicity, socioeconomic status, and ability, among others, and "provides a lens for an in-depth examination of personal experiences, relationships and contextual meanings of relations of power between individuals" [62, p. 1188].

2.2.4. Intersectionality and Influences on Social Inequity. Finally, many researchers also conduct research through the lens of intersectionality, which has been defined as the examination of the interactions of multiple forms of oppression and the outcome of these interactions with regard to power [50, 67, 68]. This research has allowed for further understanding of the differential effects that weight bias has on social equality with regard to gender, race, socioeconomic status, and sexual orientation [66, 67]. Many researchers have maintained that weight bias is "deeply gendered" and "that body size matters *differently* for men and women in the identity positions available to them" [31, p. 159]. Nurka [55] asserted that a slender body is one of the demands of "good womanhood" and that it is connected with feminine identity and success (p. 168). Weight bias and its intersections have been described by researchers from the non-weight-centric perspective as contributing to an oppressive social context for individuals with large bodies, where large bodies are visual representations for immorality [49, 69].

In addition to acknowledging that weight bias contributes to an oppressive social context, researchers have identified other consequences of dominant weight discourses for women with large bodies, including weight-based harassment and social exclusion [30], disordered relationships with food [70], the draining of women's energy and resources with regard to seeking weight loss and fad diets [58], normalizing female body anxiety [55], and the reinforcement of the cultural belief that women should control their desires [71].

2.3. Health at Every Size. Health at every size (HAES) has been described as a non-weight-centric, transdisciplinary movement [18, 19] comprising researchers from all disciplinary backgrounds, who approach weight bias through the consideration of weight and the position that societal obsessions with thinness and dieting are unhealthy and do not allow for natural body diversity [72]. Rather than focusing on weight loss, the HAES paradigm focuses on health promotion and improving the emotional, physical, and spiritual well-being of individuals of all sizes [18, 58]. Specifically, researchers from this area promote self-acceptance, body diversity, and improved health behaviours regardless of size, such as engaging in physical activity for pleasure and intuitive eating behaviours [18, 58]. HAES researchers have critically examined and challenged weight-related assumptions and the use of body mass index (BMI) as an indicator of health and have provided evidence for the need for a paradigm shift within health care [18, 73]. More specifically, HAES interventions do not focus on weight as an outcome; rather, behavioural health indices such as intuitive eating, body esteem, and psychological functioning are more relevant measures of success [74, 75].

Although the HAES paradigm is relatively new, with the majority of research published beginning in the year 2000 [76], researchers from this perspective have commented on the potential clinical application of the HAES paradigm [72, 73], the application of HAES to public health [19, 76] and dietetics [77], and have examined the long-term effects of HAES interventions [78]. When conducting research within the paradigm, HAES researchers tend to use language consistent with both perspectives when referring to both weight (e.g., *overweight*, *obesity*, and *fat*) and individuals with large bodies (e.g., *obese person* and *fat person*) [18, 19, 79], as well as the term *people of size* [80].

2.3.1. "Healthism". HAES researchers have approached the understanding of weight bias through a critical examination of "healthism." Researchers have stated that healthism has cemented discourses of health and weight as being under the almost exclusive control of the individual, who is viewed as having the responsibility and obligation to strive for the perfect body [79, 81]. This healthism, and the accompanying fitness movement, prescribes specific practices and beliefs that serve to "externally regulate individual and collective bodies as well as reinforce the internalization of bodily self-control in the name of health" [79, p. 358]. Further, researchers have asserted that the dominant healthism discourse and the strive for bodily perfection intentionally exclude the consideration of the social determinants of health, such as socioeconomic status, employment status, education, lack of access to physical activity, and lack of access to health care [79, 82].

2.3.2. Consequences of Weight Bias. HAES researchers have maintained that the discourses of health and weight that contribute to weight bias have significant consequences for individuals with large bodies, including being regarded as unattractive and unhealthy [79], demotivating healthy behaviours [18], and avoidance of health care [83]. Through this perspective, weight bias is regarded as, in part, responsible for "reinforcing and privileging slimness in a culture that promotes health at one size" [18, p. 358]. Further, healthism and weight bias also serve to decontextualize health from the structural and social forces that impact people's lives, with serious consequences for the health care and health outcomes of individuals with large bodies [79, 82].

2.4. Summary. The above review of the three emerging perspectives and approaches in weight bias research suggested that each perspective approaches discussion of weight bias from a unique point of view. However, similarities among these perspectives exist with regard to how weight bias is conceptualized and understood. In addition there are similarities and differences between the perspectives with regard to how weight bias is termed, the consequences of weight bias, and how these consequences influence social inequity. Table 1 presents a summary of this discussion.

3. Social Determinants of Weight: A Fourth Perspective for Consideration?

In the early 2000s, research in public health and epidemiology began to rapidly multiply [84], with researchers consistently documenting the social and environmental disparities in health [85]. Diez Roux and Mair [85] discussed the trends driving the increased interest in neighbourhoods and health. First, they posited that researchers have increasingly recognized that explanations focusing solely on the responsibility of the individual for ill-health are inadequate and fail to capture the complex social and structural factors that contribute to weight. Second, Diez Roux and Mair [85] suggested that

Table 1: Summary of similarities and differences identified among research areas.

Research perspective	Language used	Theoretical position	Consequences identified	Weight-based social inequity
Weight-centric	Obesity Obese person Person with obesity	Attribution theory Thin-ideal internalization Social comparison theory	Depression Anxiety Stress Binge-eating Low physical activity motivation Patient-provider relationship	Gender Patient quality of care
Health-centric	Fat/fatness Fat person	Critical analysis of obesity discourses Critical fat studies Feminist poststructuralism Intersectionality	Oppressive social context Harassment Social exclusion Female body anxiety Draining of female energy	Gender Race SES Sexual orientation
Health at every size	Obese/fat Fat person Obese person	Critical analysis of "healthism"	Reinforcing & privileging thinness Decontextualize health Demotivates health behaviour Avoidance of health care	

researchers have experienced a renewed interest in examining the causes of social inequities in health, including but not limited to differences between racial and ethnic groups. Third, researchers and policy makers have increasingly begun to consider the health effects of policies such as housing or urban planning policies [85].

Results from research investigating the social and environmental disparities in weight have suggested that factors including socioeconomic status, the neighbourhood environment, race and ethnicity, gender, and level of education all influence disparities in weight [86, 87]. Researchers from various countries around the world have observed that the rates of obesity are highest among individuals from nondominant racial and/or ethnic backgrounds as well as individuals of low socioeconomic status [87, 88]. In addition to these factors, researchers have also suggested that having a low level of educational attainment and being female also play a significant role in the social patterning of weight [89, 90]. Finally, these researchers have also examined the role of the neighbourhood environment with regard to weight disparity and have suggested that neighbourhoods with lower density of sports facilities and supermarkets, lower availability of fair-priced healthy food, and decreased walkability, as well as greater perceived hazards, show an increase in the incidence of obesity [84, 86]. Congruent with the lens of intersectionality, the highest rates of obesity occur among the most disadvantaged individuals—those who experience disadvantage in two or more areas of inequity [88].

Although the majority of epidemiology researchers documenting the disparities with regard to weight have focused discussion on overweight and obesity specifically, some researchers have also discussed the impact of these social disparities with regard to weight bias [91]. In their literature review on the relationship between gender, socioeconomic status, and obesity, Broom and Warin [92] suggested that women have the most to lose from social and economic disparities in weight, especially with regard to weight bias in employment. Faeh et al. [93] conducted a longitudinal study of education, income, and occupational class on obesity and suggested that, together with disparities in weight, the increased "mediatization" of the thin-ideal could strengthen weight bias and discrimination in the workplace, especially for women. Given the social and psychological health consequences associated with weight bias, researchers have concluded that the increasing disparities in weight are a critical public health problem, adding cumulative disadvantage to vulnerable individuals [91, 94]. As such, we would argue that one of the fundamental concepts that could bind competing perspectives on weight bias is an examination of social justice.

4. Weight Bias as a Social Justice Issue

Although the research areas reviewed above may differ with regard to the theoretical lens used to understand weight bias and the language used and identify different consequences and social inequities resulting from weight bias, each research area has recognized weight bias as an important social issue. Despite this recognition, however, weight bias has yet to be widely discussed as an important *social justice* issue.

Although the term social justice is not often used when discussing weight bias, a strong history of research from each perspective described above has situated it as such. Researchers have documented the many negative assumptions and stereotypes based on body weight [3] have demonstrated that weight bias has increased in recent decades [2] and have consistently established the systematic occurrence of weight bias within society, such as within the media, health care, education, employment, and interpersonal relationships [3]. Researchers have also pointed to the broad social forces that continue to reinforce the power and privilege given to thinness, which serve to deny natural body diversity [14, 30, 62, 67, 79]. Results have also documented the significant physical and mental health consequences of being victims of weight bias and discrimination [3, 79]. Finally, researchers have established the influence of weight bias on social inequity, with differences in disparity influenced by gender, race, socioeconomic status, and sexual orientation [66, 67], which may especially influence access to, and quality of, health care [47]. In our collective effort towards weight-based equality, it may seem as though *social justice*, a term used to describe the value emphasizing equitable opportunity, action to amend systemic oppression, and participation of all individuals in order to aid them in achieving maximum potential [95, 96], has been missing from our research.

In recent years, few researchers have recognized weight bias as an important social justice issue to be addressed in research, policy, and practice [13, 49, 69, 97]. In discussing weight bias as a social justice issue, van Amsterdam [31] recognized that differences in ability, race, and gender have previously been framed as solely biological in nature to justify systemic oppression and that social justice activism has resulted in the recognition of these categorizations as socially constructed.

Previous researchers have stated that weight bias is "socially sanctioned bigotry" [70, p. 250] and that "if we care about social justice, we need to figure out whether the suffering of fat people in virtue of violating the thinness norm is permissible" [50, p. 221]. Young [70] argued that the greater social system and the "perpetrators" of weight bias are unable to adequately and effectively discuss weight without putting thinness on a pedestal and that obesity discourse "has eluded one of the greatest political, social, and cultural movements of the twentieth (and late nineteenth) century–feminism" (p. 250-251). We assert that social justice must be placed at the forefront of the discussion of weight bias, rather than as an indirect or subtle recognition. We echo Young's [70] statement that "there is no authentic, credible space where the oppression associated with fat, can be spoken about" (p. 251) and call for such credible spaces to be carved out in weight bias literature. It is in the direction of naming weight bias as a social justice issue that we invite continued debate between disciplines and an effort to find common ground to address the societal and structural inequalities that impact people with large bodies.

5. Conclusion

Although each of the different perspectives taken among weight bias researchers has unique approaches to understanding and examining weight bias; each perspective recognizes weight bias as an important social issue surrounding a discourse of weight as being within individual control. Each perspective has also identified specific social and individual consequences of weight bias, as well as the ways in which weight bias is related to social inequities. Our review of the common perspectives taken in weight bias research revealed differences in how weight bias is termed, conceptualized, and understood. However, it also revealed areas of convergence. Most notably, there is consensus among each perspective that weight bias is influenced by the pervasive belief that weight is within individual control. There is also consensus that weight bias has negative consequences ranging from individual health consequences to social oppression and that these consequences influence social inequity when intersected with gender, race, SES, and sexual orientation. Perhaps the consideration of such similarities, increased attention to social and structural inequalities, and openness to differing perspectives on language, including the use of both person-first and identity-first language, can fuel the future of research in weight bias to occur in a space where divergent views are respected in the name of social justice.

Although limited, previous researchers have also called for increased interdisciplinarity with regard to weight bias research and activism [69, 79]. Mansfield and Rich [79] stated that obesity discourse can be critically examined from multiple perspectives, but that those who critique discourse "are united by a common commitment and desire towards challenging dominant approaches to health which are solely weight-centric" (p. 359-360). They propose that researchers, practitioners, and policy makers who critique obesity discourse need to work across artificial barriers. They argue that increased involvement with the knowledge and perspectives of diverse fields may benefit weight bias activism [79]. Clare and colleagues [69] proposed that such integration may be fostered through applied interdisciplinarity, which focuses on strategically utilizing the knowledge and skills of various areas regarded as stakeholders of a specific issue.

In this discussion, we have invited researchers to recognize weight bias as an important social justice issue and to consider ways that our unique and combined efforts might address the aversive conditions under which body size is demarcated in our society as a space for the maltreatment and oppression of people. In addition, we called for researchers from various areas to work across professional boundaries in a joined effort for social change. Working towards increased interdisciplinarity between the various research areas and increased recognition of weight bias as an important social justice issue will serve people of every size.

Competing Interests

The authors declare that they have no competing interests.

Acknowledgments

This work was supported by two grants through the Werklund School of Education Office of Research: A Powerful New Ideas in Education grant and a Team Collaboration grant. Dr. Alberga was previously supported by Eyes High Postdoctoral Fellowship from the University of Calgary and is currently supported by a Banting CIHR Postdoctoral Fellowship.

References

[1] C. S. Crandall, "Prejudice against fat people: ideology and self-interest," *Journal of Personality and Social Psychology*, vol. 66, no. 5, pp. 882–894, 1994.

[2] T. Andreyeva, R. M. Puhl, and K. D. Brownell, "Changes in perceived weight discrimination among Americans, 1995-1996 through 2004–2006," *Obesity*, vol. 16, no. 5, pp. 1129–1134, 2008.

[3] R. M. Puhl and C. A. Heuer, "The stigma of obesity: a review and update," *Obesity*, vol. 17, no. 5, pp. 941–964, 2009.

[4] J. A. Swift, S. Hanlon, L. El-Redy, R. M. Puhl, and C. Glazebrook, "Weight bias among UK trainee dietitians, doctors, nurses and

nutritionists," *Journal of Human Nutrition and Dietetics*, vol. 26, no. 4, pp. 395–402, 2013.

[5] E. L. Kenney, S. L. Gortmaker, K. K. Davison, and S. B. Austin, "The academic penalty for gaining weight: a longitudinal, change-in-change analysis of BMI and perceived academic ability in middle school students," *International Journal of Obesity*, vol. 39, no. 9, pp. 1408–1413, 2015.

[6] R. A. Carels, J. Rossi, J. Borushok et al., "Changes in weight bias and perceived employability following weight loss and gain," *Obesity Surgery*, vol. 25, no. 3, pp. 568–570, 2015.

[7] A. A. Brewis, D. J. Hruschka, and A. Wutich, "Vulnerability to fat-stigma in women's everyday relationships," *Social Science & Medicine*, vol. 73, no. 4, pp. 491–497, 2011.

[8] J. H. Yoo, "No Clear winner: effects of *The Biggest Loser* on the stigmatization of obese persons," *Health Communication*, vol. 28, no. 3, pp. 294–303, 2013.

[9] A. Janet Tomiyama, E. S. Epel, T. M. McClatchey et al., "Associations of weight stigma with cortisol and oxidative stress independent of adiposity," *Health Psychology*, vol. 33, no. 8, pp. 862–867, 2014.

[10] L. R. Vartanian and S. A. Novak, "Internalized societal attitudes moderate the impact of weight stigma on avoidance of exercise," *Obesity*, vol. 19, no. 4, pp. 757–762, 2011.

[11] L. E. Durso, J. D. Latner, M. A. White et al., "Internalized weight bias in obese patients with Binge Eating Disorder: associations with eating disturbances and psychological functioning," *International Journal of Eating Disorders*, vol. 45, no. 3, pp. 423–427, 2012.

[12] K. C. Fettich and E. Y. Chen, "Coping with obesity stigma affects depressed mood in African-American and white candidates for bariatric surgery," *Obesity*, vol. 20, no. 5, pp. 1118–1121, 2012.

[13] R. M. Puhl and C. A. Heuer, "Obesity stigma: important considerations for public health," *American Journal of Public Health*, vol. 100, no. 6, pp. 1019–1028, 2010.

[14] A. C. Saguy and K. W. Riley, "Weighing both sides: morality, mortality, and framing contests over obesity," *Journal of Health Politics, Policy and Law*, vol. 30, no. 5, pp. 869–921, 2005.

[15] R. Colls and B. Evans, "Challenging assumptions: re-thinking 'the obesity problem'," *Geography*, vol. 95, no. 2, pp. 99–105, 2010.

[16] American Psychological Association, *Publication Manual of the American Psychological Association*, American Psychological Association, Washington, DC, USA, 6th edition, 2010.

[17] D. S. Dunn and E. E. Andrews, "Person-first and identity-first language: developing psychologists' cultural competence using disability language," *American Psychologist*, vol. 70, no. 3, pp. 255–264, 2015.

[18] L. Bacon and L. Aphramor, "Weight science: evaluating the evidence for a paradigm shift," *Nutrition Journal*, vol. 10, article 9, 2011.

[19] A. Bombak, "Obesity, health at every size, and public health policy," *American Journal of Public Health*, vol. 104, no. 2, pp. e60–e67, 2014.

[20] L. O'Hara and J. Gregg, "Don't diet: adverse effects of the weight-centered health paradigm," in *Modern Dietary Fat Intakes in Disease Promotion*, F. De Meester, S. Zibadi, and R. R. Watson, Eds., pp. 431–441, Springer, New York, NY, USA, 2010.

[21] T. L. Tylka, R. A. Annunziato, D. Burgard et al., "The weight-inclusive versus weight-normative approach to health: evaluating the evidence for prioritizing well-being over weight loss," *Journal of Obesity*, vol. 2014, Article ID 983495, 18 pages, 2014.

[22] R. M. Puhl and K. D. Brownell, "Psychosocial origins of obesity stigma: toward changing a powerful and pervasive bias," *Obesity Reviews*, vol. 4, no. 4, pp. 213–227, 2003.

[23] R. M. Puhl, J. D. Latner, K. M. King, and J. Luedicke, "Weight bias among professionals treating eating disorders: attitudes about treatment and perceived patient outcomes," *International Journal of Eating Disorders*, vol. 47, no. 1, pp. 65–75, 2014.

[24] D. P. Miller, J. G. Spangler, M. Z. Vitolins et al., "Are medical students aware of their anti-obesity bias?" *Academic Medicine*, vol. 88, no. 7, pp. 978–982, 2013.

[25] K. S. O'Brien, J. D. Latner, D. Ebneter, and J. A. Hunter, "Obesity discrimination: the role of physical appearance, personal ideology, and anti-fat prejudice," *International Journal of Obesity*, vol. 37, no. 3, pp. 455–460, 2013.

[26] J. M. Burmeister, A. E. Kiefner, R. A. Carels, and D. R. Musher-Eizenman, "Weight bias in graduate school admissions," *Obesity*, vol. 21, no. 5, pp. 918–920, 2013.

[27] M. Forhan and X. Ramos Salas, "Inequities in healthcare: a review of bias and discrimination in obesity treatment," *Canadian Journal of Diabetes*, vol. 37, no. 3, pp. 205–209, 2013.

[28] S. M. Phelan, J. F. Dovidio, R. M. Puhl et al., "Implicit and explicit weight bias in a national sample of 4,732 medical students: the medical student CHANGES study," *Obesity*, vol. 22, no. 4, pp. 1201–1208, 2014.

[29] M. E. Jensen, E. A. Pease, K. Lambert et al., "Championing person-first language: a call to psychiatric mental health nurses," *Journal of the American Psychiatric Nurses Association*, vol. 19, no. 3, pp. 146–151, 2013.

[30] C. Rice, "Becoming 'the fat girl': acquisition of an unfit identity," *Women's Studies International Forum*, vol. 30, no. 2, pp. 158–174, 2007.

[31] N. van Amsterdam, "Big fat inequalities, thin privilege: an intersectional perspective on 'body size'," *European Journal of Women's Studies*, vol. 20, no. 2, pp. 155–169, 2013.

[32] B. Weiner, R. P. Perry, and J. Magnusson, "An attributional analysis of reactions to stigmas," *Journal of Personality and Social Psychology*, vol. 55, no. 5, pp. 738–748, 1988.

[33] L. R. Vartanian, T. Trewartha, and E. J. Vanman, "Disgust predicts prejudice and discrimination toward individuals with obesity," *Journal of Applied Social Psychology*, vol. 46, pp. 369–375, 2015.

[34] J.-P. Chaput, Z. M. Ferraro, D. Prud'Homme, and A. M. Sharma, "Widespread misconceptions about obesity," *Canadian Family Physician*, vol. 60, no. 11, pp. 973–975, 2014.

[35] J. Falbe, A. A. Cadiz, N. K. Tantoco, H. R. Thompson, and K. A. Madsen, "Active and healthy families: a randomized controlled trial of a culturally tailored obesity intervention for latino children," *Academic Pediatrics*, vol. 15, no. 4, pp. 386–395, 2015.

[36] R. M. Puhl, M. B. Schwartz, and K. D. Brownell, "Impact of perceived consensus on stereotypes about obese people: a new approach for reducing bias," *Health Psychology*, vol. 24, no. 5, pp. 517–525, 2005.

[37] N. Donaghue and A. Clemitshaw, "I'm totally smart and a feminist... and yet I want to be waif': exploring ambivalence towards the thin ideal within the fat acceptance movement," *Women's Studies International Forum*, vol. 35, pp. 415–425, 2012.

[38] R. A. Leit, H. G. Pope, and J. J. Gray, "Cultural expectations of muscularity in men: the evolution of Playgirl centerfolds," *International Journal of Eating Disorders*, vol. 29, no. 1, pp. 90–93, 2001.

[39] C. V. Wiseman, J. J. Gray, J. E. Mosimann, and A. H. Ahrens, "Cultural expectations of thinness in women: an update," *International Journal of Eating Disorders*, vol. 11, no. 1, pp. 85–89, 1992.

[40] P. Klaczynski, D. B. Daniel, and P. S. Keller, "Appearance idealization, body esteem, causal attributions, and ethnic variations in the development of obesity stereotypes," *Journal of Applied Developmental Psychology*, vol. 30, no. 4, pp. 537–551, 2009.

[41] K. S. O'Brien, S. Daníelsdóttir, R. P. Ólafsson, I. Hansdóttir, T. G. Fridjónsdóttir, and H. Jónsdóttir, "The relationship between physical appearance concerns, disgust, and anti-fat prejudice," *Body Image*, vol. 10, no. 4, pp. 619–623, 2013.

[42] K. S. O'Brien, J. A. Hunter, J. Halberstadt, and J. Anderson, "Body image and explicit and implicit anti-fat attitudes: the mediating role of physical appearance comparisons," *Body Image*, vol. 4, no. 3, pp. 249–256, 2007.

[43] L. Festinger, "A theory of social comparison processes," *Human Relations*, vol. 7, no. 2, pp. 117–140, 1954.

[44] B. R. Levy and C. E. Pilver, "Residual stigma: psychological distress among the formerly overweight," *Social Science & Medicine*, vol. 75, no. 2, pp. 297–299, 2012.

[45] P. M. Brochu and M. A. Morrison, "Implicit and explicit prejudice toward overweight and average-weight men and women: testing their correspondence and relation to behavioral intentions," *Journal of Social Psychology*, vol. 147, no. 6, pp. 681–706, 2007.

[46] S. Palmer and A. Rutland, "Do children want skinny friends? The role of 'weight' in children's friendship preferences and inter-group attitudes," *Anales de Psicologia*, vol. 27, no. 3, pp. 698–707, 2011.

[47] F. Mold and A. Forbes, "Patients' and professionals' experiences and perspectives of obesity in health-care settings: a synthesis of current research," *Health Expectations*, vol. 16, no. 2, pp. 119–142, 2013.

[48] A. R. Sutin, Y. Stephan, and A. Terracciano, "Weight discrimination and risk of mortality," *Psychological Science*, vol. 26, no. 11, pp. 1803–1811, 2015.

[49] C. Cooper, "Fat studies: mapping the field," *Sociology Compass*, vol. 4, no. 12, pp. 1020–1034, 2010.

[50] G. M. Eller, "On fat oppression," *Kennedy Institute of Ethics Journal*, vol. 24, no. 3, pp. 219–245, 2014.

[51] J. A. Gailey, "Fat shame to fat pride: fat women's sexual and dating experiences," *Fat Studies*, vol. 1, no. 1, pp. 114–127, 2012.

[52] S. Satinsky, B. Dennis, M. Reece, S. Sanders, and S. Bardzell, "My 'fat girl complex': a preliminary investigation of sexual health and body image in women of size," *Culture, Health and Sexuality*, vol. 15, no. 6, pp. 710–725, 2013.

[53] J. L. Graves and S. Kwan, "Is there really 'more to love'? Gender, body, and relationship scripts in romance-based reality television," *Fat Studies*, vol. 1, no. 1, pp. 47–60, 2012.

[54] M. Kargbo, "Toward a new relationality: digital photography, shame, and the fat subject," *Fat Studies*, vol. 2, no. 2, pp. 160–172, 2013.

[55] C. Nurka, "Moderation, reward, entitlement: the 'obesity epidemic' and the gendered body," *Fat Studies*, vol. 3, no. 2, pp. 166–178, 2014.

[56] L. Downing Peters, "You are what you wear: how plus-size fashion figures in fat identity formation," *Fashion Theory*, vol. 18, no. 1, pp. 45–71, 2014.

[57] E. Cameron, "Toward a fat pedagogy: a study of pedagogical approaches aimed at challenging obesity discourse in post-secondary education," *Fat Studies*, vol. 4, no. 1, pp. 28–45, 2014.

[58] M. C. McHugh and A. E. Kasardo, "Anti-fat prejudice: the role of psychology in explication, education and eradication," *Sex Roles*, vol. 66, no. 9-10, pp. 617–627, 2012.

[59] P. Watkins and A. Doyle Hugmeyer, "Teaching about eating disorders from a fat studies perspective," *Transformations: The Journal of Inclusive Scholarship and Pedagogy*, vol. 23, no. 2, pp. 171–182, 2012.

[60] H. Keane, "Feminism and the complexities of gender and health," *Australian Feminist Studies*, vol. 29, no. 80, pp. 180–188, 2014.

[61] A. K. Yancey, J. Leslie, and E. K. Abel, "Obesity at the crossroads: feminist and public health perspectives," *Signs*, vol. 31, no. 2, pp. 425–443, 2006.

[62] M. Aston, S. Price, S. F. L. Kirk, and T. Penney, "More than meets the eye. Feminist poststructuralism as a lens towards understanding obesity," *Journal of Advanced Nursing*, vol. 68, no. 5, pp. 1187–1194, 2012.

[63] J. L. Fikkan and E. D. Rothblum, "Is fat a feminist issue? exploring the gendered nature of weight bias," *Sex Roles*, vol. 66, no. 9-10, pp. 575–592, 2012.

[64] P. Vincent Roehling, "Fat is a feminist issue, but it is complicated: commentary on fikkan and rothblum," *Sex Roles*, vol. 66, no. 9-10, pp. 593–599, 2012.

[65] S. Shaw and J. Lee, "Women's studies: perspectives and practices," in *Women's Voices, Feminist Visions: Classic and Contemporary Readings*, S. Shaw and J. Lee, Eds., pp. 1–14, McGraw Hill, Boston, Mass, USA, 4th edition, 2009.

[66] N. Donaghue, "The moderating effects of socioeconomic status on relationships between obesity framing and stigmatization of fat people," *Fat Studies*, vol. 3, no. 1, pp. 6–16, 2014.

[67] C. Pausé, "X-static process: intersectionality within the field of fat studies," *Fat Studies*, vol. 3, no. 2, pp. 80–85, 2014.

[68] K. Davis, "Intersectionality as buzzword: a sociology of science perspective on what makes a feminist theory successful," *Feminist Theory*, vol. 9, no. 1, pp. 67–85, 2008.

[69] M. M. Clare, E. A. Ardron-Hudson, and J. Grindell, "Fat in school: applied interdisciplinarity as a basis for consultation in oppressive social context," *Journal of Educational and Psychological Consultation*, vol. 25, no. 1, pp. 45–65, 2015.

[70] M. Young, "One size fits all: disrupting the comsumerized, pathologized, fat female form," *Feminist Media Studies*, vol. 5, no. 2, pp. 249–252, 2005.

[71] J. C. Chrisler, "'Why can't you control yourself?' Fat should be a feminist issue," *Sex Roles*, vol. 66, no. 9-10, pp. 608–616, 2012.

[72] W. C. Miller, "The weight-loss-at-any-cost environment: how to thrive with a health-centered focus," *Journal of Nutrition Education and Behavior*, vol. 37, supplement 2, pp. S89–S93, 2005.

[73] L. B. Brown, "Teaching the 'health at every size' paradigm benefits future fitness and health professionals," *Journal of Nutrition Education and Behavior*, vol. 41, no. 2, pp. 144–145, 2009.

[74] E. Borkoles, S. Carroll, P. Clough, and R. C. J. Polman, "Effect of a non-dieting lifestyle randomised control trial on psychological well-being and weight management in morbidly obese pre-menopausal women," *Maturitas*, vol. 83, pp. 51–58, 2016.

[75] L. Humphrey, D. Clifford, and M. N. Morris, "Health at every size college course reduces dieting behaviors and improves intuitive eating, body esteem, and anti-fat attitudes," *Journal of Nutrition Education and Behavior*, vol. 47, no. 4, pp. 354–360.e1, 2015.

[76] T. L. Penney and S. F. L. Kirk, "The health at every size paradigm and obesity: missing empirical evidence may help push the reframing obesity debate forward," *American Journal of Public Health*, vol. 105, no. 5, pp. e38–e42, 2015.

[77] J. Brady, J. Gingras, and L. Aphramor, "Theorizing health at every size as a relational–cultural endeavour," *Critical Public Health*, vol. 23, no. 3, pp. 345–355, 2013.

[78] V. Provencher, C. Bégin, A. Tremblay et al., "Health-at-every-size and eating behaviors: 1-year follow-up results of a size acceptance intervention," *Journal of the American Dietetic Association*, vol. 109, no. 11, pp. 1854–1861, 2009.

[79] L. Mansfield and E. Rich, "Public health pedagogy, border crossings and physical activity at every size," *Critical Public Health*, vol. 23, no. 3, pp. 356–370, 2013.

[80] D. Burgard, "What is 'health at every size'?" in *The Fat Studies Reader*, E. D. Rothblum and S. Solovay, Eds., pp. 42–53, New York University Press, New York, NY, USA, 2009.

[81] M. Featherstone, "The body in consumer culture," in *The Body: Social Process and Cultural Theory*, M. Featherstone, M. Hepworth, and B. Turner, Eds., pp. 170–197, Sage, London, UK, 1991.

[82] L. O'Hara and J. Gregg, "The war on obesity: a social determinant of health," *Health Promotion Journal of Australia*, vol. 17, no. 3, pp. 260–263, 2006.

[83] N. K. Amy, A. Aalborg, P. Lyons, and L. Keranen, "Barriers to routine gynecological cancer screening for White and African-American obese women," *International Journal of Obesity*, vol. 30, no. 1, pp. 147–155, 2006.

[84] J. L. Black and J. Macinko, "Neighborhoods and obesity," *Nutrition Reviews*, vol. 66, no. 1, pp. 2–20, 2008.

[85] A. V. Diez Roux and C. Mair, "Neighborhoods and health," *Annals of the New York Academy of Sciences*, vol. 1186, pp. 125–145, 2010.

[86] G. Abbott, K. Backholer, A. Peeters, L. Thornton, D. Crawford, and K. Ball, "Explaining educational disparities in adiposity: the role of neighborhood environments," *Obesity*, vol. 22, no. 11, pp. 2413–2419, 2014.

[87] N. Krieger, A. Kosheleva, P. D. Waterman, J. T. Chen, J. Beckfield, and M. V. Kiang, "50-year trends in US socioeconomic inequalities in health: US-born Black and White Americans, 1959–2008," *International Journal of Epidemiology*, vol. 43, no. 4, pp. 1294–1313, 2014.

[88] A. Drewnowski, "Obesity, diets, and social inequalities," *Nutrition Reviews*, vol. 67, supplement 1, pp. S36–S39, 2009.

[89] F. Garawi, K. Devries, N. Thorogood, and R. Uauy, "Global differences between women and men in the prevalence of obesity: is there an association with gender inequality?" *European Journal of Clinical Nutrition*, vol. 68, no. 10, pp. 1101–1106, 2014.

[90] D. Howel, E. Stamp, T. J. Chadwick, A. J. Adamson, and M. White, "Are social inequalities widening in generalised and abdominal obesity and overweight among English adults?" *PLoS ONE*, vol. 8, no. 11, Article ID e79027, 2013.

[91] J. A. Ailshire and J. S. House, "The unequal burden of weight gain: An intersectional approach to understanding social disparities in BMI trajectories from 1986 to 2001/2002," *Social Forces*, vol. 90, no. 2, Article ID sor001, pp. 397–423, 2011.

[92] D. H. Broom and M. Warin, "Gendered and class relations of obesity: confusing findings, deficient explanations," *Australian Feminist Studies*, vol. 26, no. 70, pp. 453–467, 2011.

[93] D. Faeh, J. Braun, and M. Bopp, "Prevalence of obesity in Switzerland 1992–2007: the impact of education, income and occupational class," *Obesity Reviews*, vol. 12, no. 3, pp. 151–166, 2011.

[94] A. Zajacova and S. A. Burgard, "Body-weight and health from early to mid-adulthood: a longitudinal analysis," *Journal of Health and Social Behavior*, vol. 51, no. 1, pp. 92–107, 2010.

[95] N. Arthur and S. Collins, "Social justice and culture infused counselling," in *Culture Infused Counselling*, N. Arthur and S. Collins, Eds., pp. 139–164, Counselling Concepts, Calgary, Canada, 2010.

[96] E. M. Vera and S. L. Speight, "Multicultural competence, social justice, and counseling psychology: expanding our roles," *Counseling Psychologist*, vol. 31, no. 3, pp. 253–272, 2003.

[97] B. J. Cardinal, A. R. Whitney, M. Narimatsi, N. Hubert, and B. J. Souza, "Obesity bias in the gym: an under-recognized social justice, diversity, and inclusivity issue," *Journal of Physical Education, Recreation & Dance*, vol. 85, no. 6, pp. 3–6, 2014.

10

Body Size Misperception and Overweight or Obesity among Saudi College-Aged Females

Jumanah Albeeybe,[1] Abdulaziz Alomer,[2] Tasneem Alahmari,[1] Nawal Asiri,[1] Reema Alajaji,[1] Reem Almassoud,[1] and Hazzaa M. Al-Hazzaa[3]

[1]*College of Medicine, King Saud University, P.O. Box 7805, Riyadh 11472, Saudi Arabia*
[2]*Department of Orthopedics, King Saud University Medical City, King Saud University, P.O. Box 7805, Riyadh 11472, Saudi Arabia*
[3]*Lifestyle and Health Research, Health Science Research Center, Princess Nourah Bint Abdulrahman University, P.O. Box 93216, Riyadh 11673, Saudi Arabia*

Correspondence should be addressed to Hazzaa M. Al-Hazzaa; halhazzaa@hotmail.com

Academic Editor: David H. St-Pierre

The aim of the study was to investigate the associations between perceived and desired body size and overweight and obesity among college-aged females. A multistage stratified cluster random sample was used to select 907 healthy females from a major Saudi public university. The Stunkard Figure Rating Scale (FRS) was used for body size assessment. Overweight/obesity classification was based on BMI less than or equal to/greater than 25 kg/m^2. Overweight plus obesity prevalence was 28.1%. There were significant differences between females with overweight/obesity and those without overweight/obesity in both perceived and desired body size scores. Compared with only 4% of females without overweight/obesity, 37% of the participants with overweight/obesity scored higher than five (median) in the FRS. The perceived body size correlated more strongly with many of the selected variables than did the desired body size, especially with BMI ($r = 0.679$; $p < 0.001$), body weight ($r = 0.652$; $p < 0.001$), and weight loss attempts ($r = 0.466$; $p < 0.001$). Also, there was a significant relationship between BMI and weight loss attempts ($r = 0.370$; $p < 0.001$). BMI and weight loss attempts appear to predict the perceived body size and the discrepancy between perceived and desired body size scores. Psychosocial and lifestyle factors that might influence female's body misperception need to be addressed in future studies.

1. Introduction

The prevalence of obesity is increasing worldwide [1]. Such an increase in the prevalence of obesity represents a major public health challenge [1, 2]. Obesity is well recognized to associate with variety of chronic diseases [3]. Women's obesity in Saudi Arabia is considered among the highest in the world [4]. Efforts to combat this problem need to consider all behavioral aspects that are associated with overweight and obesity. One important component of behavioral change is the recognition of excess body weight and its related health risks. Perceiving their own body size correctly is considered an important motivation for taking action and engaging in healthy lifestyle behaviors [5]. Body size perception refers to the image that people form of their physical appearance in their mind and represents the degree to which individuals are satisfied with their body weight and shape. It is a multidimensional concept involving and influenced by biological, psychological, social, and cultural determinants [6].

Body dissatisfactions are common among college-aged women, as many female students tend to perceive their bodies to be considerably heavier than their actual body weight status [7, 8]. In a large sample of participating American females between 11 and 21 years, it was found that 25.1% of normal-weight females perceived themselves as overweight [9]. In addition, a 13-year cohort follow-up study revealed that women with obesity who perceived themselves as normal weight gained a considerable amount of weight, while those who correctly perceived themselves as obese had lost a significant weight from their excess body weight [10]. On the contrary, overweight perception was found to associate with higher risk of future weight gain among adults from the United States and UK [11], while body size satisfaction appears to provide some protection against excessive weight gain and binge eating [12].

Variation in body dissatisfaction related to weight status by ethnic groups has also been recognized, as African American with overweight/obesity [13] and Arab [14] adolescents who perceived themselves as underweight were more likely to gain body weight. The high occurrence of negative BI among young females represents a real concern and can influence weight status and development of body shape dissatisfaction. BI dissatisfaction has been shown to associate with a number of unhealthy behaviors such as unsafe dieting, lower self-esteem, eating disorders, and depressive symptoms [15–17].

Cultural and social influences appear to impact body image perception, weight norms, obesity, and body shape dissatisfaction and may consequently increase susceptibility to eating disorders [18–20]. Traditional cultures are thought to have protective effects against the development of eating disorders, whereas exposure to western culture may increase such risks through exposure to values communicated by media and peer contacts [21, 22]. Indeed, culture-specific influences such as faith was recently shown to have a protective effect against body dissatisfaction and excessive dieting in Bulgarian women [23]. Further, sub-Saharan African women tend to accept their body size more than white females [22]. In some African countries, like Ghana, although overweight was considered undesirable by most adult women, some weight gain was admired, considered beautiful by women and was perceived as a sign of financial prosperity by their family and friends [24]. Among a nationally representative US sample, it was shown that body weight perception did vary by sex and race/ethnicity, and that American White girls were more likely to perceive objectively lower weights as "about the right weight" compared to young African Americans, Asian American, or Native Americans girls [25]. This may explain why normal-weight young white females in the USA, who were more likely to engage in dieting, use diet products and exercise to lose weight than normal-weight African American or Hispanic females [26].

There is amble evidence accumulated within the last decade indicating that body weight concerns, dissatisfaction, and/or eating disturbances are fairly widespread among young Arab women [27–29]. A recently published research involving a large sample of Arab females attending university in five Arab countries including Bahrain, Egypt, Jordan, Oman, and Syria revealed that one-third of the females were dissatisfied with their body weight status [30]. In addition, earlier reports on body size perceptions among young women from an urban health center in eastern Saudi Arabia showed that a substantial proportion of them either overestimated (28.6%) or underestimated (28.9%) their actual body weight [31]. However, due to recent globalization and adoption of western lifestyle and eating behaviors by many developing countries including Saudi Arabia and neighboring Gulf States, the attitudes towards body weight and weight perception may have changed, shifting to a preference for thin body size [14, 32, 33]. Understanding different factors that promote body satisfaction across racial and ethnic groups is an important tool that may facilitate adopting healthy lifestyle behaviors, improve effective obesity prevention interventions, and prevent body weight dissatisfaction and eating disorders. With this background, the aim of the present study was to investigate the associations between self-perceived and desired body size and levels of overweight or obesity among a representative sample of Saudi college-aged females. Information on body size perception in relation to overweight and obesity among young Saudi females has been fairly limited.

2. Methods

2.1. Participants and Study Design. Saudi college-aged females who were attending King Saud University (KSU) during the academic year 2015/2016 comprised the study population. KSU is a major comprehensive public university located in the city of Riyadh, the capital of the country. Students attending King Saud University come from all regions of the country. A multistage stratified cluster random sampling technique was used to select the desired sample. In the first stage, a systematic random sampling procedure was used to select three colleges from within three major types of colleges within the university; humanity, health sciences, and science and computer science colleges. Then, female students within each selected college were chosen randomly through cluster sampling as the class or course group represented the cluster. The selection process made certain to include classes from each of the 4 or 5 years of study in each college.

Assuming an obesity prevalence of 20% among college students, with a confidence level of 95% and an amount of error of 2.5%, the sample size was determined as 783 students. Adding to that 15% for clustered design effect and missing data, the target sample size was calculated as 901 participating females. The ethical committee in the College of Medicine at King Saud University approved the study protocol and procedures. Written consent forms were also obtained from all the participating females.

Body weight was measured to the nearest 100 g, with minimal clothing and without shoes, using a calibrated portable medical scale (Seca Scale Model 770, Seca, Hamburg, Germany). Height was measured to the nearest cm with the subject in the full standing position without shoes using a calibrated portable measuring rod. The body mass index (BMI) was calculated as body weight in kilograms divided by squared height in meters. Participants were classified as overweight/obese ($BMI \geq 25\,kg/m^2$) or nonoverweight/nono bese ($BMI < 25\,kg/m^2$).

2.2. Body Size Assessment. For the body size assessment, we used the Stunkard Figure Rating Scale (FRS) images [34].

The body image scores were calculated in two ways: first, the student's perception of her actual body size based on the 9 silhouettes figures (called perceived body size), and second, the image that the student desires to look like from the same 9 figure images (called desired body size). Then, each figure was given a corresponding BMI score according to a previous study that has linked the actual BMI values to the FRS BI scores using a large sample size of adult females [35]. Finally, three main discrepancy (difference) scores were calculated: first, the discrepancy between perceived and desired body size scores, which represented body dissatisfaction; second, the discrepancy between the actual BMI and the BMI value corresponding to the perceived body size score, which represented body size misperception; and third, the discrepancy between the actual BMI and the BMI value corresponding to the desired body size score.

2.3. Data and Statistical Analysis. The data entered into a coded SPSS data entry sheet were checked and analyzed by IBM SPSS software, version 22. Descriptive statistics (mean, SD, or frequency) were obtained for selected anthropometric and demographic variables. Females with overweight/obesity versus those without overweight/obesity were classified based on BMI values of less than or equal to/greater than 25 kg/m^2. In addition, cross tabulation with chi-square tests was used to calculate the proportions (percentage) of perceived and desired body size scores selected by Saudi females with or without overweight/obesity. The T-test with independent samples was used to test the differences between participants with overweight/obesity versus those without overweight/obesity in the following body size discrepancy scores: discrepancy between perceived and desired body size scores, discrepancy between BMI values corresponding to perceived and desired body size scores, discrepancy between actual BMI values and BMI corresponding to perceived body size scores, and discrepancy between actual BMI values and BMI corresponding to desired body size scores. The relationships between selected variables were also tested using Pearson's correlation coefficients. Finally, linear regression analysis with stepwise method was used to predict the perceived body size scores, desired body size scores, and the discrepancy between perceived and desired body size scores, as dependent variables with anthropometric and demographic variables as predictors. The following variables were entered in the regression analyses: age, weight, height, BMI, father education, mother education, family income, weight-loss attempt, number of obese kids in the family, and parents' obesity. In all of the tests performed, we used alpha level of <0.05 as the level of significance.

3. Results

The total number of the sample was 907 healthy females. The majority (59.6%) of the college-aged females are of normal weight; however, overweight (20.4%) plus obesity (7.7%) prevalence reached 28.1%, while the proportion of females with underweight was 12.3%. Table 1 presents the participants' characteristics as a whole and relative to overweight/obesity status. The females with overweight/obesity are slightly older than those without overweight/obesity. There were no significant differences between the two groups in body height, father education, mother education, or family income. However, females with overweight/obesity have significantly more obese siblings in the family and more parental obesity. There were significantly more attempts to lose weight by the Saudi females with overweight/obesity compared with those without overweight/obesity.

The proportions (%) of perceived and desired body size scores selected by the Saudi females with or without overweight/obesity relative to the 9 FRS scores as well as the corresponding normative and actual BMI values are presented in Table 2. There were significant differences between participants with overweight/obesity and those without overweight/obesity in both perceived and desired body size scores; however, the perceived body size scores are much more pronounced in the females with overweight/obesity compared to those without overweight/obesity. 37% of the girls with overweight/obesity as opposed to only 4% of those without overweight/obesity scored higher than a score of 5 (median score) on FRS. In addition, females with overweight or obesity who gave themselves a score of 5 or higher on the Stunkard Figure Rating Scale more closely resembled their actual BMI values than those who perceived themselves as having less than a score of 5. The overwhelming majority (>87%) of females (with and without overweight/obesity) desired a score of lower than 5, which corresponds to a BMI value less than 26.2 kg/m^2 [35]. In general, higher proportion of females with overweight/obesity underestimated their body size scores compared to those without overweight/obesity.

Table 3 shows perceived and desired body size scores, actual BMI, and some computed discrepancy scores among Saudi females with overweight/obesity and those without overweight/obesity. There are significant differences between the two groups in each of these measured and calculated variables. Of particular interest is the pronounced differences between the actual BMI and BMI value corresponding to the desired body size in the females with overweight/obesity (-8.5 ± 5.2 or -28.9%) compared to those without overweight/obesity (-0.30 ± 3.1 or -1.4%). When calculating the BMI values corresponding to perceived body size scores based on the normative BMI from a previous study [35], females with overweight/obesity underestimated their actual BMI by -2.5 ± 2.5 kg/m^2 (8.5%), while those participants without overweight/obesity slightly overestimated their BMI by $+0.40 \pm 2.5$ kg/m^2 (1.9%).

The correlation coefficient analyses of selected variables showed that perceived body size scores correlated significantly with the BMI ($r = 0.679$; $p < 0.001$), the BMI value corresponding to perceived body size ($r = 0.968$; $p < 0.001$), and the number of weight-loss attempts by the participating females ($r = 0.466$; $p < 0.001$), whereas desired body size scores revealed significant associations with BMI ($r = 0.089$; $p = 0.008$) and the BMI value corresponding to desired body size ($r = 0.951$; $p < 0.001$). In addition, there is a significant moderate relationship between the BMI and the number of

Table 1: Participants' characteristics according to overweight/obesity levels.

Variable	All (N = 905)	Overweight/obese (N = 254)	Nonoverweight/nonobese (N = 651)	p value*
Age (years)	20.9 ± 1.8	21.4 ± 1.3	20.8 ± 1.5	**<0.001**
Weight (kg)	58.8 ± 14.0	74.5 ± 15.1	52.7 ± 7.2	**<0.001**
Height (cm)	158.8 ± 5.7	159.0 ± 7.8	158.7 ± 5.6	0.462
Body mass index (kg/m^2)	23.3 ± 5.1	29.4 ± 5.1	20.9 ± 2.4	**<0.001**
Father's education (%)				
High school or less	—	44.9	41.5	
University degree	—	38.6	39.5	0.755
Postgraduate degree	—	16.5	19.0	
Mother's education (%)				
High school or less	—	48.1	53.6	
University degree	—	43.2	40.2	0.349
Postgraduate degree	—	8.7	6.2	
Family income (%)				
5000 SR or less	—	5.5	7.4	
5001–10,000 SR	—	15.4	10.1	
10,001–15,000 SR	—	13.8	16.7	
15,001–20,000 SR	—	16.1	17.5	0.260
20,001–25,000 SR	—	15.0	15.2	
25,001+ SR	—	34.3	33.0	
Obese kids in the family (%)				
None	—	29.8	55.6	
1-2	—	45.6	35.6	**<0.001**
3+	—	24.6	8.8	
Parent obesity (%)				
None obese	—	49.2	59.4	
Obese mother	—	22.4	21.0	
Obese father	—	12.6	11.5	**0.002**
Both are obese	—	15.7	8.0	
Weight-loss attempt (%)				
No attempt	—	16.5	52.4	
Tried but failed	—	13.8	5.7	**<0.001**
Tried and succeeded	—	69.7	41.9	

Data are given as mean ± standard deviation or percentage; *T-test for independent samples or chi-square tests for the proportion; SR = Saudi Riyal (1 U$ = 3.75 SR).

Table 2: The proportions (%) of perceived and desired body size scores selected by Saudi females with and without overweight/obesity relative to the 9 FRS scores and the normative corresponding and actual body mass index (BMI) values.

FRS	Normative corresponding BMI values*	Perceived body size score				Desired body size score			
		Overweight/ obese		Nonoverweight/ nonobese		Overweight/ obese		Nonoverweight/ nonobese	
		%	BMI	%	BMI	%	BMI	%	BMI
1	18.3	1.6	27.4	6.6	18.3	2.4	29.9	5.5	20.9
2	19.3	5.1	28.1	30.0	19.7	34.3	28.4	38.4	21.0
3	20.9	5.9	26.8	29.5	21.1	40.9	29.5	41.3	20.9
4	23.1	23.6	27.8	27.0	22.2	20.5	30.4	12.1	20.5
5	26.2	26.8	27.8	4.9	22.2	1.2	31.1	2.2	20.4
6	29.9	22.8	30.3	1.7	22.4	0.4	29.9	0.2	21.5
7	34.3	9.4	34.0	0.3	20.5	0.3	30.7	0.2	23.1
8	38.6	4.3	36.9	0.0	—	0.0	—	0.0	—
9	45.4	0.5	44.1	0.0	—	0.0	—	0.1	23.8
Total		100		100		100		100	
>5		37%		4%		0.7%		0.5%	
p value**			**<0.001**				**0.027**		

*Corresponding BMI values were from [35]; **chi-square tests for the differences in proportions between females with overweight/obesity and those without overweight/obesity; FRS = Stunkard Figure Rating Scale.

TABLE 3: Perceived and desired body size scores, actual BMI, and some selected computed discrepancy scores among Saudi females with and without overweight/obesity.

Variable	All	Overweight/ obese	Nonoverweight/ nonobese	p value*
Perceived body size score	3.6 ± 1.5	5.0 ± 1.5	3.0 ± 1.1	**<0.001**
Desired body size score	2.7 ± 0.89	2.9 ± 0.88	2.7 ± 0.90	**0.007**
Actual (measured) BMI	23.3 ± 5.1	29.4 ± 5.1	20.9 ± 2.4	**<0.001**
BMI corresponding to perceived body size score**	22.9 ± 1.5	26.9 ± 4.9	21.3 ± 2.4	**<0.001**
BMI corresponding to desired body size score**	20.7 ± 1.9	20.9 ± 1.8	20.6 ± 1.9	**0.033**
Difference between perceived and desired body size scores	−0.82 ± 1.5	−2.1 ± 1.4	−0.31 ± 1.3	**<0.01**
Percent difference (%)	−25.0	−42.0	−10.0	
Difference between BMI corresponding to perceived and desired body size scores	2.2 ± 4.1	−6.0 ± 4.6	−0.70 ± 2.8	**<0.01**
Percent difference (%)	−9.6	−22.3	−3.3	
Difference between actual BMI and BMI corresponding to perceived body size score	−0.40 ± 3.6	−2.5 ± 5.1	+0.40 ± 2.5	**<0.001**
Percent difference (%)	−1.7	−8.5	+1.9	
Difference between actual BMI and BMI corresponding to desired body size scores	−2.6 ± 5.3	−8.5 ± 5.2	−0.30 ± 3.1	**<0.001**
Percent difference (%)	−11.2	−28.9	−1.4	

*T-test for independent samples; **based on [35].

weight-loss attempts ($r = 0.370$; $p < 0.001$). Family income did not show any significant relationship with the perceived BMI ($r = 0.039$; $p = 238$) or with desired body size ($r = -0.051$; $p = 0.123$). In addition, perceived body size scores have low but significant correlation with parent obesity ($r = -0.107$; $p < 0.001$).

Finally, Table 4 presents the results of multiple linear regression analyses for the prediction of some selected dependent variables (perceived and desired body size scores and the discrepancy between perceived and desired body size scores). The BMI and the number of weight-loss attempts appear to predict the abovementioned dependent variables. Model 2 of these predictors shows that the common variances when predicting perceived body size and the discrepancy between perceived and desired body size scores, using BMI values and the number of weight loss attempts as predictors, amounted to 51% and nearly 47%, respectively.

4. Discussion

The present study reported perceived and desired body size findings relative to overweight and obesity among a large and representative sample of Saudi college females from a public multidisciplinary higher education institute in central Saudi Arabia, where students come from all over the country. The overweight plus obesity rate among the study's participants was 28.1%. Such an average value for our college female sample is much lower than the national prevalence of overweight plus obesity among Saudi adults, which was reported to be 61.5% [4]. However, our sample was much younger than that reported in the national prevalence. In addition, the findings of this study showed a certain extent of imprecise perception of body size in both groups of college females. A considerable proportion of the Saudi females with overweight/obesity underestimated their body size scores, while a smaller proportion of those without overweight/obesity underestimated their body size scores. Such observed findings seem consistent with many previous studies [14, 33, 36–39]. In addition, a study conducted on university students from 7 European countries showed that weight ideals were rather uniform across the European countries, with female students being more likely to perceive themselves as too fat at normal BMI values [40]. Interestingly, Korean women had lower discrepancies between their current and ideal (desired) body weight than US women had, leading to the conclusion that Korean women were more satisfied with their body weight [41].

Previous local studies about body image perception among young Saudi females had mixed results. A cross-sectional study involving 663 university female students from Southeastern Saudi Arabia showed a 23% agreement between the perceived and desired body image [33]. However, in our study of college females, the common variance between perceived and desired body size was only 8%. Another study in Eastern Saudi Arabia that used the Body Shape Questionnaire and included 368 female and male students from King Faisal University revealed that only 9.4% of females with overweight plus obesity were dissatisfied with their body shape. Interestingly, the study showed that more females in the normal weight were dissatisfied (22.7%) with their body shape [32]. Furthermore, the majority of the Saudi women attending gymnasium classes in the city of Hail in Northern Saudi Arabia identified their own body shape as being overweight, but they chose the "normal weight" figures as the image they wanted to look like [42]. In the neighboring state of Bahrain, a significant discrepancy between adolescents' perception of body weight and actual BMI was found. There was a propensity for Bahraini teenagers with overweight and obesity to underestimate their weight status, and more than half of the girls expressed dissatisfaction with their current body weight

Table 4: Results of multiple linear regression analyses for the prediction of selected dependent variables.

Dependent variable	Predictor variables*	Standardized coefficient (beta)	p value	R^2
Perceived body size scores				
Model 1	Body mass index	0.679	<0.001	0.461
Model 2	Body mass index	0.587	<0.001	0.514
	Weight-loss attempt	0.248	<0.001	
Discrepancy between perceived and desired body size scores				
Model 1	Body mass index	0.622	<0.001	0.387
Model 2	Body mass index	0.511	<0.001	0.465
	Weight-loss attempt	0.301	<0.001	
Desired body size scores				
Model 1	Body weight	0.104	0.002	0.011
Model 2	Body weight	0.136	<0.001	0.019
	Weight-loss attempt	−0.095	0.007	

*Variables entered into the prediction equation (step-wise method): age, weight, height, BMI, father education, mother education, family income, weight-loss attempt, number of obese kids in the family, and parents' obesity.

[14]. In a comparative study involving university students aged 17–32 years from five Arab countries (Bahrain, Egypt, Jordan, Oman, and Syria), it was found that 65–87% of Arab college females preferred a thinner body size or a figure rating of 1–3 in the FRS [29].

Results of the present study showed that there were significant differences between perceived and desired body size scores relative to female's overweight and obesity status. Of particular interest is the pronounced differences between the actual BMI and BMI value corresponding to desired body size among college females with overweight/obesity ($8.5 \pm 5.2\ kg/m^2$) versus those without overweight/obesity ($0.30 \pm 3.1\ kg/m^2$). Similar findings were reported for young females from diverse ethnicity in different countries around the world, showing significant differences between their actual and desired (ideal) body shape and resulting in a fairly high level of body size dissatisfaction [38, 39, 43–45]. Analysis of data from large national prospective cohort in the United States involving 16,882 participants aged 9–18-year-olds showed that girls above 50th BMI percentile reported greater dissatisfaction than girls below the 50th BMI percentile [37]. The study also found that younger youth with overweight and obesity were reporting the greatest body weight concern; however, among older females, healthy weight became increasingly associated with greater weight and body shape concern [37]. It is interesting that body size misperception may occasionally provide some protection against future weight gain, as overweight or obesity misperception among youth from the United States was found to predict lesser future weight gain [46]. In addition, young women with obesity who correctly perceived themselves as obese had lost significant weight from their excess body weight [10]. Moreover, overweight adolescent girls with body dissatisfaction gained more body weight five years later [47].

Having a positive body image is important for young females because it is believed to affect their self-esteem. Research has found a fairly strong relationship between low self-esteem and body-size dissatisfaction [48] Negative body image was also shown as a strong predictor of eating disorders [16]. Using the exercise and self-esteem model as a guiding framework, results support the notion that, to improve body image, perceived changes to the body size are more important than actual changes [49]. However, it has been argued that body weight perception is independent of the actual weight status, as the participants who have been given values of their body weight before rating their body shape still reported inaccurate perceptions of their body size [36]. Moreover, a qualitative study conducted on young women from two different weights revealed that women experience a significant emphasis on overweight issues with a trend towards appearance rather than health [50]. The young women showed strong views on the cultural definitions of normal body weight and described the conflict between cultural norms and their perceptions of body size and health as a likely factor negatively influencing well-being, weight-balance, and motivation to alter lifestyle [50]. Indeed, in the Internet era, females in particular are exposed to mixed messages about body image promotion. One message is coming from the global mass media and weight loss industries and another one from health awareness movements that is encouraging females to accept a healthy body image regardless of body shape [51]. In either direction, such a message may have a negative or positive influence on future control of body weight and obesity prevention among females.

The current findings revealed a positive relationship between the BMI values corresponding to perceived body size scores and the actual BMI values ($r = 0.697$; $p < 0.001$). Such normative values linking the actual BMI to the FRS body image scores have been previously established for adult females [35]. Our results also indicated a significant moderate association between perceived body size rating and the number of weight-loss attempts. This may reflect the notion that some females who were trying to lose weight appeared more realistic about perceiving their body size, and this may play a role in weight control behaviors. Parental obesity also had a low but significant correlation with the perception of body size, which may point out to the influence of home environment on the perception of body weight images. In addition, the present findings did not show any significant relationship between family income and perceived or desired body size. However, results from the first international body project survey about body weight ideals and body dissatisfaction in 10 major world regions revealed that body dissatisfaction and desire for thinness are commonplace in high socioeconomic status settings across the world [52]. In contrast, a research studying African American adolescents concluded that socioeconomic status is correlated neither with the BMI value nor with the self-perception of body weight [53]. Furthermore, in a comparative study between three countries, the perceived body image and weight control behavior differed among adolescents in Lithuania, Croatia, and the USA, and the correlation between body size and BMI was 0.85 [54]. Similar correlation ($r = 0.85$) was reported between body size, using Stunkard nine-level figures, and BMI in American young women between the ages of 18 and 44 years [55]. The discrepancy between ideal and actual body size was also found to be significant in Dutch young women with Morocco or Turkish ethnicity, and that the perceived body size was correlated with the BMI in these females, as Spearman's correlation coefficient was at 0.73 [39].

The results of multiple linear regression analyses indicated that the BMI and the number of weight-loss attempts, but not family income or parents' education levels, appear to strongly predict perceived body size scores as well as the discrepancy between perceived and desired body size scores. However, a local cross-sectional study involving university female students from Southeastern Saudi Arabia showed physical activity, family income, fathers' level of education, numbers of owned cars, and the kind of residence were positively associated with the desire to be thin, whereas the number of sisters and the number of household cars were correlated positively with the desire to be heavy [33]. Further, a study conducted on adult residents of Nairobi slums indicated that the major predictors of underestimation of body weight among overweight and obese respondents were age and sex, but marital status and education were not significantly associated with the likelihood of BMI underestimation [56]. Among female students attending Kuwait University, the perceived body image and a desire to be thinner were strongly related to body-image dissatisfaction, and the addition of age, marital status, physical activity, dieting behavior, parental education, and family size did not significantly alter the findings [57].

4.1. Strengths and Limitations of the Study. The present study has several strengths and limitations. The strengths of the current investigation include having a large and representative sample of Saudi college-aged females selected from a diversified and large public university and the use of well-validated and widely used instruments for the assessment of the body image (body size). A further strength of our study is that weight and height values were actually measured and not reported by the participants. On the other hand, the first limitation of the present study is the cross-sectional design, which cannot imply a casual relationship between body size rating and the BMI or which factor influenced the other first. Second, the selected body size measure in the present study is not a comprehensive one, and it provides a partial assessment of women's body size concerns. Third, our data were generated from a sample of college-aged females living in an urban area, and therefore the findings may not be generalized to other sittings or segments of the Saudi population, such as working women, less-educated females, different age groups, or those living in rural areas.

5. Conclusion

Our findings indicate that a considerable proportion of college females, especially those with overweight or obesity, have underestimated their perceived body size. This means that female college students with a BMI $\geq 25.0\,kg/m^2$ seem more likely to present with body size dissatisfaction than those peers without overweight/obesity. Such findings may point out to the sociocultural influences and media pressure that emphasized body thinness among young females. Body size misperception among Saudi females with obesity is concerning. Therefore, it is recommended that psychosocial and lifestyle factors that might influence body misperception among Saudi females to be addressed in future studies. In addition, efforts to prevent body size dissatisfaction needs to begin early before the college age as part of both obesity and eating disorder prevention programs. Finally, our study contributes to the small existing literature on body image perception in relation to obesity in Saudi young females.

Authors' Contributions

Hazzaa M. Al-Hazzaa, Abdulaziz Alomer, and Tasneem Alahmari were responsible for the study concept. Jumanah Albeeybe, Tasneem Alahmari, Nawal Asiri, Reema Alajaji, and Reem Almassoud collected the data. Statistical analyses were performed by Hazzaa M. Al-Hazzaa. Jumanah Albeeybe and Hazzaa M. Al-Hazzaa drafted the paper. All authors critically read and approved the final draft.

Acknowledgments

The authors thank the students who assisted them in the data collection. Appreciation is also extended to all of the females who took part in this study. This study was funded by Students' Research Funds provided by the Deanship for Scientific Research, King Saud University.

References

[1] M. Ng, T. Fleming, M. Robinson et al., "Global, regional, and national prevalence of overweight and obesity in children and adults during 1980-2013: a systematic analysis for the global

burden of disease study 2013," *The Lancet*, vol. 384, no. 9945, pp. 766–781, 2014.

[2] World Health Organization, *Global Recommendations on Physical Activity for Health*, WHO Press, Geneva, Switzerland, 2010.

[3] D. P. Guh, W. Zhang, N. Bansback, Z. Amarsi, C. L. Birmingham, and A. H. Anis, "The incidence of co-morbidities related to obesity and overweight: a systematic review and meta-analysis," *BMC Public Health*, vol. 9, p. 88, 2009.

[4] Z. A. Memish, C. E. Bcheraoui, M. Tuffaha et al., "Obesity and associated factors-Kingdom of Saudi Arabia, 2013," *Preventing Chronic Disease*, vol. 11, p. E174, 2014.

[5] T. Baranowski, K. W. Cullen, T. Nicklas, D. Thompson, and J. Baranowski, "Are current health behavioral change models helpful in guiding prevention of weight gain efforts?," *Obesity Research*, vol. 11, pp. 23S–43S, 2003.

[6] J. Geller, S. Srikameswaran, S. J. Cockell, and S. L. Zaitsoff, "Assessment of shape- and weight-based self-esteem in adolescents," *International Journal of Eating Disorders*, vol. 28, no. 3, pp. 339–345, 2000.

[7] J. Wardle, A. M. Haase, and A. Steptoe, "Body image and weight control in young adults: international comparisons in university students from 22 countries," *International Journal of Obesity*, vol. 30, no. 4, pp. 644–651, 2006.

[8] Z. Yager and J. A. O'Dea, "Prevention programs for body image and eating disorders on university campuses: a review of large, controlled interventions," *Health Promotion International*, vol. 23, no. 2, pp. 173–189, 2008.

[9] E. M. Perrin, J. Boone-Heinonen, A. E. Field, T. Coyne-Beasley, and P. Gordon-Larsen, "Perception of overweight and self-esteem during adolescence," *International Journal of Eating Disorders*, vol. 43, pp. 447–454, 2010.

[10] E. Lynch, K. Liu, G. S. Wei, B. Spring, C. Kiefe, and P. Greenland, "The relation between body size perception and change in body mass index over 13 years: the coronary artery risk development in young adults (CARDIA) study," *American Journal of Epidemiology*, vol. 169, no. 7, pp. 857–866, 2009.

[11] E. Robinson, J. M. Hunger, and M. Daly, "Perceived weight status and risk of weight gain across life in US and UK adults," *International Journal of Obesity*, vol. 39, no. 12, pp. 1721–1726, 2015.

[12] K. R. Sonneville, J. P. Calzo, N. J. Horton, J. Haines, S. B. Austin, and A. E. Field, "Body satisfaction, weight gain and binge eating among overweight adolescent girls," *International Journal of Obesity*, vol. 36, no. 7, pp. 944–949, 2012.

[13] Y. Wang, H. Liang, and X. Chen, "Measured body mass index, body weight perception, dissatisfaction and control practices in urban, low-income African American adolescents," *BMC Public Health*, vol. 9, p. 183, 2009.

[14] A. M. Al-Sendi, P. Shetty, and A. O. Musaiger, "Body weight perception among Bahraini adolescents," *Child: Care, Health and Development*, vol. 30, no. 4, pp. 369–376, 2004.

[15] R. Ohring, J. A. Graber, and J. Brooks-Gunn, "Girls' recurrent and concurrent body dissatisfaction: correlates and consequences over 8 years," *International Journal of Eating Disorders*, vol. 31, no. 4, pp. 404–415, 2002.

[16] A. R. Sepulveda, J. A. Carrobles, A. Gandarillas, J. Poveda, and V. Pastor, "Prevention program for disturbed eating and body dissatisfaction in a Spanish university population: a pilot study," *Body Image*, vol. 4, no. 3, pp. 317–328, 2007.

[17] E. Stice, "Risk and maintenance factors for eating pathology: a meta-analytic review," *Psychological Bulletin*, vol. 128, no. 5, pp. 825–848, 2002.

[18] P. C. Evans and A. R. McConnell, "Do racial minorities respond in the same way to mainstream beauty standards? Social comparison processes in Asian, Black, and White women," *Self and Identity*, vol. 2, no. 2, pp. 153–167, 2003.

[19] M. E. Gluck and A. Geliebter, "Racial/ethnic differences in body image and eating behaviors," *Eating Behaviors*, vol. 3, no. 2, pp. 143–151, 2002.

[20] P. K. Keel and K. L. Klump, "Are eating disorders culture bound syndromes? Implications for conceptualizing their etiology," *Psychological Bulletin*, vol. 129, no. 5, pp. 747–769, 2003.

[21] A. J. Pumariega, "Body dissatisfaction among Hispanic and Asian-American girls," *Journal of Adolescence Health*, vol. 21, no. 1, p. 1, 1997.

[22] Z. Mciza, J. H. Goedecke, N. P. Steyn et al., "Development and validation of instruments measuring body image and body weight dissatisfaction in South African mothers and their daughters," *Public Health Nutrition*, vol. 8, no. 5, pp. 509–519, 2005.

[23] R. A. Angelova and V. Utermohlen, "Culture-specific influences on body image and eating distress in a sample of urban Bulgarian women: the roles of faith and traditional fasting," *Eating Behaviors*, vol. 14, no. 3, pp. 386–389, 2013.

[24] R. N. O. Aryeetey, "Perceptions and experiences of overweight among women in the Ga East District, Ghana," *Frontiers in Nutrition*, vol. 3, p. 13, 2016.

[25] M. A. Martin, A. L. May, and M. L. Frisco, "Equal weights but different weight perceptions among U.S. adolescents," *Journal of Health Psychology*, vol. 15, no. 4, pp. 493–504, 2010.

[26] Y. M. Chao, E. M. Pisetsky, L. C. Dierker et al., "Ethnic differences in weight control practices among U.S. adolescents from 1995 to 2005," *International Journal of Eating Disorders*, vol. 41, no. 2, pp. 124–133, 2008.

[27] H. Al Sabbah, C. Vereecken, Z. Abdeen, E. Coats, and L. Maes, "Associations of overweight and of weight dissatisfaction among Palestinian adolescents: findings from the National Study of Palestinian schoolchildren (HBSC-WBG2004)," *Journal of Human Nutrition and Dietetics*, vol. 22, no. 1, pp. 40–49, 2009.

[28] T. Y. Mousa, H. A. Al-Domi, R. H. Mashal, and M. A. Jibri, "Eating disturbances among adolescent school girls in Jordan," *Appetite*, vol. 54, no. 1, pp. 196–201, 2010.

[29] A. O. Musaiger, "Body size preferences among young women in five Arab countries: a cross-cultural study," *International Journal of Adolescent Medicine and Health*, vol. 26, no. 3, pp. 417–421, 2014.

[30] A. O. Musaiger and M. Al-Mannai, "Role of obesity and media in body weight concern among female university students in Kuwait," *Eating Behaviors*, vol. 14, no. 2, pp. 229–232, 2013.

[31] P. Rasheed, "Perception of body weight and self-reported eating and exercise behavior among obese and non-obese women in Saudi Arabia," *Public Health*, vol. 112, no. 6, pp. 409–414, 1998.

[32] H. H. AL-Otaibi, S. L. Nassef, and T. A. Raouf, "Body shape dissatisfaction, weight status and physical activity among a sample university students in Saudi Arabia," *Food and Nutrition Sciences*, vol. 4, no. 6, pp. 616–625, 2013.

[33] A. Khalaf, A. Westergren, V. Berggren, Ö. Ekblom, and H. M. Al-Hazzaa, "Perceived and ideal body image in young women in south western Saudi Arabia," *Journal of Obesity*, vol. 2015, Article ID 697163, 7 pages, 2015.

[34] A. J. Stunkard, T. I. Sorenson, and F. Schulsinger, "Use of the Danish adoption register for the study of obesity and thinness," in *The Genetics of Neurological and Psychiatric Disorders*,

S. Kety, L. R. Rowland, R. L. Sidman, and S. W. Matthysse, Eds., pp. 115–120, Raven Press, New York, NY, USA, 1983.

[35] C. M. Bulik, T. D. Wade, A. C. Heath, N. G. Martin, A. J. Stunkard, and L. J. Eaves, "Relating body mass index to figural stimuli: population-based normative data for Caucasians," *International Journal of Obesity and Related Metabolic Disorders*, vol. 25, no. 10, pp. 1517–1524, 2001.

[36] H. Alwan, B. Viswanathan, F. Paccaud, and P. Bovet, "Is accurate perception of body image associated with appropriate weight-control behavior among adolescents of the Seychelles," *Journal of Obesity*, vol. 2011, Article ID 817242, 8 pages, 2011.

[37] J. P. Calzo, K. R. Sonneville, J. Haines, E. A. Blood, A. E. Field, and S. B. Austin, "The development of associations among body mass index, body dissatisfaction, and weight and shape concern in adolescent boys and girls," *Journal of Adolescent Health*, vol. 51, no. 5, pp. 517–523, 2012.

[38] K. Maximova, J. J. McGrath, T. Barnett, J. O'Loughlin, G. Paradis, and M. Lambert, "Do you see what I see? Weight status misperception and exposure to obesity among children and adolescents," *International Journal of Obesity*, vol. 32, no. 6, pp. 1008–1015, 2008.

[39] M. Nicolaou, C. Doak, R. Dam, K. Hosper, J. Seidell, and K. Stronks, "Body size preference and body weight perception among two migrant groups of non-Western origin," *Public Health Nutrition*, vol. 11, no. 12, pp. 1332–1341, 2008.

[40] R. T. Mikolajczyk, A. E. Maxwell, W. El Ansari, C. Stock, J. Petkeviciene, and F. Guillen-Grima, "Relationship between perceived body weight and body mass index based on self-reported height and weight among university students: a cross-sectional study in seven European countries," *BMC Public Health*, vol. 10, p. 40, 2010.

[41] J. Jung and S. Lee, "Cross-cultural comparisons of appearance self-schema, body image, self-esteem, and dieting behavior between Korean and U.S. women," *Family and Consumer Sciences Research Journal*, vol. 34, no. 4, pp. 350–365, 2006.

[42] A. A. Ben-Ammar and M. A. Al-Holy, "Body image and lifestyle attitudes of female gymnasium users in Saudi Arabia," *Nutrition and Food Science*, vol. 43, no. 4, pp. 365–373, 2013.

[43] S. Grogan, "Body image and health: contemporary perspectives," *Journal of Health Psychology*, vol. 11, no. 4, pp. 523–530, 2006.

[44] R. Kowner, "Japanese body image: structure and esteem scores in a cross-cultural perspective," *International Journal of Psychology*, vol. 37, no. 3, pp. 149–159, 2002.

[45] K. Lunnar, E. H. Wertheim, J. K. Thompson, S. J. Paxton, F. McDonald, and K. S. Halvaarson, "Across-cultural examination of weight–related teasing, body image, and eating disturbance in Swedish and Australian samples," *International Journal of Eating Disorders*, vol. 28, no. 4, pp. 430–435, 2000.

[46] K. R. Sonneville, I. B. Thurston, C. E. Milliren, R. C. Kamody, H. C. Gooding, and T. K. Richmond, "Helpful or harmful? Prospective association between weight misperception and weight gain among overweight and obese adolescents and young adults," *International Journal of Obesity*, vol. 40, no. 2, pp. 328–332, 2016.

[47] P. van den Berg and D. Neumark-Sztainer, "Fat'n happy 5 years later: is it bad for overweight girls to like their bodies?," *Journal of Adolescent Health*, vol. 41, no. 4, pp. 415–417, 2007.

[48] P. A. van den Berg, J. Mond, M. Eisenberg, D. Ackard, and D. Neumark-Sztainer, "The link between body dissatisfaction and self-esteem in adolescents: similarities across gender, age, weight status, race/ethnicity, and socioeconomic status," *Journal of Adolescent Health*, vol. 47, no. 3, pp. 290–296, 2010.

[49] K. A. Martin Ginis, D. McEwan, A. R. Josse, and S. M. Phillips, "Body image change in obese and overweight women enrolled in a weight-loss intervention: the importance of perceived versus actual physical changes," *Body Image*, vol. 9, no. 3, pp. 311–317, 2012.

[50] A. S. Sand, N. Emaus, and O. Lian, "Overweight and obesity in young adult women: a matter of health or appearance? The Tromsø study: fit futures," *International Journal of Qualitative Studies on Health and Well-being*, vol. 10, no. 1, p. 29026, 2015.

[51] M. A. Martin, M. L. Frisco, and A. L. May, "Gender and race/ethnic differences in inaccurate weight perceptions among U. S. adolescents," *Womens Health Issues*, vol. 19, no. 5, pp. 292–299, 2009.

[52] V. Swami, D. A. Frederick, T. Aavik et al., "The attractive female body weight and female body dissatisfaction in 26 countries across 10 world regions: results of the international body project I," *Personality and Social Psychology Bulletin*, vol. 36, no. 3, pp. 309–325, 2010.

[53] W. G. Johnson, K. J. Rohan, and A. A. Kirk, "Prevalence and correlates of binge eating in white and African American adolescents," *Eating Behaviors*, vol. 3, no. 2, pp. 179–189, 2002.

[54] A. Zaborskis, G. Petronyte, L. Sumskas, M. Kuzman, and R. J. Iannotti, "Body image and weight control among adolescents in Lithuania, Croatia, and the United States in the context of global obesity," *Croatian Medical Journal*, vol. 49, no. 2, pp. 233–242, 2008.

[55] M. E. Thoma, M. L. Hediger, R. Sundaram et al., "Comparing apples and pears: women's perceptions of their body size and shape," *Journal of Womens Health*, vol. 21, no. 10, pp. 1074–1081, 2012.

[56] R. Ettarh, S. Van de Vijver, S. Oti, and C. Kyobutungi, "Overweight, obesity, and perception of body image among slum residents in Nairobi, Kenya, 2008-2009," *Preventing Chronic Disease*, vol. 10, p. E212, 2013.

[57] Y. Kabir, T. A. Zafar, and C. Waslien, "Relationship between perceived body image and recorded body mass index among Kuwaiti female university students," *Women & Health*, vol. 53, no. 7, pp. 693–705, 2013.

11

Association between Sleep Habits and Metabolically Healthy Obesity in Adults

Thirumagal Kanagasabai, Ramandeep Dhanoa, Jennifer L. Kuk, and Chris I. Ardern

School of Kinesiology and Health Science, York University, Toronto, ON, Canada

Correspondence should be addressed to Chris I. Ardern; cardern@yorku.ca

Academic Editor: Terry Huang

Higher body mass index (BMI) increases the risk of cardiometabolic diseases, but nearly a third of the people living with obesity (BMI: $\geq 30\,kg/m^2$) are metabolically healthy (MHO). Extreme sleep durations and poor sleep quality are associated with higher bodyweight and cardiometabolic dysfunction, but the full extent to which sleep habits may help differentiate those with MHO versus metabolically abnormal obesity (MAO) is not yet known. Data from the U.S. National Health and Nutritional Examination Survey 2005–08 was used (BMI: $\geq 30\,kg/m^2$; ≥ 20 y; $N = 1,777$). The absence of metabolic syndrome was used to define MHO. Those with MHO tended to be younger, female, Non-Hispanic Black, never smokers, more physically active, and with less physician diagnosed sleep disorders than MAO. Neither sleep duration nor overall sleep quality was related to MHO in crude or multivariable adjusted analyses; however, reporting "almost always" to having trouble falling asleep (OR (95% CI): 0.40 (0.20–0.78)), waking up during the night (0.38 (0.17–0.85)), feeling unrested during the day (0.35 (0.18–0.70)), and feeling overly sleepy during the day (0.35 (0.17–0.75)) was related to lower odds of MHO. Selected sleep quality factors, but not sleep quantity or overall sleep quality, are associated with the MHO phenotype.

1. Introduction

Despite the well-known complications of excess body fat [1, 2] emerging research suggests that up to 30% of people living with obesity (body mass index of $\geq 30\,kg/m^2$) are metabolically healthy (MHO) [3]. MHO individuals may also be insulin-sensitive [4] and have a similar mortality risk as metabolically healthy normal bodyweight individuals [5, 6]. However, the existence of the MHO phenotype as a distinct entity, particularly over time, remains controversial [7]. Indeed, a recent meta-analysis suggests that, with longer follow-up, MHO individuals are at a 24% greater risk of cardiovascular events and all-cause mortality compared to the metabolically healthy normal-weight people whereas metabolically *unhealthy* individuals are at similarly elevated morbidity and mortality risks regardless of their body weight class [8]. Therefore, identifying factors that help maintain the metabolic health of individuals living with higher bodyweight may help reduce their morbidity and mortality risks.

Unique determinants that differentiate MHO and metabolically abnormal obesity (MAO) are largely unknown. However, lifestyle factors such as physical activity, weight history [9–11], dietary habits [3, 12, 13], and systematic inflammation and location of fats storage [14] have been found to differ between MHO and MAO. Sleep is another potential behavior that can vary between MHO and MAO phenotypes; however, in the only two studies conducted thus far, one found no difference in self-reported sleep duration between MHO and MAO [15], and the other found higher sleep duration in MHO women (MHO: 7.6 h versus MAO: 7.0 h), but not men [3]. Neither study [3, 15] evaluated the relationship between sleep quality alongside sleep duration and MHO. They either focused on middle-aged adults [3] or were limited by the application of ethnic-specific waist circumference cut-offs to a Korean sample [15]. To date, the relationship between sleep habits and the MHO phenotype amongst the U.S. adult population has yet to be studied. The primary purpose of this study was to, therefore, estimate the relationship between sleep duration and quality factors of MHO versus MAO in free-living U.S. adults.

2. Subjects and Methods

2.1. Sample. Data for this analysis was derived from the U.S. National Health and Nutrition Examination Survey (NHANES). Briefly, NHANES is a series of cross-sectional studies designed to assess the health and nutritional status of the U.S. population and includes demographic, socioeconomic, dietary, and health-related information in the interview component and medical, dental, and physiological information in the physical examination component [16]. Approximately 5,000 individuals are sampled through a complex probability cluster design on an annual basis. As a result, the NHANES 2005–2008 cycles had an initial sample of 20,497 people. Exclusions were made in sequence for age (<20 y: $n = 9{,}583$), BMI (<30 kg/m^2: $n = 13{,}499$), pregnancy ($n = 136$), missing metabolic syndrome (MetS) components or implausible values ($n_{\text{triglycerides}} = 241$, $n_{\text{blood pressure}} = 95$, $n_{\text{waist circumference}} = 177$, $n_{\text{HDL cholesterol}} = 91$, and $n_{\text{fasting plasma glucose}} = 1{,}686$), and sleep duration ($n = 7$), leaving a final analytic sample of 1,777.

2.2. Metabolically Healthy Obesity and Metabolically Abnormal Obesity. The Joint Interim Statement for MetS was used as the indicator of cardiometabolic health in those living with obesity based on the BMI cut-off of ≥30 kg/m^2 [17]. That is, those with ≤2 MetS components were classified as MHO: elevated waist circumference: men: ≥102 cm, women: ≥88 cm; elevated fasting triglycerides (≥1.69 mM) or medication; low HDL cholesterol: men: <1.04 mM, women: <1.29 mM, or medication; elevated systolic (≥130 mmHg) and/or diastolic (≥85 mmHg) blood pressure or medication; and elevated fasting plasma glucose (≥5.6 mM) or medication [10, 17]. Those with ≥3 of the above measures were classified as MAO [17].

2.3. Sleep Habits. NHANES administered the Sleep Disorders Questionnaire to individuals aged ≥16 y to assess typical sleep habits for the past month [16]. The Sleep Disorders Questionnaire contains items from two previously validated sleep questionnaires [18]. Information on the typical sleep duration (hours (h) per night) on weekdays or workdays was collected as whole numbers [1 to 11 and ≥12 h] from a single question ["How much sleep do you usually get at night on weekdays or workdays?"] [16]. The responses were categorized as ≤4, 5-6, 7-8, and ≥9 h per night [19, 20]. Overall sleep quality was determined from six questions that were used to obtain information on the sleeping habits of the participants in the past month: "How often did you have trouble falling asleep?"; "How often did you wake up during the night and had trouble getting back to sleep?"; "How often did you wake up too early in the morning and were unable to get back to sleep?"; "How often did you feel unrested during the day, no matter how many hours of sleep you have had?"; "How often did you feel excessively or overly sleepy during the day?"; and "How often did you not get enough sleep?" Responses to each question [0 = never; 1 = rarely (1 time a month); 2 = sometimes (2–4 times a month); 3 = often (5–15 times a month); and 4 = almost always (16–30 times a month)] were summed to obtain the overall sleep quality score, which was then categorized as good (0 to <3); fair (3 to <7); poor (7 to <12); and very poor (≥12 to 24) [21, 22].

2.4. Covariates. Age (20 to <40 y, 40 to <65 y, and ≥65 y), sex, ethnicity (Non-Hispanic White, Non-Hispanic Black, Mexican American, and Other), annual household income, education, alcohol intake, smoking history, leisure-time physical activity, and physician diagnosed sleep disorder were considered as covariates [10, 23]. Smoking was categorized as current, past (if smoked ≥100 cigarettes in one's life but not a current smoker), or never (if smoked <100 cigarettes in one's life) [10]. Educational attainment was categorized as <high school, high school, and college; income as <$20,000, $20,000–44,999, and ≥$45,000; and alcohol intake as 0, <3, and ≥3 drinks per day [23]. For leisure-time physical activity (PA), the metabolic equivalent (MET) scores provided by NHANES were used to calculate MET min/week, which were then categorized as no reported PA data, low PA (1 to 499 MET min/week), and guideline adherence (≥500 MET min/week) [10, 24]. Physician diagnosed sleep disorders were obtained from a single question ["Have you ever been told by a doctor or other health professional that you have a sleep disorder?"] [16].

2.5. Statistics. Mean and 95% confidence interval (CI) for continuous variables and percentage and 95% CI for categorical variables were determined for MHO versus MAO. Differences in demographic and behavioral characteristics were assessed with independent t-test and χ^2 tests, as appropriate. The mean sleep duration and overall sleep quality score were compared by sex and MHO status. Logistic regression was subsequently used to estimate the odds ratio (OR, 95% CI) for MHO. The crude OR of MHO (OR_c), odds of MHO adjusting for age, sex, ethnicity, education, income, smoking, alcohol, and leisure-time physical activity (OR_{adj}), and the odds of MHO additionally adjusting for physician diagnosed sleep disorder (OR_{adj2}) were estimated. The moderating effects of age, sex, and physician diagnosed sleep disorder on the overall relationship were also explored. All analyses were weighted with the medical exam sample weights using SAS v9.3 (Cary, NC, U.S.). Statistical significance was set at α of 0.05.

3. Results

Table 1 shows the sample characteristics, grouped by metabolic health status. Overall, 28.3% of the adults living with obesity had MHO. MHO individuals tended to be more active, younger, female, and never smokers and were also less likely to be have a physician diagnosed sleep disorder or belong to the Non-Hispanic White ethnic group ($p < 0.05$). MHO and MAO individuals did not differ in education ($p = 0.05$), income ($p = 0.16$), or alcohol intake ($p = 0.05$). The mean (95% CI) sleep duration between MHO and MAO was also not significantly different (MHO: 6.63 (6.47, 6.78) versus MAO: 6.70 (6.62, 6.78) hours); however, MHO had a slightly

Table 1: Characteristics of the sample adult (≥20 y, obesity: BMI ≥ 30 kg/m^2) population.

Characteristics	MHO (n = 484)	MAO (n = 1,293)	p value
Age (mean (95% CI))	42.3 (40.3, 44.4)	51.0 (50.7, 53.3)	<0.05
Age (% (95% CI))			
≥20 to <40 y	49.8 (43.9, 55.7)	20.7 (17.1, 24.4)	
≥40 to <65 y	40.9 (35.6, 46.2)	58.9 (55.4, 62.5)	<0.05
≥65 y	9.3 (6.0, 12.6)	20.3 (17.3, 23.4)	
Sex			
Males	39.2 (32.8, 45.7)	49.0 (45.7, 52.3)	<0.05
Females	60.8 (54.3, 67.2)	51.0 (47.7, 54.3)	
Ethnic			
Non-Hispanic White	58.6 (49.0, 68.3)	71.8 (66.4, 77.2)	
Non-Hispanic Black	21.5 (14.4, 28.6)	13.0 (9.5, 16.5)	<0.05
Mexican American	9.7 (5.3, 14.2)	7.1 (4.8, 9.5)	
Other	10.1 (6.3, 14.0)	8.1 (5.3, 10.6)	
Education			
<High school	19.1 (15.5, 22.6)	22.2 (18.8, 25.6)	
High school	22.1 (16.3, 28.0)	27.6 (24.1, 31.1)	NS
College	58.8 (53.6, 64.0)	50.2 (45.1, 55.3)	
Income			
<$20,000	14.4 (10.9, 17.9)	18.7 (15.7, 21.7)	
$20,000–44,999	30.8 (25.3, 36.2)	29.9 (25.5, 34.3)	NS
≥$45,000	54.9 (49.0, 60.7)	51.4 (46.4, 56.4)	
Smoking			
Never	58.9 (53.3, 64.5)	49.2 (45.7, 52.8)	
Current Smoker	17.1 (13.0, 21.3)	19.9 (16.7, 23.0)	<0.05
Past smoker	23.9 (20.0, 27.9)	30.9 (27.7, 34.1)	
Alcohol			
0 drinks/day	31.7 (26.0, 37.3)	38.7 (35.1, 42.3)	
<3 drinks/day	45.1 (39.4, 50.7)	42.2 (38.9, 45.5)	NS
≥3 drinks/day	23.2 (18.8, 27.7)	19.1 (16.5, 21.7)	
Leisure-time physical activity			
No reported PA	64.6 (57.7, 71.5)	70.1 (65.3, 75.0)	
1–499 MET min/w	10.5 (7.6, 13.3)	12.1 (9.3, 14.8)	<0.05
≥500 MET min/w	24.9 (20.1, 29.8)	17.8 (14.1, 21.5)	
Sleep hour			
≤4 h	4.6 (2.8, 6.3)	7.3 (5.4, 9.2)	
5-6 h	39.6 (34.7, 44.5)	34.1 (30.5, 37.7)	NS
7-8 h	50.9 (45.8, 56.0)	52.5 (48.9, 56.1)	
≥9 h	4.9 (2.6, 7.3)	6.1 (4.7, 7.4)	
Sleep quality			
Good (<3)	18.4 (14.0, 22.7)	17.6 (14.8, 20.4)	
Fair (≥3 to <7)	23.8 (19.8, 27.8)	21.3 (17.8, 24.7)	NS
Poor (≥7 to <12)	29.9 (24.2, 35.5)	27.3 (23.4, 31.2)	
Very poor (≥12 to 24)	28.0 (23.7, 32.2)	33.8 (30.4, 37.2)	
Physician diagnosed sleep disorder			
No	90.1 (86.3, 94.0)	83.8 (80.7, 86.8)	<0.05
Yes	9.9 (6.0, 13.7)	16.2 (13.2, 19.3)	

Mean (95% CI) for continuous variables and % (95% CI) for categorical variables. MHO is metabolically healthy obesity, based on the Joint Interim Statement of metabolic syndrome. $p < 0.05$, two-sided; independent t-test or χ^2, as appropriate. NS is not significant.

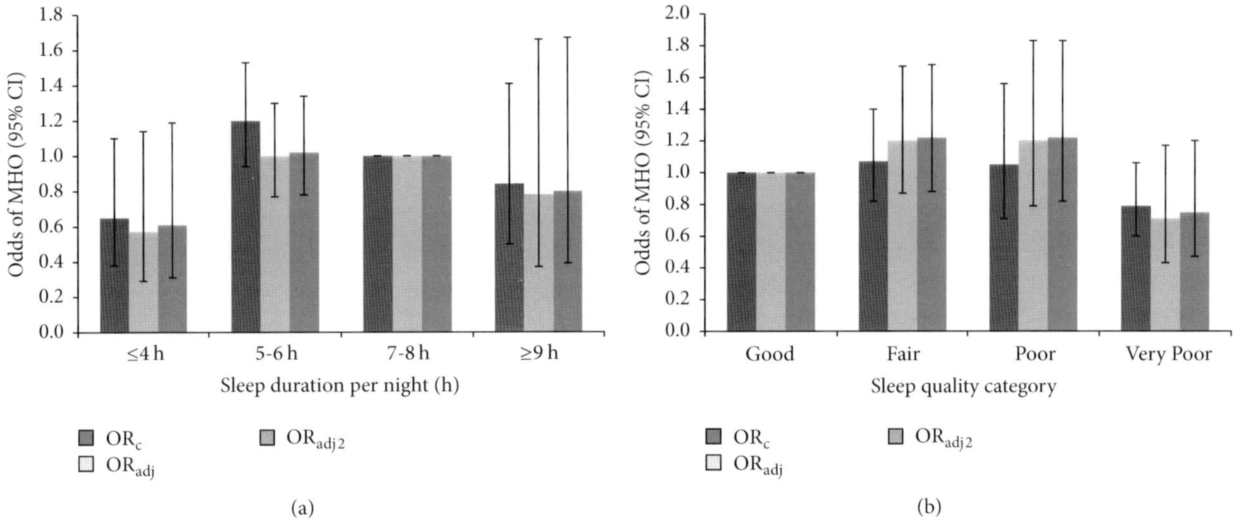

FIGURE 1: The odds of metabolically healthy obesity by sleep duration (a) and sleep quality (b) categories. Modeled for MHO (i.e., absence of metabolic syndrome according to the Joint Interim Statement, ≤2 cardiometabolic dysfunctions). Responses to sleep quality habit questions were summed to obtain the overall sleep quality, which were categorized as good (0 to <3); fair (3 to <7); poor (7 to <12); and very poor (≥12 to 24). OR_c is crude, OR_{adj} adjusted for age, sex, ethnicity, education, income, smoking, alcohol, and leisure-time physical activity, and OR_{adj2} additionally adjusted for physician diagnosed sleep disorder. MHO is metabolically healthy obesity in people with BMI of ≥30 kg/m^2. All models were not significant.

lower overall sleep quality score (8.34 (7.84, 8.83)) than MAO individuals (9.11 (8.69, 9.53)).

In crude and fully adjusted models, sleep duration and overall sleep quality were not related to MHO (Figure 1), and no significant interactions (e.g., age, sex, and physician diagnosed sleep disorder) were found (all $p > 0.05$). When individual sleep quality questions were assessed, a significant relationship was found for four of the six questions, wherein those who reported "almost always" (versus "never") had lower odds of MHO (e.g., "How often did you have trouble falling asleep?"; "How often did you wake up during the night and had trouble getting back to sleep?"; "How often did you feel unrested during the day, no matter how many hours of sleep you have had?"; and "How often did you feel excessively or overly sleepy during the day?") (Figure 2). Only two sleep quality questions were not associated with MHO (i.e., "How often did you wake up too early in the morning and were unable to get back to sleep?" and "How often did you not get enough sleep?"). However, no significant relationships between the sleep parameters and the individual cardiometabolic components were found (data not shown).

4. Discussion

To our knowledge, this is the first population-based analysis to examine both sleep duration and sleep quality factors as they relate to MHO in free-living adults. Descriptively, MHO individuals reported slightly better overall sleep quality, but neither sleep duration nor overall sleep quality was associated with the odds of MHO in fully adjusted models. Nonetheless, regularly waking up during the night, feeling unrested during the day, feeling overly sleepy during the day, and trouble falling asleep were associated with lower odds of MHO. Therefore, our study provides novel evidence that specific sleep quality measures, but not sleep duration, are associated with the cardiometabolic health of people living with obesity.

4.1. Sleep Duration. Of the two previous studies that characterized the MHO versus MAO phenotype by sleep duration, one found a difference in women only [3], while the other supports our finding of no association [15]. In the study by Hankinson et al. [3] MHO women slept 7.6 h per day while MAO women slept 7.0 h. This is in contrast to our finding of no difference and may be attributed in part to Hankinson et al.'s [3] more conservative classification of MHO as the complete absence of diagnosed cardiometabolic abnormalities (versus the absence of preclinical Joint Interim Statement diagnostic cut-offs) [17] and their use of a slightly older sample. Although MHO tends to be younger than MAO and we did not find age was a moderator, the intersection of sleep and age requires further study [25], as both sleep duration and quality decrease [26], while cardiometabolic risk increases with age [27].

Further, chronic sleep deprivation promotes weight gain by altering specific endocrine pathways, such as leptin and ghrelin, that control appetite [28]. Sleep loss is also associated with higher preference for foods rich in fats and carbohydrates that promote weight gain [29]. Elevated sympathetic nervous system activity and higher inflammation have also been linked with poor sleep and obesity [30]. However, in the MHO phenotype, these potential mechanisms may remain intact while they may be compromised in the MAO phenotype [31]. Additionally, experimental evidence suggests that sleep loss results in metabolic consequences, including reduced nocturnal utilization of glucose that can promote insulin resistance and elevate diabetes risk in otherwise

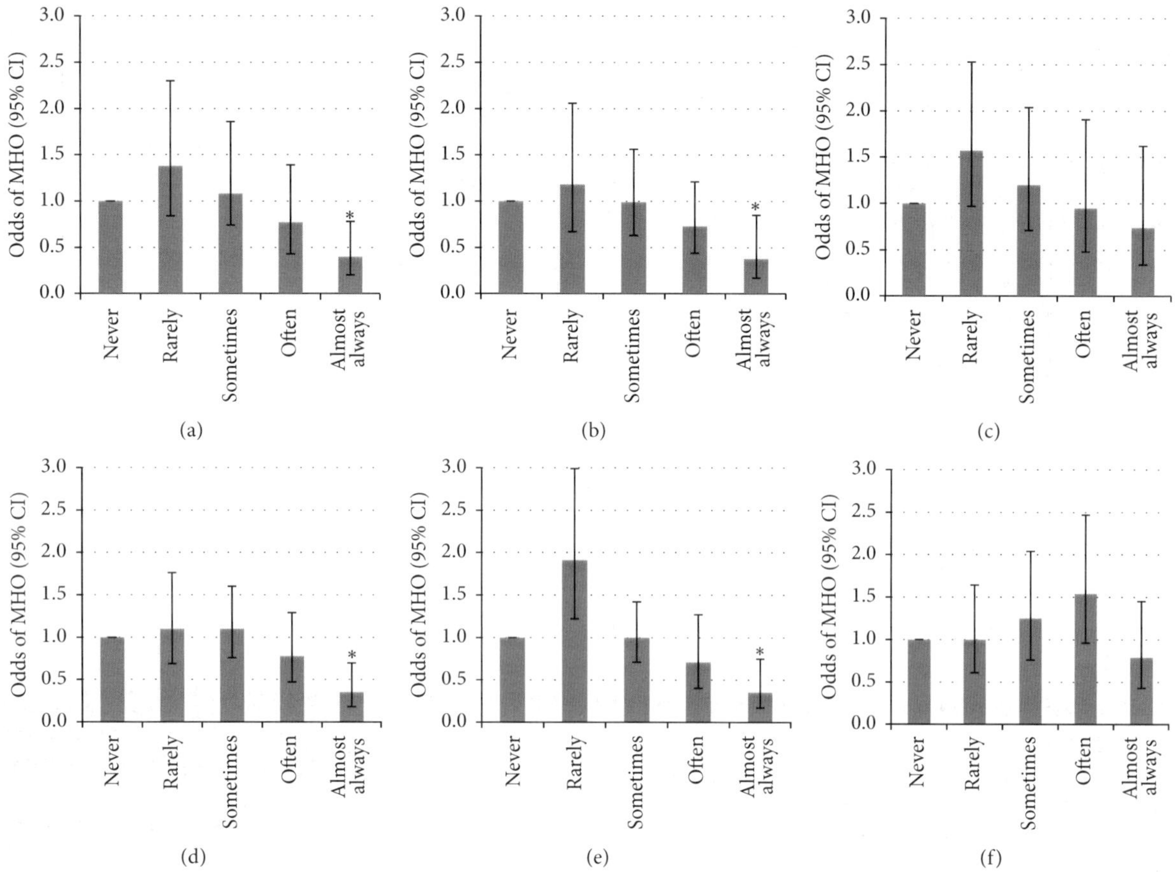

FIGURE 2: The odds of metabolically healthy obesity for each sleep quality question. (a) "How often did you have trouble falling asleep?"; (b) "How often did you wake up during the night and had trouble getting back to sleep?"; (c) "How often did you wake up too early in the morning and were unable to get back to sleep?"; (d) "How often did you feel unrested during the day, no matter how many hours of sleep you have had?"; (e) "How often did you feel excessively or overly sleepy during the day?"; and (f) "How often did you not get enough sleep?" Modeled for MHO (i.e., absence of metabolic syndrome according to the Joint Interim Statement, ≤ 2 cardiometabolic dysfunctions) adjusting for age, sex, ethnicity, education, income, smoking, alcohol, leisure-time physical activity, and physician diagnosed sleep disorder. Responses for each question were as follows: never; rarely (1 time a month); sometimes (2–4 times a month); often (5–15 times a month); and 4, almost always (16–30 times a month). MHO is metabolically healthy obesity in people with BMI of $\geq 30\ kg/m^2$. *Significant difference.

healthy individuals [28, 32]. A disproportionate number of individuals with diagnosed sleep disorders also have cardiometabolic dysfunction and obesity [33]. Therefore, although adequate sleep may be one of the common features that differentiate the MHO phenotype from the MAO phenotype, because of the complex interaction between sleep, obesity, and cardiometabolic dysfunction, the directionality of this relationship is not yet clear.

4.2. Sleep Quality. Results of this study suggest that select sleep quality measures, but not overall sleep quality, are associated with cardiometabolic health. These findings are supported by findings that poor sleep quality factors are related to obesity [34, 35], blood pressure [36], and glucose dysregulation [37, 38]. Indeed, individuals with obesity tend to have lower sleep quality and are more likely to experience a sleep disorder [39]. Mechanical [40] and physiological mechanisms [41] related to excess bodyweight could account in part for this decrease in sleep quality; however, whether obesity/higher bodyweight causes the decrease in sleep quality or vice versa remains unclear [30].

It remains to be seen whether overall sleep quality or efficiency, waking up during the night, daytime sleepiness, trouble falling asleep, sleep latency, or a combination of these factors is essential for cardiometabolic health and is an area in need of further study [21, 42]. Nonetheless, our study provides a new perspective on the complications of individuals with obesity in that MHO individuals have slightly better overall sleep quality than those with MAO, and selected sleep quality factors help predict the MHO phenotype. In our study, regularly reporting waking up during the night (i.e., 16–30 times a month), feeling unrested during the day, feeling overly sleepy during the day, and trouble falling asleep were moderately associated with the MHO phenotype [43]. However, some chronic conditions, for example, diabetes, hypertension, obesity (the clinical diagnosis), and depression, are also associated with fragmented sleep, insomnia, and excessive daytime sleepiness [44, 45].

Therefore, further research in this area is needed to better understand the relationship between various sleep quality factors and cardiometabolic health amongst those living with obesity/higher bodyweight.

4.3. Limitations. Several limitations exist with our study. First, due to the cross-sectional nature of our study, we cannot infer a causal relationship between sleep habits and MHO. Second, we were unable to assess the relationship between changing sleep patterns and napping within a 24 h period, which may give a better depiction of the sleep-MHO relationship. It is also possible that some yet to be assessed combination of sleep quantity and quality is a better predictor of MHO. Other cardiometabolic risk factors, such as percent body fat, HOMA-IR, and LDL-cholesterol, may also be indicators of the MHO phenotype but they were not included in our definition. Our definition for MHO compares favorably with much of the current literature, but MHO has been defined with many different definitions [46]. Further, we used self-reported sleep habits, which were susceptible to recall and healthy responder biases. Finally, we did not consider any other diseases (e.g., depression, coronary heart disease) or circumstances, such as shift-work, that affect sleep and circadian rhythm [47, 48]. Given the limitations of this study and current knowledge on the relationship between sleep and the MHO phenotype, research using objective measures of sleep within a longitudinal framework is needed. Particularly, studies to assess the importance of changing sleep patterns as they relate to the MHO versus MAO phenotypes are needed. Future research in this area should also quantify the contributions of other diseases and circumstances (mentioned above) to the sleep-MHO relationship.

5. Conclusions

Experiencing regular disturbances in sleep quality, but not overall sleep quality or sleep duration, is associated with MHO. Further studies in other populations living with obesity (i.e., higher bodyweight) are needed to confirm our findings.

Competing Interests

The authors have no conflict of interests to declare.

Acknowledgments

This work was funded by a research grant (no. 131594) from the Canadian Institute of Health Research.

References

[1] P. T. James, "Obesity: the worldwide epidemic," *Clinics in Dermatology*, vol. 22, no. 4, pp. 276–280, 2004.

[2] M. Blüher, "The distinction of metabolically 'healthy' from 'unhealthy' obese individuals," *Current Opinion in Lipidology*, vol. 21, no. 1, pp. 38–43, 2010.

[3] A. L. Hankinson, M. L. Daviglus, L. V. Horn et al., "Diet composition and activity level of at risk and metabolically healthy obese american adults," *Obesity*, vol. 21, no. 3, pp. 637–643, 2013.

[4] G. Calori, G. Lattuada, L. Piemonti et al., "Prevalence, metabolic features, and prognosis of metabolically healthy obese italian individuals: the cremona study," *Diabetes Care*, vol. 34, no. 1, pp. 210–215, 2011.

[5] J. L. Kuk and C. I. Ardern, "Are metabolically normal but obese individuals at lower risk for all-cause mortality?" *Diabetes Care*, vol. 32, no. 12, pp. 2297–2299, 2009.

[6] M. Hamer and E. Stamatakis, "Metabolically healthy obesity and risk of all-cause and cardiovascular disease mortality," *Journal of Clinical Endocrinology and Metabolism*, vol. 97, no. 7, pp. 2482–2488, 2012.

[7] M. Hamer, J. A. Bell, S. Sabia, G. D. Batty, and M. Kivimäki, "Stability of metabolically healthy obesity over 8 years: the English longitudinal study of ageing," *European Journal of Endocrinology*, vol. 173, no. 5, pp. 703–708, 2015.

[8] C. K. Kramer, B. Zinman, and R. Retnakaran, "Are metabolically healthy overweight and obesity benign conditions?: a systematic review and meta-analysis," *Annals of Internal Medicine*, vol. 159, no. 11, pp. 758–769, 2013.

[9] S. M. Camhi, M. E. Waring, S. B. Sisson, L. L. Hayman, and A. Must, "Physical activity and screen time in metabolically healthy obese phenotypes in adolescents and adults," *Journal of Obesity*, vol. 2013, Article ID 984613, 10 pages, 2013.

[10] T. Kanagasabai, N. A. Thakkar, J. L. Kuk, J. R. Churilla, and C. I. Ardern, "Differences in physical activity domains, guideline adherence, and weight history between metabolically healthy and metabolically abnormal obese adults: a cross-sectional study," *International Journal of Behavioral Nutrition and Physical Activity*, vol. 12, article 64, 2015.

[11] K. J. Smith, E. Bessell, C. G. Magnussen, T. Dwyer, and A. J. Venn, "Does youth adiposity, or change in adiposity from youth to adulthood, predict metabolically healthy obesity in adulthood?" *Pediatric Obesity*, vol. 11, no. 5, pp. 349–353, 2016.

[12] C. M. Phillips, "Metabolically healthy obesity: definitions, determinants and clinical implications," *Reviews in Endocrine and Metabolic Disorders*, vol. 14, no. 3, pp. 219–227, 2013.

[13] S. M. Camhi, E. Whitney Evans, L. L. Hayman, A. H. Lichtenstein, and A. Must, "Healthy eating index and metabolically healthy obesity in U.S. adolescents and adults," *Preventive Medicine*, vol. 77, pp. 23–27, 2015.

[14] I. Alam, T. P. Ng, and A. Larbi, "Does inflammation determine whether obesity is metabolically healthy or unhealthy? the aging perspective," *Mediators of Inflammation*, vol. 2012, Article ID 456456, 14 pages, 2012.

[15] J. Y. Ryu, J. S. Lee, H. C. Hong et al., "Association between body size phenotype and sleep duration: Korean National Health and Nutrition Examination Survey v (KNHANES V)," *Metabolism: Clinical and Experimental*, vol. 64, no. 3, pp. 460–466, 2015.

[16] National Center for Health Statistics, "NHANES—About the National Health and Nutrition Examination Survey," 2011, http://www.cdc.gov/nchs/nhanes/about_nhanes.htm.

[17] K. G. M. M. Alberti, R. H. Eckel, S. M. Grundy et al., "Harmonizing the metabolic syndrome: a joint interim statement of the international diabetes federation task force on epidemiology and prevention; National heart, lung, and blood institute; American heart association; World heart federation; International atherosclerosis society; And international association for

the study of obesity," *Circulation*, vol. 120, no. 16, pp. 1640–1645, 2009.

[18] L. Plantinga, K. Lee, L. A. Inker et al., "Association of sleep-related problems with CKD in the United States, 2005–2008," *American Journal of Kidney Diseases*, vol. 58, no. 4, pp. 554–564, 2011.

[19] A. Tamakoshi and Y. Ohno, "Self-reported sleep duration as a predictor of all-cause mortality: results from the JACC Study, Japan," *Sleep*, vol. 27, no. 1, pp. 51–54, 2004.

[20] J. E. Gangwisch, D. Malaspina, B. Boden-Albala, and S. B. Heymsfield, "Inadequate sleep as a risk factor for obesity: analyses of the NHANES I," *Sleep*, vol. 28, no. 10, pp. 1289–1296, 2005.

[21] J. Engeda, B. Mezuk, S. Ratliff, and Y. Ning, "Association between duration and quality of sleep and the risk of pre-diabetes: evidence from NHANES," *Diabetic Medicine*, vol. 30, no. 6, pp. 676–680, 2013.

[22] T. Kanagasabai and C. I. Ardern, "Inflammation, oxidative stress, and antioxidants contribute to selected sleep quality and cardiometabolic health relationships: a cross-sectional study," *Mediators of Inflammation*, vol. 2015, Article ID 824589, 11 pages, 2015.

[23] T. Kanagasabai, J. X. Nie, C. Mason, and C. I. Ardern, "Metabolic syndrome and prevalent any-site, prostate, breast and colon cancers in the U.S. adult population: NHANES 1999–2010," *Journal of Metabolic Syndrome*, vol. 3, article no. 135, 2014.

[24] Office of Disease Prevention and Health Promotion, *Physical Activity Guidelines for Americans*, US Department of Health and Human Services, Washington, DC, USA, 2008.

[25] M. L. Unruh, S. Redline, M.-W. An et al., "Subjective and objective sleep quality and aging in the sleep heart health study," *Journal of the American Geriatrics Society*, vol. 56, no. 7, pp. 1218–1227, 2008.

[26] M. M. Ohayon, M. A. Carskadon, C. Guilleminault, and M. V. Vitiello, "Meta-analysis of quantitative sleep parameters from childhood to old age in healthy individuals: developing normative sleep values across the human lifespan," *Sleep*, vol. 27, no. 7, pp. 1255–1273, 2004.

[27] N. Khansari, Y. Shakiba, and M. Mahmoudi, "Chronic inflammation and oxidative stress as a major cause of age-related diseases and cancer," *Recent Patents on Inflammation and Allergy Drug Discovery*, vol. 3, no. 1, pp. 73–80, 2009.

[28] K. Spiegel, K. Knutson, R. Leproult, E. Tasali, and E. Van Cauter, "Sleep loss: a novel risk factor for insulin resistance and Type 2 diabetes," *Journal of Applied Physiology*, vol. 99, no. 5, pp. 2008–2019, 2005.

[29] M.-P. St-Onge, S. Wolfe, M. Sy, A. Shechter, and J. Hirsch, "Sleep restriction increases the neuronal response to unhealthy food in normal-weight individuals," *International Journal of Obesity*, vol. 38, no. 3, pp. 411–416, 2014.

[30] K. Spiegel, E. Tasali, R. Leproult, and E. Van Cauter, "Effects of poor and short sleep on glucose metabolism and obesity risk," *Nature Reviews Endocrinology*, vol. 5, no. 5, pp. 253–261, 2009.

[31] G. Plourde and A. D. Karelis, "Current issues in the identification and treatment of metabolically healthy but obese individuals," *Nutrition, Metabolism and Cardiovascular Diseases*, vol. 24, no. 5, pp. 455–459, 2014.

[32] K. Spiegel, R. Leproult, and E. Van Cauter, "Impact of sleep debt on metabolic and endocrine function," *Lancet*, vol. 354, no. 9188, pp. 1435–1439, 1999.

[33] A. Svatikova, R. Wolk, A. S. Gami, M. Pohanka, and V. K. Somers, "Interactions between obstructive sleep apnea and the metabolic syndrome," *Current Diabetes Reports*, vol. 5, no. 1, pp. 53–58, 2005.

[34] P. Lyytikäinen, T. Lallukka, E. Lahelma, and O. Rahkonen, "Sleep problems and major weight gain: a follow-up study," *International Journal of Obesity*, vol. 35, no. 1, pp. 109–114, 2011.

[35] M. Watanabe, H. Kikuchi, K. Tanaka, and M. Takahashi, "Association of short sleep duration with weight gain and obesity at 1-year follow-up: a large-scale prospective study," *Sleep*, vol. 33, no. 2, pp. 161–167, 2010.

[36] M. D. Corbalán-Tutau, J. A. Madrid, and M. Garaulet, "Timing and duration of sleep and meals in obese and normal weight women. Association with increase blood pressure," *Appetite*, vol. 59, no. 1, pp. 9–16, 2012.

[37] P. M. Nilsson, M. Rööst, G. Engström, B. Hedblad, and G. Berglund, "Incidence of diabetes in middle-aged men is related to sleep disturbances," *Diabetes Care*, vol. 27, no. 10, pp. 2464–2469, 2004.

[38] A. Barceló, F. Barbé, M. De La Peña et al., "Insulin resistance and daytime sleepiness in patients with sleep apnoea," *Thorax*, vol. 63, no. 11, pp. 946–950, 2008.

[39] L. A. Panossian and S. C. Veasey, "Daytime sleepiness in obesity: Mechanisms beyond obstructive sleep apnea—a review," *Sleep*, vol. 35, no. 5, pp. 605–615, 2012.

[40] J. P. Kirkness, A. R. Schwartz, H. Schneider et al., "Contribution of male sex, age, and obesity to mechanical instability of the upper airway during sleep," *Journal of Applied Physiology*, vol. 104, no. 6, pp. 1618–1624, 2008.

[41] U. Scherrer, D. Randin, L. Tappy, P. Vollenweider, E. Jéquier, and P. Nicod, "Body fat and sympathetic nerve activity in healthy subjects," *Circulation*, vol. 89, no. 6, pp. 2634–2640, 1994.

[42] F. P. Cappuccio, L. D'Elia, P. Strazzullo, and M. A. Miller, "Quantity and quality of sleep and incidence of type 2 diabetes: a systematic review and meta-analysis," *Diabetes Care*, vol. 33, no. 2, pp. 414–420, 2010.

[43] H. Chen, P. Cohen, and S. Chen, "How big is a big odds ratio? Interpreting the magnitudes of odds ratios in epidemiological studies," *Communications in Statistics—Simulation and Computation*, vol. 39, no. 4, pp. 860–864, 2010.

[44] E. O. Bixler, A. N. Vgontzas, H.-M. Lin, S. L. Calhoun, A. Vela-Bueno, and A. Kales, "Excessive daytime sleepiness in a general population sample: the role of sleep apnea, age, obesity, diabetes, and depression," *Journal of Clinical Endocrinology and Metabolism*, vol. 90, no. 8, pp. 4510–4515, 2005.

[45] P. Cheng, V. Pillai, H. Mengel, T. Roth, and C. L. Drake, "Sleep maintenance difficulties in insomnia are associated with increased incidence of hypertension," *Sleep Health*, vol. 1, no. 1, pp. 50–54, 2015.

[46] C. M. Durward, T. J. Hartman, and S. M. Nickols-Richardson, "All-cause mortality risk of metabolically healthy obese individuals in NHANES III," *Journal of Obesity*, vol. 2012, Article ID 460321, 12 pages, 2012.

[47] O. Van Reeth, L. Weibel, K. Spiegel, R. Leproult, C. Dugovic, and S. Maccari, "Physiology of sleep (review)-interactions between stress and sleep: from basic research to clinical situations," *Sleep Medicine Reviews*, vol. 4, no. 2, pp. 201–219, 2000.

[48] J. M. Fuller, K. K. Wong, I. Krass, R. Grunstein, and B. Saini, "Sleep disorders screening, sleep health awareness, and patient follow-up by community pharmacists in Australia," *Patient Education and Counseling*, vol. 83, no. 3, pp. 325–335, 2011.

12

Smallanthus sonchifolius (Yacon) Flour Improves Visceral Adiposity and Metabolic Parameters in High-Fat-Diet-Fed Rats

Stella Maris Honoré, Maria Virginia Grande, Jorge Gomez Rojas, and Sara Serafina Sánchez

Instituto Superior de Investigaciones Biológicas (INSIBIO), Consejo Nacional de Investigaciones Científicas y Técnicas-Universidad Nacional de Tucumán (CONICET-UNT), Chacabuco 461, T4000ILI San Miguel de Tucumán, Argentina

Correspondence should be addressed to Stella Maris Honore; smhonore@gmail.com

Academic Editor: Aron Weller

Smallanthus sonchifolius (yacon), a native plant of South America, was observed to improve lipid profile in rodents and humans. This study aimed to investigate the antiobesity properties of yacon roots in a high-fat-diet (HFD) model and the underlying mechanisms. A total of 30 Wistar male rats were divided into five groups ($n = 6$): the standard chow diet (SD) group was fed a SD; the HFD group was fed a HFD; and the HFD Y340 and HFD Y680 groups were fed a HFD plus yacon flour (340 and 680 mg FOS/kg b. w./day, respectively). HFD Y340 and HFD Y680 rats exhibited marked attenuation of weight gain, a decrease in visceral fat pad weight, a restoration of the serum lipid profile and atherogenic index in a dose-dependent manner, being the higher dose more effective ($p < 0.05$). In addition, we found that HFD Y680 rats showed lower glucose and insulin levels, improved glucose tolerance, and insulin sensitivity ($p < 0.5$). A downregulation of several adipocyte specific-transcription factors, including peroxisome proliferator-activated receptor gamma2 (PPAR-γ2), CCAAT/enhancer binding protein a (C/EBP-a) and activating protein (aP2) mRNA levels, was determined in the visceral adipose tissue of HFD Y680 rats ($p < 0.05$). An improvement of adipokine profile in HFD Y680 rats and decreased serum proinflammatory cytokine levels ($p < 0.05$) were determined by ELISA. Decreased macrophage infiltration and F4/80 and MCP-1 expression in the visceral adipose tissue of HFD Y680 rats ($p < 0.5$), together with a higher pAkt/Akt expression ($p < 0.05$) were also observed by immunofluorescence and immunoblotting. A significant increase in glucagon (Gcg) and PYY mRNA levels in distal ileum of HFD Y680 rats ($p < 0.05$) were also detected. In the second approach, we determined that yacon supplementation potentiates the effects of the HFD reversion to a standard diet. In conclusion, yacon showed antiobesity properties by inhibiting adipogenesis and improving the visceral adipose tissue function.

1. Introduction

Overweight and obesity have become a global health problem owing to their strong association with a high incidence of various chronic diseases, such as type-2 diabetes, hypertension, coronary heart disease, and other noncommunicable diseases [1]. Obesity results from an energy imbalance between calorie intake and energy expenditure. The extra energy is stored as triglyceride in adipose tissue through an adipogenic process and accumulated in ectopic sites like muscle and liver, leading to a metabolic dysfunction [2, 3].

Adipogenesis is a process of cell differentiation by which precursor mesenchymal cells give rise to mature adipose cells to fulfill a key metabolic and endocrine role. Different hormones, nutrients, and transcription factors have been shown to regulate lipid accumulation during adipocyte differentiation [4]. Furthermore, the regulation of adipogenic transcriptional factors of mRNA levels, such as peroxisome proliferator-activator receptor-γ (PPAR-γ), CCAAT/enhancer binding protein-α (C/EBP-α), and related genes (adipocyte fatty acid-binding protein: AP2; fatty acid synthase: FAS), leads to changes in the activity of key proteins involved in lipids and fatty acids metabolism, inflammation, and cell-cycle regulation [5].

During obesity, adipose tissue expansion is marked not only by an increase in white adipose tissue mass but also by morphological changes which affects adipocyte function [6, 7]. Increasing evidence indicates that the excessive fat depots, particularly visceral adiposity, are linked to a chronic low-grade inflammatory state [1, 4, 5]. Moreover, through the release of free fatty acids (FFAs) and various adipokines such as leptin, adiponectin, resistin, PAI-1, Il-1b, and TNF-α, the hypertrophic adipocytes play a role in the progression of insulin resistance [2, 8].

It is known that obesity is not always spontaneously reversible, so its treatment requires a multidisciplinary approach [9]. The combination of diet and physical activity is only effective during time in which it is practiced and the available drugs are only moderately effective and have significant adverse effects [10, 11]. Dietary supplements have been proposed to promote weight loss or appetite suppression in the management of obesity. In this sense, natural products provide a rich source for safe and effective therapeutic compounds with multiple mechanisms of action [12, 13].

Yacon (*Smallanthus sonchifolius* (Poepp and Endl.) H. Robinson) belongs to a member of Asteraceae family, which ranges through the Andean region in South America [14, 15]. Yacon roots have special features which include high water content and large amount of soluble dietary fibers, with low energy density [14]. Given their high content in fructooligosaccharides (FOSs) [16, 17] and phenolic compounds, such as chlorogenic and caffeic acids [18], yacon roots have been considered as a beneficial functional food with prebiotic properties [19–22]. FOSs are fructose oligosaccharide joined by β $(2 \rightarrow 1)$ or β $(2 \rightarrow 6)$ linkages, able to resist the hydrolysis of enzymes in the upper gastrointestinal tract. Experimental studies have demonstrated that the addition of oligofructose to the diet improves the growth of *Bifidus* and *Lactobacillus* in the colon enhancing mineral absorption and gastrointestinal metabolism in both humans and animals [16, 19]. Dietary polyphenols also modulated the growth of beneficial microbial populations, influencing the intestinal mucosa integrity and energy harvest, through endocrine and systemic metabolic signaling [23, 24].

Previous studies demonstrated that dietary yacon supplementation reduces postprandial serum triglycerides in normal rats, without toxicity or adverse nutritional effects [17]. Also, it was shown that yacon improves beta cell function and modulates the plasma insulin concentration in diabetic rats [25, 26]. Additionally, yacon roots present strong antioxidant activity and anti-inflammatory effects preventing the risks associated with metabolic diseases [27–29]. Recently, long-term consumption of yacon syrup has been shown to improve insulin resistance and reduce body weight in premenopausal women [30]. These findings raise the interesting possibility that adipose tissue could be a target organ of the yacon roots in the management of obesity. However, no data are currently available on the ability of yacon roots to affect adipose tissue.

A number of studies have shown that the diet-induced obese animal models mimic human obesity more than other models such as genetic knockout mutants [31]. For instance, rodents chronically exposed to a high-fat diet develop dyslipidemia, white adipose tissue expansion, insulin resistance, and altered metabolic regulatory hormones [32, 33] constituting a useful tool to evaluate the potential mechanisms underlying the effects of yacon on obesity.

Table 1: Chemical characterization of yacon flour.

Component	Content
Total sugar (mg/g flour)	780.0 ± 5.24
FOS (mg/g flour)	432.1 ± 2.17
Sucrose (mg/g flour)	73.3 ± 0.78
Glucose (mg/g flour)	79.6 ± 1.13
Fructose (mg/g flour)	195 ± 0.22
Total polyphenols (mg GAE/g flour)	17.02 ± 3.18

Values are presented as means ± DE ($n = 3$). GAE, gallic acid.

The current study was designed to assess efficacy of *Smallanthus sonchifolius* roots in suppressing visceral fat accumulation, ameliorate obesity-related phenotypic and biochemical markers, and provide a molecular mechanism for how yacon dietary supplementation can improve obesity in a HFD-fed-rat model. Even more is investigated if the effects of yacon are modified by the type of diet consumed.

2. Materials and Methods

2.1. Plant Material and Root Flour Preparation. The *Smallanthus sonchifolius* (yacon) (Clone LIEY97-1) roots, are cultivated locally at 550 m above the sea level, in the province of Tucumán, 27S, NW Argentina. Voucher specimens were deposited in the herbarium of "Instituto Miguel Lillo," San Miguel de Tucumán, Tucumán, Argentina (No. 600982LIL). The roots were carefully washed, peeled, sliced, and dried at 60°C in a forced air circulation oven to reduce water content. The dried material was then pulverized to obtain yacon roots flour. The powder was stored at 4°C until use.

2.2. Carbohydrate Composition and Phenolic Content of Yacon Flour. Total sugar content and carbohydrate composition of yacon flour were estimated in samples extracted with 80% ethanol at 80°C [34]. Total sugar content of yacon flour was estimated by the phenol-sulphuric acid method [35]. The extract was dried, dissolved in water, and desalted with a mixed exchange resin (Amberlite MB3, Sigma). The purified water extract was injected into an HPLC system equipped with an IR detector (Gilson 132 IR) using a RSO-oligosaccharide Ag^{++} column (Rezex) and water at 70°C as the mobile phase. Oligosaccharides peaks were identified using sucrose, glucose, fructose, and fructofuranosylnystose as external standards [25]. In the experimental designs, daily intake levels of yacon root flour were calculated with respect to the amount of FOS using doses equivalent to 340 mg FOS/Kg b. w./day [25] and 680 mg FOS/Kg b. w./day corresponding to 0.79 and 1.57 g of yacon flour/kg body weight/day, respectively.

Total polyphenol content was determined by the Folin–Ciocalteu method [36] and expressed as milligram gallic acid (GAE) equivalents per gram of flour. Results of the analysis for the yacon flour are shown in Table 1.

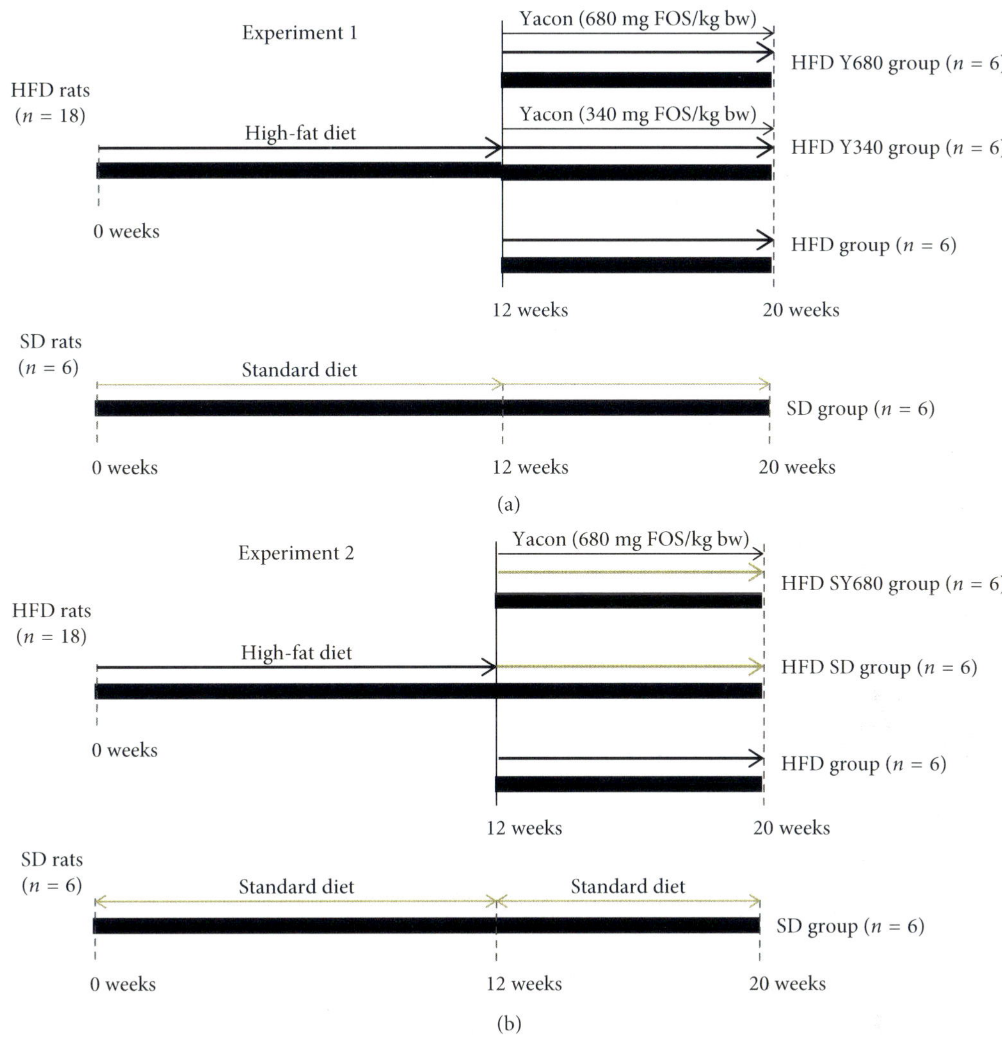

Figure 1: Experimental design. (a) Experiment 1: effects of the yacon flour on HFD-induced metabolic disease. (b) Experiment 2: effects of yacon supplementation and the reversion to a SD diet on HFD-induced metabolic disease. SD: standard diet-fed rats; HFD: high-fat-diet-fed rats; HFD SD: high-fat-diet-fed rats reversed to a SD diet; HFD SY680: high-fat-diet-fed rats reversed to a SD diet and supplemented with yacon flour (680 mg FOS/kg b.z.).

2.3. Animals and Diets. Male Wistar rats weighing 200–250 g were obtained from the colony bred at the INSIBIO (CONICET-UNT), Tucumán, Argentina. Rats were kept in a breeding room with controlled environment (temperature: 23 ± 1°C, relative humidity: 60 ± 5%, and 12 h light-dark cycle). All the experimental procedures were in strict accordance with the Guide for the Care and Use of Laboratory Animals (Institute of Laboratory Animal Resources, Commission on Life Sciences, National Research Council, National Academy Press, Washington, DC) and the local Animal Care Committee from the Universidad Nacional de Tucumán (Prot. No. 004/2017).

The experimental animals were randomly divided into two groups: the standard diet group (SD, $n = 12$) and the high-fat-diet group (HFD, $n = 36$). The SD group was fed *ad libitum*, with a standard chow diet containing 12.08 kJ/g calories: 69.5% from carbohydrates, 5.6% from fat, and 24.9% from protein (Association de Cooperativas Argentinas-S.E.N.A.S.A. No. 04-288/A). The HFD group received a standard-based diet enriched with eatable lard and carbohydrates (modified from [33]) to induce obesity and hyperlipidemia. The total calories in fat diet were 17.40 kJ/g: 35.0% from carbohydrates, 41.0% from fat, and 24.0% from protein. Both animal groups were maintained on each diet for 12 weeks. At this time, animals fed HFD reached obesity status (Figure 1).

2.4. Experimental Design

2.4.1. Experiment 1. After 12 weeks on HFD or standard chow, the animals were randomly divided into the following groups according to the treatment with or without the addition of yacon flour as a dietary supplement for 8 weeks (Figure 1).

(i) HFD Y340 group ($n = 6$), rats fed a high-fat-diet plus a tablet of yacon flour equivalent to 340 mg FOS/kg b. w.

(ii) HFD Y680 group ($n = 6$), rats fed a high-fat-diet plus a tablet of yacon flour equivalent to 680 mg FOS/kg b. w.

(iii) HFD group ($n = 6$), rats fed a high-fat-diet.

(iv) SD group ($n = 6$), rats fed standard diet.

2.4.2. Experiment 2. In a second design, after 12 weeks rats which fed standard diet continued with the same chow, while animals under HFD were changed to a standard diet with or without yacon, according to the following scheme (Figure 1).

(i) HFD SD group ($n = 6$), rats which change high-fat-diet feeding by standard diet

(ii) HFD SY group ($n = 6$) rats which change high-fat-diet feeding by fed standard diet plus a tablet of yacon flour containing 680 mg FOS/kg b. w.

(iii) HFD group ($n = 6$), rats fed a high-fat-diet.

(iv) SD group ($n = 6$), rats fed standard diet.

2.5. Morphometric and Nutritional Determinations. Animals were weighed (g) weekly throughout the experimental period. Food intakes were recorded daily as follows: food intake = initial food weight (g) – leftover food weight (g) – spilled food weight (g); energy intake = food intake (g) x total energy of the chow diet (kJ/g). The spilled food was weighed and dried after feces had been picked out. The body length (nose–anus length), thoracic circumference (immediately behind the foreleg), and abdominal circumference (immediately anterior to the forefoot) were determined in all rats at as was described previously [37]. The body weight and body length were used to determine the following anthropometrical parameters: Body mass index (BMI) = body weight (g)/length^2 (cm^2); Lee index = cube root of body weight (g)/nose-to-anus length (cm).

Nutritional parameters were calculated based on food and caloric intake: energy intake (kJ/day) = mean food consumption x dietary metabolizable energy; FER (food efficiency ratio) = (body weight gain/food intake) ×100.

2.6. Tissue Sampling. At the end of the experimental period, rats were fasted overnight and deeply anaesthetized with 1 :1 xylazin-ketamine. Blood samples were collected by cardiac puncture into EDTA-Na 4.1%-containing tubes, and plasma was separated by centrifugation at 3000 g for 10 min [25]. Blood samples were collected into plane glass tubes. After clotting, samples were centrifuged and serum was used for biochemical determinations. Liver, muscle (soleus), spleen, pancreas, and visceral (mesenteric), perirenal, and epididymal fat pads were removed and rinsed thoroughly with ice-cold saline, blotted, weighed, and fixed in 4% formaldehyde saline for histological analysis. The remaining tissues were frozen immediately and stored at −80°C until analyzed.

2.7. Biochemical Determinations. Triglycerides and total cholesterol concentrations were determined by enzymatic colorimetric methods using available commercial kits (Wiener lab Group, Argentina). The high-density lipoprotein cholesterol (HDLc) was determined after precipitation of very low-density lipoprotein (VLDL) and low-density lipoprotein (LDLc) with polyanions (dextran sulphate and magnesium chloride). LDL-cholesterol concentration was determined by a two-step homogeneous assay without precipitation. Free fatty acids were determined using available commercial kits (ab65341, Abcam, USA).

Circulating tumor necrosis factor-α (TNF-α) (RAB0479), interleukin-1β (IL-1β) (RAB0277), insulin (RAB0904) (all from SIGMA Aldrich, St. Louis, MO, USA), leptin (ab100773), and adiponectin (ab108784) (Abcam, USA) were performed using commercially available kits according to the manufacturer′s instructions.

Blood glucose concentrations were measured using a glucose meter (Roche Diagnostics GmbH, Mannheim, Germany). The HOMA-IR (Homeostasis model assessment of insulin resistance) index was calculated as [fasting glucose (mg/dl) × fasting insulin (ng/ml)/405] to assess insulin resistance [38].

2.7.1. Oral Glucose Tolerance Test (OGTT). Rats were administered orally with 50% D-glucose (2 g/kg body weight) after a 12 h fast. Blood glucose concentration was measured with a Glucometer (Accu-Check; Roche Diagnostics, GmbH, Mannheim, Germany) with blood from tail-tip bleedings at 0, 15, 30, 60, and 120 min. Area under the curve (AUC) was calculated as changes from 0 to 120 min and expressed in (mg/dl/min).

2.7.2. Insulin Tolerance Test (ITT). Rats were injected intraperitoneally with 0.75 IU/kg body weight porcine Insulin (Betasint, BETA laboratory) after a 4-hour fast. Blood glucose concentration was measured with a Glucometer (Accu-Check; Roche Diagnostics, GmbH, Mannheim, Germany) with blood from tail-tip bleedings at 0, 15, 30, and 60 min. The areas under the curve (AUC 0–60 min) were calculated.

2.7.3. Oral Fat-Loading Test. To assess postprandial increase in triglyceride, oral fat-load tests were performed at the end of 8 week of yacon diet-supplementation. Rats from the HFD Y680, HFD, and SD groups were fasted for 12 h. The HFD Y680 group received a single yacon-tablet containing 680 mg FOS/kg body weight. Thirty minutes later with 2.5 ml/kg b. w. of corn oil was given to all groups of animals. Tail blood samples were taken at 0 h and 1, 2, 3, and 4 hours after oral chow administration for the triglycerides determination. AUCs (0–4 h) were calculated in both experiments.

2.8. Histology and Immunohistochemistry. Samples from fixed visceral fat were dehydrated, embedded in paraffin, and cut into 4 μm-thick sections at 50 μm intervals. The sections were stained with hematoxylin and eosin (H&E), mounted on glass slides, and examined by optical microscopy. Images were analyzed using ImageJ software for quantification (National Institutes of Health, Bethesda, MD).

After, blocked with 10% (w/v) normal goat serum for 1 h, sections were subjected to immunohistochemical staining overnight at 4°C with a 1 : 100 dilution of a anti MCP-1 polyclonal antibody (Santa Cruz Biotechnology, USA) following by Alexa Fluor 594 antibody (Invitrogen) (1 h, at room temperature). The sections were mounted in aqueous mounting medium with antifading agents (Biomeda, Foster, CA). The specimens were analyzed using an Olympus BX80 fluorescence microscope (Olympus Optical Ltd., Tokyo) and the ImageJ software. At least 15 nonadjacent microscope fields were analyzed in each tissue.

2.9. RNA Extraction and PCR and qPCR Amplification. Total RNA was isolated from visceral adipose and intestine tissue using the RNeasy Lipid Tissue Mini Kit (Qiagen, Basel, Switzerland) and Trizol reagent (Invitrogen), respectively, according to the manufacturer's instruction. 0.5 μg RNA was reverse transcribed (RT) into first-strand cDNA using M-MLV Reverse Transcriptase (Promega, USA) and oligo (dT) primers (Invitrogen, USA). After the RT procedure, the resulting cDNAs were used for PCR and qPCR. Gene expression was evaluated using a Mastercycler personal instrument (Eppendorf, Germany) in optimized conditions and quantified using the QuantiFast SYBR Green Kit (Qiagen, Hilden, Germany) on a Lightcycler 2.0 instrument (Roche Diagnostics, Mannheim, Germany) with the following cycle conditions: 95°C for 10 seconds followed by 30 cycles of 95°C for 5 seconds and 57°C for 30 seconds. The primers used are PPARγ2 (AB019561.1) forward primer 5′-CCCTGGCAAAGCATTTGTAT-3′ and reverse primer 5′-ACTGGCACCCTTGAAAAATG-3′; C/EBP-a (NM001287 577) forward primer 5′-GGAGGGACTTAGGGAGTTGG-3′ and reverse primer 5′ GGAAACCTGGCCTGTTGTAA-3′; aP2 (U75581) forward primer 5′-GGGACCTGGAAAC TCGTCTC-3′ and reverse primer 5′-CTGACCGGAT-GACGACCAAG-3′; Gcg (NM012707.2) forward primer 50-CATTCACAGGGCACATTCAC-30 and reverse primer 50-TGACGTTTGGCAATGTTGTT-30; PYY (AB238226.1) forward primer 50-GTGGACCAGTGGTGAAGACC-30 and reverse primer 50-GGGACATGAACACACACAGC-30; β-actin (NM007393) forward primer 5′-CCGGCTTCGCG-GGCGACG-3′ and reverse primer 5′-TCCCGGCCAGC-CAGGTCC-3′. The results were normalized to β-actin mRNA levels.

2.10. Western Blotting. Visceral adipose tissues were homogenized in the whole cell lysis buffer containing 1% NP-40, 0.1% SDS, 0.5% sodium deoxycholate (SIGMA Aldrich, USA), 0.1 mM EDTA, 2 mM PMSF, a Complete Protease Inhibitor Cocktail (Roche, Germany), and supernatants were collected. An amount of 25–50 mg of protein was loaded on to 7.5% SDS polyacrylamide gels and transferred to 0.22/0.45 mm a nitrocellulose membrane (Hybond-C super; Amersham, Buckinghamshire, UK). The membrane was blocked with 5% (w/v) fat-free milk dissolved in phosphate buffered saline containing 0.05% (v/v) Tween-20 (TBST). The membrane was incubated at 4°C overnight with rabbit polyclonal antibody against Akt (1 : 100 dilution; Cell Signaling Technology Inc. Danvers, USA), p-Akt (1 : 100 dilution; Cell Signaling Technology Inc. Danvers, USA), F4/80 (1 : 100 dilution; Santa Cruz Biotech, USA), or Actin (1 : 3000 dilution; SIGMA Aldrich, USA). The washed membrane was incubated with HRP-conjugated secondary antibodies at room temperature for 1 h, and then a biotin-extrAvidin-peroxidase system (SIGMA Aldrich, USA) was used to determine signals. Band intensities were quantified by ImageJ software.

2.11. Statistical Analysis. All results are presented as the mean ± standard deviation and were analyzed with Graph Pad Prism 6.01 (San Diego, CA, USA). To assess the significance of variation, groups were compared by one-way ANOVA followed by Bonferroni's multiple comparisons test. A probability level of $p < 0.05$ was considered statistically significant.

3. Results

3.1. Yacon Improves Morphometric and Feeding Parameters in HFD-Fed Rats. Rats fed a high-fat diet greatly increased the body weight compared to the SD group ($p < 0.05$). The average growth rate for rats on the HFD was 19.7 g/week while rats on a SD-chow were merely 10.2 g/week. At 12 weeks, the body weight of HFD rats resulted around 20% higher compared with SD-fed rats ($p < 0.05$) (Figure 2(a)). Yacon flour supplementation to the HFD rats for the following 8 weeks significantly reduced the final body weight in a dose-dependent manner ($p < 0.05$) (Figures 2(a) and 2(b)). An improvement in the morphometric parameters was also observed in supplemented rats (Supplemental data, Table S1). Yacon significantly reduced the food intake leading to a lower energy intake ($p < 0.05$) (Figures 2(c) and 2(d)). Food efficiency ratio (FER) was also reduced in both tested doses compared with the HFD group ($p < 0.05$) (Figure 2(e)).

3.2. Yacon Improves Lipid Serum Profiles in HFD-Fed Rats. Fasting triglycerides (TG), low-density lipoprotein (LDLc), and free fatty acids levels were increased in HFD-fed rats compared with the SD group, whereas high-density lipoproteins (HDLc) were reduced ($p < 0.05$). Yacon significantly reduced triglycerides and free fatty acids concentrations in both doses tested with a higher effect at 680 mg FOS/kg b. w. ($p < 0.05$), evidencing a dose-dependent effect on these parameters. No effect on total cholesterol levels was observed ($p > 0.05$). Interestingly, yacon flour significantly decreased LDLc and increased HDLc values at the dose of 680 mg FOS/kg b. w, improving the TG/HDLc index ($p < 0.05$) (Table 2).

3.3. Yacon Improves Body Composition of HFD-Fed Rats. Table 3 shows the effects of yacon flour consumption on relative organ weights. HFD-fed rats exhibited an increase in

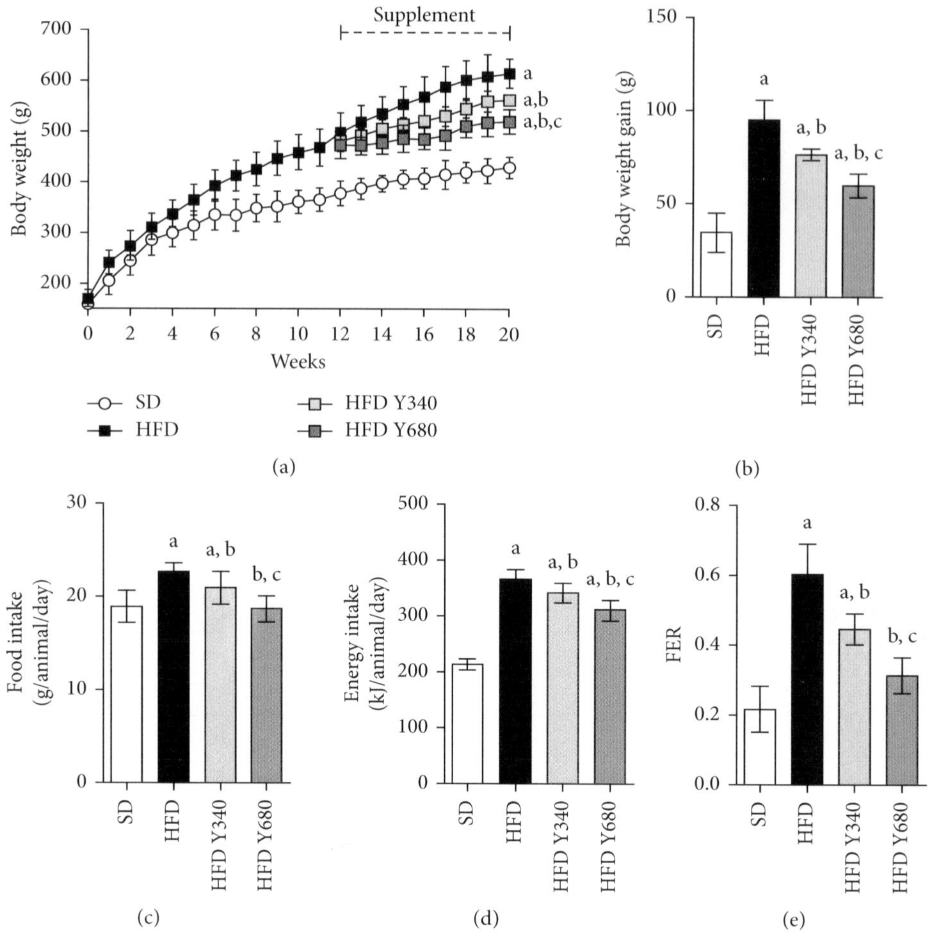

FIGURE 2: Effect of yacon flour on HFD-fed rats after 8 weeks of supplementation. (a) Time course of body weight in rats fed standard diet (SD) or high-fat diet (HFD) supplemented or not with yacon flour (340 or 680 mg FOS/kg body weight: HFD Y340 and HFD Y680, respectively). (b) Body weight gain. (c) Food intake. (d) Energy intake. (e) Feed efficiency ratio (FER). Data are mean ± standard deviation ($n = 6$/group). $^{a}p < 0.05$ vs. SD group, $^{b}p < 0.05$ vs. HFD group, $^{c}p < 0.05$ vs. HFD Y340 group.

hepatic mass and a decrease in the cecum and muscle ($p < 0.05$). Administration of yacon supplement reduced the liver mass in HFD rats in both tested doses ($p < 0.05$). Only the dose of 680 mg FOS/kg b. w. was able to increase significantly the cecum weight. There was no alteration in the soleus weight after yacon supplementation ($p > 0.05$). No significant changes were observed for the spleen and pancreas in all the studied groups.

Yacon supplementation significantly reduced the total fat weight in HFD-fed rats at a dose of 680 mg FOS/kg b. w. ($p < 0.05$). However, only a tendency to decrease was shown at 340 mg FOS/kg b. w. dose. Interestingly, differences in fat deposition in terms of epididymal, perirenal, and mesenteric pads, were observed after yacon supplementation. Yacon considerably reduced visceral pad weight in both doses tested, with a maximum effect at 680 mg FOS/kg b. w. ($p < 0.05$) (Table 3). However, epididymal and retroperitoneal pads deposition decreased only at a higher dose of 680 mg FOS/kg b. w. ($p < 0.05$) (Table 3). These data led us to believe that visceral fat may be a target of yacon effects.

3.4. Yacon Modulates Adipocyte Size and Gene Expression in Adipose Tissue. At the cellular level, obesity is characterized by an increase in the number (hyperplasia) and size of individual adipocytes that have differentiated from preadipocyte in fat depots [5]. Histological analysis from visceral adipose tissue sections stained with H&E revealed that high-fat feeding increased fat deposits and adipocytes size in the HFD animals. Interestingly, yacon supplement (680 mg FOS/kg b. w.) resulted in reduced fat deposits and smaller adipocytes in visceral pad, with similar size to those observed in SD-fed rat (Figures 3(a) and 3(b)).

To analyze if yacon could modulate the expression of genes involved in adipogenesis in visceral fat, the amount of PPAR-γ2, a major transcription regulator of adipogenic process, was measured in supplemented HFD-fed rats. The expressions of PPAR-γ2, as well as their downstream targets, C/EBPa and aP2, were significantly decreased in HFD Y680-fed rats ($p < 0.05$) (Figures 3(c)–3(e)). These data imply a role of yacon on avoiding visceral adipose tissue expansion induced by diet.

Table 2: Effects of yacon supplement on serum lipid profile of HFD-fed rats.

	SD	HFD	HFD Y340	HFD Y680
Triglyceride (mg/dl)	64.1 ± 5.0	195.8 ± 12.1[a]	98.5 ± 2.4[b]	83.0 ± 4.1[b]
Total cholesterol (mg/dl)	70.2 ± 14.1	86.2 ± 26.0	80.2 ± 32.0	79.1 ± 18.0
HDLc (mg/dl)	48.0 ± 5.1	32.4 ± 10.3[a]	40.6 ± 14.2	50.3 ± 7.2[b]
LDLc (mg/dl)	13.6 ± 8.2	44.2 ± 9.5[a]	27.2 ± 8.1	19.3 ± 6.5[b]
TG/HDLc index	1.33 ± 0.11	6.09 ± 1.04[a]	2.47 ± 0.07[b]	1.67 ± 0.16[b,c]
Free fatty acid (mmol/l)	0.76 ± 0.11	1.10 ± 0.13[a]	0.96 ± 0.05[b]	0.84 ± 0.07[b,c]

Values are means ± standard deviation (n = 6 rats/group). [a]$p < 0.05$ compared to the SD group. [b]$p < 0.05$ compared to the HFD group.

Table 3: Effects of yacon supplement on organs weights of HFD-fed rats.

	SD	HFD	HFD Y340	HFD Y680
Total fat pad (% b. w.)	3.40 ± 0.69	6.44 ± 0.67[a]	5.54 ± 0.53	3.61 ± 0.95[b]
Epididymal fat pad (% b. w.)	1.47 ± 0.13	2.18 ± 0.20[a]	1.94 ± 0.26	1.42 ± 0.22[b]
Perirenal fat pad (% b. w.)	1.06 ± 0.26	2.55 ± 0.37[a]	2.15 ± 0.23	1.47 ± 0.31[b]
Visceral fat pad (% b. w.)	0.86 ± 0.23	1.71 ± 0.18[a]	1.33 ± 0.12[b]	0.72 ± 0.22[b]
Muscle (soleus) (% b. w.)	1.35 ± 0.07	0.98 ± 0.20[a]	1.20 ± 0.19	1.18 ± 0.26
Liver (% b. w.)	2.66 ± 0.13	3.10 ± 0.18[a]	2.51 ± 0.11[b]	2.47 ± 0.12[b]
Spleen (% b. w.)	0.13 ± 0.01	0.12 ± 0.02	0.13 ± 0.01	0.13 ± 0.03
Pancreas (% b. w.)	0.43 ± 0.11	0.43 ± 0.12	0.49 ± 0.02	0.58 ± 0.06
Cecum (% b. w.)	0.23 ± 0.02	0.16 ± 0.02[a]	0.20 ± 0.03	0.28 ± 0.04[b,c]

Values are means ± standard deviation (n = 6 rats/group). [a]$p < 0.05$ compared to the SD group. [b]$p < 0.05$ compared to the HFD group; [c]$p < 0.05$ compared to the HFD Y340 group. Fat pad weights are expressed as the sum of visceral, retroperitoneal, and epididymal weights. b. w., body weight.

3.5. Yacon Reduces Inflammation in Visceral Adipose Tissue of HFD-Fed Rats. It is known that excessive adipose tissue expansion leads to adipose macrophage infiltration and metabolic dysfunction contributing to low-grade local and systemic inflammation [2]. In this way, we analyzed whether yacon could modulate inflammatory markers in visceral fat and serum. MCP-1 expression levels and the macrophage biomarker F4/80 were significantly elevated in the visceral adipose tissue of HFD-fed rats compared with SD rats ($p < 0.05$). Yacon supplementation reduced the expression of the mentioned markers in HFD-fed animals (Figures 4(a)–4(c)). In accordance with this fact, yacon also reduced the circulating level of proinflammatory cytokines TNF-α and IL-1β levels in HFD-fed animals (Figures 4(d) and 4(e)).

Additionally, adiponectin and leptin have been implicated in adipose tissue dysfunction [6]. Therefore, the effect of yacon on modulating these adipokine levels in HFD rats was evaluated. High leptin and low adiponectin levels were observed in HFD-fed ($p < 0.05$). Yacon supplementation significantly decreased the leptin and increased the adiponectin concentrations in HFD-fed rats, restoring the leptin/adiponectin ratio ($p < 0.05$) (Figures 4(f)–4(h)).

3.6. Yacon Improves Metabolic Parameters in HFD-Fed Rats. Estimation of blood glucose, insulin, and HOMA-IR index in the experimental groups is depicted in Figure 5. The results showed that high-fat feeding led to alterations in glucose homeostasis inducing a significant increase in the fasting serum glucose and insulin levels, accompanied by the increased HOMA-IR index ($p < 0.05$). Yacon supplementation significantly decreased fasting glucose and insulin levels resulting in a lower HOMA-IR index compared with HFD rats ($p < 0.05$) (Figures 5(a)–5(c)).

In addition, during OGTT, SD rats increased the blood glucose level to a maximum, 15 min after the oral glucose loading, and then declined to the basal value (Figure 5(a)). Whereas, glucose peak in HFD rats was higher at 15 min and remained high over the 120 min. Interestingly, yacon supplementation elicited a significant decrease in the blood glucose level at 15 min and beyond when compared with HFD rats (Figure 5(d)). The AUC was significantly increased in the HFD group compared to the SD group ($p < 0.05$), but decreased in the yacon-treated group ($p < 0.05$). Moreover, the ITT showed that the blood glucose levels after insulin injection in the SD- and HFD Y680-fed groups were lower than those in HFD rats ($p < 0.05$), indicating that yacon improved glucose tolerance and insulin resistance in HFD rats (Figure 5(e)).

Changes in protein expression of Akt, the most important molecule of the insulin signaling in target organs, were measured using Western blot analysis (Figure 5(f)). Akt protein expression was similar in the visceral adipose tissue of all the analyzed groups ($p > 0.05$). However, while Akt phosphoryation in the visceral adipose tissue of HFD rats was lower compared to SD rats ($p < 0.05$), yacon supplementation increased the phosphoryation levels of this protein, in HFD rats leading to higher p-Akt/Akt and pAkt/Insulin ratios ($p < 0.05$) (Figures 5(g)).

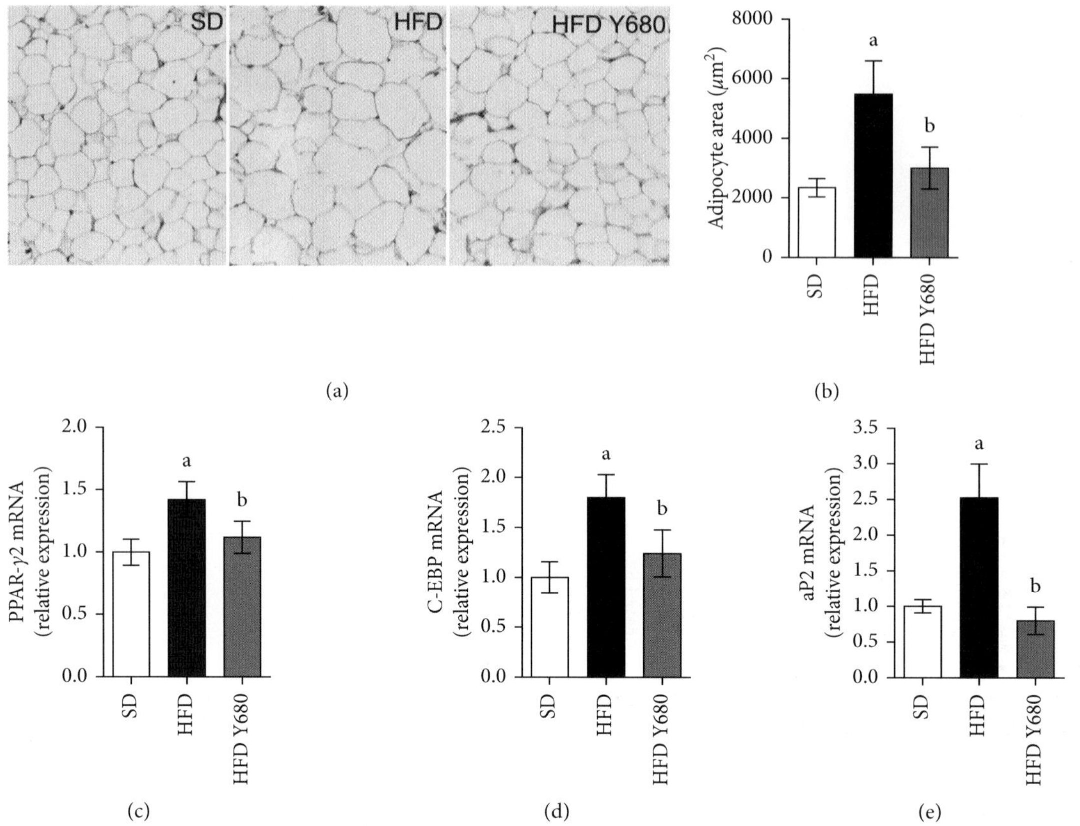

FIGURE 3: Effects of yacon flour on the adipose tissue of HFD-fed rats and adipogenesis-related genes. (a) Representative photomicrographs of visceral adipose tissue sections stained with H&E (original magnification 126X). (b) Adipocytes size in visceral adipose tissue. qPCR analysis of visceral fat from rats fed standard diet (SD) or high-fat diet (HFD) supplemented or not with yacon flour (680 mg FOS/kg body weight: HFD Y680) after 8 weeks of treatment: PPAR-γ2: peroxisome proliferator-activated receptor gamma2 (c); C/EBP-a: CCAA-T/enhancer-binding protein (d); aP2: activating protein 2 (e). Data were normalized to Actin mRNA and expressed as fold change over the SD rats. Values are presented as mean ± standard deviation of triplicate qPCR analysis ($n = 6$/group). $^{a}p < 0.05$ vs. SD, $^{b}p < 0.05$ vs. HFD.

3.7. Yacon Improves Glucagon and PYY mRNA Expression in HFD-Fed Rats. It is well established that high-fat diet impairs gastrointestinal peptides secretion, implicated in appetite control and insulin release [31]. Then, we assessed whether yacon effects are related to changes in incretins expression. The mRNA levels of glucagon (Gcg), the precursor of glucagon-like peptide-1 (GLP-1) and the peptide tyrosine tyrosine (PYY) in distal ileum of the HFD-fed rats were significantly reduced compared to those of the SD-fed rats ($p < 0.05$). Dietary supplementation with yacon strongly increased Gcg and PYY expression of HFD-fed rats, recovering the mRNA levels ($p < 0.05$). The data concerning to the expression of intestinal peptides are shown in Figure 6.

3.8. Yacon Decreases Serum Triglyceride Levels after Oral Fat-Loading. Lipid intestinal uptake is a crucial step for obesity progression and hyperlipidemia. In order to assess whether the yacon modifies lipid absorption at the intestinal level, we perform an oral triglyceride loading test. Figure S1 (Supplementary materials) shows the serum triglyceride values of the different experimental groups after oral oil loading. HFD rats showed a sharp increment of triglycerides at 30 min, reaching a maximum peak at 1h and then decreasing to triglyceride baseline value at 4 h. In contrast, the serum triglycerides curve of HFD Y680 rats did not increase considerably from the baseline, being similar to that from SD rats. These data indicate that yacon attenuates diet-induced obesity in rats by decreasing fat absorption.

3.9. Yacon Improves the Effects of the Reversion to Standard Diet. To identify whether the yacon supplementation potentiate the effects of the HFD reversion to a standard diet, we performed a second experimental design. We found that all of the parameters analyzed were improved after HFD rats turned to SD feeding for 8 weeks (Supplementary materials, Table S1). Interestingly, yacon consumption strongly reduced the final body weight and the body weight gain in the HFD SY680 group compared to HFD SD only (Figures 7(a) and 7(b)). Consistently, body and visceral adipose weight were significantly lower in HFD SY680-fed rats when compared with all the other groups (Figures 7(c) and 7(d)). Rats in the HFD SY680 group showed lower food intake than HFD SD rats, which resulted in a reduced energy intake and FER (Supplementary materials, Figure S2). Serum triglyceride levels of HFD SY680 rats were also significantly reduced when compared to HFD SD- or to SD-fed rats (Figure 7(e)).

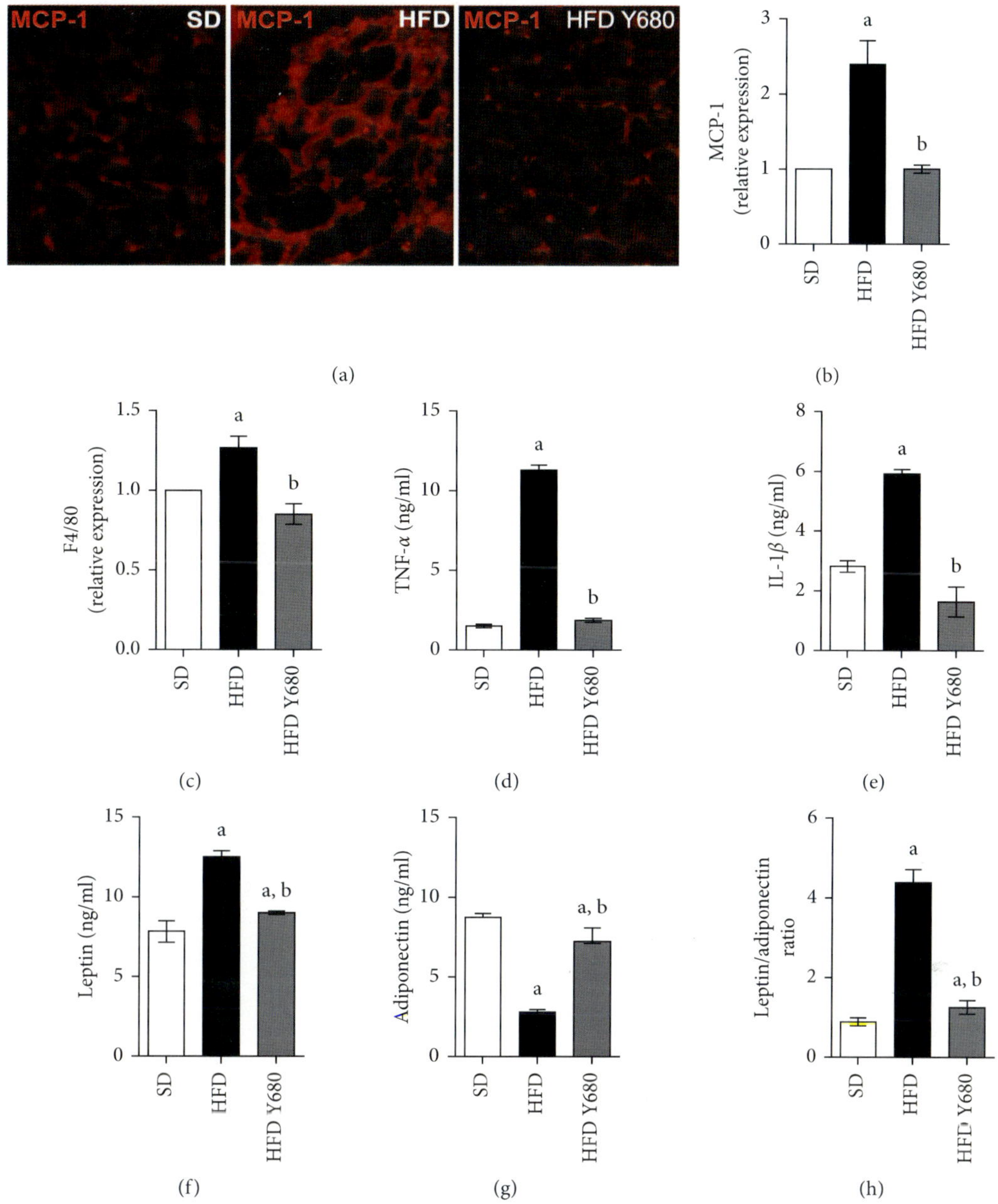

FIGURE 4: Effects of yacon flour on inflammatory markers in HFD-fed rats. (a) Representative sections of visceral fat stained with MCP-1 from rats fed standard diet (SD) or high-fat diet (HFD) supplemented or not with yacon flour (680 mg FOS/kg body weight: HFD Y680) (original magnification 126X). (b) Staining score, assigned to each section according to the MCP-1 levels. (c) F4/80 protein expression of in visceral fat by western blotting. (d, e) Serum TNF-α and IL-1β concentrations determined by ELISA. (f, g) Plasma leptin and adiponectin concentrations. (h) Leptin/adiponectin ratio. Data are mean ± standard deviation ($n = 6$/group). $^{a}p < 0.05$ vs. SD, $^{b}p < 0.05$ vs. HFD.

In accordance with this finding, fasting glucose, glucose tolerance, and insulin resistance were also improved being the blood glucose concentrations similar to those of the SD rats during the glucose challenges (Figures 7(f) and 7(g)).

4. Discussion

Nutritional strategies represent alternatives to pharmaceutical approaches for reducing hyperglycemia and body weight [13]. Thus, the identification of novel foods that promote satiety or reduce energy density provides an interesting tool in managing obesity and its associated comorbidities [6, 13].

Here, we report an interesting effect of yacon root flour, a natural product rich in FOS and phenolic compounds, as a dietary supplement. The addition of yacon flour to a high-fat diet, at doses of 340 and 680 mg FOS/kg b. w./day, was effective in reducing body weight, in a dose-dependent manner. This effect was more pronounced when yacon was accompanied by a standard diet. Moreover, regional fat depots analysis showed primarily fat loss from the visceral pads, a known critical factor in reducing overall disease risk, including type-2 diabetes development [38]. Furthermore, *in vivo* effects of yacon roots on lipid metabolism included a significant reduction in serum triglycerides, VLDLc, and

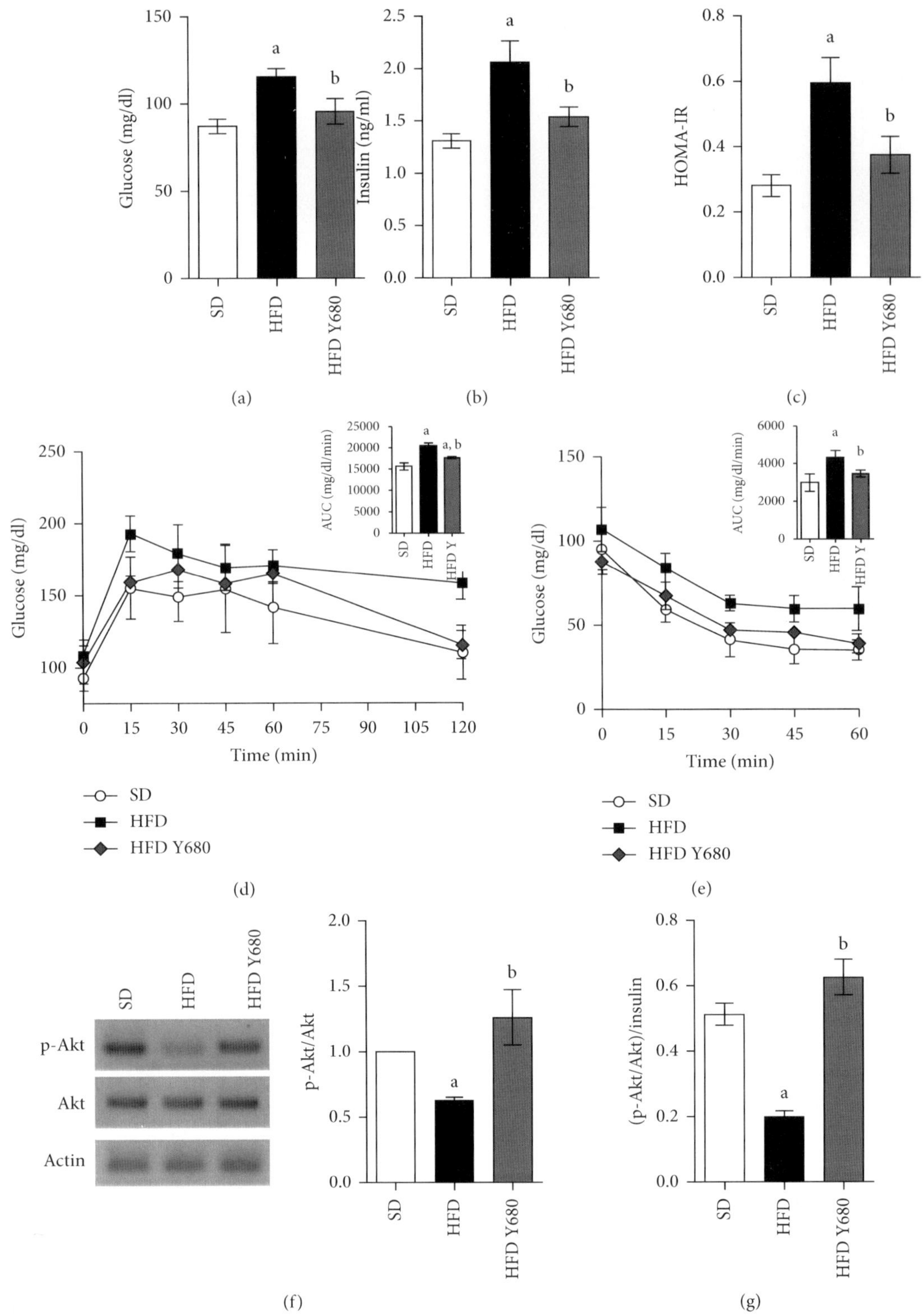

FIGURE 5: Effects of yacon flour on HFD-induced metabolic disease. (a) Fasting glucose concentrations at the end of experiment. (b) Time course of glycemia in response to oral glucose overload (2 g/kg body weight) at 8 weeks (insert: area under the curve of blood glucose following glucose overload). (c) Time course of glycemia following a single intraperitoneal (i.p.) injection of insulin (0.75 U/kg b. w.) after 8 weeks of yacon supplementation (insert: area under the curve of blood glucose following insulin injection). (d) Fasting plasma insulin concentrations at the end of experiment. (e) Homeostasis model assessment of insulin resistance (HOMA-IR) index. (f) Akt and p-Akt protein expressions in visceral fat by western blotting. The mean value of SD-fed rats was set at 1. (g) p-Akt/Insulin ratio. Data are expressed as the mean ± standard deviation ($n = 6$/group). $^{a}p < 0.05$ vs. SD, $^{b}p < 0.05$ vs. HFD. SD: standard diet-fed rats; HFD: high-fat-diet-fed rats; HFD SD: high-fat-diet-fed rats reversed to a SD chow; HFD SY680: high-fat-diet-fed rats reversed to a SD chow and supplemented with yacon flour (680 mg FOS/kg b. w.).

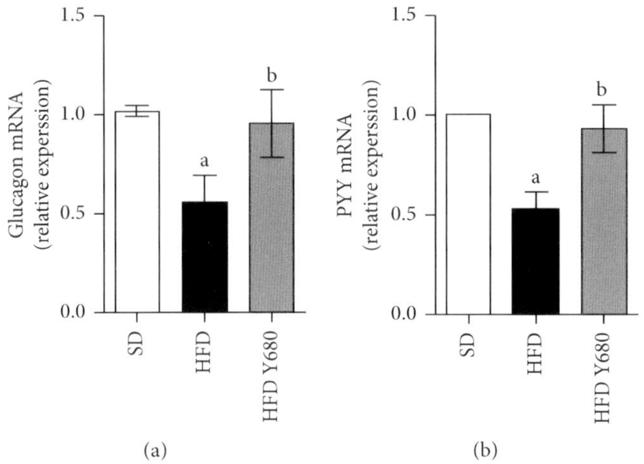

FIGURE 6: Effects of yacon flour on intestinal mRNA levels of proglucagon and PYY in HFD-fed rats. Proglucagon: Gcg (a) and polypeptide YY: Pyy (b) mRNA expression in intestinal samples of rats fed standard diet (SD) or high-fat diet (HFD) supplemented or not with yacon flour (680 mg FOS/kg body weight: HFD Y680) after 8 weeks of treatment. Data were normalized to Actin mRNA and expressed as fold change over the SD rats. Values are presented as mean ± standard deviation of triplicate PCR analysis ($n = 6$/group). $^{a}p < 0.05$ vs. SD, $^{b}p < 0.05$ vs. HFD. SD: standard diet-fed rats; HFD: high-fat-diet-fed rats; HFD SD: high-fat-diet-fed rats reversed to a SD chow; HFD SY680: high-fat-diet-fed rats reversed to a SD chow and supplemented with yacon flour (680 mg FOS/kg b. w.).

free fatty acids towards a healthy atherogenic index in HFD-fed rats, with a higher effect at 680 mg FOS/kg b. w.

One of the mechanisms by which the yacon root triggers weight loss seems to be a decrease in energy intake, given our observation of a lower food intake after yacon supplementation. Dietary fiber is known to attenuate food intake through different mechanisms that include the displacement of certain nutrients in the diet by the fiber; the inhibition of food absorption in the small intestine; and modification of satiety hormone response with appetite reduction [39]. It is well recognized that FOS could also be a fermentable substrate for the colon microbiota, being low polymerization FOS (DP2-10) the most used by *Bifidobacterium* spp. and *Lactobacillus* spp. [16]. Bifidobacteria have been shown to be beneficial to the health of the host and to be correlated with a lean state [40]. Bacterial fermentation of FOS in the cecum and proximal colon has been shown to produce short chain fatty acids such as acetate, propionate and butyrate. In addition, dietary polyphenols directly or indirectly impact on gut function, decreasing pathogenic bacterial growth and promoting the production of the microbial short chain fatty acids by beneficial microbial populations [23]. These carboxylic acids, especially butyrate, are also capable of stimulating the L-cells of the intestinal mucosa increasing the secretion of gut hormones that are involved in appetite regulation [41]. It has been reported that inulin-type fructans fermentation increase the production of the anorexigenic hormones glucagon-like peptide-1 (GLP-1) and peptide YY (PYY) in rodents affecting the food intake and energy expenditure [42, 43]. Consistently, in the present work, we reported an increased expression of Gcg (the GLP-1 precursor) and PYY genes in the distal ileum of yacon supplemented HFD rats. In concordance, increased GLP-1 levels in the colon and in serum were shown when yacon roots were administered to diabetic rats [25]. Thus, FOS and phenolic compounds present in yacon flour could be able to decrease body weight in HFD rats, through the central action of GLP-1 and PYY.

Chronic consumption of a high-fat diet has been shown to produce obesity characterized by a separate or simultaneous increase in adipocyte number and size [2]. Yacon roots had a significant effect on the reduction of visceral adipose tissue mass and adipocyte size. The expansion of adipose tissue begins when differentiated adipocytes rapidly respond to nutrient excess acting as lipid-synthesizing and lipid storing cells [5]. The differentiation of preadipocytes involves a highly regulated and coordinated cascade of transcription factors, where PPAR-γ and C/EBPa play a central role [4, 44]. PPAR-γ2 is the major regulator of adipogenesis and is also required for the maintenance of the adipocyte differentiated state [45]. PPAR-γ2, a splicing isoform of PPAR-γ, is selectively expressed in the adipose tissues. In powerful synergy with C/EBPa, PPAR-γ2 controls adipocyte differentiation and lipid metabolism by regulating transcription factors such as aP2 and lipogenic/lipolytic genes and thus enhances the efficiency of lipid utilization [46, 47]. aP2 is a carrier protein for fatty acids mainly expressed in adipocytes and macrophages and plays an important role in the development of insulin resistance and metaflammation [45]. In our study, the mRNA levels of the transcription factor PPAR-γ2 and its target genes C/EBPa and aP2 increased in the visceral adipose tissue of the HFD-fed rats. Similarly, previous reports indicated that PPAR-γ2 mediates high-fat-diet-induced adipocyte differentiation and adipocyte hypertrophy to generate large adipocytes and insulin resistance in obese patients [48] and in animal models [49]. Thus, decreased PPAR-γ, C/EBPa, and aP2 expression in visceral adipose tissue by yacon supplement may suppress adipogenesis, enhancing insulin sensitivity, and lowering blood lipid concentrations. Similarly, it has been reported that inulin-type fructans have an effect on differentiation and triglyceride accumulation in adipocytes through a decrease in PPARγ-activated processes [50].

Increased adiposity during obesity greatly influences insulin sensitivity, glucose and lipid metabolism, and inflammation [3, 8, 45]. In the present study, rats long exposed to high-fat diet developed a hyperglycemic state associated with insulin resistance and/or glucose intolerance. Adiponectin is the most abundantly adipokine expressed in adipose tissue with pleiotropic insulin-sensitizing effects. It has been shown that it reduces hepatic glucose production and stimulates glucose uptake and fatty acid oxidation in skeletal muscle [51]. Leptin, another adipokine, regulates weight balance, glucose, and lipids metabolism [52]. While adiponectin levels reduce in response to excessive fat depots, plasma leptin concentrations are positively associated with the amount of body fat [53]. In our study, yacon supplement to obese animals modified adiponectin and leptin plasma

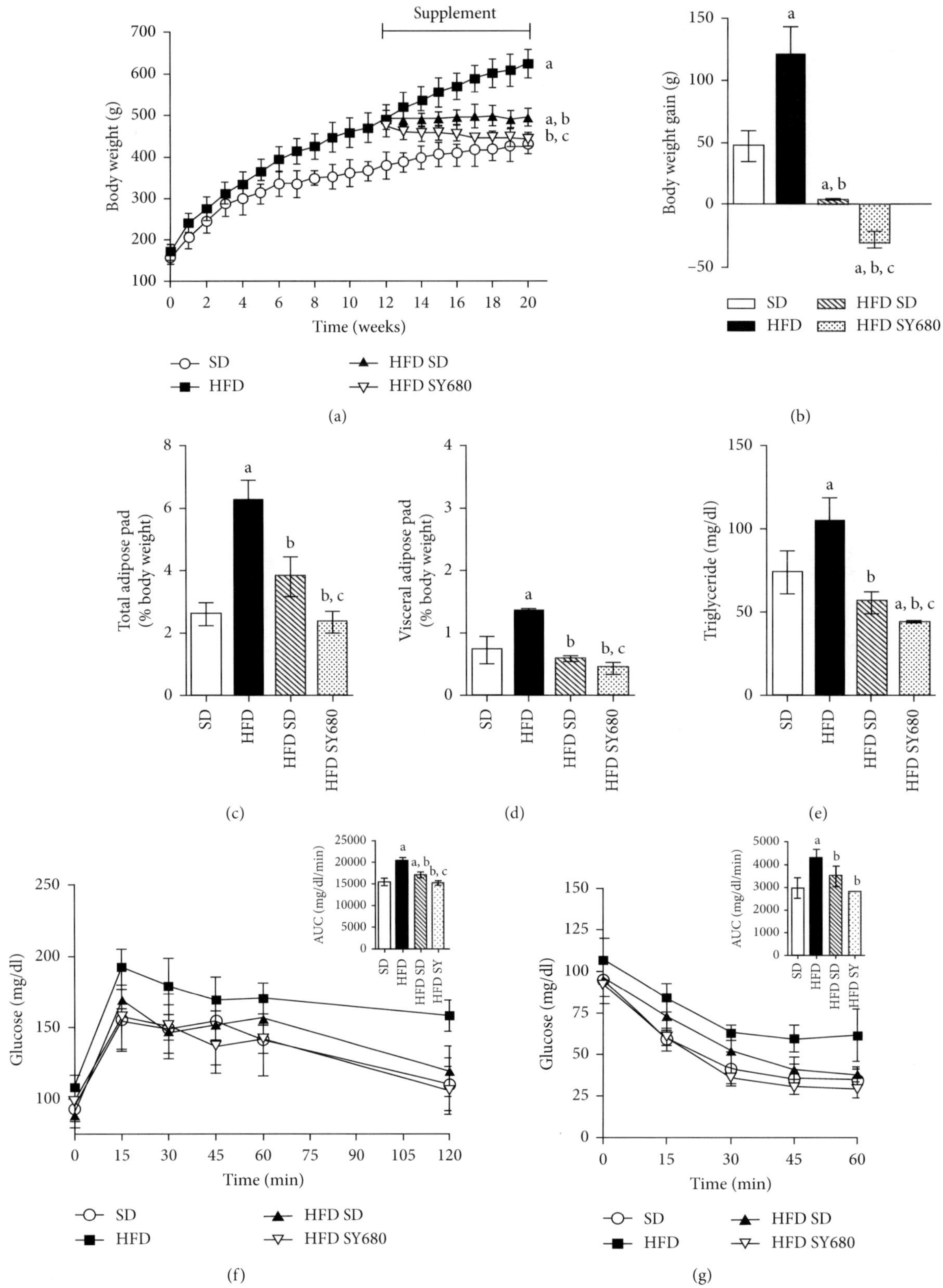

FIGURE 7: Effects of yacon supplement and the reversion to a SD chow on HFD-induced metabolic disease. (a) Body weight. (b) Body weight gain. (c) Total fat weight. (d) Visceral fat pad weight. (e) Fasting triglyceride concentrations. (f) Time course of glycemia in response to oral glucose overload (2 g/kg body weight) at 8 weeks (insert: area under the curve of blood glucose following glucose overload). (g) Time course of glycemia following a single intraperitoneal (i.p.) injection of insulin (0.75 U/kg b. w.) (insert: area under the curve of blood glucose following insulin injection). Data are mean ± standard deviation ($n = 6$/group). $^{a}p < 0.05$ vs. SD, $^{b}p < 0.05$ vs. HFD, $^{c}p < 0.05$ vs. HFD SD. SD: standard-diet-fed rats; HFD: high-fat-diet-fed rats; HFD SD: high-fat-diet-fed rats reversed to a SD chow; HFD SY680: high-fat-diet-fed rats reversed to a SD chow and supplemented with yacon flour (680 mg FOS/kg b.w.).

concentrations increasing adiponectin/leptin ratio. Thus, the improved glucose tolerance and insulin action in obese rats after yacon supplementation may lead us to suggest that this beneficial effect could be mediated by adipokines modulation as was suggested previously [54]. Moreover, releasing GLP-1 from intestinal L-cells directly into the portal vein could also represent an additional mechanism related to yacon FOS-improved glucose homeostasis [55]. On the other hand, phenolic compounds are been involved in the regulation of postprandial glycemia and glucose tolerance also modulating gastrointestinal hormone secretion [56].

Obesity is now considered as a chronic inflammatory state linked to an abnormal cytokine production and the activation of inflammatory signaling pathways in adipose tissue [1, 3, 5]. The excess of nutrients induces the accumulation of macrophages, through the monocyte chemoattractant protein-1 (MCP-1), and is implicated in the development and maintenance of obesity-induced adipose tissue inflammation [57]. In the present study, we described an increased expression of MCP-1 and the macrophage marker F4/80 in the adipose tissue of obese animals which was significantly reduced by yacon supplement. This allows us to suggest that inhibition of MCP-1 by yacon supplement could lead to a low level of macrophage infiltration contributing to reduce adipose tissue inflammation improving insulin resistance and metabolic state. Moreover, our results also demonstrated that yacon treatment significantly decreased circulating levels of proinflammatory cytokines TNF-α and IL-1β in HDF-rats. This fact could be related to lower levels of TNFα, IL-1β, and MCP1 in the adipose tissues of supplemented HFD rats. Furthermore, it has been established that inflammatory cytokines TNF-α and IL-6 inhibit the expression of insulin signaling mediators in adipose tissue leading to a worsening of whole-body insulin resistance and glucose intolerance [1, 3]. Our results demonstrated that long-term yacon supplementation ameliorates abnormal insulin signaling cascades in the visceral adipose tissue of HFD rats by enhancing the phosphorylation level of the Akt protein, the pAkt/Akt ratio, and pAkt/Insulin ratio. In agreement with this, Satoh et al. [58] using a euglycemic-hyperinsulinemic clamp procedure demonstrated that yacon diet improved hepatic insulin sensitivity by increasing liver Akt activation in Zucker fa/fa rats.

High-fat diet is considered a direct cause in the development of dyslipidemia during obesity [31, 32]. The data obtained in the present study demonstrated that yacon flour administered to obese rats improved the lipids profile, reducing triglycerides and LDLc. It is interesting to note that the beneficial effects in lipids metabolism are more evident when yacon supplementation is accompanied by a standard diet. As previously reported by us, yacon roots exhibit a lipid lowering effect, mainly reducing serum triglycerides and VLDLc levels, in normal and diabetic rats [17, 25]. Moreover, in human studies, we demonstrate that yacon syrup lowers plasma lipid concentrations and decreases glycemia in patients with insulin resistance [30]. The triglyceride lowering effect could explain at least in part the inhibition of *de novo* fatty acid synthesis and downregulation of lipogenic enzymes as has been suggested for oligofructose [59]. In addition, it is well known that soluble dietary fibers delay fat absorption as we observed during the fat load test, contributing to the hypolipidemic effects of yacon.

On the other hand, the lack of significant changes in total cholesterol levels in our study may be explained by the short supplement-time and/or the concentration of FOS utilized in our study. Reductions in cholesterol have only been found with long-term feeding of oligofructose in relatively high doses [60]. Additionally, the presence chlorogenic and caffeic acid in yacon roots could also contribute to the hypolipidemic effect observed after yacon supplement [18]. It was established that caffeic acid, particularly chlorogenic acid, improves lipid metabolism in high-fat-diet-induced obese mice [61].

5. Conclusion

The data presented in this study suggest that yacon may act by different ways to suppress body weight gain, food intake, FER levels, weight and size of adipose tissue, and serum levels of triglyceride and improve adipokine profile in HFD-fed rats. These results can be associated with the decrease in adipogenesis related to mRNA expression of PPAR-γ, C/EBPa, and aP2. The high content of nondigestible fermentable fibers present in yacon roots as FOS together with phenolic compounds could be largely responsible for the beneficial effects observed. This simple dietary intervention appears to be capable of improving obesity outcomes regardless of susceptibility to an obesogenic nutritional environment. Hence, yacon roots can be considered a potent and useful functional food.

Authors' Contributions

SMH and SSS were Career Investigators of CONICET.

Acknowledgments

This research was supported by PIP 2015 (no. 183) (CONICET Argentina), PIUNT D549-2 (SCAIT-UNT, Argentina), PICT 2013 (no. 1949), and PICT-2017 (no. 3941) (ANPCyT, Argentina) grants to SSS and SMH. We wish to thank to Dr. Afredo Grau, Regional Ecology Institute (UNT, Argentina), for supplying yacon roots and Dr. Alejandra Kortsarz for skilled technical assistance with FOS estimation. MVG and JGR received CONICET fellowship.

yacon improves nutritional parameters after HFD rats turned to a SD feeding. (

References

[1] G. S. Hotamisligil, "Inflammation, metaflammation and immunometabolic disorders," *Nature*, vol. 542, no. 7640, pp. 177–185, 2017.

[2] R. N. Redinger, "Fat storage and the biology of energy expenditure," *Translational Research*, vol. 154, no. 2, pp. 52–60, 2009.

[3] A. Engin, "The pathogenesis of obesity-associated adipose tissue inflammation," in *Advances in Experimental Medicine and Biology*, vol. 960, pp. 221–245, Springer, Berlin, Germany, 2017.

[4] Q. Q. Tang and M. D. Lane, "Adipogenesis: from stem cell to adipocyte," *Annual Review of Biochemistry*, vol. 81, no. 1, pp. 715–736, 2012.

[5] J. M. Rutkowski, J. H. Stern, and P. Scherer, "The cell biology of fat expansion," *Journal of Cell Biology*, vol. 208, no. 5, pp. 501–512, 2015.

[6] T. D. Cummins, C. R. Holden, B. E. Sansbury et al., "Metabolic remodeling of white adipose tissue in obesity," *American Journal of Physiology-Endocrinology and Metabolism*, vol. 307, no. 3, pp. E262–E277, 2014.

[7] N. Abate, A. E. Sumner, and M. S. Chandalia, "Manifestations of adipose tissue dysfunction," *Journal of Obesity*, vol. 2013, Article ID 940275, 1 pages, 2013.

[8] P. S. Patel, E. D. Buras, and A. Balasubramanyam, "The role of the immune system in obesity and insulin resistance," *Journal of Obesity*, vol. 2013, Article ID 616193, 9 pages, 2013.

[9] American College of Cardiology/American Heart Association Task Force on Practice Guidelines and Obesity Expert Panel, "Expert panel report: guidelines (2013) for the management of overweight and obesity in adults," *Obesity*, vol. 22, no. S2, pp. S41–410, 2014.

[10] M. Glandt and I. Raz, "Present and future: pharmacologic treatment of obesity," *Journal of Obesity*, vol. 2011, p. 636181, 2011.

[11] A. Velazquez and C. M. Apovian, "Updates on obesity pharmacotherapy," *Annals of the New York Academy of Sciences*, vol. 1411, no. 1, pp. 106–119, 2018.

[12] A. Grandone, A. Di Sessa, G. R. Umano, R. Toraldo, and E. M. Del Giudice, "New treatment modalities for obesity," *Best Practice & Research Clinical Endocrinology & Metabolism*, vol. 32, no. 4, pp. 535–549, 2018.

[13] N. N. Sun, T. Y. Wu, and C. F. Chau, "Natural dietary and herbal products in anti-obesity treatment," *Molecules*, vol. 21, no. 10, p. 1351, 2016.

[14] J. Seminario, M. Valderrama, and I. Manrique, *El yacon: fundamentos para el aprovechamiento de un recurso promisorio*, CIP, Universidad Nacional de Cajamarca, Agencia Suiza para el desarrollo y la Cooperación (COSUDE), Lima, Peru, 2003, http://www.cipotato.org/market/pdfdocs/yacon_fundamentos_password.pdf.

[15] S. M. Honoré, S. B. Genta, and S. S. Sanchez, "*Smallanthus sonchifolius* (yacon) leaves: an emerging source of compounds for diabetes management," *Journal of Research in Biology*, vol. 5, no. 5, pp. 21–42, 2015.

[16] R. Pedreschi, D. Campos, G. Noratto, R. Chirinos, and L. Cisneros-Zevallos, "Andean yacon root (*Smallanthus sonchifolius* Poepp. Endl) fructooligosaccharides as a potential novel source of prebiotics," *Journal of Agricultural and Food Chemistry*, vol. 51, no. 18, pp. 5278–5284, 2003.

[17] S. B. Genta, W. M. Cabrera, A. Grau, and S. S. Sánchez, "Subchronic 4-month oral toxicity study of dried *Smallanthus sonchifolius* (yacon) roots as a diet supplement in rats," *Food and Chemical Toxicology*, vol. 43, no. 11, pp. 1657–1665, 2005.

[18] J. Lachman, E. C. Fernandez, and M. Orzak, "Yacon [*Smallanthus sonchifolia* (Poepp. et Endl.) H. Robinson] chemical composition and use: a review," *Plant, Soil and Environment*, vol. 49, no. 6, pp. 283–290, 2003.

[19] M. B. Roberfroid, "Inulin-type fructans: functional food ingredients," *Journal of Nutrition*, vol. 137, no. 11, pp. 2493S–2502S, 2007.

[20] M. Geyer, I. Manrique, L. Degen, and C. Beglinger, "Effect of yacon (*Smallanthus sonchifolius*) on colonic transit time in healthy volunteers," *Digestion*, vol. 78, no. 1, pp. 30–33, 2008.

[21] Md Vaz-Tostes, M. L. Viana, M. Grancieri et al., "Yacon effects in immune response and nutritional status of iron and zinc in preschool children," *Nutrition*, vol. 30, no. 6, pp. 666–672, 2014.

[22] M. F. Gomes da Silva, A. P. Dionísio, A. A. F. Carioca et al., "Yacon syrup: food applications and impact on satiety in healthy volunteers," *Food Research International*, vol. 100, pp. 460–467, 2017.

[23] G. Williamson and M. N. Clifford, "Role of the small intestine, colon and microbiota in determining the metabolic fate of polyphenols," *Biochemical Pharmacology*, vol. 139, pp. 24–39, 2017.

[24] M. Dueñas, I. Muñoz-González, C. Cueva et al., "A survey of modulation of gut microbiota by dietary polyphenols," *BioMed Research International*, vol. 2015, Article ID 850902, 15 pages, 2015.

[25] N. C. Habib, S. M. Honoré, S. B. Genta, and S. S. Sánchez, "Hypolipidemic effect of *Smallanthus sonchifolius* (yacon) roots on diabetic rats: biochemical approach," *Chemico-Biological Interactions*, vol. 194, no. 1, pp. 31–39, 2011.

[26] G. O. Oliveira, C. P. Braga, and A. A. Fernandes, "Improvement of biochemical parameters in type 1 diabetic rats after the roots aqueous extract of yacon [*Smallanthus sonchifolius* (Poepp.& Endl.)] treatment," *Food and Chemical Toxicology*, vol. 59, pp. 256–260, 2013.

[27] N. C. Habib, C. Serra-Barcellona, S. M. Honoré, S. B. Genta, and S. S. Sánchez, "Yacon roots (*Smallanthus sonchifolius*) improve oxidative stress in diabetic rats," *Pharmaceutical Biology*, vol. 53, no. 8, pp. 1183–1193, 2015.

[28] S. Sousa, J. Pinto, C. Rodrigues et al., "Antioxidant properties of sterilized yacon (*Smallanthus sonchifolius*) tuber flour," *Food Chemistry*, vol. 188, pp. 504–509, 2015.

[29] G. T. Delgado, R. Thomé, D. L. Gabriel, W. M. Tamashiro, and G. M. Pastore, "Yacon (*Smallanthus sonchifolius*)-derived fructooligosaccharides improves the immune parameters in the mouse," *Nutrition Research*, vol. 32, no. 11, pp. 884–892, 2012.

[30] S. Genta, W. Cabrera, N. Habib et al., "Yacon syrup: beneficial effects on obesity and insulin resistance in humans," *Clinical Nutrition*, vol. 28, no. 2, pp. 182–187, 2009.

[31] M. Tschöp and M. L. Heiman, "Rodent obesity models: an overview," *Experimental and Clinical Endocrinology & Diabetes*, vol. 109, no. 6, pp. 307–319, 2001.

[32] C. Marques, M. Meireles, S. Norberto et al., "High-fat diet-induced obesity rat model: a comparison between Wistar and Sprague-Dawley rat," *Adipocyte*, vol. 5, no. 1, pp. 11–21, 2015.

[33] R. Zhang, J. Zhou, M. Li et al., "Ameliorating effect and potential mechanism of *Rehmannia glutinosa* oligosaccharides on the impaired glucose metabolism in chronic stress rats fed with high-fat diet," *Phytomedicine*, vol. 21, no. 5, pp. 607–614, 2014.

[34] C. J. Pollock, "Oligosaccharide intermediates of fructan synthesis in *Lolium temulentum*," *Phytochemistry*, vol. 21, no. 10, pp. 2461–2465, 1982.

[35] M. Dubois, K. Gilles, J. K. Hamilton, P. A. Rebers, and F. Smith, "Colorimetric method for determinations of sugars and related substances," *Analytical Chemistry*, vol. 28, no. 3, pp. 350–356, 1956.

[36] A. L. Waterhouse, "Polyphenolics: determination of total phenolics," in *Current Protocols in Food Analytical Chemistry*, R. E. Wrolstad, Ed., pp. 11–18, Wiley, New York, NY, USA, 2002.

[37] E. L. Novelli, Y. S. Diniz, C. M. Galhardi et al., "Anthropometrical parameters and markers of obesity in rats," *Laboratory Animals*, vol. 41, no. 1, pp. 111–119, 2007.

[38] D. W. Stovall, A. P. Bailey, and L. M. Pastore, "Assessment of insulin resistance and impaired glucose tolerance in lean women with polycystic ovary syndrome," *Journal of Women's Health*, vol. 20, no. 1, pp. 37–43, 2011.

[39] J. L. Slavin, "Dietary fiber and body weight," *Nutrition*, vol. 21, no. 3, pp. 411–418, 2005.

[40] G. Musso, R. Gambino, and M. Cassader, "Gut microbiota as a regulator of energy homeostasis and ectopic fat deposition: mechanisms and implications for metabolic disorders," *Current Opinion in Lipidology*, vol. 21, no. 1, pp. 76–83, 2010.

[41] I. Kaji, S. Karaki, and A. Kuwahara, "Short-chain fatty acid receptor and its contribution to glucagon-like peptide-1 release," *Digestion*, vol. 89, no. 1, pp. 31–36, 2014.

[42] P. D. Cani, A. M. Neyrinck, N. Maton, and N. M. Delzenne, "Oligofructose promotes satiety in rats fed a high-fat diet: involvement of glucagon-like Peptide-1," *Obesity Research*, vol. 13, no. 6, pp. 1000–1007, 2005.

[43] J. A. Parnell and R. A. Reimer, "Weight loss during oligofructose supplementation is associated with decreased ghrelin and increased peptide YY in overweight and obese adults," *American Journal of Clinical Nutrition*, vol. 89, no. 6, pp. 1751–1759, 2009.

[44] S. R. Farmer, "Transcriptional control of adipocyte formation," *Cell Metabolism*, vol. 4, no. 4, pp. 263–273, 2006.

[45] R. Stienstra, C. Duval, M. Muller, and S. Kersten, "PPARs, obesity, and inflammation," *PPAR Research*, vol. 2007, Article ID 95974, 10 pages, 2007.

[46] W. T. Festuccia, M. Laplante, M. Berthiaume, Y. Gelinas, and Y. Deshaies, "PPAR gamma agonism increases rat adipose tissue lipolysis, expression of glyceride lipases, and the response of lipolysis to hormonal control," *Diabetologia*, vol. 49, no. 10, pp. 2427–2436, 2006.

[47] D. Li, F. Zhang, X. Zhang et al., "Distinct functions of PPARγ isoforms in regulating adipocyte plasticity," *Biochemical and Biophysical Research Communications*, vol. 481, no. 1-2, pp. 132–138, 2016.

[48] F. Diraison, E. Dusserre, H. Vidal, M. Sothier, and M. Beylot, "Increased hepatic lipogenesis but decreased expression of lipogenic gene in adipose tissue in human obesity," *American Journal of Physiology-Endocrinology and Metabolism*, vol. 282, no. 1, pp. E46–E51, 2002.

[49] S. Kim, Y. Jin, Y. Choi, and T. Park, "Resveratrol exerts anti-obesity effects via mechanisms involving down-regulation of adipogenic and inflammatory processes in mice," *Biochemical Pharmacology*, vol. 81, no. 11, pp. 1343–1351, 2011.

[50] E. M. Dewulf, P. D. Cani, A. M. Neyrinck et al., "Inulin-type fructans with prebiotic properties counteract GPR43 overexpression and PPARγ-related adipogenesis in the white adipose tissue of high-fat diet-fed mice," *Journal of Nutritional Biochemistry*, vol. 22, no. 8, pp. 712–722, 2011.

[51] E. Hu, P. Liang, and B. M. Spiegelman, "AdipoQ is a novel adiposespecific gene dysregulated in obesity," *Journal of Biological Chemistry*, vol. 271, no. 18, pp. 10697–10703, 1996.

[52] H. Cui, M. López, and K. Rahmouni, "The cellular and molecular bases of leptin and ghrelin resistance in obesity," *Nature Reviews Endocrinology*, vol. 13, no. 6, pp. 338–351, 2017.

[53] K. G. Park, K. S. Park, M. J. Kim et al., "Relationship between serum adiponectin and leptin concentrations and body fat distribution," *Diabetes Research and Clinical Practice*, vol. 63, no. 2, pp. 135–142, 2004.

[54] M. V. Grande, S. S. Sánchez, and S. M. Honoré, "Dietary supplementation with *Smallanthus sonchifolius* (yacon) flour improves visceral adiposity and metabolic parameters in high-fat diet fed rats," *Medicina*, vol. 77, no. 1, p. 445, 2017.

[55] R. A. Reimer and J. C. Russell, "Glucose tolerance, lipids, and GLP-1 secretion in JCR:LA-cp rats fed a high protein fiber diet," *Obesity*, vol. 16, no. 1, pp. 40–46, 2008.

[56] Z. Bahadoran, P. Mirmiran, and F. Azizi, "Dietary polyphenols as potential nutraceuticals in management of diabetes: a review," *Journal of Diabetes & Metabolic Disorders*, vol. 12, no. 1, p. 43, 2013.

[57] H. Kanda, S. Tateya, Y. Tamori et al., "MCP-1 contributes to macrophage infiltration into adipose tissue, insulin resistance, and hepatic steatosis in obesity," *Journal of Clinical Investigation*, vol. 116, no. 6, pp. 1494–1505, 2006.

[58] H. Satoh, M. T. Audrey Nguyen, A. Kudoh, and T. Watanabe, "Yacon diet (*Smallanthus sonchifolius*, Asteraceae) improves hepatic insulin resistance via reducing Trb3 expression in Zucker fa/fa rats," *Nutrition & Diabetes*, vol. 3, no. 5, p. e70, 2013.

[59] N. M. Delzenne and N. Kok, "Effects of fructans-type prebiotics on lipid metabolism," *American Journal of Clinical Nutrition*, vol. 73, no. 2, pp. 456S–458S, 2001.

[60] M. Beylot, "Effects of inulin-type fructans on lipid metabolism in man and in animal models," *British Journal of Nutrition*, vol. 93, no. 1, pp. S163–S168, 2005.

[61] A. S. Cho, S. M. Jeon, M. J. Kim et al., "Chlorogenic acid exhibits anti-obesity property and improves lipid metabolism in high-fat diet-induced-obese mice," *Food and Chemical Toxicology*, vol. 48, no. 3, pp. 937–943, 2010.

13

The Role of Race and Gender in Nutrition Habits and Self-Efficacy: Results from the Young Adult Weight Loss Study

Janna D. Stephens,[1] Andrew Althouse,[2] Alai Tan,[1] and Bernadette Mazurek Melnyk[1]

[1] *The Ohio State University College of Nursing, Columbus, OH, USA*
[2] *Heart and Vascular Institute, University of Pittsburgh Medical Center, Pittsburgh, PA, USA*

Correspondence should be addressed to Janna D. Stephens; stephens.653@osu.edu

Academic Editor: Aron Weller

Overweight and obesity are a massive public health problem and young adults are at high risk for gaining weight once they enter a college. This study sought to examine gender and race as they relate to nutrition habits and self-efficacy in a population of diverse young adults from the Young Adult Weight Loss Study. Participants ($N = 62$) were 29% males, 38.7% white, 33.8% Asian, and 12.9% African American. Males had lower self-efficacy for healthy eating (mean score = 92.5, SD = 17.1) compared to females (mean = 102.3, SD = 13.7, $p = 0.02$). Males had higher consumption of sodium compared to females (4308 versus 3239 milligrams/day, $p = 0.01$). There were no significant differences across racial subgroups in self-efficacy for healthy eating ($p = 0.67$) or self-efficacy for exercise ($p = 0.61$). Higher self-efficacy scores for healthy eating were significantly associated with less total sodium ($r = -0.37$, $p = 0.007$), greater fruit consumption, and less saturated fat. Our results indicate that weight loss interventions should be individualized and that there may be specific areas to target that are different for men and women. Additional larger studies should be conducted to confirm if racial differences exist across nutrition habits and self-efficacy and to confirm gender differences noted in this study.

1. Introduction

Overweight/obesity is a major public health concern in the United States (US) as reported by the most recent National Health and Nutrition Examination Survey (NHANES), with 60.3% of adults aged 20–39 years being overweight (BMI 25.0–29.9) or obese (BMI $\geq$ 30) [1]. Certain subgroups of the population have higher rates of overweight/obesity; for example, non-Hispanic blacks are reported to have a rate of 71.9% among those aged 20–39 years [1]. Obesity has been linked to many significant health concerns, including hypertension, type 2 diabetes, coronary heart disease, stroke, osteoarthritis, certain types of cancer, and mortality [2, 3].

The transition out of high school to college or an independent setting has been identified as a critical time for establishing healthy lifestyle habits as individuals are traditionally more independent and they experience major changes in their overall habits, including eating and exercise [3–8]. A recent report from the American College Health Association indicated that less than 5% of college students consume 5 or more servings of fruit/vegetables per day and 80% report not meeting the Physical Activity Guidelines for Americans [9]. In addition, this newfound independence can lead to a lack of self-efficacy for healthy eating and exercise [6, 10, 11]. Being overweight/obese during these transition years seriously increases the probability that these youth will remain overweight.

We sought to characterize factors associated with self-efficacy for healthy eating and self-efficacy for exercise in a group of young adults from the Young Adult Weight Loss (YAWL) Study.

2. Methods

2.1. Study Design. This descriptive study used baseline data collected from the YAWL randomized controlled trial testing a weight loss intervention in young adults who were overweight or obese [12]. The full details and methods of the YAWL randomized controlled trial are described elsewhere [12]. For the purposes of this study, we examined the distribution and correlations of specific baseline data collected including healthy eating self-efficacy, exercise self-efficacy, nutrition knowledge, exercise habits, and healthy eating habits.

2.2. Sample and Setting. In the YAWL study those who met the inclusion criteria (BMI 25–40 kg/m^2, aged 18–25 years, and owning an iPhone or Android device) were eligible to participate. Participants were recruited in and around a university setting on the east coast, although participants were not required to be a college or university student. Recruitment methods consisted of flyers/posters, social media posts, email announcements, and word of mouth. Sixty-two participants consented to be in the study. For the purposes of this study, all 62 individuals who had baseline data were included in the analysis.

2.3. Measures and Instruments. Data was collected at the baseline study visit and entered into the Research Electronic Data Capture (REDCap) application, a secure, web-based application. Height and weight were measured by research personnel with the participant in light clothing. All questionnaires were collected on paper and pencil, except the Automated Self-Administered 24-Hour Recall (ASA24), which was collected via the participant's computer immediately following the baseline visit. Physical activity was assessed using the Godin Leisure-Time Exercise Questionnaire, dietary habits were assessed using the ASA-24, nutritional knowledge was measured with the nutrition knowledge survey, and self-efficacy was measured for both healthy eating and physical activity.

The Godin Leisure-Time Exercise Questionnaire is self-administered and assesses a total score for strenuous, moderate, and mild activity over a 7-day period as well as assessing the time spent in activity long enough to work up a sweat [13]. The ASA24 is a web-based, automated self-administered 24-hour recall of foods. The ASA24 provides analysis on calories, nutrients, and food group estimates [14]. Information obtained from the ASA-24 included caloric intake, food pyramid equivalents, and nutrients from all foods reported according to the Food and Nutrient Database for Dietary Studies [14]. For the purposes of this study, we examined total fiber, sodium, saturated fat, fruit servings, and vegetable servings per day.

The Self-Efficacy for Healthy Eating Scale was a 13-item questionnaire that explored a person's belief in their ability to make better food choices in given situations. The Self-Efficacy for Exercise Scale was a 14-item questionnaire assessing an individual's belief in their ability to perform physical activity in given situations. Scores were calculated by adding each item score together to achieve an overall total score. The nutrition knowledge survey assesses knowledge on food consumption from sodium to fat to overall healthy meals [15]. This survey was scored by adding the numbers that were correct together to achieve a total score out of a maximum 40 points.

2.4. Statistical Analysis. Descriptive statistics were used to summarize sample characteristics and baseline measures of healthy eating self-efficacy, exercise self-efficacy, nutrition knowledge, exercise habits, and healthy eating habits by gender and racial groups. t-test and analysis of variance were used to test whether there was significant between-group difference in these baseline measures. Pearson correlation coefficients were used to examine the pair-wise associations between BMI, healthy eating self-efficacy, exercise self-efficacy, nutrition knowledge, exercise habits, and healthy eating habits. All significance tests were two-sided with significant level at 0.05. We used SAS 9.4 (SAS Institute®, Cary, NC) for the analysis.

3. Results

Participants ($N = 62$) were 18–25 years old, 29% males, 38.7% white, 33.8% Asian, and 12.9% African American. The overall median age was 20.0 (18.0–25.0) years, median BMI was 28.5 kg/m^2 (25.0–40.4), and median waist circumference was 93.8 cm (81.0–120.0) [12]. The sample was 90% current college student. Overall, 79% of participants were iPhone users while 21% of participants were Android users.

Males had lower self-efficacy for healthy eating (mean score = 92.5, SD = 17.1) when compared to females (mean = 102.3, SD = 13.7, and $p = 0.02$) but there was no gender difference in self-efficacy for exercise ($p = 0.95$). Males had higher consumption of sodium when compared to females (4308 versus 3239 milligrams/day, $p = 0.01$). There were no significant differences across racial subgroups in self-efficacy for healthy eating ($p = 0.67$) or self-efficacy for exercise ($p = 0.61$). There were no significant gender or racial differences in nutrition knowledge scores, although males and whites scored higher on average. Also, there were no significant differences across racial subgroups in healthy eating habits, although whites consumed more added sugars and more sodium than other racial subgroups. See Table 1 for full results.

We also examined the relationship between baseline BMI, self-efficacy for healthy eating and exercise, physical activity, and nutrition habits (Table 2). Higher self-efficacy scores for healthy eating were significantly associated with less total sodium ($r = -0.37$, $p = 0.007$), less saturated fat ($r = -0.48$, $p < 0.001$), and greater fruit consumption ($r = 0.284$, $p = 0.04$). Self-efficacy for exercise was associated with 7-day exercise habits ($r = 0.280$, $p = 0.03$). There was no significant association between self-efficacy and total fiber intake, total vegetable intake, or added sugar intake.

There was an association between fiber intake and other eating habits. Fiber intake was significantly associated with sodium consumption ($r = 0.294$, $p = 0.03$), fruit serving consumption ($r = 0.487$, $p < 0.001$), and vegetable serving consumption ($r = 0.431$, $p = 0.001$). In addition, vegetable serving consumption was associated with fruit serving consumption ($r = 0.430$, $p = 0.001$), and sodium consumption

TABLE 1: Mean (SD) by sex and race/ethnicity.

	Male ($n = 18$)	Female ($n = 44$)	p value[$]	White ($n = 24$)	Black ($n = 8$)	Asian ($n = 21$)	Other ($n = 9$)	p value[¥]
Healthy eating self-efficacy	92.5 (17.1)	102.3 (13.7)	**0.02**	101.3 (16.7)	102.1 (11.1)	96.1 (14.3)	99.8 (17.9)	0.67
Exercise self-efficacy	85.7 (22.5)	85.4 (20.5)	0.95	88.5 (24.7)	85.4 (18.1)	80.4 (19.7)	89.6 (15.5)	0.61
Godin leisure time score	42.1 (24.4)	31.9 (19.2)	0.08	34.0 (24.9)	31.1 (22.2)	36.0 (19.1)	38.1 (17.5)	0.92
Nutrition knowledge	28.8 (4.1)	28.1 (3.6)	0.47	29.3 (4.3)	27.5 (3.5)	27.5 (3.5)	28.4 (2.7)	0.40
Total fiber (g)	13.4 (6.6)	15.4 (10.1)	0.48	17.0 (10.9)	16.9 (11.9)	12.5 (7.7)	13.5 (5.1)	0.49
Total sodium (mg)	4308 (1646)	3239 (1203)	**0.01**	3682 (1411)	3499 (1372)	3509 (1583)	3254 (1197)	0.90
Total saturated fat (g)	33.0 (16.1)	25.4 (14.0)	0.11	26.4 (16.1)	31.1 (21.6)	26.6 (13.7)	29.4 (9.9)	0.85
Vegetable servings/day	1.4 (1.1)	1.3 (1.3)	0.81	1.5 (1.0)	0.6 (0.7)	1.5 (1.5)	1.2 (1.2)	0.39
Fruit servings/day	0.7 (1.0)	1.3 (1.6)	0.24	0.9 (1.0)	1.9 (1.1)	1.0 (2.1)	1.1 (1.0)	0.55
Total added sugar (g)	9.8 (10.3)	11.0 (9.2)	0.70	13.9 (11.1)	10.2 (6.9)	7.0 (7.7)	11.6 (8.5)	0.21

[$] *t*-test.
[¥] ANOVA.

was associated with total saturated fat ($r = 0.633$, $p < 0.001$) and vegetable serving consumption ($r = 0.405$, $p = 0.003$).

BMI was marginally associated with sugar consumption ($r = 0.29$, $p = 0.04$) and fruit consumption ($r = 0.26$, $p = 0.07$) and not associated with healthy eating self-efficacy, exercise self-efficacy, nutrition knowledge, exercise habits, and other healthy eating habits.

4. Discussion

The results presented in this paper are from a unique study examining the use of a Smartphone application and text messaging for weight loss in a diverse group of young adults.

Studies report that as many as 68% of first-year college students gain weight [16]. Both males and females have been reported to gain a substantial amount of weight, which significantly increases their BMI and percent body fat over a 4-year period [16]. A recent meta-analysis concluded that weight gain is significant in college students, even beyond the first year, with students gaining up to 20.2 pounds (9.20 kg) over four years [17]. In recent studies reporting a positive relationship between healthy beliefs and behaviors, results tend to be reported as a whole, rather than broken down by gender and race [18, 19]. Therefore, there may be key differences between groups that, if identified, could lead to more successful intervention programs.

Our current study sought to examine results based on gender and race reported. Overall, males had a lower self-efficacy for healthy eating and consumed more sodium on average than females. The lower self-efficacy and subsequent poorer nutritional habits indicate that males may need an intervention that focuses specifically on increasing self-efficacy for healthy eating before researchers can expect to see any significant changes in nutritional habits. It is interesting to note that males scored higher than females on the nutrition knowledge survey in our study. This could indicate that males have the knowledge needed to eat healthy and yet recognize that they cannot commit to healthy eating behaviors, thus leading to lower self-efficacy scores. However, in similar studies conducted in college students, no differences were noted in nutrition knowledge scores between males and females, but reports show that those who score better on nutrition knowledge have healthier eating habits [20, 21]. This information could be used in tailoring interventions in that males could receive less education but more assistance with adherence.

In addition, cultural differences exist that may affect weight perception in late adolescents and young adults. Studies report that black females believe a larger amount of weight is gained normally during college compared to their white counterparts and some identify themselves as normal weight when they are overweight or obese; therefore these characteristics may act to mediate the effects of a weight loss intervention [22, 23]. It is important to note that there is limited research which focuses on race and weight in this population. Of the 49 studies in a recent meta-analysis, only 2 (4%) of the studies were not conducted with predominately Caucasian samples [17]. Of the remaining 47 studies, 40 (85%) had samples comprised of ≥75% Caucasian subjects [17].

Our results from examining racial subgroups by self-efficacy scores indicated no significant differences. Therefore, it appears that the racial groups from the YAWL study had similar beliefs in their ability to perform exercise and healthy eating habits. However, nutritional habits, although not significant, were poorer in whites than other racial subgroups. Other studies conducted had similar results reporting poorer nutrition for whites compared to African Americans and Hispanics [24]. Whites consumed more sodium and added sugars. A more in-depth approach to examining nutrition habits should be performed across racial subgroups. Intervention materials, specifically text messages focusing on healthy eating, may be better tailored to specific nutrients for certain groups. For example, from the current analysis, it appears that white males should receive messages that focus predominately on sodium consumption. In addition, we were limited by the information we obtained from the ASA24. In the future, it may be beneficial to look at whole

Table 2: Correlation matrix (method: Pearson correlation).

Variable	Pearson correlation coefficient ($N = 62$)									
	BMI	Healthy eating self-efficacy	Exercise self-efficacy	Godin leisure time score	Nutrition knowledge	Total fiber (g)	Total sodium (mg)	Total saturated fat	Total vegetable servings per day	Total fruit servings per day
BMI	1.000	—	—	—	—	—	—	—	—	—
Healthy eating self-efficacy	0.002	1.000	—	—	—	—	—	—	—	—
Exercise self-efficacy	−0.069	0.312*	1.000	—	—	—	—	—	—	—
Godin leisure time score	−0.074	−0.020	0.280*	1.000	—	—	—	—	—	—
Nutrition knowledge	0.019	−0.014	0.170	0.093	1.000	—	—	—	—	—
Total fiber (g)	0.010	0.086	0.236	−0.092	0.249	1.000	—	—	—	—
Total sodium (mg)	−0.013	−0.371**	−0.196	−0.136	0.133	0.294*	1.000	—	—	—
Total saturated fat	−0.060	−0.481***	−0.172	−0.194	0.080	0.248	0.633***	1.000	—	—
Total vegetable servings per day	−0.054	0.080	0.091	−0.017	0.225	0.431***	0.405**	0.053	1.000	—
Total fruit servings per day	0.256	0.284*	0.144	−0.066	0.123	0.487***	0.052	−0.128	0.430**	1.000
Total added sugars	0.288*	−0.101	−0.011	−0.292*	−0.074	0.257	0.040	0.188	−0.203	0.032

*$p < 0.05$, **$p < 0.01$, and ***$p < 0.001$.

foods consumed across racial subgroups to better identify differences in diet that could possibly be related to culture.

Self-efficacy for healthy eating scores was significantly associated with better eating habits. In addition, self-efficacy for exercise was associated with better exercise habits. With these results, it appears that self-efficacy could be a prime target area for interventions leading to healthier lifestyle habits. It may be beneficial for researchers to focus on building self-efficacy of a certain behavior before asking a participant to perform that behavior.

Results from the current analysis could contribute to the refinement of the intervention utilizing a Smartphone application and text messaging for weight loss in diverse young adults by providing more information on how to individualize and personalize pieces of the intervention package. Perhaps the structure of weight loss interventions in the young adult population should begin with a period of efficacy building followed by a period of behavior change to see maximum results. Program(s) with that structure should be evaluated in a subsequent randomized controlled trial.

There were several limitations to this analysis. A small sample size of $N = 62$ individuals was analyzed. In addition, all data collected on diet and exercise was self-report. Finally, this study was conducted on a single campus located on the east coast. A larger randomized controlled trial should be conducted with long-term outcomes to determine if these results are reproducible in a larger, diverse sample. Also, instruments should be used to collect direct data on exercise and eating habits rather than relying on self-report.

5. Conclusion

The results from this secondary analysis of the YAWL study indicate that self-efficacy for healthy eating and that for exercise are important factors related to healthy eating and exercise behaviors. Although no racial differences were noted, there were gender differences that should be considered when planning future interventions. A larger randomized controlled trial is needed to evaluate the results from this analysis.

References

[1] C. L. Ogden, M. D. Carroll, B. K. Kit, and K. M. Flegal, "Prevalence of childhood and adult obesity in the United States, 2011-2012," *JAMA—Journal of the American Medical Association*, vol. 311, no. 8, pp. 806–814, 2014.

[2] P. Kopelman, "Health risks associated with overweight and obesity," *Obesity Reviews*, vol. 8, no. 1, pp. 13–17, 2007.

[3] D. A. Anderson, J. R. Shapiro, and J. D. Lundgren, "The freshman year of college as a critical period for weight gain: an initial evaluation," *Eating Behaviors*, vol. 4, no. 4, pp. 363–367, 2003.

[4] H. J. Wengreen and C. Moncur, "Change in diet, physical activity, and body weight among young-adults during the transition from high school to college," *Nutrition Journal*, vol. 8, no. 1, article 32, 2009.

[5] M. C. Nelson, M. Story, N. I. Larson, D. Neumark-Sztainer, and L. A. Lytle, "Emerging adulthood and college-aged youth: an overlooked age for weight-related behavior change," *Obesity*, vol. 16, no. 10, pp. 2205–2211, 2008.

[6] J. Stephens, G. Moscou-Jackson, and J. K. Allen, "Young adults, technology, and weight loss: a focus group study," *Journal of Obesity*, vol. 2015, Article ID 379769, 6 pages, 2015.

[7] S. E. Lowery, S. E. Robinson Kurpius, C. Befort et al., "Body image, self-esteem, and health-related behaviors among male and female first year college students," *Journal of College Student Development*, vol. 46, no. 6, pp. 612–623, 2005.

[8] M. L. Greaney, F. D. Less, A. A. White et al., "College students' barriers and enablers for healthful weight management: a qualitative study," *Journal of Nutrition Education and Behavior*, vol. 41, no. 4, pp. 281–286, 2009.

[9] American College Health Association, "National college health assessment II: undergraduate student reference group executive summary," 2015.

[10] T. Smith-Jackson and J. J. Reel, "Freshmen women and the "freshman 15": perspectives on prevalence and causes of college weight gain," *Journal of American College Health*, vol. 60, no. 1, pp. 14–20, 2012.

[11] C. K. Nikolaou, C. R. Hankey, and M. E. J. Lean, "Weight changes in young adults: a mixed-methods study," *International Journal of Obesity*, vol. 39, no. 3, pp. 508–513, 2015.

[12] J. D. Stephens, A. M. Yager, and J. Allen, "Smartphone technology and text messaging for weight loss in young adults: a Randomized controlled trial," *Journal of Cardiovascular Nursing*, vol. 32, no. 1, pp. 39–46, 2017.

[13] G. Godin and R. J. Shephard, "Godin leisure time exercise questionniare," *Medicine and Science in Sports and Exercise*, pp. S36–S38, 1997.

[14] A. F. Subar, S. I. Kirkpatrick, B. Mittl et al., "The automated self-administered 24-hour dietary recall (ASA24): a resource for researchers, clinicians, and educators from the national cancer institute," *Journal of the Academy of Nutrition and Dietetics*, vol. 112, no. 8, pp. 1134–1137, 2012.

[15] A. M. Jones, C. Lamp, M. Neelon et al., "Reliability and validity of nutrition knowledge questionnaire for adults," *Journal of Nutrition Education and Behavior*, vol. 47, no. 1, pp. 69–74, 2015.

[16] S. Gropper, K. Simmons, L. Connell, and P. Ulrich, "Changes in body weight, composition, and shape: a 4-year study of college students," *Applied Physiology, Nutrition, and Metabolism*, vol. 37, pp. 1118–1123, 2012.

[17] M. V. Fedewa, B. M. Das, E. M. Evans, and R. K. Dishman, "Change in weight and adiposity in college students: a systematic review and meta-analysis," *American Journal of Preventive Medicine*, vol. 47, no. 5, pp. 641–652, 2014.

[18] B. M. Melnyk, L. Small, D. Morrison-Beedy et al., "Mental health correlates of healthy lifestyle attitudes, beliefs, choices, and behaviors in overweight adolescents," *Journal of Pediatric Health Care*, vol. 20, no. 6, pp. 401–406, 2006.

[19] B. Mazurek Melnyk, C. Slevin, L. Militello, J. Hoying, A. Teall, and C. Mcgovern, "Physical health, lifestyle beliefs and behaviors, and mental health of entering graduate health professional students: evidence to support screening and early intervention," *Journal of the American Association of Nurse Practitioners*, vol. 28, no. 4, pp. 204–211, 2016.

[20] J. Kolodinsky, J. R. Harvey-Berino, L. Berlin, R. K. Johnson, and T. W. Reynolds, "Knowledge of current dietary guidelines and food choice by college students: better eaters have higher knowledge of dietary guidance," *Journal of the American Dietetic Association*, vol. 107, no. 8, pp. 1409–1413, 2007.

[21] N. Yahia, C. A. Brown, M. Rapley, and M. Chung, "Level of nutrition knowledge and its association with fat consumption among college students," *BMC Public Health*, vol. 16, no. 1, article 1047, 2016.

[22] M. A. White, P. D. Martin, R. L. Newton et al., "Mediators of weight loss in a family-based intervention presented over the internet," *Obesity Research*, vol. 12, no. 7, pp. 1050–1059, 2004.

[23] J. B. Webb, P. Butler-Ajibade, S. A. Robinson, and S. J. Lee, "Weight-gain misperceptions and the third-person effect in Black and White college-bound females: potential implications for healthy weight management," *Eating Behaviors*, vol. 14, no. 3, pp. 245–248, 2013.

[24] E. Zang, N. Barrett, and L. Cohen, "Differences in nutritional risk factors for breast cancer among new york city white, hispanic, and black college students," *Ethnicity & Disease*, vol. 4, no. 1, pp. 28–40, 1994.

14

Overweight and Obesity in Schoolchildren: Hierarchical Analysis of Associated Demographic, Behavioral, and Biological Factors

Cézane P. Reuter,[1] Elza D. de Mello,[2] Priscila T. da Silva,[3] Tássia S. Borges,[4] Elisa I. Klinger,[3] Silvia I. R. Franke,[1] and Andréia R. de M. Valim[5]

[1]*Physical Education and Health Department, Postgraduate Program in Health Promotion, University of Santa Cruz do Sul (UNISC), 96.815-900 Santa Cruz do Sul, RS, Brazil*
[2]*Postgraduate Program in Child & Adolescent Health, Federal University of Rio Grande do Sul (UFRGS), 90.035-003 Porto Alegre, RS, Brazil*
[3]*Postgraduate Program in Health Promotion, University of Santa Cruz do Sul (UNISC), 96.815-900 Santa Cruz do Sul, RS, Brazil*
[4]*School of Dentistry, Lutheran University Center of Palmas (CEULP-ULBRA), 77.019-900 Palmas, TO, Brazil*
[5]*Biology and Pharmacy Department, Postgraduate Program in Health Promotion, University of Santa Cruz do Sul (UNISC), 96.815-900 Santa Cruz do Sul, RS, Brazil*

Correspondence should be addressed to Cézane P. Reuter; cpreuter@hotmail.com

Academic Editor: Eliot Brinton

Studies focused on the mechanisms involved in the development of obesity in children and adolescents have reported associations between this condition and birth weight, sedentary lifestyle, and hereditary conditions. However, few studies have simultaneously evaluated these factors. This cross-sectional study aims to identify demographic, behavioral, and biological factors associated with overweight/obesity in children and adolescents. 381 schoolchildren aged seven to 17 years were included in the study to evaluate the associations between overweight/obesity and biological factors (including family history of obesity, birth weight, and the fat mass and obesity-associated (FTO) rs9939609 polymorphism), demographic variables (including gender and age), and behavioral variables (including physical activity and/or sports participation). The results of this study showed that there was a lower prevalence of obesity in schoolchildren aged 11–17 years (PR: 0.89; $p = 0.004$). Obesity was more prevalent in children whose father (PR: 1.24; $p < 0.001$) and maternal grandmother (PR: 1.16; $p = 0.019$) were obese. Higher prevalence rates of obesity were also identified in schoolchildren who were overweight at birth (PR: 1.18; $p = 0.002$) and carriers of the obesity risk genotype (PR: 1.13; $p = 0.016$). Biological factors, such as family history of obesity, overweight at birth, and the presence of the fat mass and obesity-associated rs9939609 polymorphism were associated with the prevalence of obesity in children and adolescents.

1. Introduction

The mechanisms underlying the development of obesity in children and adolescents have been the topic of intense research, and studies are perpetually indicating different sets of factors that may be associated with these conditions [1]. Recent studies have suggested a relationship between birth weight, obesity, and sedentary lifestyle [1, 2]. In addition, it has been suggested that birth weight may be explained by hereditary factors and associated with maternal body mass index (BMI) and paternal eating behaviors. These factors constitute important health aspects that may lead to an increased risk of developing an altered metabolic profile [3, 4].

In this way, the use of birth weight as a health determinant has been increasingly supported because it allows for a set of data related to health outcomes, mainly in childhood and adolescence, to be predicted [5]. Previous studies have indicated that high birth weight infants are 2.5 times more likely to become obese children and adolescents [6]. In addition, adolescents with either high or low birth weight are at increased risk of developing insulin resistance, hyperleptinemia, adiposity, and metabolic disorders [7].

Similarly, the results of the Healthy Lifestyle in Europe by Nutrition in Adolescence (HELENA) study, which included 3,528 children from European cities, suggested that children in the 9-year-old age group with a low physical fitness level were at elevated risk of developing cardiovascular risk factors such as obesity and overweight [8].

Epidemiological studies of other mechanisms involved in genetic inheritance have noted that the FTO gene polymorphism may be associated with obesity, and data suggest that children and adolescents with FTO gene polymorphism rs9939609, especially with the AA and AT risk allele, may be more likely to become obese [9, 10]. Therefore, exploring and ascertaining associations between the behaviors of children and parents may be an efficient manner in which to reduce the prevalence of diseases associated with the development of obesity in this population. Thus, the present study aimed to identify demographic, behavioral, and biological factors associated with overweight/obesity in children and adolescents.

2. Materials and Methods

This cross-sectional study included a sample of 381 schoolchildren aged seven to 17 years from nine schools in urban and rural areas of the city of Santa Cruz do Sul, Rio Grande do Sul State, southern Brazil. The study sample was of convenience, with a draw in each classroom for the election of the students participating. The study was approved by the Committee of Ethics in Research with Human Beings of the University of Santa Cruz do Sul (UNISC) under protocol number 2959/11, in accordance to Declaration of Helsinki. All parents or guardians signed the free and informed consent form.

The G*Power 3.1 program (Heinrich-Heine-Universität Düsseldorf, Germany) was used to calculated the sample size needed for a Poisson regression (presence versus absence of obesity as a dependent variable). Using the calculation parameters recommended by Faul et al. [11], we determined that a minimum sample of 372 students would be required to detect an effect size of 0.30 at a power ($1-\beta$) of 0.80 and significance level of $\alpha = 0.05$.

We used the BMI to evaluate the presence of overweight/obesity, which was calculated using the following formula: BMI = weight/(stature)2. The values obtained using this formula were classified according to the cutoff points established by the World Health Organization [12] Subsequently, we classified subjects into the following two categories: low weight/normal weight and overweight/obesity. Demographic variables (sex and age) were self-reported by the schoolchildren and later validated via data obtained from the school. Subsequently, age was classified into the following two categories: child (up to 12 years) and adolescent (up to 18 years), as established by the Child and Adolescent Statute [13]. This choice of age group assumed to perform a comparison between ages and observe what would be more related to BMI. In this way, knowing the influences of age, we may act on prevention and health promotion programs, focusing mainly on major influencers. Maternal education was self-reported by parents. The evaluated behavioral variable was participation in physical/sports activities, as reported by the school. A questionnaire adapted from that of Barros and Nahas [14] was used, with categories comprising "never," "sometimes/almost always," and "always."

To identify potentially associated biological factors, family history of obesity (father, mother, siblings, and maternal and paternal grandparents), and birth weight were evaluated via a questionnaire completed by the parents of the students. Birth weight, obtained in grams, was later classified as "underweight/insufficient weight," "adequate weight," and "overweight," according to the Puffer and Serrano classification [15].

In addition, the presence of the rs9939609 polymorphism in the fat mass and obesity-associated gene (FTO) gene was evaluated. The rs9939609 polymorphism was selected because it has been found to have a higher allelic frequency in the target population of the study, which was predominantly Caucasian [16, 17]. Deoxyribonucleic acid (DNA) was extracted from whole blood samples containing ethylenediaminetetraacetic acid (EDTA) using the Qiagen Kit (QIAamp DNA Blood Mini Kit, Qiagen, Germany) and subsequently quantitated using the Qubit® 2.0 fluorometer (Invitrogen, Carlsbad, CA, USA). Polymorphism genotyping was carried out via real-time polymerase chain reactions (PCRs), which were performed in a 96-well format in a total of 5 μl reaction volume using 10 ng of genomic DNA and VIC®/FAM™ dye tagged TaqMan probes (Applied Biosystems, Foster City, CA, USA) in StepOnePlus (Applied Biosystems, Foster City, CA, USA). The number of cycles and the temperature used for the PCRs were determined according to the manufacturer's recommendations. All genotyping was performed in duplicate, showing an accuracy of 100%. The Hardy–Weinberg equilibrium was tested ($p > 0.05$).

Data analysis was performed using SPSS 23.0 for Windows software (IBM, USA). First, descriptive analyses of the exposure and outcome variables were performed, and absolute and relative values were calculated. In the multivariate analysis, a Poisson regression was used, which has demonstrated robust variance (prevalence ratio (PR) with 95% confidence interval). A hierarchical model was used for the analysis, and the variables were categorized into the following groups, which are organized from the most distal level (furthest from the outcome) and to the most proximal level (closest to the outcome): (a) sociodemographic (sex, age, and maternal education); (b) behavioral (physical/sports activity); and (c) biological (familial obesity, birth weight, and FTO rs9939609). For the final models, the exposures were entered into the model by level and selected via backward stepwise selection (variables with $p < 0.20$ were included in the multivariable analysis). Variables with $p < 0.05$ in the final model were considered statistically significant.

Table 1: Sample characteristics ($n = 381$).

Variables	n (%)
Sex	
Male	189 (49.6)
Female	192 (50.4)
Age group	
Children	134 (35.2)
Adolescents	247 (64.8)
BMI	
Low weight/normal weight	245 (64.3)
Overweight/obesity	136 (35.7)
Birth weight	
Underweight/insufficient weight	117 (30.7)
Adequate weight	229 (60.1)
Overweight	35 (9.2)
FTO rs9939609	
TT	162 (42.5)
AT/AA	219 (57.5)
Maternal education	
≤4 years	121 (32.5)
5 to 11 years	204 (54.8)
≥12 years	47 (12.7)

BMI: body mass index; FTO: fat mass and obesity-associated gene.

3. Results and Discussion

The descriptive characteristics of the sample are presented in Table 1. Of the 381 students evaluated, 50.4% were female, and the prevalence of overweight/obesity was 35.7%. The obesity risk allele (A) was present in 57.5% of the students.

Table 2 presents the associations between the evaluated demographic, behavioral, and biological factors and overweight/obesity in schoolchildren. We observed that overweight/obesity was less prevalent (PR: 0.89; $p < 0.001$) in adolescents than children. Several biological factors, such as having an obese father (PR: 1.24; $p < 0.001$) and maternal grandmother (PR: 1.16; $p = 0.01$), being overweight at birth (PR: 1.18; $p < 0.001$), and having the obesity risk genotype (AA) rs9939609 polymorphism (PR: 1.13; $p = 0.01$) were associated with greater overweight/obesity prevalence rates in schoolchildren.

4. Discussion

Our findings describe the associations observed between demographic and biological factors and overweight/obesity. In this study, a lower prevalence of obesity was identified in adolescents (PR: 0.89; $p = 0.004$). Although recent studies have also reported there to be high prevalence rates of obesity in both children and adolescents [18, 19], similar findings were found in a study recently conducted by Jagadesan et al., which reported there to be a lower prevalence of obesity in adolescents, suggesting that the prevalence of overweight and obesity did not increase with age in the evaluated population, except for a small increase observed between 10 and 12 years of age [20]. However, it has been reported that obese children and adolescents may be more likely to remain obese during adulthood [21]. In addition, current evidence points to a 47% increase in the prevalence of obesity in children between 1980 and 2013 [22]. These data demonstrate the need to develop and direct more complex actions and research to prevent obesity in early childhood. Although in our sample the highest percentage of examined have been teenagers, these showed a smaller percentage of obesity. This result may have been influenced by the wide age range of subjects of this study, which involve children and adolescents; however, statistical analysis was performed in order to avoid/reduce effects of possible/any confounding variable.

Our results showed a higher prevalence of the FTO genotype in students with the risk allele (A) for obesity (57.5%). The results of a study previously carried out in Santa Cruz do Sul suggested that a high prevalence of obesity has been maintained in children and adolescents, and of students with the AA genotype, 57.4% were overweight/obese [16]. Meng and coworkers noted that polymorphisms in the FTO gene (rs62048402 and rs9939609) had significant effects on BMI [23]. Thus, these data emphasize the contribution of genetic factors in the etiology of obesity [24–26], which has been further supported by findings indicating that the heritability of BMI can vary from 30 to 70% [25].

In addition, our findings showed that students with the AA genotype had a 13% greater prevalence of obesity. Therefore, the results of this study support the existence of associations between the variants of the FTO gene and obesity. Similar estimates were identified for variants of the FTO gene in a study of 15,580 Chinese children aged seven to 18 years from the cities of Beijing, Tianjin, Chongqing, Hangzhou, Shanghai, and Nanning. The study indicated that participants with allele A (AA and AT) had a higher prevalence of obesity (OR: 1.47 and OR: 3.32, respectively). In addition, obesity-related metabolic traits, such as increased BMI; waist circumference; hip circumference; and triglyceride, low-density lipoprotein cholesterol (LDL-c), and glucose and decreased high-density lipoprotein cholesterol (HDL-c) levels, were more frequently identified in participants with the AT or AA genotype than participants with the TT genotype [10]. However, this result needs to be further investigated.

The results of the study suggest there to be an association between obesity/obesity in children and adolescents and familial history of diabetes, with schoolchildren who had an obese father and obese maternal grandmother having 24% and 16% greater prevalence rates of overweight/obesity, respectively. Similar findings were previously observed in Tuscany, Italy, where the results of a cross-sectional study of 1,751 children between eight and nine years of age suggested that the prevalence of obesity among children with mothers of normal weight was only 1.4%, whereas the prevalence of obesity among children with obese mothers was 30.3%. Similarly, the prevalence of obesity among children with normal weight fathers was 4%, and the prevalence of obesity among children with obese fathers was 23.9% [27]. In the cities of Catania and Sicily, Italy, the results of a cross-sectional study involving 1,521 children and adolescents suggested that excess birth weight (≥4.0 kg; OR: 1.83; $p < 0.05$), overweight or obese mother (OR: 2.33, $p < 0.0001$), obese father (OR: 1.68; $p < 0.001$), and low/medium parental education level (OR: 1.72; $p < 0.005$) were associated with increased odds of youth obesity

TABLE 2: Crude and adjusted analyses of the prevalence of obesity and associated factors.

Variables	Crude model (CI 95%)	*p*	Adjusted model (CI 95%)	*p*
Level 1: sociodemographic				
Sex				
Male	1.00		1.00	
Female	0.95 (0.89–1.02)	0.23	0.95 (0.89–1.02)	0.20
Age group				
Children	1.00		1.00	
Adolescents	0.88 (0.82–0.95)	0.00	0.89 (0.83–0.96)	0.00
Maternal education				
≤4 years	0.93 (0.83–1.05)	0.29	0.95 (0.84–1.07)	0.44
5 to 11 years	1.00 (0.89–1.11)	0.99	1.00 (0.89–1.11)	0.98
≥12 years	1.00		1.00	
Level 2: behavioral				
Physical/sports activity				
Never	1.00 (0.90–1.11)	0.970	1.00 (0.90–1.11)	0.94
Sometimes/almost always	1.03 (0.95–1.12)	0.364	1.04 (0.96–1.12)	0.33
Always	1.00		1.00	
Level 3: biological				
Obese father				
Yes	1.25 (1.09–1.44)	0.001	1.24 (1.08–1.41)	0.00
No	1.00		1.00	
Obese mother				
Yes	1.06 (0.93–1.20)	0.366	0.92 (0.81–1.05)	0.25
No	1.00		1.00	
Obese siblings				
Yes	0.92 (0.65–1.29)	0.634	0.93 (0.62–1.38)	0.72
No	1.00		1.00	
Obese maternal grandmother				
Yes	1.15 (1.02–1.31)	0.021	1.16 (1.02–1.32)	0.01
No	1.00		1.00	
Obese maternal grandfather				
Yes	1.13 (0.95–1.36)	0.156	1.02 (0.83–1.26)	0.80
No	1.00		1.00	
Obese paternal grandmother				
Yes	1.05 (0.90–1.23)	0.484	0.95 (0.81–1.12)	0.58
No	1.00		1.00	
Obese paternal grandfather				
Yes	1.11 (0.97–1.43)	0.085	1.00 (0.81–1.23)	0.99
No	1.00		1.00	
Birth weight				
Underweight/insufficient weight	0.94 (0.87–1.02)	0.149	0.94 (0.87–1.02)	0.18
Overweight	1.17 (1.05–1.31)	0.004	1.18 (1.06–1.31)	0.00
Adequate weight	1.00		1.00	
FTO rs9939609				
TT	1.00		1.00	
AT	0.96 (0.89–1.04)	0.393	0.95 (0.89–1.03)	0.26
AA*	1.17 (1.06–1.30)	0.002	1.13 (1.02–1.25)	0.01

*Obesity risk genotype; CI: confidence interval; FTO: fat mass and obesity-associated gene; Poisson regression analysis with presence of overweight/obesity evaluated as outcome variable.

development. In addition, breastfeeding was identified as a protective factor (OR: 0.64; $p < 0.0005$) [28].

Our results also indicated that schoolchildren who were overweight at birth had an 18% higher prevalence of overweight/obesity than schoolchildren who had a normal weight at birth. These findings provide additional evidence supporting the presence of a relationship between birth weight and overweight/obesity. A study carried out with 470 schoolchildren in Salvador, Bahia, showed that high birth weight was associated with high BMI and complications such as obesity, changes in lipid profile, and cardiovascular diseases [2]. Thus, the authors have previously argued that both low birth weight and high birth weight may be associated with elevated health risks among schoolchildren [29]. However, underweight/insufficient weight at birth was not associated with overweight/obesity in our study.

A study conducted in Michigan, USA, with two to five-year-old children and their mothers showed similar findings, indicating that newborn children with a BMI above the 90th percentile had a 2.5-fold higher prevalence of obesity [7]. In adolescents, high birth weight has been reported to be associated with cardiovascular risk factors, such as obesity and high blood pressure [2]. Thus, the findings of the present study demonstrated that birth weight was associated with obesity in childhood and adolescence, which may allow for the early identification of metabolic risk and birth weight variations that could trigger cardiometabolic complications during later stages of life. However, it is important to note that birth weight variations should not be considered as a cause of health compromises in isolation, given the innumerable opportunities for changes in lifestyle.

Thus, the datasets used in our study helped provide increased understanding regarding the complexity of the etiology of obesity in children and adolescents. In general, our data provided further evidence suggesting that the control and management of obesity requires a holistic and interdisciplinary view that respects the individualities of each child and that offers conditions within which effective changes can be made, including hereditary factors, biological, and lifestyle factors. However, it should be noted that the study had limitations. Because it was a cross-sectional study, it was not possible to establish causality. In addition, the birth weight, physical activity participation, and BMI variables were self-reported by parents, which may have biased the observed associations. Also, the weeks of gestation were not evaluated, being considered an important vies of the study. However, the study utilized a very broad approach in assessing conditions related to the health of children and adolescents and identifying factors relevant to the health of Brazilian children. In addition, the results of the study suggest that new analyses involving the collection of physical activity data through objective evaluations should be performed to better understand this association.

5. Conclusion

Biological factors, such as family history of obesity, including paternal and matrilineal obesity, overweight at birth, and the presence of the fat mass and obesity-associated rs9939609 polymorphism, were associated with the presence of overweight/obesity in children and adolescents.

Acknowledgments

We are grateful for the contribution of Professor Miria Suzana Burgos (in memoriam) to this study and for all her dedication and coordination of the study "School Health."

References

[1] T. Zhang, L. Cai, L. Ma et al., "The prevalence of obesity and influence of early life and behavioral factors on obesity in Chinese children in Guangzhou," *BMC Public Health*, vol. 16, no. 954, pp. 1–13, 2016.

[2] M. A. C. A. Sousa, I. S. B. Guimarães, C. Daltro et al., "Association between birth weight and cardiovascular risk factors in adolescents," *Arquivos Brasileiros de Cardiologia*, vol. 101, no. 1, pp. 9–17, 2013.

[3] A. Diemert, S. Lezius, M. Pagenkemper et al., "Maternal nutrition, inadequate gestational weight gain and birth weight: results from a prospective birth cohort," *BMC Pregnancy and Childbirth*, vol. 16, no. 224, pp. 1–9, 2016.

[4] Y. Slyvka, Y. Zhang, and F. V. Nowak, "Epigenetic effects of paternal diet on offspring emphasis on obesity," *Endocrine*, vol. 48, no. 1, pp. 36–46, 2015.

[5] C. W. Moscetti and N. P. Pronk, "Invisible seams: preventing childhood obesity through an improved obstetrics-pediatrics care continuum," *Preventive Medicine Reports*, vol. 5, pp. 1–3, 2017.

[6] S. H. Mehta, M. Kruger, and R. J. Sokol, "Being too large for gestational age precedes childhood obesity in African Americans," *American Journal of Obstetric and Gynecology*, vol. 204, no. 3, pp. 1–10, 2011.

[7] B. K. Stansfield, M. E. Fain, J. Bhatia et al., "Nonlinear relationship between birth weight and visceral fat in adolescents," *Journal of Pediatrics*, vol. 174, pp. 185–92, 2015.

[8] L. B. Andersen, A. Bugge, M. Dencker et al., "The association between physical activity, physical fitness and development of metabolic disorders," *International Journal of Pediatric Obesity*, vol. 6, no. S1, pp. 29–34, 2011.

[9] L. L. Quan, H. Wang, Y. Tian et al., "Association of fat-mass and obesity-associated gene FTO rs9939609 polymorphism with the risk of obesity among children and adolescents: a meta-analysis," *European Review for Medical and Pharmacological Sciences*, vol. 19, no. 4, pp. 614–623, 2015.

[10] M. Yang, Y. Xu, L. Liang et al., "The effects of genetic variation in FTO rs9939609 on obesity and dietary preferences in Chinese Han children and adolescents," *PLoS One*, vol. 9, no. 8, Article ID e104574, 2014.

[11] F. Faul, E. Erdfelder, A. Buchner et al., "Statistical power analyses using G*Power 3.1:Tests for correlation and regression analyses," *Behavior Research Methods*, vol. 41, no. 4, pp. 1149–1160, 2009.

[12] World Health Organization, WHO 2007, *Growth Reference Data for 5-19 Years*, 2007, http://www.who.int/growthref/en/.

[13] Brasil, *Estatuto da Criança e do Adolescente (ECA)*, 2012, http://9cndca.sdh.gov.br/legislacao/Lei8069.pdf.

[14] M. V. G. Barros and M. V. Nahas, *Medidas da atividade física: teoria e aplicação em diversos grupos populacionais*, Midiograf, Londrina, Brazil, 2003.

[15] R. R. Puffer and C. V. Serrano, *Patterns of Birth Weight*, PAHO Scientific Publication, Vol. 504, PAHO Scientific Publication, Washington, DC, USA, 1987.

[16] C. P. Reuter, M. S. Burgos, J. C. Bernhard et al., "Association between overweight and obesity in schoolchildren with rs9939609 polymorphism (FTO) and family history for obesity," *Jornal de Pediatria*, vol. 92, no. 5, pp. 493–498, 2016.

[17] I. Carvalho Filho and L. Monasterio, "Immigration and the origins of regional inequality: Government-sponsored European migration to Southern Brazil before World War I," *Regional Science and Urban Economics*, vol. 42, no. 5, pp. 794–807, 2012.

[18] S. V. Pawar, A. S. Choksey, S. S. Jain et al., "Overweight and obesity in 4 schools of Mumbai," *Journal of Clinical and Diagnostic Research*, vol. 10, no. 3, 2016.

[19] B. Camarinha, P. Graça, and P. J. Nogueira, "Prevalence of pre-obesity/obesity in pre and basic school children at Vila Nova de Gaia, Portugal," *Acta Medica Portuguesa*, vol. 29, no. 1, pp. 31–40, 2016.

[20] S. Jagadesan, R. Harish, P. Miranda et al., "Prevalence of overweight and obesity among school children and adolescents in Chennai," *Indian Pediatrics*, vol. 51, pp. 544–549, 2014.

[21] World Health Organization, *Population-Based Approaches to Childhood Obesity Prevention*, WHO, Geneva, Switzerland, 2012.

[22] J. A. Snethen, M. E. Broome, P. Treisman et al., "Effective weight loss for children: a meta-analysis of intervention studies 2002–2015," *Worldviews on Evidence-Based Nursing*, vol. 13, no. 4, pp. 294–302, 2016.

[23] X. R. Meng, J. Y. Song, J. Ma et al., "Association study of childhood obesity with eight genetic variants recently identified by genome-wide association studies," *Pediatric Research*, vol. 76, no. 3, pp. 310–315, 2014.

[24] C. F. Silva, M. R. Zandoná, M. R. Vitolo et al., "Association between a frequent variant of the FTO gene and anthropometric phenotypes in Brazilian children," *BMC Medical Genetics*, vol. 14, no. 4, pp. 1–8, 2013.

[25] C. G. Bell, A. J. Walley, and P. Froguel, "The genetics of human obesity," *Nature Reviews Genetics*, vol. 6, no. 3, pp. 221–234, 2005.

[26] K. Schousboe, G. Willemsen, K. O. Kyvik et al., "Sex differences in heritability of BMI: a comparative study of results from twin studies in eight countries," *Twin Research*, vol. 6, no. 5, pp. 409–421, 2003.

[27] G. Lazzeri, A. Pammolli, V. Pilato et al., "Relationship between 8/9-yr-old school children BMI, parents' BMI and educational level: a cross sectional survey," *Nutrition Journal*, vol. 10, pp. 1–8, 2011.

[28] C. Parrino, F. Vinciguerra, N. La Spina et al., "Influence of early-life and parental factors on childhood overweight and obesity," *Journal of Endocrinological Investigation*, vol. 39, no. 11, pp. 1315–1321, 2016.

[29] L. C. Pellanda, "Trajectories of cardiovascular health: life course epidemiology in Brazil," *Arquivos Brasileiros de Cardiologia*, vol. 102, no. 5, pp. 418-419, 2014.

15

Gestational Weight Gain Intervention Impacts Determinants of Healthy Eating and Exercise in Overweight/Obese Pregnant Women

Abigail M. Pauley,[1] Emily Hohman,[2] Jennifer S. Savage,[2] Daniel E. Rivera,[3] Penghong Guo,[3] Krista S. Leonard,[1] and Danielle Symons Downs[1,4]

[1]*Exercise Psychology Laboratory, Department of Kinesiology, The Pennsylvania State University, University Park, State College, PA, USA*
[2]*Center for Childhood Obesity Research, Department of Nutritional Sciences, College of Health and Human Development, The Pennsylvania State University, University Park, PA, USA*
[3]*School for Engineering of Matter, Transport, Energy, Arizona State University, Tempe, AZ, USA*
[4]*Department of Obstetrics and Gynecology, College of Medicine, The Pennsylvania State University, Hershey, PA, USA*

Correspondence should be addressed to Danielle Symons Downs; dsd11@psu.edu

Academic Editor: Sharon Herring

High gestational weight gain (GWG) in overweight/obese pregnant women increases maternal-fetal complications. We conducted a 6-week GWG intervention based on an energy balance model that includes theories of planned behavior (TPB) and self-regulation constructs to promote exercise and healthy eating motivation and behaviors. The purposes of this proof-of-concept feasibility study were to examine: (1) the energy balance model constructs over the intervention, and (2) pre-post intervention, weekly, and dose-response changes in study constructs. *Methods.* Overweight/obese pregnant women ($N = 17$) were randomized to 1 of 6 conditions, increasing in intensity, and included varied combinations of components (exercise sessions, healthy eating demonstrations, etc.). Exercise and healthy eating TPB (attitude, subjective norm, perceived behavioral control, intention), and self-regulation (prospective, retrospective) constructs were collected weekly. Exercise behavior, energy intake, and GWG were collected daily. *Results.* We observed: (a) significant increases in exercise TPB constructs, healthy eating attitude (limit unhealthy foods), exercise/healthy eating retrospective self-regulation; (b) significant decrease in healthy eating subjective norm (limit unhealthy foods); (c) trending increases for healthy eating perceived behavioral control (limit unhealthy foods), healthy eating prospective self-regulation, and energy intake; (d) significantly higher active time, steps, and energy expenditure at W3 relative to other weeks; (e) no significant increase in GWG; and, (f) a dose response effect such that women in more intensive dosages had greater gains in exercise and healthy eating perceived behavioral control (eat healthy/limit unhealthy foods). *Conclusion.* Brief exposure to a theoretically-driven, GWG intervention resulted in changes to exercise and healthy eating TPB and self-regulation motivational determinants, no significant increase in GWG, and suggests intervention intensity can strengthen perceived ability to engage in exercise/healthy eating behaviors; offering initial proof-of-concept for the intervention to regulate GWG in overweight/obese pregnant women. Future research will test this intervention over the course of pregnancy to understand long-term impact on maternal-fetal health outcomes.

1. Introduction

Over half of all overweight and obese pregnant women gain weight in excess of the current gestational weight gain (GWG) recommendations [1, 2]. This is problematic because high GWG increases the risk for preterm delivery, gestational diabetes, vascular disease, hypertensive disorders of pregnancy, and postpartum weight retention [1]. Even more alarming, high GWG elevates the risk for fetal morbidity including macrosomia (i.e., birth weight >4,000 g regardless of gestational age), birth trauma (e.g., shoulder dystocia), and longer hospital stays [1, 3]. Data from the National Vital Statistics System [2] indicate that a high percentage of overweight (61%) and obese (55%) women are at greater risk for exceeding the IOM GWG guidelines (i.e., total weight gain: 15–25 pounds for overweight; 11–20 pounds for obese) and therefore warrant intervention to effectively manage GWG for optimal maternal and fetal health.

Of particular concern, the rate of overweight/obese pregnant women exceeding GWG guidelines is predicted to increase given the lack of a "gold standard" intervention or clinical treatment [4]. Furthermore, the majority of interventions that aimed to reduce GWG in overweight/obese pregnant women have either yielded minimal effects or have been unsuccessful altogether [5–9]. However, information can be learned from the few effective studies. Vesco et al. [10] conducted a group-based weight management intervention in obese pregnant women using an energy-reduced DASH diet, recommendation of 30 minutes of moderate physical activity, and individual and group education sessions. They observed lower GWG in the intervention group from baseline (7–21 weeks gestation) through follow-up (34 weeks gestation) compared to the control group. Sagedal et al. [11] conducted an intervention where pregnant women received dietary counseling and twice-weekly exercise classes. They observed lower mean GWG in the intervention group compared to controls who received routine prenatal care. Despite these findings, the majority of participants in both studies still exceeded the IOM GWG recommendations. Sagedal et al. [11] also reported the proportion of women who exceeded the IOM GWG guidelines did not differ between condition, suggesting that a more intensive intervention approach (e.g., individually tailored exercise and dietary guidance) addressing the unique needs of overweight/obese women is needed to effectively manage GWG [4, 11, 12].

Given this premise, we developed an individually tailored GWG intervention to manage weight in overweight/obese pregnant women based on a model of energy balance that includes the theories of planned behavior (TPB) and self-regulation [13–19]. The TPB aims to explain behavior through underlying constructs of attitude (positive or negative evaluation of the behavior), subjective norm (perceived social support to engage in the behavior), and perceived behavioral control (ease or difficulty in performing the behavior), which influence intention (person's level of motivation) to perform or not perform a behavior such as exercise or healthy eating [20]. Self-regulation is the ability for a person to work towards a goal by monitoring and managing thoughts, feelings, and behaviors, which is critical to changing behaviors such as exercise and healthy eating [21, 22]. Targeting both the TPB constructs and self-regulation simultaneously within an intervention can strengthen the likelihood of changing behavior, especially when the intervention is individually tailored based on the participant's level of the construct, for example, using strategies such as daily self-monitoring, positive encouragement, and reinforcement for a woman with low perceived behavioral control for exercising and eating healthy.

Previous work by Symons Downs et al. [23] established the utility to increase exercise determinants in pregnant women with gestational diabetes, but there is little research that has examined the associations between TPB and self-regulation constructs among pregnant women within the context of a GWG management intervention, especially in overweight/obese pregnant women. Thus, we conducted a brief, 6-week trial of an intervention focusing on exercise and healthy eating motivation and behaviors to manage GWG in overweight/obese pregnant women [18, 19]. The overall goal of this proof-of-concept trial was to establish feasibility of the intervention components and the extent to which the TPB and self-regulation constructs motivated overweight/obese pregnant women to engage in exercise and healthy eating behaviors (as exercise and healthy eating are essential for regulating GWG). The purposes of this feasibility study were to (1) descriptively examine the energy balance model constructs over the 6-week pilot intervention and (2) examine pre-post intervention, weekly, and dose-response changes in the study constructs. Since the intervention period was brief, and intervention behavior change often takes longer than 6 weeks, we anticipated to observe changes in the underlying TPB and self-regulation motivational determinants without our energy balance model rather than observing changes in behavior (exercise, healthy eating, and GWG) [24]. We also expected to observe a dose-response effect such that the TPB and self-regulation constructs would improve with an increase in intervention dosage intensity. Our future research will test this GWG intervention in a larger trial over the course of pregnancy to understand long-term changes in exercise, healthy eating, and GWG as well as impact on additional maternal-infant outcomes.

2. Methods

2.1. Participants. Overweight/obese pregnant women ($N = 17$; M age = 29.4 years, SD = ± 5.6) were recruited using on-site clinic (e.g., speaking with potential participants after a prenatal appointment) and community (e.g., ads, flyers, and word of mouth) methods in locations in Central Pennsylvania. Women were randomized to 1 of 6 intervention dosages, which increased in intensity, for 6 weeks using a statistician-developed scheme placing an equal distribution of overweight and obese women in each dosage (Figure 1). Inclusion criteria were first pregnancy (no prior full-term (≥37 weeks gestation) births), between 12 and 28 weeks gestation, 18–45 years old, body mass index (BMI) ≥ 25, English-speaking, and no contraindications to exercise or eating healthy foods [25, 26]. Physician's consent was obtained from the women's obstetrics and gynecology providers prior to enrollment.

2.2. Study Design

2.2.1. Baseline and Follow-Up Assessments. Participants were met at the University's Clinical Research Center, explained study procedures, and obtained informed consent.

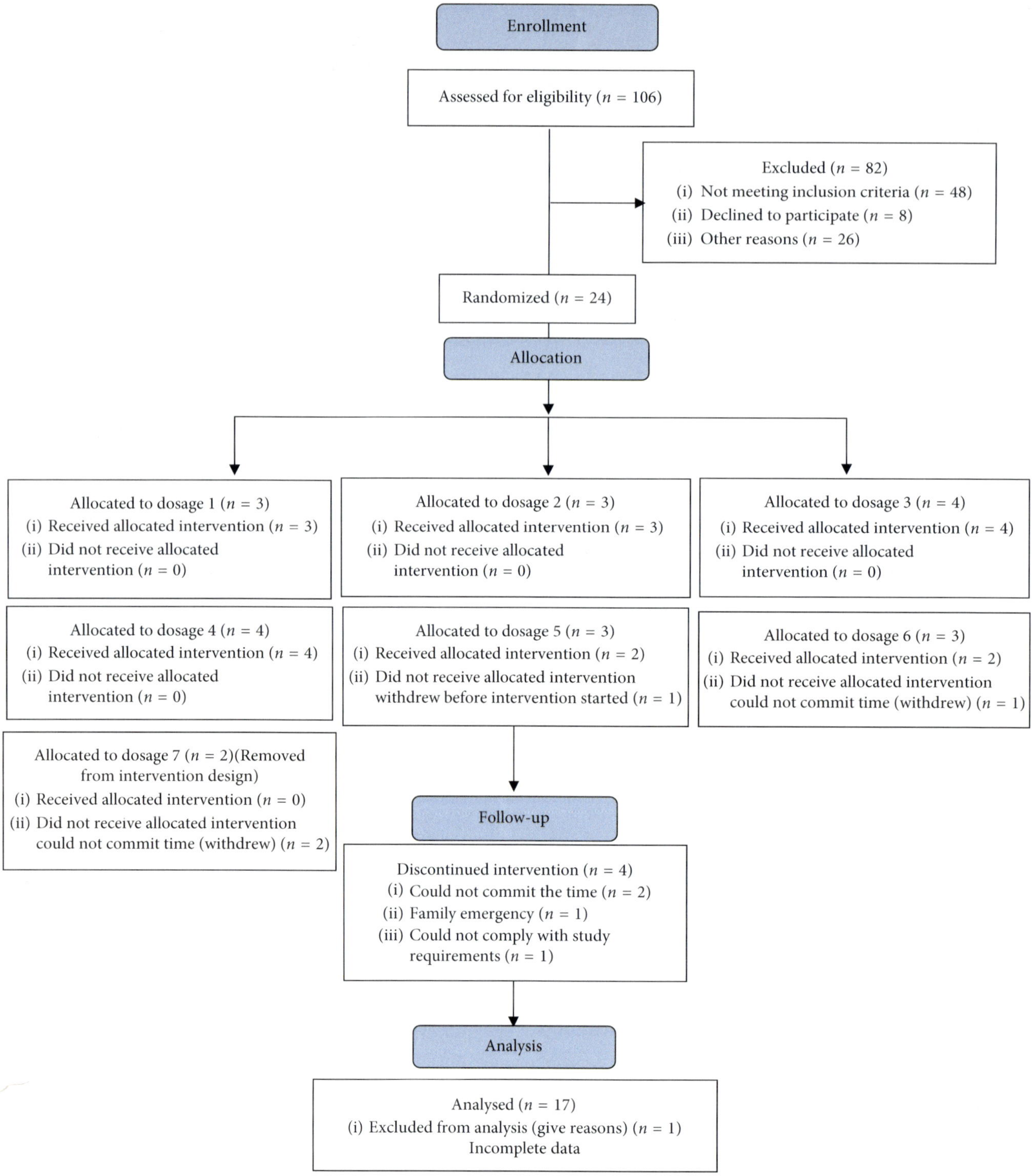

Figure 1: Consort recruitment table.

Eligible and interested women completed a brief medical exam to ensure safety for participation followed by measures of their height, weight, and blood pressure. During the baseline assessment, women also completed self-reported measures of exercise and healthy eating TPB (attitude, subjective norm, perceived behavioral control, and intention) and self-regulation (prospective and retrospective) constructs and personal demographics (e.g., age and BMI). Women were given instructions on how to complete self-reported measures using an online data capture system (REDCap; [27]). Women were given a wrist-worn exercise activity monitor (to measure active time, energy expenditure in kcal, and steps), Wi-Fi weight scale, and instructions on how to use these devices as well as how to complete diet records using a smartphone app for three days during baseline. During the intervention, women completed weekly measures of the exercise and healthy eating TPB and self-regulation constructs and daily measures exercise behavior (wrist-worn activity monitor) and weight (Wi-Fi scale); energy intake was assessed three days/week using the smartphone app for dietary record intake, but for the current analyses, a back-calculation method was used for energy intake (described below). The same procedures (not including the medical exam and technology trainings) were used to collect data at the follow-up assessment.

2.2.2. Intervention. Intervention dosages were based on principles of behavior change, TPB, and self-regulation [20, 28, 29], content from past successful interventions [23, 30], and initial prototype development feedback from pregnant women. Intervention dosages were built upon one another in a "step-up" design for intensity such that Dosage 1 included the "baseline intervention" with education on principles of exercise, healthy eating, GWG, goal-setting, and self-monitoring. Dosage 2 included the baseline intervention (i.e., Dosage 1) + a "step-up" of 30 min of healthy eating active learning (e.g., cooking demonstrations, recipe preparation, understanding principles of portion size, and energy density). The dosages increased in intensity with added exercise sessions, self-monitoring with instructor feedback, and healthy eating meal replacements up through Dosage 6. We originally designed the intervention with seven dosages; however, feedback from women during prototype development found this dosage to be too intensive, so we removed it from the study design. Figure 2 illustrates the six intervention dosages that were tested in this study.

2.3. Measures. Study measures of exercise and healthy eating TPB and self-regulation were collected weekly for six weeks (i.e., week 1 = baseline, weeks 2–5 of intervention, and week 6 = follow-up) via online surveys. Intensive longitudinal data inform interventions and efficacy by capturing people's lives while they are actually living [31] which is a different approach from conventional experimental/survey research. All TPB constructs were measured on a 7-point Likert scale with higher scores indicating more positive attitude, subjective norm, perceived behavioral control, and intention.

2.3.1. Exercise TPB Constructs. Attitude was assessed with 7 differential pairs (e.g., useless-useful) that described how women felt about exercising for at least 30 minutes/day of accumulated moderate physical activity on most, if not all, days of the week [32, 33]. *Subjective Norm* was assessed with three items (e.g., strongly disagree-strongly agree) measuring perceived support from important others to exercise for 30 minutes/day on most days in the following week. *Perceived Behavioral Control* was assessed with 3 items (e.g., for me to be physically active each day in the next week will be: extremely difficult/very little control/strongly disagree-extremely easy/complete control/strongly agree). *Intention* to engage in 30 minutes of exercise on most days of the week was assessed with six items (e.g., I intend to be physically active each day in the next week: strongly disagree-strongly agree). Internal consistency scores for the exercise TPB measures ranged from alpha = 0.77–0.98 from pre-post for all constructs. Compliance of the exercise TPB measures was 99%.

2.3.2. Healthy Eating TPB Constructs. Authors developed the healthy eating TPB scale by modifying the validated exercise TPB items. *Eating Attitudes* were assessed with 14 differential pairs, 7 assessing healthy eating attitudes (how women felt about eating healthy foods each day in the next week) and 7 assessing attitudes about limiting unhealthy foods (i.e., sugary beverages, eating chips, candy, baked goods, and fried foods each day in the next week). *Subjective Norm* was assessed using six items; three items measured women's perceptions of the extent to which significant others (e.g., husband, mother, and friend) provided support for them to eat healthy each day in the next week and three items assessed perceived support from others to limit unhealthy foods. *Perceived Behavioral Control* was assessed using six items; three items measured the ease or difficulty in eating healthy foods each day in the next week and three items assessed the ease or difficulty in limiting unhealthy foods each day in the next week. *Intention* was assessed using 12 items (e.g., strongly disagree/definitely not/not at all-strongly agree/definitely/very much). Three items were adapted to healthy eating from the exercise intention measure. Three items asked about women's intention to limit unhealthy foods. Three items assessed women's intention/motivation/plan to eat healthy and three items assessed intention to limit unhealthy foods each day in the next week. Internal consistency scores for the healthy eating and limiting unhealthy food TPB measures ranged from alpha = 0.73–0.98 from pre-post for all constructs. Compliance of both, the healthy eating and limiting unhealthy food TPB measures, was 99%.

2.3.3. Exercise Self-Regulation. Exercise self-regulation was assessed with 16 items to evaluate the degree to which women self-regulated their exercise behavior (e.g., if I achieve my short-term (daily or weekly) goals for exercise, I will feel proud; [28, 29, 34]). Eight items assessed prospective (i.e., in the next week) and eight items assessed retrospective (i.e., in the past week) self-regulation. Items were divided into 7 subscales: self-monitoring, goal-setting, action planning, coping planning, scheduling, cuing, and affective reaction. Internal consistency scores were excellent (alpha = 0.92–0.97) across time points. Compliance of the exercise self-regulation measure was 99%.

2.3.4. Healthy Eating Self-Regulation. Healthy eating self-regulation was assessed with 16 items to evaluate the degree to which women self-regulates their healthy eating behavior (e.g., if I achieve my short-term (daily or weekly) goals for eating healthy, I will feel proud; [28, 29]). Eight items assessed prospective and eight items assessed retrospective healthy eating self-regulation. Items were divided into 7

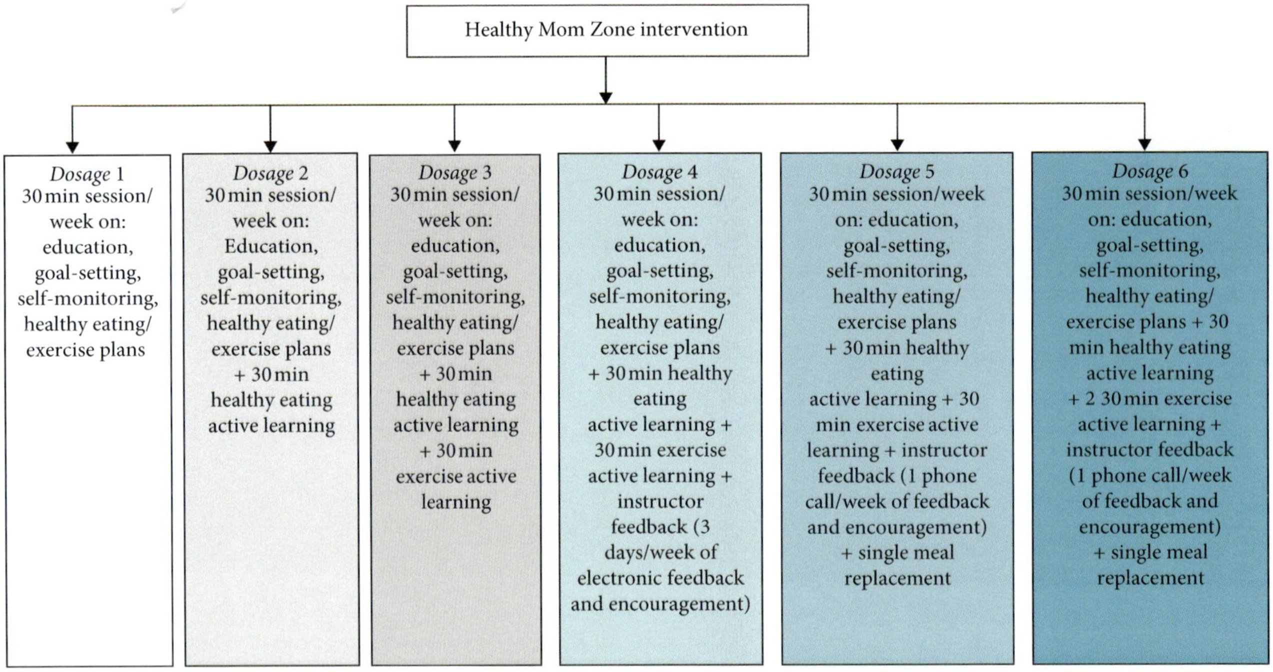

FIGURE 2: Healthy mom zone intervention dosages description.

subscales: self-monitoring, goal-setting, action planning, coping planning, scheduling, cuing, and affective reaction. Internal consistency scores ranged from alpha = 0.83–0.93 across the time points. Compliance of the healthy eating self-regulation measure was 99%.

2.3.5. Exercise Behavior. Exercise behavior was assessed using a wrist-worn activity monitor to measure daily activity time, energy expenditure, and steps [35, 36]. Women wore the activity monitor 24 hours/day over the entire intervention period. Each woman had her own wrist monitor that connected to her phone via a mobile app to use as a self-monitoring tool. Compliance with the monitors was 93%.

2.3.6. Energy Intake. Energy intake was assessed using a back-calculation equation of energy intake [16] to address concerns about under/overreporting of energy intake when using self-report (pencil and paper or smartphone app) food records [37]. In the calculation, the participant's weight and energy expenditure are used to predict energy intake. Energy intake was predicted for each day over the 6-week intervention using average kcal/day.

2.3.7. GWG. GWG was assessed daily using a Wi-Fi scale over the 6-week study period. Women weighed themselves each day as soon as they woke up. The scale transmitted weights automatically to secure participant online accounts; online data were accessed and stored in REDCap. Compliance with the scale was 87%.

2.4. Data Analysis. Descriptive statistics were used to examine study means, standard deviations, and frequencies. Changes in TPB and self-regulation scores from baseline to follow-up were calculated with *t*-tests. Repeated-measures ANCOVA controlling for gestational age, dosage (1–6), and prepregnancy BMI was conducted to examine the weekly changes in the planned behavior/self-regulation constructs, exercise, energy intake, and GWG. Effects of study dosage on pre-post changes were assessed with ANOVA. Analyses were performed in SAS 9.4 (SAS Institute, Cary, NC) and SPSS 25 (IBM Corp., Armonk, New York). As this is a pilot study, the *p* value for statistically significant differences overtime was set to $p \leq 0.05$ and the *p* value for trends overtime was set to $p \leq 0.10$ [38].

3. Results

3.1. Demographics. The sample ($N = 17$) was homogenous; most participants were Caucasian, married, completed college, and had a family income of $40,000 or higher per year (Table 1). Prepregnancy BMI of participants was in the overweight range (M BMI = 29.1 kg/m^2, SD = ± 3.8, range = 24.7–39; 65% overweight, 35% obese). Women were randomized to 1 of 6 dosages: Dosage 1 $n = 3$, Dosage 2 $n = 3$, Dosage 3 $n = 4$, Dosage 4 $n = 4$, Dosage 5 $n = 2$, and Dosage 6 $n = 2$.

3.2. Pre-Post Intervention Change in Energy Balance Model Constructs. There was a significant increase in healthy eating attitude (limit unhealthy foods, $p = 0.046$) and a trend for an increase in healthy eating perceived behavioral control (limit unhealthy foods, $p = 0.06$, Figure 3). There was a significant increase in retrospective exercise and healthy eating self-regulation ($p = 0.004$, $p = 0.0001$). There were no significant changes for any of the other exercise/healthy eating TPB or self-regulation constructs, exercise and healthy eating behaviors, or GWG.

Table 1: Demographic characteristics of the study sample.

Variable	Total sample $N = 17$		
	M	SD	%
Age	29.4	5.6	
Body mass index (BMI)	29.1	3.8	
Gestational age at study start	16.4	4.5	
Weight at study start (pounds)	185.74	27.49	
Weight gain over 4-week dosage (pounds)	6.6	4.5	
Marital status			
Married			75.0
Not married living with partner			18.75
Single			6.25
Divorced			0
Race			
Caucasian			94.5
Hispanic			5.5
Education			
Graduate			23.5
College			76.5
High school			0
Family income			
$100,000			29.4
$40–$100,000			52.9
$20–$40,000			11.7
$10–$20,000			5.9

M = mean; SD = standard deviation.

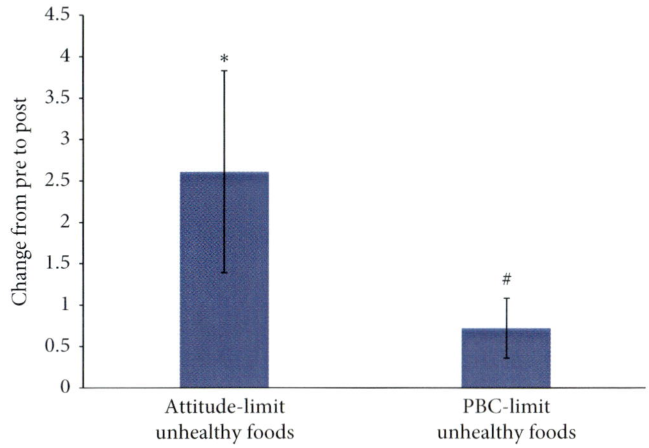

Figure 3: Change in TPB limit unhealthy eating constructs from pre- to post-assessment. Values are mean ± SE, $^*p < 0.05$, $^\#p < 0.10$.

3.3. Weekly Change in Energy Balance Model Constructs

3.3.1. Exercise TPB. The repeated-measures model for exercise attitude was significant, Wilks lambda = 0.258, $F = 4.613$, $p = 0.028$. Overall, attitude increased from W1–W6 of the intervention with significant differences at W2–W4 ($p = 0.044$) and trending differences at W2–W6 ($p = 0.078$). The repeated-measures model for exercise subjective norm was also significant, Wilks lambda = 0.271, $F = 4.301$, $p = 0.034$. Subjective norm increased from W1–W6; however, these differences did not reach statistical significance. The repeated-measures models for exercise perceived behavioral control and intention were not significant, Wilks lambda = 0.900, $F = 0.178$, $p = 0.963$, and Wilks lambda = 0.537, $F = 1.379$, $p = 0.326$, respectively. However, exercise perceived behavioral control and intention had significant differences at W2–W5 ($p = 0.014, p = 0.017$, respectively); perceived behavioral control also had trending differences at W2–W6 ($p = 0.070$; Table 2).

3.3.2. Healthy Eating TPB. The repeated-measures model for healthy eating attitude, subjective norm, perceived behavioral control, and intention was not significant, Wilks lambda = 0.487, $F = 1.687$, $p = 0.243$, Wilks lambda = 0.728, $F = 0.523$, $p = 0.753$, Wilks lambda = 0.786, $F = 0.435$, $p = 0.813$, and Wilks lambda = 0.388, $F = 2.522$, $p = 0.118$, respectively. There were no significant changes across weeks. The repeated-measures models for healthy eating attitude, perceived behavioral control, and intention (limit unhealthy foods) were not significant, Wilks lambda = 0.493, $F = 1.646$, $p = 0.253$, Wilks lambda = 0.553, $F = 0.969$, $p = 0.503$, and Wilks lambda = 0.631, $F = 0.934$, $p = 0.507$, respectively. There were no significant changes across weeks. The repeated-measures model for healthy eating subjective norm (limit unhealthy foods) was significant, Wilks lambda = 0.094, $F = 9.659$, $p = 0.013$. Subjective norm decreased from W1–W6; however, these differences did not reach statistical significance (Table 2).

3.3.3. Exercise and Healthy Eating Self-Regulation. The repeated-measures model for exercise self-regulation prospective was not significant, Wilks lambda = 0.744, $F = 0.549$, $p = 0.736$; there were no significant differences across weeks. The repeated-measures model for exercise self-regulation retrospective was also not significant, Wilks lambda = 0.566, $F = 1.227$, $p = 0.379$. However, significant weekly increases were observed from W2–W4, W2–W5, and W2–W6 ($p = 0.028, 0.023, 0.043$, respectively). The repeated-measures model for healthy eating self-regulation prospective trended toward significance, Wilks lambda = 0.358, $F = 2.873$, $p = 0.089$. Healthy eating self-regulation prospective increased from W1–W6; however, these differences were not statistically significant. The repeated-measures model for healthy eating self-regulation retrospective was not significant, Wilks lambda = 0.542, $F = 1.350$, $p = 0.335$. However, significant week increases were observed from W1–W3, W1–W4, W1–W6, and W2–W4 ($p = 0.017, 0.014, 0.016, 0.043$, respectively) and a trending increase was observed at W1–W5 ($p = 0.079$) (Table 3).

3.3.4. Exercise and Healthy Eating Behavior. The repeated-measures model for active time was not significant, Wilks lambda = 0.494, $F = 1.024$, $p = 0.490$; however, there were significant differences at W2-W3, W3-W4, and W3–W6 ($p = 0.007, p < 0.001, p < 0.001$, respectively) and trending differences at W3–W5 ($p = 0.086$) such that W3 had significantly higher active time (e.g., 96 min) compared to the other weeks (e.g., 72 min on average). The repeated-measures models for step and active kcal were also not

Table 2: Exercise and healthy eating theory of planned behavior repeated measures.

	Week 1		Week 2		Week 3		Week 4		Week 5		Week 6		Wilks lambda	F	Partial eta squared	p value
	M	SD	M	SD	M	SD	M	SD	M	SD	M	SD				
TPB exercise attitude (N = 16)	6.08	0.83	6.09	0.67	6.31	0.60	6.32	0.68	6.22	0.70	6.32	0.79	**0.258**	**4.613**	**0.742**	**0.028*****
TPB exercise subjective norm (N = 16)	5.75	1.24	5.77	1.12	5.88	1.39	6.04	1.24	5.9	1.17	5.96	1.19	**0.271**	**4.301**	**0.729**	**0.034*****
TPB exercise perceived behavioral control (N = 16)	5.27	1.04	4.29	0.89	5.35	1.04	5.17	1.16	5.56	0.98	5.38	0.97	0.900	0.178	0.100	0.963
TPB exercise intention (N = 16)	5.41	1.39	5.23	0.97	5.58	1.00	5.33	1.1	5.67	0.99	5.44	1.21	0.537	1.379	0.463	0.326
TPB healthy eating attitude (N = 16)	6.30	0.695	6.30	0.41	6.37	0.55	6.36	0.57	6.40	0.64	6.47	0.59	0.487	1.687	0.513	0.243
TPB healthy eating subjective norm (N = 15)	6.29	0.93	6.18	1.10	6.04	1.11	6.16	1.17	6.02	1.23	6.04	1.27	0.728	0.523	0.272	0.753
TPB healthy eating perceived behavioral control (N = 16)	5.75	0.68	6.79	0.75	5.85	0.69	5.81	1.2	5.92	0.63	6.02	0.75	0.786	0.435	0.214	0.813
TPB healthy eating intention (N = 16)	5.92	0.98	6.05	0.74	6.07	0.83	5.93	0.87	6.01	0.86	6.13	0.93	0.388	2.522	0.612	0.118
TPB limit healthy eating attitude (N = 16)	5.92	0.85	6.19	0.58	6.21	0.6	6.20	0.65	6.19	0.68	6.32	0.64	0.493	1.646	0.507	0.253
TPB limit healthy eating subjective norm (N = 13)	6.41	0.81	6.23	0.92	6.05	1.10	6.15	1.18	6.10	0.81	6.00	1.34	**0.094**	**9.659**	**0.906**	**0.013*****
TPB limit healthy eating perceived behavioral control (N = 14)	5.64	0.86	5.98	0.83	5.83	0.87	5.62	1.13	5.74	0.83	5.88	0.82	0.553	0.969	0.447	0.503
TPB limit healthy eating intention (N = 16)	5.56	1.28	5.78	1.03	5.74	0.91	5.65	0.89	5.73	0.96	5.85	0.95	0.631	0.934	0.369	0.507

$^*p < 0.05$; $^\#p < 0.10$.

significant, Wilks lambda = 0.877, F = 0.169, p = 0.965, and Wilks lambda = 0.841, F = 0.189, p = 0.954, respectively. However, steps and active kcal at W3 were significantly higher than at W6 (p = 0.013, p = 0.006, respectively). The repeated-measures model for energy intake trended toward significance, Wilks lambda = 0.003, F = 73.617, p = 0.088. Overall, energy intake increased from W1–W6 of the intervention by 197 kcal; however, these weekly differences were not statistically significant (Table 4).

3.3.5. GWG. The repeated-measures model for GWG was not significant, Wilks lambda = 0.521, F = 1.150, p = 0.430, and there were no significant changes across weeks (Table 5). GWG did not significantly increase over the 6-week intervention; observation of mean GWG across the weeks showed a similar pattern of approximately 1.1 pound change/week over the study period.

3.4. Dose-Response Change in Energy Balance Model Constructs. There was a positive relationship between study dosage and pre-post change in exercise perceived behavioral control (p = 0.07; Figure 4(c)), healthy eating perceived behavioral control (p = 0.03; Figure 4(a)), healthy eating perceived behavioral control for limiting unhealthy foods (p = 0.03; Figure 4(b)), healthy eating intention (p = 0.04), and healthy eating intention for limiting unhealthy foods (p = 0.03). In other words, women randomized to receive dosages at higher intensities had greater intention to eat healthy/limit unhealthy foods and their perception of eating healthy/limiting unhealthy foods and exercising was more positive. There were no significant dose-response pre-post changes in exercise and healthy eating self-regulation, exercise and healthy eating behaviors, or GWG.

4. Discussion

The objectives of this feasibility study were to descriptively examine the energy balance model constructs over the 6-week pilot intervention and examine pre-post intervention, weekly, and dose-response change in the study constructs. Overall, we found that brief exposure to the theoretically driven, GWG intervention resulted in significant changes to some of the exercise and healthy eating TPB and self-regulation motivational determinants, an increase in exercise behaviors at W3 of the intervention, and no significant changes to energy intake or GWG, supporting the initial proof-of-concept of the intervention among overweight/obese pregnant women. We also observed a dose-response effect such that an increase in intervention dosage was associated with greater exercise and healthy eating perceived control. These findings are further discussed below.

In partial support of our assumption, the intervention resulted in changes to some of the TPB and self-regulation motivational determinants over the intervention period. More specifically, we observed significant increases in

Table 3: Exercise and healthy eating self-regulation repeated measures.

	Week 1		Week 2		Week 3		Week 4		Week 5		Week 6		Wilks lambda	F	Partial eta squared	p value
	M	SD	M	SD	M	SD	M	SD	M	SD	M	SD				
Exercise prospective (N = 16)	40.63	6.69	37.55	6.28	35.88	6.66	37.19	8.71	38.06	8.66	36.5	8.85	0.744	0.549	0.265	0.736
Exercise retrospective (N = 16)	28.00	9.32	30.81	8.78	33.97	7.63	35.49	10.54	36.35	9.71	36.04	10.47	0.566	1.227	0.434	0.379
Healthy eating prospective (N = 16)	39.33	8.05	36.56	6.23	36.19	7.19	38.21	7.15	37.85	8.51	38.38	8.1	**0.358**	**2.873**	**0.642**	**0.089**$^{\#}$
Healthy eating retrospective (N = 16)	25.87	9.70	31.25	9.45	34.03	7.13	36.63	8.24	34.56	9.83	37.13	9.25	0.542	1.350	0.458	0.335

$^{*}p < 0.05$; $^{\#}p < 0.10$.

Table 4: Exercise and healthy eating behavior repeated measures.

	Week 1		Week 2		Week 3		Week 4		Week 5		Week 6		Wilks lambda	F	Partial eta squared	p value
	M	SD	M	SD	M	SD	M	SD	M	SD	M	SD				
Active time (N = 13)	75.05	23.1	71.27	27.76	96.38	34.60	73.95	31.16	65.68	30.27	71.72	29.04	0.494	1.024	0.506	0.490
Steps (N = 14)	7674	2688	7917	3323	8582	2997	8235	3345	7205	3228	7042	2794	0.877	0.169	0.123	0.965
Energy expenditure (N = 13)	467.2	202.2	447.4	236.5	507.4	218.3	497.9	251.3	405.3	234.4	411.7	212.8	0.841	0.189	0.159	0.954
Energy intake (N = 9)	2755	928	2780	475	2935	541	2732	668	2887	550	2952	593	**0.003**	**73.62**	**0.997**	**0.088**$^{\#}$

$^{*}p < 0.05$; $^{\#}p < 0.10$.

Table 5: Change in GWG repeated measures.

	ΔW1-W2		ΔW2-W3		ΔW3-W4		ΔW4-W5		ΔW5-W6		Wilks lambda	F	Partial eta squared	p value
	M	SD	M	SD	M	SD	M	SD	M	SD				
GWG (N = 12)	1.50	1.17	0.65	1.48	1.08	0.94	1.00	0.87	1.59	0.85	0.521	1.150	0.479	0.430

$^{*}p < 0.05$; $^{\#}p < 0.10$. Weight is measured in pounds.

exercise attitude, subjective norm, perceived behavioral control, and intention, healthy eating attitude (limit unhealthy foods) and exercise/healthy eating retrospective self-regulation, a trend toward significance for an increase in healthy eating perceived behavioral control (limit unhealthy foods) and healthy eating prospective self-regulation. These findings are consistent with our past research among pregnant women with gestational diabetes [23], and they suggest that brief exposure to the intervention can positively impact how women feel about exercise and healthy eating.

These findings also illustrate a positive impact on women's perceived ability and self-regulation for exercise and healthy eating, which in turn can have a positive impact on these behaviors to help better regulate GWG. More specifically, the intervention education and skills (including exercise and healthy eating action plans) taught to the women along with the use of mHealth tools (e.g., Wi-Fi scale, wrist-worn activity monitor, and smartphone app for intake served as both intervention self-regulatory tools and behavioral measures) positively influenced women's retrospective and prospective self-regulation. These findings also suggest that women felt more comfortable with regulating their exercise and eating behaviors from week to week and were able to think about setting goals and action plans in advance of an upcoming week. These findings are promising for the future intervention that will require women to self-regulate exercise and healthy eating behaviors over the duration of pregnancy to regulate their weight gain. While we did not find significant pre-post intervention change in exercise perceived behavioral control and intention, there were significant increases in exercise perceived behavioral control and intention from W2–W5 and a trend toward significance for exercise perceived behavioral control from W2–W6. This suggests that the accumulation of the education and skills learned over the course of the short intervention period provided the women with tools to manage perceived barriers and improve their intention for exercise. These weekly findings are promising for the design of the future intervention as they may be replicated over a longer intervention period. Similarly, with a trend toward

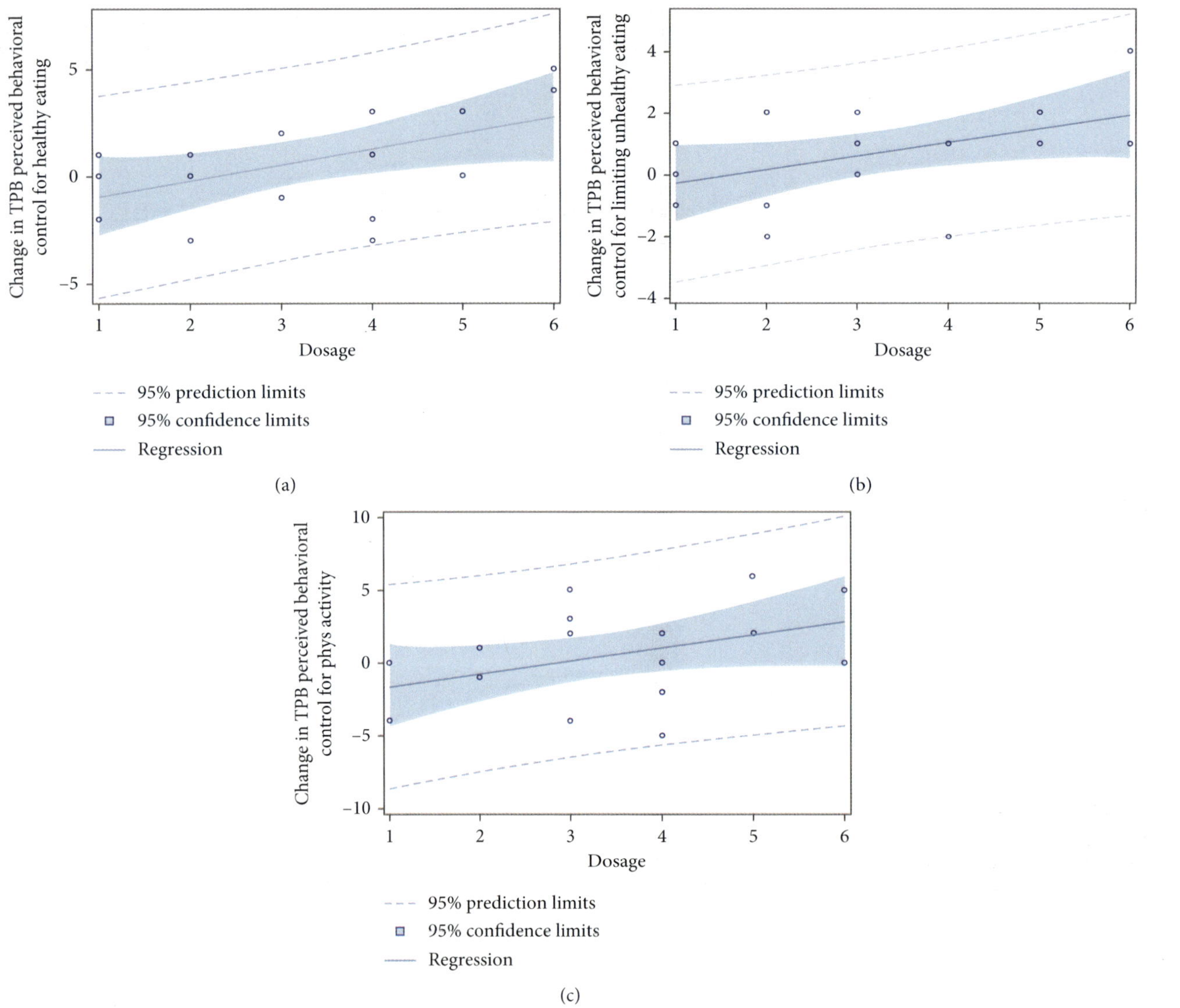

FIGURE 4: Intervention dose was positively associated with pre-post change in perceived behavioral control for (a) healthy eating ($p = 0.03$), (b) limiting unhealthy eating ($p = 0.03$), and (c) exercise ($p = 0.07$).

significance for perceived behavioral control (limit unhealthy foods), the program content appears to provide women with useful strategies to overcome key barriers to eating healthy foods and improved their perceived ability to reduce consumption of unhealthy foods. The positive findings for increases in exercise perceived behavioral control and healthy eating perceived behavioral control (limit unhealthy foods) are particularly important for designing interventions as perceived behavioral control is a strong determinant of behavior in pregnant women [32] and will play a key role in the future intervention to manage GWG over the entire course of pregnancy.

Moreover, while we found increases in exercise subjective norm and healthy eating attitude (limit unhealthy foods), we interestingly observed a significant decrease in healthy eating subjective norm (limit unhealthy foods) over the intervention period. One explanation for these findings may be that women are exposed to intervention content on strategies to exercise and eat healthy, and this content partly focuses on the role that friends and family have in supporting these behaviors. While the women themselves may have improved their own feelings about the benefits of exercise and eating healthy through the intervention exposure, it is possible that some of the women also gained insight to barriers in their support system to eating healthy (e.g., husband or family poor eating habits) that decreased their subjective norm for limiting unhealthy foods. Future research is needed to better understand these normative influences for limiting unhealthy foods; additional intervention content on social influences may be needed in the future larger intervention to help women overcome these barriers.

Although we did not assume that brief exposure of the intervention would result in significant changes to exercise and healthy eating behaviors, we nevertheless observed some interesting findings. For example, although exercise activity time at W6 of the intervention was slightly lower (71 min) compared to W1 (75 min), exercise activity time was considerably higher at W3 (96 min) compared to all other weeks (e.g., range 65–75 min), and there was a significant increase in time from W2-W3. A similar pattern was observed for activity steps and energy expenditure kcal with the highest observed values at W3 of the intervention. It is possible that women started to feel more comfortable with the intervention by W3, and this resulted in a spike in their activity, but then they may have encountered some barriers (e.g., soreness or fatigue from exercise; thinking they were doing "too much too fast") that led to a decline in activity following W3. Even though the exercise sessions recommend activity within the guidelines (150 min/week of moderate intensity aerobic activity [25, 26]), the recommendation may have been perceived to be more intense by some than it actually was. Given that intervention exposure longer than six weeks is generally needed to see impact on behavioral changes [24], and we did not obtain weekly feedback on the women regarding specific exercise barriers, some caution is warranted with interpreting these findings. However, considering these findings in combination with the promising evidence for the positive effects of the intervention on the exercise motivational determinants, there is proof-of-concept for the intervention impacting exercise behaviors. Future research is needed to test this assumption over a longer period of time during pregnancy to understand changes in exercise as a result of the intervention.

Moreover, while energy intake trended toward a significant increase over the study period, it is important to note that (a) pregnant women are supposed to increase their energy intake in pregnancy and adjust it relative to their activity level [39], and (b) the observed increase from W1 to W6 was only a difference of approximately 200 kcal. In other words, there is proof-of-concept for the intervention to regulate energy intake such that it did not lead to a significant increase in kcal over the study period. Also, caloric needs for pregnant women differ across the trimesters, so the increase in kcal could be related to the range in gestational age of the participants [39] (e.g., gestational age at study start ranged from 12 to 25 weeks and at study end, ranged from 18 to 31 weeks). Increases in caloric needs over the course of pregnancy need to be taken into consideration when developing interventions to manage GWG. Future research is needed to understand the impact of our intervention on energy intake over the entire pregnancy and in relation to GWG. Furthermore, although we did not anticipate to find any significant differences in GWG, it is nevertheless important to note that we did not observe a significant increase in GWG over the course of the intervention period. The average change in GWG from week to week was ~1.1 pounds. Although this rate of change is higher than is recommended for overweight/obese pregnant women (e.g., average range of 0.4–0.7 pounds per week after the 1st trimester for overweight and obese, respectively; [1]), it is promising that we did not observe any large spikes in weight gain for most of the women. Future research is needed to test our intervention over the entire pregnancy to fully understand the impact on GWG.

Also, in partial support of our assumption, we observed a dose-response pre-post change in exercise perceived behavioral control, healthy eating perceived behavioral control, healthy eating perceived behavioral control (limit unhealthy foods), healthy eating intention, and healthy eating intention (limit unhealthy foods) but not exercise or healthy eating attitude or subjective norm. The dose-response change in exercise perceived behavioral control is important to highlight because with the higher dosage, the woman's perceived ease to exercise increases as they are provided with the tools to perform the behavior and know it is safe. With the feeling of increased ease to exercise, women are more likely to continue with exercise, which in turn will help manage energy balance for healthy weight gain throughout pregnancy. Similarly, the dose-response in perceived behavioral control healthy eating and healthy eating (limit unhealthy food) suggests that with a higher intervention dosage, there is greater perceived ease of eating healthy and limiting unhealthy foods. Higher intervention dosages included more intensive education materials, greater number of cooking demonstrations, and meal replacements, which provided women with the perceived resources and skills to make it easier to eat healthy and limit unhealthy foods. Also, in higher dosages, women had greater intention to eat healthy foods and to limit unhealthy foods. Coupled with the positive increase in attitude to limit unhealthy foods from pre- to post-intervention, and the trend for an increase in perceived behavioral control to limit unhealthy foods, these findings illustrate proof-of-concept for our intervention dosages. This is particularly important as our future intervention trial will be adapted over the entire pregnancy to help women adjust to their individual needs. For example, if a woman is successfully regulating her weight gain and staying within her GWG goals, she will continue with the baseline intervention (e.g., similar to Dosage 1 in this study). However, if another woman is struggling with regulating her GWG within her goals, the intervention will be adapted (i.e., made more intensive by increasing the dosage as illustrated in dosages 2–6 in this study) in 3- to 4-week cycles to manage GWG [19]

5. Implications for Practice and/or Policy

These study findings are important for clinical practice as they illustrate the importance of targeting motivational determinants for behavior change in addition to exercise and healthy eating to regulate GWG. Clinicians may want to consider talking with their overweight/obese prenatal patients more specifically about their attitudes, feelings, and barriers to making behavioral changes to better regulate their weight gain. Strengths of this study include the theoretically driven basis of the intervention, focus on overweight/obese women, population in need of managing GWG for healthy maternal and infant outcomes, randomized study design, and impact of the intervention on several outcomes after brief exposure. This study is also one of the first interventions to target both TPB and self-regulation constructs in an energy balance model for regulating GWG in overweight/obese pregnant women. These strengths are important for developing future interventions as well as disseminating information when helping pregnant women to regulate their GWG.

Limitations of this study include a small sample size with a homogenous sample (e.g., married, middle to upper class, Caucasian), which limits generalizability. Future research will aim to broaden generalizability of our study findings. Also, given the short duration of the intervention, we did not anticipate to see significant behavioral changes in exercise, energy intake, or GWG. Future research will need to examine the impact of the intervention on these behavioral targets over the full duration of pregnancy. Furthermore, although the healthy eating TPB measures were adapted from the validated exercise TPB measures, future research is needed to validate these items within our energy balance model.

6. Conclusions

Brief exposure to a theoretically driven, GWG intervention based on a model of energy balance resulted in significant increases to exercise and healthy eating motivational determinants, an increase in exercise in the middle of the intervention, and no significant changes to energy intake or GWG, supporting the initial proof-of-concept of the intervention among overweight/obese pregnant women. Future research will test this intervention in a larger trial over the entire duration of pregnancy to understand its impact on regulating GWG and maternal-infant health.

Disclosure

A poster related to this manuscript was presented at Obesity Week on November 11, 2016 (An Individually Tailored Gestational Weight Gain Intervention Impacts Determinants of Healthy Eating and Exercise Behaviors in Overweight and Obese Pregnant Women). The content is solely responsibility of the authors and does not necessarily represent the official views of the NIH.

Acknowledgments

The authors would like to acknowledge the assistance of the Healthy Mom Zone team who assisted with participant recruitment and data collection for this study. The project described was supported by the National Center for Advancing Translational Sciences and National Institutes of Health, through Grants UL1 TR000127 and TR002014. Support for this work has been provided by the National Heart, Lung, and Blood Institute (NHLBI) of the National Institutes of Health through Grant 1 R01 HL119245-01.

References

[1] Institute of Medicine, *Weight Gain during Pregnancy: Reexamining the Guidelines*, National Academies Press, Washington, DC, USA, 2009.

[2] National Vital Statistics System, "*QuickStats:* gestational weight gain among women with full-term, singleton births, compared with recommendations—48 States and the District of Columbia," *Morbidity and Mortality Weekly Report*, vol. 65, no. 40, p. 1121, 2016.

[3] J. M. Vernini, J. B. Moreli, C. G. Magalas, R. A. Cosat, M. V. Rudge, and I. M. Calderon, "Maternal and fetal outcomes in pregnancies complicated by overweight and obesity," *Reproductive Health*, vol. 13, no. 1, p. 100, 2016.

[4] D. S. Downs, "Obesity in special populations," *Primary Care: Clinics in Office Practice*, vol. 43, no. 1, pp. 109–120, 2016.

[5] J. M. Dodd, D. Turnbull, A. J. McPhee et al., "Antenatal lifestyle advice for women who are overweight or obese: LIMIT randomised trial," *BMJ*, vol. 348, article g1285, 2014.

[6] I. Guelinckx, R. Devlieger, P. Mullie, and G. Vansant, "Effect of lifestyle intervention on dietary habits, physical activity, and gestational weight gain in obese pregnant women: a randomized controlled trial," *American Journal of Clinical Nutrition*, vol. 91, no. 2, pp. 373–380, 2010.

[7] M. Hawkins, M. Hosker, B. H. Marcus et al., "A pregnancy lifestyle intervention to prevent gestational diabetes risk factors in overweight Hispanic women: a feasibility randomized controlled trial," *Diabetic Medicine*, vol. 32, no. 1, pp. 108–115, 2015.

[8] R. A. Krukowski, D. S. West, M. DiCarlo, M. A. Cleves, M. E. Saylors, and A. Andres, "Association of gestational weight gain expectations and advice on actual weight gain," *Obstetrics and Gynecology*, vol. 129, no. 1, pp. 76–82, 2017.

[9] L. Poston, A. L. Briley, S. Barr et al., "Developing a complex intervention for diet and activity behaviour change in obese pregnant women (the UPBEAT trial); assessment of behavioural change and process evaluation in a pilot randomised controlled trial," *BMC Pregnancy and Childbirth*, vol. 13, p. 148, 2013.

[10] K. K. Vesco, N. Karanja, J. C. King et al., "Efficacy of a group-based dietary intervention for limiting gestational weight gain among obese women: a randomized trial," *Obesity*, vol. 22, no. 9, pp. 1989–1996, 2014.

[11] L. Sagedal, N. Øverby, E. Bere et al., "Lifestyle intervention to limit gestational weight gain: the Norwegian fit for delivery randomised controlled trial," *BJOG: An International Journal of Obstetrics and Gynaecology*, vol. 124, no. 1, pp. 97–109, 2017.

[12] R. A. Krukowski, D. West, M. DiCarlo et al., "A behavioral intervention to reduce excessive gestational weight gain," *Maternal and Child Health Journal*, vol. 21, no. 3, pp. 485–491, 2016.

[13] Y. Dong, D. E. Rivera, D. M. Thomas et al., "A dynamical systems model for gestational weight gain behavioral interventions," in *Proceedings of the 2012 American Control Conference*, pp. 4059–4064, Montreal, QC, Canada, June 2012, PMID: 24309837.

[14] Y. Dong, D. E. Rivera, D. S. Downs, J. S. Savage, D. M. Thomas, and L. M. Collins, "Hybrid model predictive control for optimizing gestational weight gain behavioral interventions," in *Proceedings of the 2013 American Control Conference*, pp. 1970–1975, Washington, DC, USA, June 2013, PMID: 24336314, PMCID: PMC3856197.

[15] Y. Dong, S. Deshpande, D. E. Rivera, D. S. Downs, and J. S. Savage, "Hybrid model predictive control for sequential decision policies in adaptive behavioral interventions," in *Proceedings of the 2014 American Control Conference*, pp. 4198–4203, Portland, OR, USA, June 2014, ISBN: 978-1-4799-3271-9, PMID: 25635157, PMCID: PMC4307847.

[16] P. Guo, D. E. Rivera, D. S. Downs et al., "Semi-physical identification and state estimation of energy intake for interventions to manage gestational weight gain," in *Proceedings of the 2016 American Control Conference*, pp. 1271–1276, Boston, MA, USA, July 2016, PMID: 27570366 PMCID: PMC5001697.

[17] J. S. Savage, D. S. Downs, Y Dong, D. E. Rivera, and L. C. Collins, "Control systems engineering for optimizing a prenatal weight gain intervention to regulate infant birth weight," *American Journal of Public Health*, vol. 104, no. 7, pp. 1247–1254, 2014.

[18] D. Symons Downs, J. S. Savage, D. E. Rivera et al., "Influence of a feasibility study on the design of an individually-tailored, adaptive intervention to manage weight in overweight and obese pregnant women," *Annals of Behavioral Medicine*, vol. 51, no. S1, pp. S1451–S1452, 2017.

[19] D. Symons Downs, J. S. Savage, D. E. Rivera et al., "Individually tailored, adaptive intervention to manage gestational weight gain: protocol for a randomized controlled trial in women with overweight and obesity," *JMIR Research Protocols*, vol. 7, no. 6, p. e150, 2018.

[20] I. Ajzen, "The theory of planned behavior," *Organizational Behavior and Human Decision Processes*, vol. 50, no. 2, pp. 179–211, 1991.

[21] C. S. Carver and M. F. Scheier, *On the Self-Regulation of Behavior*, Cambridge University Press, Cambridge, UK, 1998.

[22] H. Leventhal, D. Nerenz, and D. Steele, "Illness representations and coping with health threats," in *A Handbook of Psychology and Health*, A. Baum and J. Singer, Eds., vol. 4, pp. 219–252, Erlbaum, Hillsdale, NJ, USA, 1984.

[23] D. S. Downs, J. M. Dinallo, L. L. Birch, I. M. Paul, and J. S. Ulbrecht, "Randomized face-to-face vs. home exercise interventions in pregnant women with gestational diabetes," *Psychology of Sport and Exercise*, vol. 30, pp. 73–81, 2017.

[24] B. Fjeldsoe, M. Neuhaus, E. Winkler, and E. Eakin, "Systematic review of maintenance of behavior change following physical activity and dietary interventions," *Health Psychology*, vol. 30, no. 1, pp. 99–109, 2011.

[25] ACOG Committee on Obstetric Practice, "ACOG Committee opinion no. 267: exercise during pregnancy and the postpartum period," *Obstetrics and Gynecology*, vol. 99, no. 1, pp. 171–173, 2002.

[26] ACOG Committee on Obstetric Practice, "ACOG Committee opinion no. 650: physical activity and exercise during pregnancy and the postpartum period," *Obstetrics and Gynecology*, vol. 126, no. 6, pp. e135–e142, 2015.

[27] P. A. Harris, R. Taylor, R. Thielke, J. Payne, N. Gonzalez, and J. G. Conde, "Research electronic data capture (REDCap)—a metadata-driven methodology and workflow process for providing translational research informatics support," *Journal of Biomedical Informatics*, vol. 42, no. 2, pp. 377–381, 2009.

[28] P. S. Petosa, *Use of social cognitive theory to explain exercise behavior among adults*, Ph.D. dissertation, The Ohio State University, Columbus, OH, USA, 1993.

[29] F. F. Sniehotta, R. Schwarzer, U. Scholz, and B. Schüz, "Action planning and coping planning for long-term lifestyle change: theory and assessment," *European Journal of Social Psychology*, vol. 35, no. 4, pp. 565–576, 2005.

[30] The Diabetes Prevention Program (DPP) Research Group, "The diabetes prevention program (DPP)," *Diabetes Care*, vol. 25, no. 12, pp. 2165–2171, 2002.

[31] T. A. Walls and J. L. Schafer, *Models for Intensive Longitudinal Data*, Oxford University Press, Oxford, UK, 2006.

[32] D. S. Downs and H. A. Hausenblas, "Exercising for two: Examining pregnant women's second trimester exercise intention and behavior using the framework of the theory of planned behavior," *Women's Health Issues*, vol. 13, no. 6, pp. 222–228, 2003.

[33] D. Symons Downs and H. A. Hausenblas, "Exercising during pregnancy and postpartum: an elicitation study using the framework of the theory of planned behavior," *Journal of Midwifery and Women's Health*, vol. 49, no. 2, pp. 138–144, 2004.

[34] M. R. Umstattd, R. Motl, S. Wilcox, R. Saunders, and M. Watford, "Measuring physical activity self-regulation strategies in older adults," *Journal of Physical Activity and Health*, vol. 6, no. S1, pp. S105–S112, 2009.

[35] T. Ferguson, A. V. Rowlands, T. Olds, and C. Maher, "The validity of consumer-level, activity monitors in healthy adults worn in free-living conditions: a cross-sectional study," *International Journal of Behavioral Nutrition and Physical Activity*, vol. 12, no. 1, pp. 1–9, 2015.

[36] F. A. Storm, B. W. Heller, and C. Mazzà, "Step detection and activity recognition accuracy of seven physical activity monitors," *PLoS One*, vol. 10, no. 3, Article ID e0118723, 2015.

[37] S. W. Lichtman, K. Pisarska, E. R. Berman et al., "Discrepancy between self reported and actual caloric intake and exercise in obese subjects," *New England Journal of Medicine*, vol. 327, no. 27, pp. 1893–1898, 1992.

[38] M. A. Hertzog, "Considerations in determining sample size for pilot studies," *Research in Nursing & Health*, vol. 31, no. 2, pp. 180–191, 2008.

[39] M. A. Kominiarek and P. Rajan, "Nutrition recommendations in pregnancy and lactation," *Medical Clinics of North America*, vol. 100, no. 6, pp. 1199–1215, 2016.

16

The Chronic Effect of Interval Training on Energy Intake: A Systematic Review and Meta-Analysis

Jenna Taylor, Shelley E. Keating, David J. Holland, Jeff S. Coombes, and Michael D. Leveritt

School of Human Movement and Nutrition Sciences, The University of Queensland, St. Lucia, Brisbane, QLD 4072, Australia

Correspondence should be addressed to Jenna Taylor; j.kirchner@uq.edu.au

Academic Editor: R. Prager

Single bouts of acute exercise do not appear to increase subsequent energy intake (EI), even when energy deficit is large. However, studies have shown a compensatory effect on EI following chronic exercise, and it remains unclear whether this is affected by exercise intensity. We investigated the chronic effect of high-intensity interval training (HIIT) and sprint interval training (SIT) on EI when compared with moderate-intensity continuous training (MICT) or no exercise (CON). Databases were searched until 13 March 2017 for studies measuring EI in response to chronic exercise (≥4 weeks of duration) of a high-intensity interval nature. Meta-analysis was conducted for between-group comparisons on EI (kilojoules) and bodyweight (kg). Results showed large heterogeneity, and therefore, metaregression analyses were conducted. There were no significant differences in EI between HIIT/SIT versus MICT ($P = 0.282$), HIIT/SIT versus CON ($P = 0.398$), or MICT versus CON ($P = 0.329$). Although bodyweight was significantly reduced after HIIT/SIT versus CON but not HIIT/SIT versus MICT (in studies measuring EI), this was not clinically meaningful (<2% mean difference). In conclusion, there is no compensatory increase in EI following a period of HIIT/SIT compared to MICT or no exercise. However, this review highlights important methodological considerations for future studies.

1. Introduction

Obesity is a now a global epidemic with the prevalence of overweight and obesity estimated as 39% of the world's population [1]. Increasing energy expenditure through exercise to manage obesity is a logical approach. However, when compared to dietary restriction, exercise is often portrayed as a somewhat "futile method for weight loss" because exercise interventions commonly lead to less than expected weight loss [2, 3]. Indeed, it is generally accepted that exercise requires concomitant dietary modification for significant weight loss (>5% reduction) [4, 5].

The modest effect of exercise interventions on weight loss is likely a result of individual variability in response to intervention [3]. Proposed mechanisms for less than expected weight loss in some individuals may be explained by reduced exercise adherence [4], decreased spontaneous physical activity [2], overestimation of weight loss from predictive equations [6], and automatic metabolic adaptations that lower the energy expenditure [2]. A comprehensive review of these factors has been presented elsewhere [2]. Dietary compensation factors that could increase caloric intake and result in less than expected weight loss with exercise include biological changes driving appetite [7], changes in food preferences and food reward [8], and other psychological dietary behaviours (e.g., restraint and disinhibition) [9, 10].

There is now a general consensus that acute moderate-intensity aerobic exercise does not increase absolute energy intake [11, 12], even when energy deficit is large [13]. However, there is still uncertainty about the effect of mode and intensity of acute exercise on appetite and energy intake response. There is also less agreement about the effect of higher-intensity exercise and chronic exercise on energy intake. Donnelly and colleagues found that long-term exercise did not result in a compensatory increase in energy intake [12], while a partial compensation (+30%) in energy intake with chronic exercise has been demonstrated following 7 days [14] and 14 days [15].

There is much interest in the effect of high-intensity interval training (HIIT) or sprint interval training (SIT) on weight loss and specifically whether exercise intensity influences appetite and energy intake. Regarding fat loss, results to date are conflicting with studies showing a superior effect of HIIT [16–18], superior effect of MICT [19, 20], and similar effects [21–26]. A recent meta-analysis found no significant differences between HIIT/SIT and MICT on total fat mass or total body fat percentage [27] and that body fat reduction tended to favor MICT if it produced a greater energy expenditure.

The evidence regarding the effect of exercise intensity on appetite and energy intake is also conflicting [26, 28–31]. Appetite is a physical desire for food, mediated by central and peripheral systems (including secretion of hormones via the gastrointestinal tract) that influence both psychological (desire and enjoyment) and physiological (hunger and satiety) states that affect energy intake. In terms of acute studies, only one study [28] has found a significant reduction in ad libitum energy intake following HIIT compared with MICT, despite no differences in perceived appetite. Other studies have found no group differences in energy intake with [30, 32] or without [29, 33] changes in appetite. Following chronic exercise, Sim et al. [26] found a clinically meaningful improvement in appetite regulation following 12 weeks of HIIT but not for MICT and CON. This study measured appetite regulation as ad libitum energy intake following a preload meal. Alkahtani et al. [31] also found an effect of exercise intensity on dietary compensation following a 4-week intervention, with HIIT decreasing intake of fat by 16% and decreasing exercise-induced preference for high-fat, nonsweet foods. The moderate-intensity group increased fat intake by 38% and showed an increase in exercise-induced preference for high-fat, nonsweet foods. Panissa et al. [24] found no group differences in energy intake or appetite after 6 weeks of training.

Acute suppression of appetite from exercise may be due to changes in appetite-regulating hormones, by simultaneously suppressing acylated ghrelin (orexigenic hormone) and increasing peptide YY (anorexigenic hormone) up to 9 hours after exercise [34]. However, despite appetite being suppressed in the hours following exercise, total daily energy intake appears to be unaffected [35]. Therefore, acute appetite suppression may not necessarily translate into decreased volitional caloric intake [13, 36, 37]. Long-term adaptations that may influence appetite and energy intake include changes in psychological eating behaviours (restraint, desire, and food preferences) and improvements in insulin sensitivity. Insulin levels have been shown to improve satiety and reduce energy intake; however, this effect is blunted in people with insulin resistance [38]. Therefore, exercise protocols producing enhanced insulin sensitivity such as HIIT compared with MICT [39] may offer greater improvements in appetite regulation and energy intake [26].

Given the importance of obesity management and the interest in HIIT, we sought to determine what effect this time-efficient exercise option may have on energy intake. HIIT/SIT is often considered time efficient, when greater or comparable health and fitness benefits to MICT are produced with less time commitment [19].

The purpose of this study was to conduct a systematic review with a meta-analysis of randomized controlled trials to determine the chronic effect of HIIT/SIT on energy intake when compared with MICT or no exercise (CON) in an adult population. Understanding the impact of exercise intensity on energy intake would assist in developing more targeted and effective exercise protocols for weight management in the future.

2. Methods

This systematic review has been designed and presented in accordance with the Preferred Reporting Items for Systematic Reviews and Meta-Analyses (PRISMA) Statement [40].

2.1. Eligibility Criteria. Full-text, randomized controlled trials in English peer-reviewed journals were eligible for inclusion in this systematic review and meta-analysis if energy intake was measured in response to chronic exercise training of a high intensity, or sprint interval nature, compared with MICT or no exercise. Specifically, HIIT was characterized by an exercise intensity of 85–95% peak heart rate (HR_{peak}), or 80–95% peak oxygen consumption (VO_{2peak}) or peak work rate. SIT was characterized by an exercise intensity relating to all-out sprint, or ≥100% VO_{2peak} or peak power. These are consistent with recently proposed classifications for interval training [41]. Eligibility of studies was not restricted by duration of intervals or all-out sprints. In comparison, MICT was characterized as exercise performed continuously at a steady state, within the intensity range of 60–75% HR_{peak}, 40–64% VO_{2peak}, or 40–59% heart rate reserve (HRR) [42, 43]. Energy intake (measured as kilojoules or calories) was required to be measured before and after the exercise intervention. There was no restriction placed on assessment methods for energy intake. Therefore, if the study reported energy intake, it was included in the meta-analysis. To be considered a chronic exercise intervention, duration was required to be ≥4 weeks. Studies were excluded if participants were children or adolescents or if participants were provided with individual dietary prescription or medical weight loss aids.

2.2. Search Strategy. The search strategy involved major databases (PubMed, Scopus, and EMBASE/MEDLINE) and the following search terms in title/abstract/keywords: "exercise" OR "training" AND "interval" OR "intermittent" OR "sprint" OR "low volume" AND "energy intake" OR "caloric intake" OR "body composition" OR "bodyweight", AND "week/s" OR "month/s". Additional search criteria were applied to retrieve studies published in English and to eliminate reviews and studies involving animals. The last search was conducted on March 13, 2017.

2.3. Data Extraction. Full-text versions were independently assessed for eligibility criteria and quality by 2 investigators (Jenna Taylor and Michael D. Leveritt) and coded as "yes" or "no." If a discrepancy in coding between authors was presented, a discussion took place until the result was unanimous. An independent researcher was available if a unanimous decision could not be reached. The outcome measures used were energy intake in kilojoules. If data were reported in kilocalories, these were converted to kilojoules using a conversion factor of 4.18 kilojoules per kilocalorie. The secondary outcome measure of bodyweight in kilograms was also extracted from the studies reporting energy intake. Data on participant characteristics and other aspects of study methodology (including exercise interventions and energy intake method) were also extracted into table format.

2.4. Study Quality. Quality of the included studies was assessed by a modified Physiotherapy Evidence Database (PEDro) Scale [44]. The original 11-point scale includes items for eligibility criteria, random allocation, concealment of allocation, baseline comparability, blinding of subjects, blinding of therapists, blinding of assessors, adequate follow-up, intention to treat analysis, between-group statistical comparisons, and reporting of point estimates and variability. The scale was modified to include an additional 4 criteria that may have impact on the primary outcome: exercise training supervision, reporting of exercise adherence, measurement of habitual physical activity, and estimation/calculation of energy expenditure. Additionally, the scale was modified to exclude 2 criteria that are technically challenging in interval training exercise interventions: blinding of subjects and blinding of therapists. Therefore, the modified scale included 13 criteria with one point awarded for each.

2.5. Meta-Analyses. All analyses were conducted using the Comprehensive Meta-Analysis software (Version 3, Biostat, Englewood, NJ). Methods for meta-analysis and metaregression were based on recommendations for continuous outcomes from the Cochrane Handbook for Systematic Reviews [45].

For the primary analysis, a between-group meta-analysis was conducted by pooling energy intake for HIIT/SIT compared with MICT, HIIT/SIT compared with CON, and MICT compared with CON. The between-trial standardized mean difference or effect size, 95% confidence interval (CI), and P values were calculated using a random effect model. We presumed a correlation of 0.7 between outcomes measured within each comparison group. Hedge's g was used to measure the effect size due to small sample sizes of the included studies. Heterogeneity was assessed via the Cochran Q-test (significance determined at the level of significance $P = 0.1$) and quantified with the I^2 statistic to determine how much of the variability between studies is due to heterogeneity rather than chance. For the secondary analysis, the same methods and comparisons were used for bodyweight data. Publication bias and small-study effect was assessed by visual inspection of funnel plot asymmetry (precision versus effect size) using Egger's test and by calculating the P value of Egger's intercept. Metaregression analyses were performed to examine the relationships between effect size estimates and the following covariates: (1) duration of intervention, (2) the total number of exercise sessions, (3) age, (4) sex, (5) baseline body mass index (BMI), (6) metabolic disease, (7) energy intake collection method, and (8) study quality.

3. Results

Results of the search strategy and study selection are outlined in Figure 1. A total of 1618 studies were retrieved using the aforementioned search strategy with 1094 studies remaining following removal of duplicates. During title and abstract screening, 974 studies were excluded, leaving a total of 119 studies for full-text analysis. Of the 119 studies, English full-text versions were available for 92 studies. After exclusions, 17 studies remained following full-text analysis, with 6 authors being contacted for energy intake data [20, 25, 26, 46–48]. Of the authors contacted, one study had not measured energy intake [25], leaving 16 studies to be included in the meta-analysis. One of the contacted authors reported that their energy intake data were published elsewhere [49], and therefore, this paper was used in the analysis.

3.1. Participant Characteristics. Participant characteristics are summarized in Table 1. Data were reported for a total of 475 participants in the included studies (159 HIIT, 64 SIT, 165 MICT, and 87 CON). The mean age of participants ranged from 20 to 55 years. Six studies recruited only males [17, 21, 23, 26, 47, 50], six studies had only females [18, 20, 24, 51–53], and four studies recruited both males and females [19, 46, 49, 54]. Only one study mentioned timing of the menstrual cycle [18], and no studies reported the use of oral contraceptives. Most studies used healthy individuals [18–21, 24, 26, 46, 50–54], with four studies recruiting participants with metabolic syndrome [17, 23, 49] or type 2 diabetes [47]. Only one study recruited active participants [53]. All other studies recruited inactive participants.

3.2. Study Methodology Characteristics. Exercise intervention characteristics are detailed in Table 1. Sixteen studies were included in the meta-analysis with a total of 12 HIIT groups, 13 MICT groups, 4 SIT groups, and 7 CON (no exercise) groups. Due to the small number of SIT groups, these were combined with HIIT for analysis, giving a total of 16 HIIT/SIT groups.

Large heterogeneity of protocols existed within the HIIT/SIT groups, with some studies using high-intensity intervals of <30 seconds [18, 26, 46, 47, 50, 52], 30–60 seconds [19, 21, 24, 51, 54], 2 minutes [17, 53], 3 minutes [23], and 4 minutes [20, 49]. On the contrary, the intensity of exercise prescribed for HIIT was consistent at 85–95% VO_{2peak} or HR_{peak}. The only exception was the SIT studies that employed workloads of 120% VO_{2peak} [19], 170% VO_{2peak} [26], or "all-out sprinting" [47, 51]. MICT groups were also relatively similar with regard to exercise intensity with prescriptions in the range of 50–70% VO_{2peak} or HR_{peak}.

Participants exercised at a frequency of 4 days per week [17, 52, 54] or 3 days per week [18–21, 23, 24, 26, 46, 47, 49–51, 53],

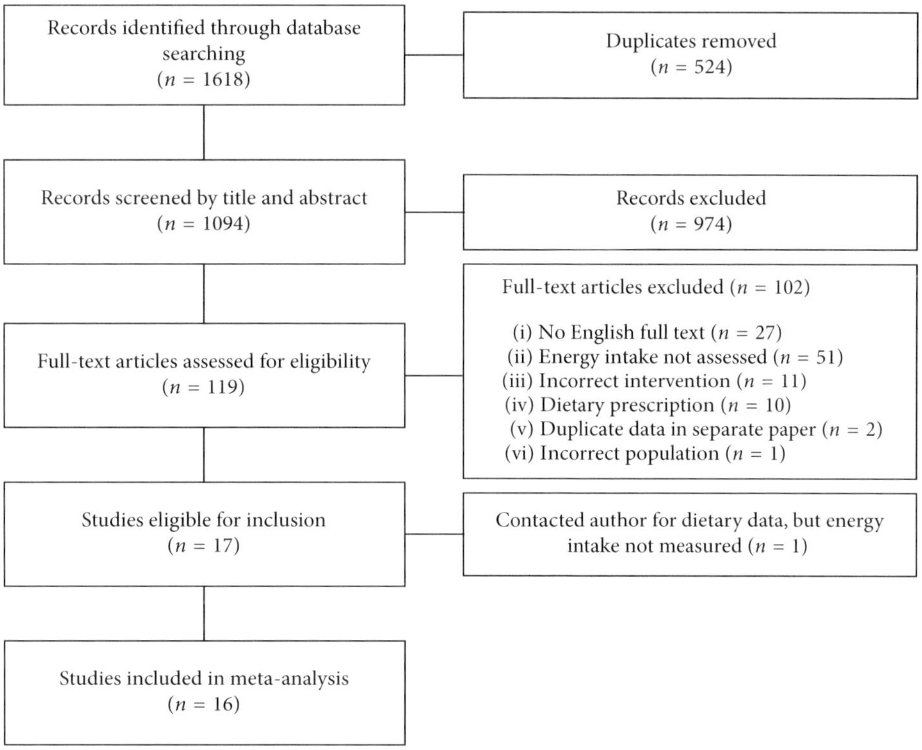

FIGURE 1: Flowchart of study selection.

with duration of exercise <30 minutes per day [21, 24, 47, 50–53] or 30–50 minutes per day [17–20, 23, 26, 49, 54]. Nine studies [17, 18, 20, 21, 24, 26, 46, 51, 54] reported using various methods to create "isocaloric" or "work-matched" protocols for HIIT and MICT. Most studies reported supervision of training [17, 19, 23, 24, 26, 46–48, 50, 51, 53, 54]; however, adherence to training intensities was poorly reported. Only one study confirmed adherence to the prescribed intensity of training protocols [17]. Three studies reported a significant difference in average training workload between groups but did not discuss whether this adhered with the intended intensity [18, 26, 47, 50]. One study reported no significant difference in average training HR between groups [52], and the remaining 11 studies made no mention of average training intensity or adherence [19–21, 23, 24, 46, 49, 51, 53, 54].

Studies also varied in their measurement of daily energy intake. The majority of studies used self-reported food diaries for 3 days [18, 19, 23, 24, 46, 47, 50, 52, 53] or 7 days [54]. Other studies used a self-administered diet history [21] or food frequency questionnaires [17, 20, 49]. One study used an ad libitum test meal with known composition and then used the self-reported weighed food diary for remainder of the day [26], and one study used the automated 24-hour diet recall method over 3 days [51].

All studies except Earnest et al. [17] included means and standard deviations of daily energy intake before and after the intervention. Earnest et al. [17] reported the mean and standard deviation of baseline energy intake and change scores for postintervention energy intake.

3.3. Study Quality. Using the modified PEDro Scale, six studies scored ≤8/13 [18, 20, 21, 24, 50, 52] and ten studies scored ≥8/13 [17, 19, 23, 26, 46, 47, 49, 51, 53, 54]. All included studies randomly allocated participants to groups, reported statistical comparisons between groups for the primary outcome, and reported point estimates and variability. Only one study reported blinding the assessor [19]. Details of study quality scores are presented in Table 2. As the majority of studies scored ≥8, metaregression was performed to assess the study quality; however, the results showed no significance.

3.4. Meta-Analyses. The between-group analyses for the primary analysis on energy intake are presented as HIIT/SIT versus MICT (Figure 2), HIIT/SIT versus CON (Figure 3), and MICT versus CON (Figure 4). There were no significant differences in energy intake for any comparison groups, including HIIT/SIT versus MICT ($P = 0.282$), HIIT/SIT versus CON ($P = 0.398$), or MICT versus CON ($P = 0.329$), or with subgroup analyses for HIIT and SIT. There was evidence of moderate heterogeneity for HIIT/SIT versus MICT ($I^2 = 50\%$), high heterogeneity for HIIT/SIT versus CON ($I^2 = 92\%$), and low heterogeneity for MICT versus CON ($I^2 = 0\%$). Due to the heterogeneity of studies, metaregression was performed but found no effect of study duration, the total number of exercise sessions, age, sex, baseline BMI (>30 $kg{\cdot}m^{-2}$), metabolic disease (compared with healthy participants), energy intake collection method, or study quality (≤8 or ≥8). Outcomes of the metaregression are presented in Table 3. The between-group analyses for the

TABLE 1: Participant and intervention characteristics of included studies.

Reference	Population	Age (years)	BMI (kg/m^2)	Duration (weeks)/sessions	HIIT/SIT protocol	MICT protocol	CON	Energy intake method
Ruffino et al. [47]	Male T2DM inactive	55	30.6	8/24 HIIT and 40 MICT	SIT: $n = 16$; cycling, supervised ~2 × 30 sec (all-out sprint) with 4 min active recovery. Total duration = ~10 min	$n = 16$; cycling, supervised continuous (40–55% HRR). Total duration = 30 min	N/A	3-day food diary
Higgins et al. [51]	Female healthy inactive	20	30.3	6/18	SIT: $n = 29$; cycling, supervised ~5–7 × 30 sec (all-out sprint) with 4 min active recovery. Total duration = ~25–38 min	$n = 23$; cycling, supervised continuous (60–70% HRR). Total duration = 20–30 min	N/A	24-hour recalls (3 days, automated)
Sim et al. [26]	Male healthy inactive	30	27.2	12/36	SIT: $n = 12$; cycling, supervised 10 × 15 sec (170% VO_{2peak}) with 60 sec active recovery (30% VO_{2peak}). Total duration = 30–45 min	$n = 12$; cycling, supervised continuous (60% VO_{2peak}). Total duration = 30–45 min	$n = 10$	2-day food diary
Keating et al. [19]	Male/female healthy inactive	43	28.3	12/36	SIT: $n = 13$; cycling, supervised 6 × 30–60 sec (120% VO_{2peak}) with 2-3 min active recovery. Total duration = 20–24 min	$n = 13$; cycling, supervised continuous (50–65% VO_{2peak}). Total duration = 36–48 min	$n = 12$	3-day food diary
Kong et al. [52]	Female healthy inactive	20	25.7	5/20	HIIT: $n = 10$; cycling 60 × 8 sec (90% VO_{2max}) with 12 sec active recovery. Total duration = ~20 min	$n = 8$; cycling continuous (65% VO_{2peak}). Total duration = 40 min	N/A	3-day food diary
Martins et al. [46]	Male/female healthy inactive	34	33.3	12/36	HIIT: $n = 16$; cycling, supervised ~60 × 8 sec (85–90% VO_{2max}) with 12 sec passive rest. Total duration = 20 min	$n = 14$; cycling, supervised continuous (70% VO_{2peak}). Total duration = 32 min	N/A	3-day food diary
Panissa et al. [24]	Female healthy untrained	28	24.6	6/18	HIIT: $n = 11$; unknown mode, supervised 15 × 1 min (90% HR_{max}) with 30 sec active recovery (60% HR_{max}). Total duration = 22 min	$n = 11$; unknown mode, supervised continuous (70% HR_{max}). Total duration = 29 min	N/A	3-day food diary
Matsuo et al. [23]	Male metabolic syndrome inactive	48	27.6	8/24	HIIT: $n = 13$; cycling, supervised 3 × 3 min (85% VO_{2peak}) with 2 min active recovery (50% VO_{2peak}). Total duration = 18 min	$n = 13$; cycling, supervised continuous (65% VO_{2peak}). Total duration = 45 min	N/A	3-day food diary (weighed)
Sasaki et al. [21]	Male healthy inactive	NR	23.9	4/12	HIIT: $n = 12$; cycling 10 × 1 min (85% VO_{2max}) with 30 sec passive rest. Total duration = 14 min	$n = 12$; cycling continuous (45% VO_{2peak}). Total duration = 22 min	N/A	Self-administered diet history questionnaire

Table 1: Continued.

Reference	Population	Age (years)	BMI (kg/m^2)	Duration (weeks)/sessions	HIIT/SIT protocol	MICT protocol	CON	Energy intake method
Earnest et al. [17]	Male metabolic syndrome inactive	48	30.9	6/18	HIIT: n = 21; treadmill, supervised 8 × 2 min (90–95% VO_{2max}) with 2 min active recovery (50% VO_{2max}). Total duration = 12 kcal/kg/week	n = 16; treadmill, supervised continuous (50–70% VO_{2max}). Total duration = 12 kcal/kg/week	N/A	Food frequency questionnaire
Eimarieskandari et al. [20]	Female healthy inactive	22	29.6	8/24	HIIT: n = 7; treadmill 4 × 4 min (85–95% HR_{peak}) with 3 min active recovery (50–70% HR_{2peak}). Total duration = 33 min	n = 7; treadmill continuous (50–70% HR_{peak}). Total duration = 36–41 min	N/A	7-day diet questionnaire
Wallman et al. [54]	Male/female healthy inactive	42	30.5	8/32	HIIT: n = 8; cycling, supervised 10 × 60 sec (90% VO_{2peak}) with 2 min active recovery (30% VO_{2peak}). Total duration = 30 min	n = 8; cycling, supervised continuous (50–65% VO_{2peak}). Total duration = 30 min	n = 8	7-day food diary
Trapp et al. [18]	Female healthy inactive	20	23.2	15/45	HIIT: n = 15; cycling 60 × 8 sec (85% VO_{2max}) with 12 sec active recovery. Total duration = 20 min	n = 15; cycling continuous (60% VO_{2peak}). Total duration = 40 min	n = 15	3-day food diary
Heydari et al. [50]	Male healthy inactive	25	29.0	12/36	HIIT: n = 20; cycling, supervised 60 × 8 sec (85–90% HR_{peak}) with 12 sec active recovery. Total duration = 20 min	N/A	n = 18	3-day food diary
Stensvold et al. [49]	Male/female metabolic syndrome inactive	50	31.8	12/36	HIIT: n = 11; treadmill, supervised 4 × 4 min (90–95% HR_{peak}) with 3 min active recovery (70% HR_{peak}). Total duration = 43 min	N/A	n = 10	Food frequency questionnaire
Walter et al. [53]	Female healthy active	22	23.6	6/18	HIIT: n = 19; cycling, supervised 5 × 2 min (90–100% HR_{max}) with 1 min passive rest. Total duration = 19 min	N/A	n = 11	24-hour recalls (3 days, manual)

BMI: body mass index; HIIT: high-intensity interval training; SIT: sprint interval training; HR_{peak}: peak heart rate; VO_{2peak}: peak oxygen consumption; MICT: moderate-intensity continuous training; CON: control.

Table 2: Study quality.

Study	1	2	3	4	5	6	7	8	9	10	11	12	13	Total
Earnest et al. [17]	1	1	1	1	0	1	0	1	1	1	1	1	1	11
Eimarieskandari et al. [20]	1	1	0	1	0	1	0	1	1	0	0	0	0	6
Heydari et al. [50]	0	1	0	1	0	0	0	1	1	1	0	0	0	5
Higgins et al. [51]	1	1	0	1	0	1	0	1	1	1	1	1	1	10
Keating et al. [19]	1	1	1	1	1	1	1	1	1	1	1	1	0	12
Kong et al. [52]	1	1	0	1	0	0	0	1	1	0	0	1	1	7
Martins et al. [46]	1	1	0	1	0	0	0	1	1	1	1	1	1	9
Matsuo et al. [23]	1	1	1	1	0	1	0	1	1	1	1	0	1	10
Panissa et al. [24]	1	1	0	0	0	1	0	1	1	1	0	0	0	6
Ruffino et al. [47]	1	1	0	1	0	0	0	1	1	1	1	1	0	8
Sasaki et al. [21]	0	1	0	1	0	0	0	1	1	0	0	1	0	5
Sim et al. [26]	1	1	1	1	0	1	0	1	1	1	1	1	0	10
Stensvold et al. [49]	1	1	1	1	0	1	0	1	1	1	0	0	0	8
Trapp et al. [18]	0	1	0	1	0	0	0	1	1	0	0	0	1	5
Wallman et al. [54]	0	1	0	1	0	1	0	1	1	1	0	1	1	8
Walter et al. [53]	1	1	0	1	0	1	1	1	1	1	0	0	0	8

Modified PEDro criteria: (1) eligibility criteria were specified; (2) participants were randomly allocated to groups; (3) allocation was concealed; (4) groups were similar at baseline; (5) blinding of assessors; (6) measures of at least one key outcome were obtained from more than 85% of participants allocated to groups; (7) intention to treat analysis: data for at least one key outcome were analyzed by "intention to treat"; (8) the results of between-group statistical comparisons are reported for the primary outcome; (9) the study provides the point measures and measures of variability for at least one key outcome; (10) exercise training was supervised; (11) exercise adherence was reported; (12) habitual physical activity was measured; (13) energy expenditure of exercise training was estimated/calculated and reported.

Study name	Comparison	Effect size (95% CI)	*P* value
Matsuo et al. [23]	HIIT versus MICT	−0.118 (−0.863 to 0.627)	
Sasaki et al. [21]	HIIT versus MICT	0.396 (−0.385 to 1.177)	
Panissa et al. [24]	HIIT versus MICT	−0.221 (−1.012 to 0.571)	
Wallman et al. [54]	HIIT versus MICT	0.152 (−0.864 to 1.168)	
Eimarieskandari et al. [20]	HIIT versus MICT	−0.145 (−1.161 to 0.871)	
Earnest et al. [17]	HIIT versus MICT	−0.454 (−1.099 to 0.190)	
Kong et al. [52]	HIIT versus MICT	−0.078 (−0.964 to 0.808)	
Overall: HIIT versus MICT		−0.082 (−0.530 to 0.366)	0.720
Martins et al. [46]	SIT versus MICT	−0.080 (−0.825 to 0.665)	
Keating et al. [19]	SIT versus MICT	0.317 (−0.432 to 1.067)	
Sim et al. [26]	SIT versus MICT	0.076 (−0.697 to 0.848)	
Trapp et al. [18]	SIT versus MICT	−2.879 (−4.142 to −1.616)	
Higgins et al. [51]	SIT versus MICT	−0.382 (−0.926 to 0.162)	
Ruffino et al. [47]	SIT versus MICT	0.107 (−0.568 to 0.783)	
Overall: SIT versus MICT		−0.280 (−0.745 to 0.186)	0.239
Overall: HIIT/SIT versus MICT		−0.177 (−0.500 to 0.146)	0.282

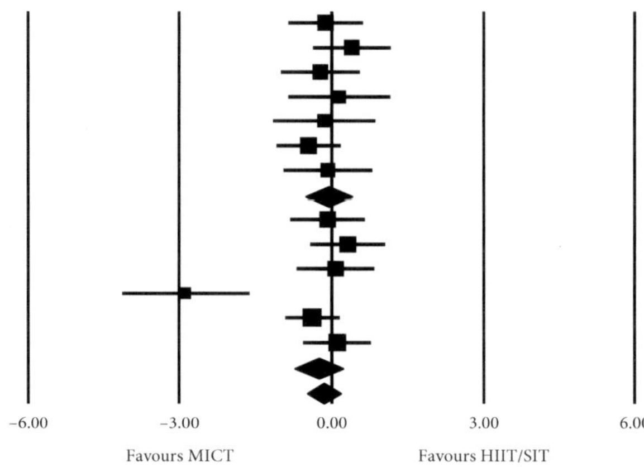

Figure 2: Meta-analysis for the comparison of HIIT/SIT versus MICT on energy intake. HIIT: high-intensity interval training, SIT: sprint interval training, MICT: moderate-intensity continuous training, and CI: confidence interval.

Study name	Comparison	Effect size (95% CI)	*P* value
Wallman et al. [54]	HIIT versus CON	0.116 (−0.840 to 1.071)	
Heydari et al. [50]	HIIT versus CON	0.108 (−0.463 to 0.679)	
Stensvold et al. [49]	HIIT versus CON	0.560 (−0.280 to 1.399)	
Walter et al. [53]	HIIT versus CON	−1.222 (−2.008 to −0.436)	
Overall: HIIT versus CON		−0.112 (−1.376 to −1.152)	0.862
Keating et al. [19]	SIT versus CON	0.267 (−0.495 to 1.030)	
Sim et al. [26]	SIT versus CON	0.672 (−0.160 to 1.503)	
Trapp et al. [18]	SIT versus CON	−3.898 (−5.198 to −2.598)	
Overall: SIT versus CON		−0.843 (−2.339 to 0.652)	0.269
Overall: HIIT/SIT versus CON		−0.417 (−1.382 to 0.549)	0.398

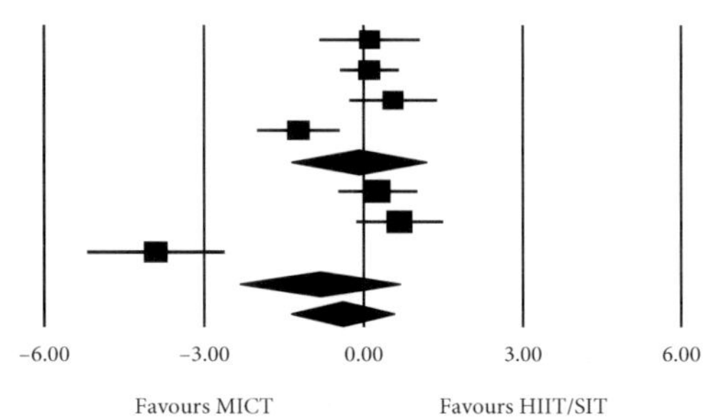

Figure 3: Effect of HIIT/SIT versus CON on energy intake. HIIT: high-intensity interval training, SIT: sprint interval training, CON: control, and CI: confidence interval.

Study name	Comparison	Effect size (95% CI)	*P* value
Keating et al. [19]	MICT versus CON	0.058 (−0.700 to 0.817)	
Sim et al. [26]	MICT versus CON	−0.443 (−1.261 to 0.375)	
Trapp et al. [18]	MICT versus CON	−0.469 (−1.307 to 0.369)	
Wallman et al. [54]	MICT versus CON	0.041 (−0.950 to 1.032)	
Overall: MICT versus CON		−0.209 (−0.629 to 0.211)	0.329

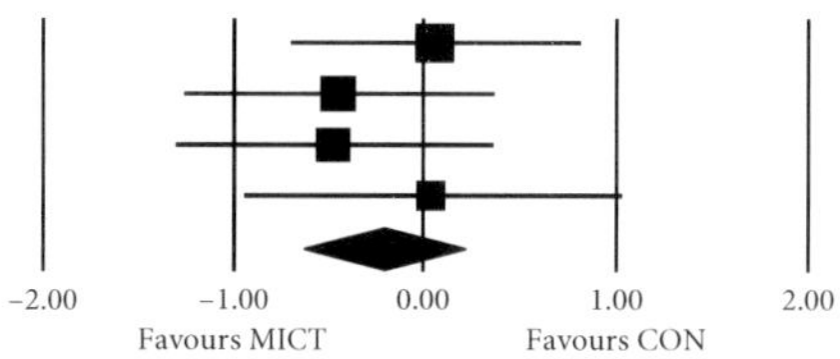

FIGURE 4: Effect of MICT versus CON on energy intake. MICT: moderate-intensity continuous training, CON: control, and CI: confidence interval.

TABLE 3: Metaregression of the pooled effect of comparisons of HIIT/SIT versus MICT on energy intake (kJ) by characteristics of studies.

Comparison	Regression coefficient (95% CI)	*P* value
HIIT/SIT versus MICT (13 studies)		
(i) Duration	−0.2043 (−1.3249 to 0.9163)	0.767
(ii) Sessions	0.0315 (−0.3807 to 0.4437)	0.881
(iii) Sex: male	−0.2832 (−1.2370 to 0.6706)	0.561
(iv) Sex: female	−0.5507 (−1.8521 to 0.7507)	0.407
(v) Age	0.0084 (−0.0468 to 0.0637)	0.765
(vi) BMI	0.0749 (−0.7328 to 0.8826)	0.858
(vii) Metabolic disease	−0.0137 (−0.9263 to 0.8990)	0.977
(viii) Energy intake method	—	0.992
(xi) Study quality	0.3190 (−0.3588 to 0.9968)	0.356
HIIT/SIT versus CON (7 studies)		
(i) Duration	−0.2043 (−1.3249 to 0.9163)	0.721
(ii) Sessions	0.0315 (−0.3807 to 0.4437)	0.881
(iii) Sex: male	1.9613 (−2.2499 to 6.1725)	0.361
(iv) Sex: female	−0.0725 (−5.6154 to 5.4704)	0.980
(v) Age	0.1078 (−0.1153 to 0.3309)	0.344
(vi) BMI	0.0305 (−2.2832 to 2.3443)	0.979
(vii) Metabolic disease	1.1265 (−2.1349 to 4.3879)	0.979
(viii) Energy intake method	—	0.826
(xi) Study quality	1.7705 (−0.3926 to 3.9337)	0.109

BMI: body mass index; HIIT: high-intensity interval training; SIT: sprint interval training; MICT: moderate-intensity continuous training; CON: control; CI: confidence interval.

secondary analysis on bodyweight are presented as HIIT/SIT versus CON (Figure 5), HIIT/SIT versus MICT (Figure 6), and MICT versus CON (Figure 7). A significant difference between groups for change in bodyweight was found for HIIT/SIT versus CON ($P = 0.011$) but not for HIIT/SIT versus MICT ($P = 0.644$) or MICT versus CON ($P = 0.246$). There was evidence of low heterogeneity for all comparisons ($I^2 = 0\%$), and therefore, metaregression was not warranted.

Finally, funnel plots and Egger's intercept showed no evidence of publication bias or small-study effect for any primary or secondary analysis comparisons.

4. Discussion

To our knowledge, this is the first systematic review with meta-analysis examining the chronic effect of interval training on energy intake when compared with MICT or no exercise. When data from studies were pooled, there were no significant differences in change in energy intake with HIIT/SIT or MICT, and the metaregression found no impact of other variables on these outcomes. Our secondary analysis found a significant reduction in bodyweight with HIIT/SIT compared to CON (in studies that measured energy intake); however, there is no significant difference in bodyweight for HIIT/SIT compared to MICT, or MICT compared to CON.

Our results are consistent with Donnelly et al. [12], who found that 94% of studies showed no effect of long-term continuous aerobic exercise on daily energy intake [12]. On the contrary, Stubbs et al. [14] and Whybrow et al. [15] have demonstrated chronic exercise (>7–14 days) results in partial compensation in energy intake (~30%) when energy expenditure from exercise is consistent in the realm of 1.5–3.0 MJ/day. Differences in energy intake compensation between our results and these studies are likely explained by the energy cost of exercise. In the included studies, participants exercised 3-4 days per week with exercise duration up to 50 minutes per day. Only 6 studies [17, 18, 23, 26, 46, 54] quantified and reported energy cost of exercise, with all equating to ≤1.5 MJ per session (including basal energy expenditure) and <4.5 MJ per week. This is vastly different from the studies showing a partial compensation in energy intake [14, 15] as participants were exercising 7 days per week for a minimum of 80 minutes/day. Stubbs et al. [14] observed that women partially compensated their energy intake (~+30%) when the daily energy cost of exercise increased to 3.4 MJ/day over 7 days (23.8 MJ/week). Furthermore, Whybrow et al. [15]

Study name	Comparison	Effect size (95% CI)	*P* value
Wallman et al. [54]	HIIT versus CON	0.075 (−0.880 to 1.030)	
Heydari et al. [50]	HIIT versus CON	0.847 (0.252 to 1.443)	
Stensvold et al. [49]	HIIT versus CON	0.183 (−0.641 to 1.007)	
Walter et al. [53]	HIIT versus CON	0.142 (−0.581 to 0.866)	
Overall: HIIT versus CON		0.395 (−0.012 to 0.801)	0.057
Keating et al. [19]	SIT versus CON	0.000 (−0.759 to 0.759)	
Sim et al. [26]	SIT versus CON	0.399 (−0.417 to 1.215)	
Trapp et al. [18]	SIT versus CON	0.885 (−0.094 to 1.676)	
Overall: SIT versus CON		0.418 (−0.073 to 0.909)	0.095
Overall: HIIT/SIT versus CON		0.404 (0.091 to 0.717)	0.011

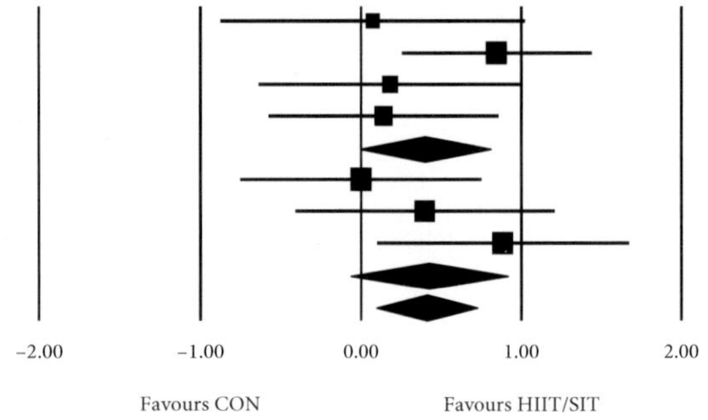

Figure 5: Meta-analysis for the comparison of HIIT/SIT versus CON on bodyweight. HIIT: high-intensity interval training, SIT: sprint interval training, CON: control, and CI: confidence interval.

Study name	Comparison	Effect size (95% CI)	*P* value
Matsuo et al. [23]	HIIT versus MICT	−0.000 (7.44 to 0.744)	
Sasaki et al. [21]	HIIT versus MICT	0.044 (−0.728 to 0.817)	
Panissa et al. [24]	HIIT versus MICT	0.094(−0.695 to 0.883)	
Wallman et al. [54]	HIIT versus MICT	0.126 (−0.889 to 1.142)	
Eimarieskandari et al. [20]	HIIT versus MICT	−0.149 (−1.165 to 0.867)	
Earnest et al. [17]	HIIT versus MICT	0.317 (−0.323 to 0.958)	
Kong et al. [52]	HIIT versus MICT	−0.227 (−1.115 to 0.662)	
Overall: HIIT versus MICT		0.064 (−0.241 to 0.370)	0.680
Martins et al. [46]	SIT versus MICT	0.179 (−0.567 to 0.925)	
Keating et al. [19]	SIT versus MICT	−0.531 (−1.289 to 0.228)	
Sim et al. [26]	SIT versus MICT	0.031 (−0.742 to 0.803)	
Trapp et al. [18]	SIT versus MICT	0.536 (−0.444 to 0.635)	
Higgins et al. [51]	SIT versus MICT	0.095 (−0.444 to 0.635)	
Ruffino et al. [47]	SIT versus MICT	−0.011 (−0.686 to 0.665)	
Overall: SIT versus MICT		0.036 (−0.251 to 0.323)	0.806
Overall: HIIT/SIT versus MICT		0.049 (−0.160 to 0.259)	0.644

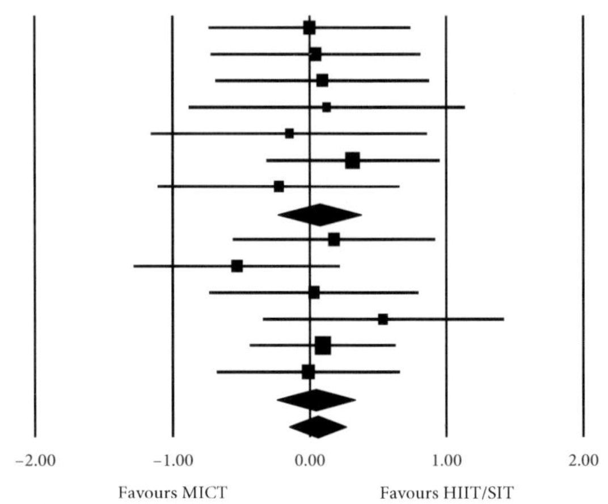

Figure 6: Effect of HIIT/SIT versus MICT on bodyweight. HIIT: high-intensity interval training, SIT: sprint interval training, MICT: moderate-intensity continuous training, and CI: confidence interval.

Study name	Comparison	Effect size (95% CI)	*P* value
Keating et al. [19]	MICT versus CON	−0.141 (−0.900 to 0.619)	
Sim et al. [26]	MICT versus CON	−0.338 (−1.151 to 0.476)	
Trapp et al. [18]	MICT versus CON	−0.491 (−1.330 to 0.348)	
Wallman et al. [54]	MICT versus CON	0.040 (−0.951 to 1.031)	
Overall: MICT versus CON		−0.248 (−0.668 to 0.171)	0.246

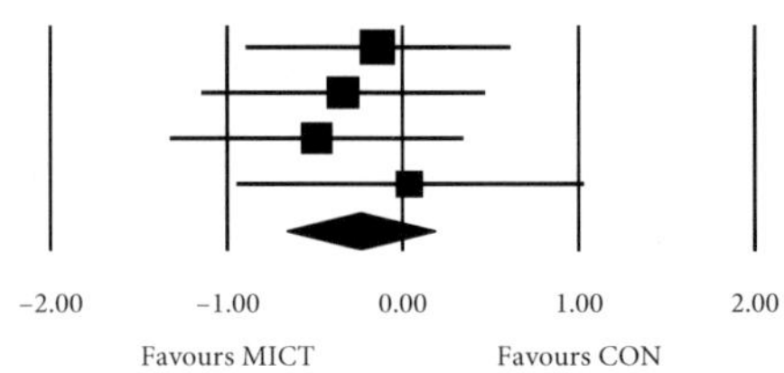

Figure 7: Effect of MICT versus CON on bodyweight. MICT: moderate-intensity continuous training, CON: control, and CI: confidence interval.

demonstrated the same in men when the daily energy cost of exercise increased to 2.8 MJ/day over 14 days (19.6 MJ/week).

Methods of quantifying energy intake in the included studies were variable and subject to potential error and bias, with most studies employing self-reported food diaries or food frequency questionnaires. Self-reported food diaries have an inherent risk of bias as the process of recording food intake can lead participants to change their eating behaviours [55]. Additionally, there is a large participant burden in keeping the record, which may lead to incomplete data. Food frequency questionnaires involve less participant burden but are designed to estimate usual dietary intake of specific food items or nutrients over time (usually 6 to 12 months) rather than daily energy intake [55]. Unfortunately, all methods of assessing energy intake are susceptible to underreporting from participants. However, 24-hour recalls have shown less underreporting (~12–20%) compared to food frequency questionnaires (~30–36%) when compared to total energy expenditure by doubly labeled water [56]. Other studies using a multiple-pass 24-hour recall method to measure energy intake have found levels of underreporting to be ~11% [57]. Using the multiple-pass 24-hour recall method on multiple days has also been shown to reduce underreporting from 30% (1 day) to 11% (2 days) and 4% (3 days) [58]. Inherent variability associated with underreporting may mean it is difficult to detect a change in studies, particularly with a small number of participants and few time points. The provision of ad libitum meals and snacks with known compositions in laboratory settings may seem to be a more accurate method to determine daily energy intake with less potential for underreporting; however, energy intake behaviours could be affected by an artificial environment, social desirability (if eating in the presence of others), and differences in desire for the types of foods provided.

There are a number of factors that could result in individual variability of energy intake compensation in response to chronic exercise, such as biological changes driving appetite [7], psychological factors (restraint and disinhibition), and changing food preferences and food reward (hedonic influence) [8]. Restraint refers to the extent to which individuals restrict their diet in order to control their body weight [59]. Disinhibition refers to the loss of restraint or self-control, which may occur in the presence of forbidden foods, alcohol, and emotional states [60]. Acute exercise has been shown to increase energy intake in unrestrained eaters and decrease energy intake in restrained eaters [61]. Whether exercise intensity influences these psychological factors remains unknown. While we recognize that the physiological stimulus of HIIT and SIT is different and hence may affect appetite and energy intake differently, our metaregression found no differences between modalities of interval training used.

Evidence is now emerging that chronic exercise may improve the sensitivity of appetite hormones to regulate appetite more effectively [62]. Although studies have shown no change in fasting anorexigenic hormones (peptide YY, pancreatic polypeptide, and glucagon-like peptide 1) following 12-week exercise interventions [26, 63, 64], Martins et al. [63] found concentrations of PYY and glucagon-like peptide 1 to be elevated to a greater extent in the exercise group following a meal. Furthermore, Sim et al. [26] have shown that HIIT for 12 weeks reduced energy intake at a test meal, following a high energy preload, thereby eluding to an improvement in appetite regulation. Similarly, fasting acylated ghrelin levels appear to increase [63] or remain stable after long-term exercise [26, 64] but are suppressed to a greater extent in the exercise group following a meal [63]. It has been hypothesized that enhanced suppression of acylated ghrelin and stimulation of anorexigenic hormones postprandial with long-term exercise may improve appetite regulation in individuals who are obese by terminating meals more rapidly and leading to longer between-meal intervals [34]. More research is needed to determine long-term effects of exercise on appetite hormones and potential influence on weight loss. As discussed earlier, other long-term adaptations such as insulin sensitivity may also influence appetite regulation.

Our results showed a significant reduction in bodyweight for HIIT only when compared with a no-exercise control; however, only studies that actually measured energy intake were included in this analysis. Therefore, it is not appropriate to make a conclusion regarding the effect of HIIT/SIT on bodyweight from this subgroup of studies. While no significant changes were observed for bodyweight in MICT versus CON, only four studies were included in the pooled analysis, which limits the ability to draw conclusions. As highlighted earlier, the effect of HIIT compared to MICT on weight loss and fat loss remains unclear. Conflicting results are likely due to a number of factors such as individual variability of outcomes and the heterogeneity of interval training protocols in terms of interval duration and total workload. Furthermore, as participant adherence to the prescribed intensity has been poorly reported, it is unclear whether participants are achieving the intensity targets and hence whether there is a significant difference between groups.

Regardless of whether weight loss targets are achieved, exercise produces an abundance of metabolic and cardiovascular health benefits, including but not limited to improvements in blood pressure, lipid profile, and fasting serum glucose [4]. Furthermore, exercise interventions have been shown to result in significant reductions in visceral adipose tissue even in the absence of changes in body mass and/or waist circumference [26, 65], which may contribute to these health benefits.

A major limitation of this review is the varying level of study quality. Only 44% of studies quantified and reported energy cost of exercise, 44% of studies reported exercise adherence, 56% of studies measured habitual physical activity levels, and 6% of studies reported adherence to training intensities. Without measuring and reporting these outcomes, it is difficult to determine the impact an exercise intervention can have on creating an energy-deficit sufficient to affect energy intake. Therefore, although it is difficult for this review to draw definitive conclusions from the results, it does highlight important methodological considerations.

In conclusion, our results found no compensatory increase in energy intake following a period of HIIT/SIT compared to MICT or no exercise. To date, no studies comparing HIIT with MICT have found significant differences in daily energy intake with time or intervention using self-recorded food diaries or food frequency questionnaires. Studies with alternative dietary assessment with less potential bias may be needed to detect significant differences in energy intake. The multiple-pass 24-hour recall method on multiple days can be associated with less underreporting and reduces potential for participant error and bias. Furthermore, it is imperative that future studies report exercise energy expenditure, exercise adherence, and habitual physical activity as total energy expenditure could significantly influence energy intake response. Additionally, to investigate whether exercise intensity influences energy intake, it is important for studies to report on adherence to the exercise protocols to determine whether participants are achieving the target intensities. Finally, HIIT versus MICT studies investigating individual variation in energy intake and the effect on psychological factors (restraint and disinhibition) and food preferences may provide further insight into long-term changes in eating behaviour with exercise.

Abbreviations

HIIT: High-intensity interval training
SIT: Sprint interval training
MICT: Moderate-intensity continuous training
VO_{2peak}: Peak oxygen consumption
HR_{peak}: Peak heart rate
PEDro: Physiotherapy Evidence Database

BMI: Body mass index
CI: Confidence interval.

Authors' Contributions

Jenna Taylor and Jeff S. Coombes were responsible for study conception. All authors contributed to study design and data collection. Jenna Taylor was responsible for manuscript writing. All authors contributed to critical revision of the manuscript and approved the final version.

Acknowledgments

Jenna Taylor was supported by the National Health and Medical Research Council of Australia and the Australian Government via a research higher degree scholarship (1133622). Shelley E. Keating was supported by the National Health and Medical Research Council of Australia via an Early Career Research Fellowship (1122190).

References

[1] WHO, *Global Status Report on Noncommunicable Diseases 2014*, World Health Organization, Geneva, Switzerland, 2015.

[2] N. A. King, P. Caudwell, M. Hopkins et al., "Metabolic and behavioral compensatory responses to exercise interventions: barriers to weight loss," *Obesity*, vol. 15, no. 6, pp. 1373–1383, 2007.

[3] N. A. King, M. Hopkins, P. Caudwell, R. J. Stubbs, and J. E. Blundell, "Individual variability following 12 weeks of supervised exercise: identification and characterization of compensation for exercise-induced weight loss," *International Journal of Obesity*, vol. 32, no. 1, pp. 177–184, 2008.

[4] K. Shaw, H. Gennat, P. O'Rourke, and C. Del Mar, "Exercise for overweight or obesity," *Cochrane Database of Systematic Reviews*, vol. 18, no. 4, p. Cd003817, 2006.

[5] J. Stevens, K. P. Truesdale, J. E. McClain, and J. Cai, "The definition of weight maintenance," *International Journal of Obesity*, vol. 30, no. 3, pp. 391–399, 2005.

[6] D. M. Thomas, C. Bouchard, T. Church et al., "Why do individuals not lose more weight from an exercise intervention at a defined dose? An energy balance analysis," *Obesity Reviews*, vol. 13, no. 10, pp. 835–847, 2012.

[7] J. E. Blundell, C. Gibbons, P. Caudwell, G. Finlayson, and M. Hopkins, "Appetite control and energy balance: impact of exercise," *Obesity Reviews*, vol. 16, no. 1, pp. 67–76, 2015.

[8] G. Finlayson, E. Bryant, J. E. Blundell, and N. A. King, "Acute compensatory eating following exercise is associated with implicit hedonic wanting for food," *Physiology & Behavior*, vol. 97, no. 1, pp. 62–67, 2009.

[9] C. Martins, M. D. Robertson, and L. M. Morgan, "Effects of exercise and restrained eating behaviour on appetite control," *Proceedings of the Nutrition Society*, vol. 67, no. 1, pp. 28–41, 2008.

[10] N. A. King, K. Horner, A. P. Hills et al., "Exercise, appetite and weight management: understanding the compensatory responses in eating behaviour and how they contribute to variability in exercise-induced weight loss," *British Journal of Sports Medicine*, vol. 46, no. 5, pp. 315–322, 2012.

[11] M. M. Schubert, B. Desbrow, S. Sabapathy, and M. Leveritt, "Acute exercise and subsequent energy intake. A meta-analysis," *Appetite*, vol. 63, pp. 92–104, 2013.

[12] J. E. Donnelly, S. D. Herrmann, K. Lambourne, A. N. Szabo, J. J. Honas, and R. A. Washburn, "Does increased exercise or physical activity alter ad-libitum daily energy intake or macronutrient composition in healthy adults? A systematic review," *PLoS One*, vol. 9, no. 1, article e83498, 2014.

[13] J. A. King, M. Miyashita, L. K. Wasse, and D. J. Stensel, "Influence of prolonged treadmill running on appetite, energy intake and circulating concentrations of acylated ghrelin," *Appetite*, vol. 54, no. 3, pp. 492–498, 2010.

[14] R. J. Stubbs, A. Sepp, D. A. Hughes et al., "The effect of graded levels of exercise on energy intake and balance in free-living women," *International Journal of Obesity and Related Disorders*, vol. 26, no. 6, pp. 866–869, 2002.

[15] S. Whybrow, D. A. Hughes, P. Ritz et al., "The effect of an incremental increase in exercise on appetite, eating behaviour and energy balance in lean men and women feeding ad libitum," *British Journal of Nutrition*, vol. 100, no. 5, pp. 1109–1115, 2008.

[16] K. Karstoft, K. Winding, S. H. Knudsen et al., "The effects of free-living interval-walking training on glycemic control, body composition, and physical fitness in type 2 diabetic patients: a randomized, controlled trial," *Diabetes Care*, vol. 36, no. 2, pp. 228–236, 2013.

[17] C. P. Earnest, M. Lupo, J. Thibodaux et al., "Interval training in men at risk for insulin resistance," *International Journal of Sports Medicine*, vol. 34, no. 4, pp. 355–363, 2013.

[18] E. G. Trapp, D. J. Chisholm, J. Freund, and S. H. Boutcher, "The effects of high-intensity intermittent exercise training on fat loss and fasting insulin levels of young women," *International Journal of Obesity*, vol. 32, no. 4, pp. 684–691, 2008.

[19] S. E. Keating, E. A. Machan, H. T. O'Connor et al., "Continuous exercise but not high intensity interval training improves fat distribution in overweight adults," *Journal of Obesity*, vol. 2014, Article ID 834865, 12 pages, 2014.

[20] R. Eimarieskandari, S. Zilaeibouri, M. Zilaeibouri, and A. Ahangarpour, "Comparing two modes of exercise training with different intensity on body composition in obese young girls," *Ovidius University Annals, Series Physical Education & Sport/Science Movement and Health*, vol. 12, no. 2, pp. 473–478, 2012.

[21] H. Sasaki, T. Morishima, Y. Hasegawa et al., "4 weeks of high-intensity interval training does not alter the exercise-induced growth hormone response in sedentary men," *SpringerPlus*, vol. 3, no. 1, p. 336, 2014.

[22] H. Zhang, T. K. Tong, W. Qiu, and Y. He, "Effect of high-intensity interval training protocol on abdominal fat reduction in overweight Chinese women: a randomized controlled trial," *Kinesiology*, vol. 47, no. 1, pp. 57–66, 2015.

[23] T. Matsuo, R. So, N. Shimojo, and K. Tanaka, "Effect of aerobic exercise training followed by a low-calorie diet on metabolic syndrome risk factors in men," *Nutrition, Metabolism and Cardiovascular Diseases*, vol. 25, no. 9, pp. 832–838, 2015.

[24] V. L. G. Panissa, E. D. Alves, G. P. Salermo, E. Franchini, and M. Y. Takito, "Can short-term high-intensity intermittent training reduce adiposity?," *Sport Sciences for Health*, vol. 12, no. 1, pp. 99–104, 2016.

[25] A. E. Tjønna, S. J. Lee, O. Rognmo et al., "Aerobic interval training versus continuous moderate exercise as a treatment

for the metabolic syndrome: a pilot study," *Circulation*, vol. 118, no. 4, pp. 346–354, 2008.

[26] A. Y. Sim, K. E. Wallman, T. J. Fairchild, and K. J. Guelfi, "Effects of high-intensity intermittent exercise training on appetite regulation," *Medicine & Science in Sports & Exercise*, vol. 47, no. 11, pp. 2441–2449, 2015.

[27] S. Keating, N. A. Johnson, G. I. Mielke, and J. S. Coombes, "A systematic review and meta-analysis of interval training versus moderate-intensity continuous training on body adiposity," *Obesity Reviews*, vol. 18, no. 8, pp. 943–964, 2017.

[28] A. Y. Sim, K. E. Wallman, T. J. Fairchild, and K. J. Guelfi, "High-intensity intermittent exercise attenuates ad-libitum energy intake," *International Journal of Obesity*, vol. 38, no. 3, pp. 417–422, 2005.

[29] C. Martins, D. Stensvold, G. Finlayson et al., "Effect of moderate- and high-intensity acute exercise on appetite in obese individuals," *Medicine & Science in Sports & Exercise*, vol. 47, no. 1, pp. 40–48, 2015.

[30] K. Deighton, R. Barry, C. E. Connon, and D. J. Stensel, "Appetite, gut hormone and energy intake responses to low volume sprint interval and traditional endurance exercise," *European Journal of Applied Physiology*, vol. 113, no. 5, pp. 1147–1156, 2013.

[31] S. A. Alkahtani, N. M. Byrne, A. P. Hills, and N. A. King, "Interval training intensity affects energy intake compensation in obese men," *International Journal of Sport Nutrition & Exercise Metabolism*, vol. 24, no. 6, pp. 595–604, 2014.

[32] K. Deighton, E. Karra, R. L. Batterham, and D. J. Stensel, "Appetite, energy intake, and PYY3-36 responses to energy-matched continuous exercise and submaximal high-intensity exercise," *Applied Physiology, Nutrition, and Metabolism*, vol. 38, no. 9, pp. 947–952, 2013.

[33] S. Howe, T. Hand, D. Larson-Meyer, K. Austin, B. Alexander, and M. Manore, "No effect of exercise intensity on appetite in highly-trained endurance women," *Nutrients*, vol. 8, no. 12, p. 223, 2016.

[34] M. M. Schubert, S. Sabapathy, M. Leveritt, and B. Desbrow, "Acute exercise and hormones related to appetite regulation: a meta-analysis," *Sports Medicine*, vol. 44, no. 3, pp. 387–403, 2014.

[35] K. Deighton and D. J. Stensel, "Creating an acute energy deficit without stimulating compensatory increases in appetite: is there an optimal exercise protocol?," *Proceedings of the Nutrition Society*, vol. 73, no. 2, pp. 352–358, 2014.

[36] J. A. King, L. K. Wasse, and D. J. Stensel, "The acute effects of swimming on appetite, food intake, and plasma acylated ghrelin," *Journal of Obesity*, vol. 2011, Article ID 351628, 8 pages, 2011.

[37] K. Deighton, J. C. Zahra, and D. J. Stensel, "Appetite, energy intake and resting metabolic responses to 60 min treadmill running performed in a fasted versus a postprandial state," *Appetite*, vol. 58, no. 3, pp. 946–948, 2012.

[38] A. Flint, N. T. Gregersen, L. L. Gluud et al., "Associations between postprandial insulin and blood glucose responses, appetite sensations and energy intake in normal weight and overweight individuals: a meta-analysis of test meal studies," *British Journal of Nutrition*, vol. 98, no. 1, pp. 17–25, 2007.

[39] C. Jelleyman, T. Yates, G. O'Donovan et al., "The effects of high-intensity interval training on glucose regulation and insulin resistance: a meta-analysis," *Obesity Reviews*, vol. 16, no. 11, pp. 942–961, 2015.

[40] D. Moher, A. Liberati, J. Tetzlaff, and D. G. Altman, "Preferred reporting items for systematic reviews and meta-analyses: the PRISMA statement," *International Journal of Surgery*, vol. 8, no. 5, pp. 336–341, 2010.

[41] K. S. Weston, U. Wisløff, and J. S. Coombes, "High-intensity interval training in patients with lifestyle-induced cardiometabolic disease: a systematic review and meta-analysis," *British Journal of Sports Medicine*, vol. 48, no. 16, pp. 1227–1234, 2014.

[42] American College of Sports and Medicine, *ACSM's Guidelines for Exercise Testing and Prescription*, Lippincott Williams & Wilkins, Philadelphia, PA, USA, 9th edition, 2014.

[43] K. Norton, L. Norton, and D. Sadgrove, "Position statement on physical activity and exercise intensity terminology," *Journal of Science and Medicine in Sport*, vol. 13, no. 5, pp. 496–502, 2010.

[44] C. Sherrington, R. D. Herbert, C. G. Maher, and A. M. Moseley, "PEDro. A database of randomized trials and systematic reviews in physiotherapy," *Manual Therapy*, vol. 5, no. 4, pp. 223–226, 2000.

[45] J. Higgins and S. Green, *Cochrane Handbook for Systematic Reviews of Interventions Version 5.1.0*, The Cochrane Collaboration, Hoboken, NJ, USA, 2011.

[46] C. Martins, I. Kazakova, M. Ludviksen et al., "High-intensity interval training and isocaloric moderate-intensity continuous training result in similar improvements in body composition and fitness in obese individuals," *International Journal of Sport Nutrition and Exercise Metabolism*, vol. 26, no. 3, pp. 197–204, 2016.

[47] J. S. Ruffino, P. Songsorn, M. Haggett et al., "A comparison of the health benefits of reduced-exertion high-intensity interval training (REHIT) and moderate-intensity walking in type 2 diabetes patients," *Applied Physiology, Nutrition and Metabolism*, vol. 42, no. 2, pp. 202–208, 2017.

[48] D. Stensvold, A. E. Tjønna, E.-A. Skaug et al., "Strength training versus aerobic interval training to modify risk factors of metabolic syndrome," *Journal of Applied Physiology*, vol. 108, no. 4, pp. 804–810, 2010.

[49] D. Stensvold, S. A. Slordahl, and U. Wisloff, "Effect of exercise training on inflammation status among people with metabolic syndrome," *Metabolic Syndrome and Related Disorders*, vol. 10, no. 4, pp. 267–272, 2012.

[50] M. Heydari, J. Freund, and S. H. Boutcher, "The effect of high-intensity intermittent exercise on body composition of overweight young males," *Journal of Obesity*, vol. 2012, Article ID 480467, 8 pages, 2012.

[51] S. Higgins, M. V. Fedewa, E. D. Hathaway, M. D. Schmidt, and E. M. Evans, "Sprint interval and moderate-intensity cycling training differentially affect adiposity and aerobic capacity in overweight young-adult women," *Applied Physiology, Nutrition, and Metabolism*, vol. 41, no. 11, pp. 1177–1183, 2016.

[52] Z. Kong, S. Sun, M. Liu, and Q. Shi, "Short-term high-intensity interval training on body composition and blood glucose in overweight and obese young women," *Journal of Diabetes Research*, vol. 2016, Article ID 4073618, 9 pages, 2016.

[53] A. A. Walter, A. E. Smith, K. L. Kendall, J. R. Stout, and J. T. Cramer, "Six weeks of high-intensity interval training with and without beta-alanine supplementation for improving cardiovascular fitness in women," *Journal of Strength and Conditioning Research*, vol. 24, no. 5, pp. 1199–1207, 2010.

[54] K. Wallman, L. Plant, B. Rakimov, and A. Maiorana, "The effects of two modes of exercise on aerobic fitness and fat mass in an overweight population," *Research in Sports Medicine*, vol. 17, no. 3, p. 156, 2009.

[55] R. K. Johnson, "Dietary intake—how do we measure what people are really eating?," *Obesity Research*, vol. 10, no. 11, pp. 63S–68S, 2002.

[56] A. F. Subar, V. Kipnis, R. P. Troiano et al., "Using intake biomarkers to evaluate the extent of dietary misreporting in a large sample of adults: the open study," *American Journal of Epidemiology*, vol. 158, no. 1, pp. 1–13, 2003.

[57] A. J. Moshfegh, D. G. Rhodes, D. J. Baer et al., "US Department of Agriculture Automated Multiple-Pass Method reduces bias in the collection of energy intakes," *American Journal of Clinical Nutrition*, vol. 88, no. 2, pp. 324–332, 2008.

[58] Y. Ma, B. C. Olendzki, S. L. Pagoto et al., "Number of 24-hour diet recalls needed to estimate energy intake," *Annals of Epidemiology*, vol. 167, no. 11, p. S11, 2008.

[59] A. J. Stunkard and S. Messick, "The three-factor eating questionnaire to measure dietary restraint, disinhibition and hunger," *Journal of Psychosomatic Research*, vol. 29, no. 1, pp. 71–83, 1985.

[60] M. J. Bond, A. J. McDowell, and J. Y. Wilkinson, "The measurement of dietary restraint, disinhibition and hunger: an examination of the factor structure of the Three Factor Eating Questionnaire (TFEQ)," *International Journal of Obesity*, vol. 25, no. 6, pp. 900–906, 2001.

[61] A. Lluch, N. A. King, and J. E. Blundell, "No energy compensation at the meal following exercise in dietary restrained and unrestrained women," *British Journal of Nutrition*, vol. 84, no. 2, pp. 219–225, 2000.

[62] K. Beaulieu, M. Hopkins, J. Blundell, and G. Finlayson, "Does habitual physical activity increase the sensitivity of the appetite control system? A systematic review," *Sports Medicine*, vol. 46, no. 12, pp. 1897–1919, 2016.

[63] C. Martins, B. Kulseng, N. A. King, J. J. Holst, and J. E. Blundell, "The effects of exercise-induced weight loss on appetite-related peptides and motivation to eat," *Journal of Clinical Endocrinology and Metabolism*, vol. 95, no. 4, pp. 1609–1616, 2010.

[64] K. J. Guelfi, C. E. Donges, and R. Duffield, "Beneficial effects of 12 weeks of aerobic compared with resistance exercise training on perceived appetite in previously sedentary overweight and obese men," *Metabolism: Clinical and Experimental*, vol. 62, no. 2, pp. 235–243, 2013.

[65] S. E. Keating, D. A. Hackett, H. M. Parker et al., "Effect of aerobic exercise training dose on liver fat and visceral adiposity," *Journal of Hepatology*, vol. 63, no. 1, pp. 174–182, 2015.

17

Pilot Project to Integrate Community and Clinical Level Systems to Address Health Disparities in the Prevention and Treatment of Obesity among Ethnic Minority Inner-City Middle School Students

Jessica Rieder,[1] Agnieszka Cain,[1] Erica Carson,[1] Andrea Benya,[1] Paul Meissner,[2] Carmen R. Isasi,[3] Judith Wylie-Rosett,[3] Neal Hoffman,[1] Colleen Kelly,[1] Ellen J. Silver,[1] and Laurie J. Bauman[1]

[1]*Department of Pediatrics, Children's Hospital at Montefiore, The Pediatric Hospital for Albert Einstein College of Medicine, Bronx, NY, USA*
[2]*Department of Family and Social Medicine, Albert Einstein College of Medicine, Bronx, NY, USA*
[3]*Department of Epidemiology and Population Health, Albert Einstein College of Medicine, Bronx, NY, USA*

Correspondence should be addressed to Jessica Rieder; jrieder@montefiore.org

Academic Editor: Sharon Herring

Effective obesity prevention and treatment interventions are lacking in the United States, especially for impoverished minority youths at risk for health disparities, and especially in accessible community-based settings. We describe the launch and pilot implementation evaluation of the first year of the *B'N Fit POWER* initiative as a middle school-based comprehensive wellness program that integrates weight management programming into existing onsite preventive and clinical services. Consistent with the existing implementation science literature, we focused on both the organizational structures that facilitate communication and the development of trust among stakeholders, students, and families and the development of realistic and timely goals to implement and integrate all aspects of the program. New implementation and programming strategies were developed and tested to increase the proportion of students screened, support the linkage of students to care, and streamline the integration of program clinical and afterschool components into routine services already offered at the school. We report on our initial implementation activities using the Standards for Reporting Implementation Studies (StaRI) framework using hybrid outcomes combining the Reach element from the RE-AIM framework with a newly conceptualized Wellness Cascade.

1. Introduction

While 17% of 2–19-year-old children and adolescents are affected by obesity in the United States [1], the most severe forms of obesity have increased, particularly among adolescents and non-Hispanic blacks [2]. Low SES are 1.35 times more likely to be obese and low SES ethnic minority adolescents are less likely to live in neighborhoods supportive of physical activity than higher SES Caucasian youths [3, 4]. Despite the fact that obesity in adolescence increases the risk for many chronic conditions, effective preventive and treatment interventions are lacking, especially for minority youths at risk for health disparities [5–7].

Intensive pediatric weight management programs featuring physical activity, nutrition, and sedentary behavior reduction counseling, parental involvement, and cultural tailoring [8–11] can decrease weight and risk for developing type 2 diabetes mellitus (DM) [6, 9, 12–15], yet most are offered in highly specialized treatment centers, are demanding of patients, and require highly trained staff [16]. Effective less-intensive, large-scale public health efforts that target youths in schools or communities tend to focus on prevention of obesity and while they engage and promote healthy lifestyle behaviors for large numbers of youths, they often lack comprehensive services and many have not demonstrated favorable effects on BMI [6, 17–21].

The Bronx Nutrition and Fitness Initiative for Teens (B'N Fit) was developed in 2005 by the Children's Hospital at Montefiore (CHAM) in partnership with the Mosholu Montefiore Community Center (MMCC) as a 9-month weight-loss program to address health disparities and treat obesity in adolescents from a low-income minority community. B'N Fit was a hybrid approach which included comprehensive obesity evaluation and treatment plans in a hospital ambulatory care service venue combined with community-based nutrition and physical activity education. Barriers to retention and achieving obesity-related recommendations included low motivation to change behaviors and the home and community environment. Nonetheless, B'N Fit decreased the rate of weight gain and changed behaviors in adolescents with high rates of severe obesity (67%) and obesity-related comorbidities (57%) [22]. However, youth feedback indicated that targeting adolescents with obesity and offering the program components at sites that were not in their normal routine affected attendance and retention rates. B'N Fit was perceived to be offered at inconvenient locations and times and attending could be stigmatizing.

Translating the program to a school setting for all students was a potential solution for addressing these issues. There is an abundance of literature evaluating school-based weight management intervention effectiveness, but there is relative paucity of implementation studies addressing how programs were implemented and whether their feasibility was evaluated and the Community Preventive Task Force has found insufficiency evidence to recommend school-based obesity programs to prevent or reduce overweight and obesity among children and adolescents [23–28]. Following the Standards for Reporting Implementation Studies (StaRI) reporting framework [29], this paper describes the approach used to launch and evaluate the implementation of the *B'N Fit POWER* initiative as a school-based comprehensive program that integrates weight management into programming accessible to all students with an emphasis on strategies for sustaining such programming in a low-resource middle school setting.

2. Methods

2.1. Description of the B'N Fit POWER Initiative. The American health-care system is embracing the Triple Aim®—achieving better care for patients, better health for communities, and lower costs through health-care system improvement. It is developing new ways to integrate and coordinate services, emphasize patient engagement and patient-centered care, and develop new payment models that place value on population-based health outcomes rather than the volume of services [30]. The Clinical–Community Integration Framework as described by Dietz et al. [31] has been designed to address this needed change in the health-care system by integrating existing clinical and community services to provide improved coordination of services with an emphasis on close links between the patient and family unit as a model for preventing and treating obesity. *B'N Fit POWER* uses this framework and integrates several elements of successful intensive and school-based obesity prevention and treatment interventions by providing onsite medical care and youth-focused afterschool programming to teach and model healthy lifestyle behaviors and incorporating youth-centered outcome metrics to evaluate the program (Figure 1).

B'N Fit POWER is a voluntary multicomponent school-based wellness program that draws on Youth Development (YD) theory to emphasize adolescent strengths and promote positive adolescent development and health behaviors that lead to a healthy weight, rather than avoidance of risks and negative behaviors [32]. While studies have demonstrated that YD based curriculums, which foster a youth-centered, culturally appropriate, and psychologically safe atmosphere, can effectively decrease BMI and improve healthy lifestyle knowledge, behaviors, and attitudes; few concurrently evaluate health impact [33–38]. A school is an ideal setting to implement an integrated program with a YD emphasis because youths spend almost half of their waking hours in schools and may be more inclined to participate in activities that are supported by caring adults in their schools, especially if they have friends that also participate [19, 39]. *B'N Fit POWER's* implementation occurred at Public School/Middle School–95 (PS/MS-95), a kindergarten through 8th grade school that has both an onsite School-Based Health Center (SBHC) operated by the Montefiore School Health Program (MSHP) and an afterschool program run by the Mosholu Montefiore Community Center (MMCC). Working with existing services provided by involved stakeholders, the program offered comprehensive wellness-focused medical assessments as part of routine SBHC clinical practice, and enhanced the MMCC afterschool group-based provision of services to provide healthy lifestyle behavior change education, cooking classes, and daily physical activity opportunities (Table 1). The program incorporated onsite Wellness in the Schools (WITS) family support to cook healthy meals and the Prevention Intervention Research Center (PIRC) expertise to incorporate youth resilience and YD concepts into the program. With a USDA-funded school food program, the PS/MS-95 School is mandated to have a Wellness Council where teachers, students, parents, MSHP Community Health Organizer, and administrators collaborate to support wellness programming at the school. In partnership with the Wellness Council, *B'N Fit POWER* staff learned about the need for and interest in healthy lifestyle programming, barriers to enrollment and program engagement, and outcomes of interest.

Implementation entailed a two-year planning phase, where the B'N Fit Director met separately with the key stakeholders. The first-year quarterly meetings with the MMCC administration focused on afterschool recruitment and engagement strategies, collection of screening and program attendance data, reducing potential stigma related to a school-based obesity intervention, and the structure and curriculum content of the afterschool program. Quarterly meetings with the MSHP staff focused on developing clinical assessment tools, provision of clinical services, and collection of clinical data. Quarterly meetings with the PIRC staff

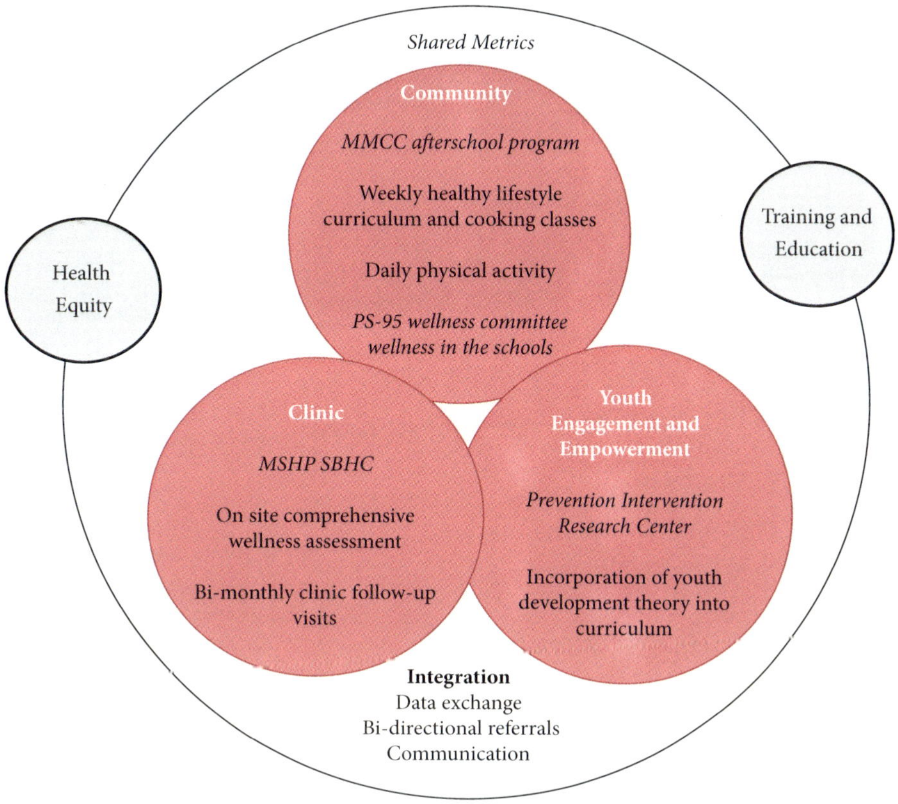

FIGURE 1: The *B'N Fit POWER* clinical and community integration framework. Adapted from the Clinical–Community Integration Framework by Dietz et al. [31].

focused on the design of the program evaluation and outcome metrics, strategies for reducing stigma, and strategies for incorporation of YD elements into the afterschool program curriculum. An initial meeting with the Principal of PS/MS-95 was also conducted to obtain permission to pilot the program in the school. During the second year, separate meetings with each of the MMCC, MSHP, and PIRC stakeholders occurred monthly to discuss the implementation strategies in more detail, and meetings with the principal occurred quarterly. Monthly meetings with the School Wellness Council began in the latter part of the second year in preparation for a fall program start, and the partnership with the WITS staff, MSHP Community Health organizer, students, and teachers focuses on engaging parents during bi-annual Family Fun Fitness Nights, developing efficient protocols for acquisition of outcome metrics, and supporting a healthy lifestyle culture at the school.

2.2. Setting/Context. The Bronx, which is the poorest urban county in the United States and least healthy county in New York State, has high ethnic diversity (54% Hispanic and 43% African-American). Childhood poverty is 43%, and school absenteeism is high, as is the prevalence of obesity [1, 40, 41]. Data from the New York City Department of Education indicate that 70.6% of PS-95 students live in households that are below 130% of the poverty level [42], and nearly half (46.9%) of all Bronx residents report feeling at risk of becoming homeless [43]. The low SES of teens living in the Bronx limits their exposure to opportunities that can make a difference in their lives and reduce health disparities compared with other teens [44]. Despite these immense barriers to attaining good health in the Bronx, the long-term presence and commitment to providing onsite health and afterschool services by the MSHP and MMCC, respectively, along with the efforts of the principal and onsite stakeholders to provide and sustain established quality health education for its students qualifies this school to implement the services of *B'N Fit POWER* with an opportunity to create an integrated program to address these disparities.

2.3. Selecting Intervention Outcome Metrics. Program outcome metrics were selected if they could be commonly utilized by all partners and if they could be accurate, credible, and reproducible measures of progress. Primary outcomes included the following: (1) Height and weight determinations done at the SBHC using a Scaletronix® scale as per routine clinic assessment. (2) The NYC Fitnessgram: the current measure of fitness for all NYC public school students (approximately 85% of NYC public school students have BMI measured annually via the NYC FitnessGram) [45]. Students are assessed in four fitness areas, cardiovascular fitness or aerobic capacity, muscle strength, muscular endurance, and flexibility, and scores are evaluated against criterion-based "Healthy Fitness Zone®" standards that indicate the level of fitness necessary for health. (3) The 51-item *B'N Fit POWER* survey data, which include assessment

Table 1: Contributing stakeholders and their role in the *B'N Fit POWER* implementation.

Stakeholders	Description	Staffing	Implementation role in *B'N Fit POWER*
Bronx Nutrition And Fitness Initiative For Teens	*Program activities*: Adolescent Weight Management Program operated out of the Children's Hospital at Montefiore	(i) 0.15 FTE Project Director* (ii) 0.5 FTE POWER Program Coordinator* (iii) Student volunteers	(i) Provision of guidelines for screening, clinical evaluation, treatment plans, and afterschool requirements (ii) Development of program metrics (iii) Integration of stakeholder efforts (iv) Conducts MMCC afterschool staff trainings to support screening process (v) Conducts height and weight screenings
Mosholu Montefiore Community Center (MMCC)	*Program activities*: operates afterschool (3–6 pm) programs in 15 sites: (i) Recreation and physical activity opportunities (ii) Educational support (iii) Enrichment and socialization (iv) Youth leadership	(i) In-kind program director (ii) In-kind youth leaders ×4 (iii) In-kind administrative staff (iv) Per diem cooking specialist* (v) Per diem exercise specialist*	(i) Supports community-led recruitment (ii) Provides afterschool group-based healthy lifestyle behavior education, cooking and gardening classes, and daily physical activity opportunities (iii) Integrates *B'N Fit POWER* into existing afterschool program structure
The Montefiore School Health Program (MSHP)	*Program activities*: operates during the school day (8 am–3 pm); provides onsite coordinated primary and preventive health care in 25 locations (i) Delivers medical, mental health, dental, and community health services	(i) In-kind primary care MD/NP (ii) In-kind social worker (iii) In-kind licensed practical nurse (iv) In-kind, community health organizer (CHO) (v) In-kind receptionist (vi) In-kind medical director	(i) Develops efficient clinic protocols (ii) Conducts comprehensive wellness medical assessments, ordering standard lab set, generates 1-page treatment plan, and supports healthy lifestyle education as part of the routine onsite clinical practice (iii) Conducts follow-up visits as per routine clinical practice to monitor progress
PS/MS-95 School And Wellness Council	*Governance activities*: USDA-funded school food program, mandated to have an onsite Wellness Council	(i) School principal (ii) MSHP CHO (iii) Education consultant (iv) PTA president (v) WITS staff (vi) Students and parents	(i) Facilitates understanding of existing healthy lifestyle programming (ii) Incorporates target behavior concepts into school wellness activities (iii) Establishes outcomes of interest
Prevention Intervention Research Center (PIRC)	*Research evaluation activities*: develop and test interventions to prevent mental health problems in children and youths with chronic health conditions	(i) In-kind Director (ii) In-kind developmental psychologist (iii) Program staff	(i) Supports program evaluation (ii) Incorporates YD concepts into the program curriculum
Wellness in the Schools (WITS)	*Program activities*: national nonprofit that teaches kids healthy habits to learn and live better	(i) In-kind onsite chefs	(i) Supports healthy menus during cooking and family events
Students and families	Students attend school, B'N Fit afterschool, and on wellness council, parents serve on PTA	(i) Student volunteers (ii) Parent volunteers	(i) Informs need for and interest in program (ii) Identifies barriers to enrollment, program engagement, and outcomes of interest

*Staff funded specifically for *B'N Fit POWER*, and all others staffing in-kind or volunteers.

Table 2: Intervention outcome metrics.

Clinical assessment	
Anthropometrics	Height and weight
Vitals	Blood pressure
Laboratory evaluation	(1) If BMI < 85th percentile—no additional labs (2) If BMI ≥ 85th percentile—lipids and HbA1c
Fitness assessment	
NYC FitnessGram	(1) Cardiovascular fitness (2) Aerobic capacity (3) Muscle strength (4) Muscular endurance (5) Flexibility
Behavioral outcomes: 51-item B'N Fit survey	
Subscales	*Number of items*
7 target behaviors	14 items in questionnaire: (1) Eat breakfast and lunch daily (2) Eat 2-3 servings of fruits a day (3) Eat 3–6 servings of vegetables a day (4) Drink 8 cups of water daily/limit sugary drinks to ≤1 cup daily (5) Sleep at least 8 hours a night (6) Get at least an hour of physical activity daily (7) Eat unhealthy snack foods or fast foods no more than weekly
Self-efficacy, outcome expectancy, school attendance and grades, nutrition knowledge, and behaviors	Total 37 items
Other	
Afterschool attendance	Daily attendance at MMCC afterschool program

of the *7 Target Behaviors*, nutrition knowledge, and outcome expectancy. The *7 Target Behaviors*, which were developed, following the Expert Committee Recommendations, USDA MyPlate dietary guidelines, and NHLBI sleep recommendations [46–48], are detailed in Table 2. Secondary outcomes include improvements in cardiovascular and diabetes risk as measured by routinely collected markers of cardiovascular disease (LDL, triglycerides, and HDL) and insulin resistance (HbA1C). Additional routinely collected outcomes include school attendance and grades, attendance at afterschool sessions tracked using the MMCC afterschool NYC Department of Youth and Community Services (DYCD) database.

2.4. Selecting Implementation Outcome Metrics. Our implementation outcome metrics employed a hybrid strategy that combined elements of the RE-AIM framework and a Wellness Adaptation of the HIV cascade. The RE-AIM approach to evaluating the public health impact of health promotion interventions is based on 5 factors: reach, efficacy, adoption, implementation, and maintenance [49]. The underlying principle of the framework is that, beyond program effectiveness, the impact of system-based, community-based, or public health interventions relates to the contribution of each evaluative dimension, but a majority of studies fail to equally discuss all elements of the model [50–52]. Additionally, we adapted the HIV Cascade, which has been used as a conceptual framework for evaluating HIV treatment programs and represents population level representation of involvement in sequential steps of HIV treatment [53]. The hybrid strategy or "Wellness Cascade" evaluates the successive steps of our program implementation by establishing (1) the proportion of students that are available to be screened; (2) the proportion of students that are diagnosed with overweight and obesity; (3) the proportion that are recruited and enrolled in the program; (4) the proportion that are compliant with program requirements and thus engage in treatment; (5) the proportion that are retained in the program and thus complete the treatment; and (6) the proportion with a successful outcome (Table 3)

2.5. Intervention Evaluation. To evaluate the feasibility of implementing the program and secondarily to evaluate its effectiveness, we designed a quasiexperimental trial of *B'N Fit POWER* to compare students receiving *B'N Fit POWER* to students who chose not to enroll in the program and receive standard of care to address the following specific aims: (1) to determine whether *B'N Fit POWER* is effective in improving fitness, healthy weight attainment, and 7 target behaviors; (2) to assess the impact of moving the B'N Fit program into a school setting on participant engagement; and (3) to assess the mediating pathways associated with program effects. Following an initial health screening, students voluntarily enrolled in *B'N Fit POWER* (Group 1) were to receive comprehensive medical assessments at the MSHP integrated with MMCC afterschool programming that incorporates a curriculum focusing on *7 Target Behaviors* during weekly leadership sessions and daily physical activity. The comparison group consisting of all other students not enrolling in *B'N Fit POWER* (Group 2) would receive the standard of care (standard MSHP and MMCC afterschool program).

Table 3: Implementation outcome metrics: Wellness Cascade.

Wellness cascade steps	Aim at each step
(1) Proportion of students *screened*	Screening all students in the school annually
(2) Proportion of students *diagnosed* with overweight or obesity	Identifying all students in the school with a BMI ≥ 85th percentile annually
(3) Proportion of students recruited and *enrolled* in the program	Recruitment aim of having at least 85% of the participants recruited annually with BMI ≥ 85th percentile
(4) Proportion of students that *engaged in treatment* and compliant with program	Aim for students to attend all clinic visits and at least 75% of afterschool sessions during the year
(5) Proportion that are retained in the program and thus *completed the treatment*	Aim for at least 75% of students retained in the program for the entire school year annually
(6) Proportion of youths that attain a *successful outcome*	Aim for at least 50% of participating youths achieve a BMI *z*-score reduction of 0.2 defined as clinically important change [54]. Aim for a 25% improvement in the attainment of 7 target behaviors

Using the MMCC Afterschool program DYCD database, an opt-out letter was sent home to all MMCC afterschool program participants who would be incoming middle school students in the 2016/2017 school year inviting them to participate in a health assessment in the spring of 2016. The screening consisted of the following: (1) height and weight assessments were done in the MSHP SBHC, and BMI was calculated by the PI and (2) NYC Fitnessgram and *B'N Fit POWER* survey data were conducted by a physical activity specialist and youth leaders during afterschool program physical activity and leadership sessions, respectively. Students then received printed materials supporting healthy diet and physical activity behaviors. In addition, to improve access for youths who were not in afterschool, BMIs of all students registered in the MSHP SBHC were reviewed as part of the electronic medical record (EMR) review. These students, if not already registered in the afterschool program, did not undergo the screening. Although open to all, students whose BMI ≥ 85th percentile for sex and age were actively recruited and approached about enrolling in the program during the course of routine interactions with both MMCC and MSHP staff as well as via telephone outreach by the B'N Fit Staff. Additionally, distribution of flyers in the SBHC and to MMCC settings and a family information session promoted awareness about the program at the school. Emphasis was placed on explaining the physical activity and health benefits of participating in *B'N Fit POWER* rather than focusing on BMI and the need for weight loss. The target enrollment was to recruit at least 85% of program participants to have a BMI ≥ 85th percentile.

Once screened as per the *B'N Fit POWER* protocol, students were invited to enroll in *B'N Fit POWER* if they were 11 to 14 years, going to be in the 6th–8th grade in the fall of 2016, able to register in both the MMCC afterschool program, and in the MSHP SBHC, and a parent or guardian was available in person or by phone for clinic visits. Students were excluded if they had a mental illness that would render them incapable of consenting for the research or complying with the *B'N Fit POWER* afterschool program protocol or had medical problems that made it unsafe for them to participate in the program. The study was approved by the Institutional Review Board. Parents signed informed consent, and HIPAA authorization and participants provided assent at their initial SBHC visit. Once enrolled in *B'N Fit POWER*, students underwent the 60-minute baseline SBHC-adapted *B'N Fit POWER* wellness assessment during the summer months. The rationale for conducting the baseline assessment over the summer was to limit the time taken out of class for the initial assessment during the school year. During the initial assessment, a brief 2-page weight history questionnaire and the *7 Target Behavior* questionnaire would be filled out by the patient and entered into the EMR that is on the Epic (onsite EMR) platform [55] by the licensed practical nurse (LPN). The parent would complete the Pediatric Symptom Checklist, a validated 17-item behavioral screen addressing internalization, externalization, and attentional domains, to also be entered into the Epic platform by the LPN. The medical provider would then review the questionnaires and conduct a brief nutrition assessment (including a 24-hour diet recall), focused physical exam, including BP assessment, and depending on their BMI and BP, the student would undergo lab evaluations that were agreed upon by MSHP staff based on cost and feasibility of obtaining in the SBHC (Table 2). As per SBHC protocol, students received onsite mental health services if the PSC17 was positive in one or more domains. At a second 15-minute follow-up visit, the provider reviewed lab work and an Epic generated 1-page treatment plan summarizing comorbidities, target behavior, and weight goal and plan to achieve target changes. Following the initial assessment, students would return every 6 to 8 weeks for a total of four additional follow-up visits to monitor their progress with target changes.

Following their initial assessment, students participated in the MMCC afterschool program which provides afterschool programming for elementary and middle school students conducted from 3 to 6 pm daily from Monday through Friday throughout the school year. Similar to the other students in the afterschool program, who are required to attend 3 hours of Leadership each week, students enrolled in B'N Fit had the option of creating their own schedule with some minimum requirements: (1) attend three hours of *B'N Fit POWER* leadership sessions which included the *B'N Fit POWER* leadership curriculum, cooking class, and core physical activity education; and (2) attend at least 5 hours of physical activity programming each week. Attendance at all afterschool activities was tracked as per routine.

2.6. Implementation Evaluation. To evaluate the implementation feasibility, we collaboratively developed a strategy to integrate program metrics into the SBHC, MMCC afterschool, and school work-flows of onsite community partners using a Plan-Do-Study-Act (PDSA) cycle that followed the school year schedule [56]. Program improvement planning was done over the summer and implemented throughout the school year. MMCC collected attendance data and SBHC collected follow-up BMI and target behavior data throughout the school year. Outcomes were analyzed over the summer to inform follow-up improvements for the fall. Entry of anthropometric, lab, and target behaviors into Epic as part of the routine clinic visit aligned with current MSHP SBHC provider practice and provided a built-in sustainable method for tracking program outcomes. Further, attendance at *B'N Fit POWER* afterschool sessions was taken as per routine in the MMCC program supporting a sustainable method for tracking attendance and compliance with *B'N Fit POWER* leadership and physical activity requirements and supported a built-in structure for the program evaluation. Existing monthly onsite Wellness Council meetings provided a forum for discussing progress at each stage of the PDSA cycle with all stakeholders.

In the following results section, we describe the strategies used to maximize and optimize the screening for overweight and obesity, establish the feasibility of diagnosing students with overweight and obesity, facilitate enrollment and linkage to care, and program implementation. Results related to efficacy, receiving and completing therapy, and attainment of successful outcomes will be discussed elsewhere.

3. Implementation Results

3.1. Screening, Diagnosis, and Enrollment into the Program. We recruited students from the SBHC and MMCC afterschool programs. In the spring of 2016, 204 students in 5th–7th grade were registered in afterschool and 91 students completed screening during afterschool program hours, and of these, 42 (46%) met BMI criteria (BMI ≥ 85th percentile). An additional 63 students identified from the SBHC EMR review met BMI criteria. Of approximately 420 middle school students attending the school, we were able to obtain screening BMI data on 154 youths (37%), and of these, 105 met the BMI criteria of having a BMI ≥ 85th percentile. Of these students diagnosed with overweight or obesity, 55 (52%) were interested in the program (45 referred through MMCC; 10 referred through SBHC) (Figure 2). Of these, 35 registered in both SBHC and MMCC and completed signed parent consent and child assent. Of the 35 youths with IRB consent, 30 (86%) had a BMI ≥ 85 percentile for sex and age (Figure 2).

3.2. Process Evaluation of Screening, Diagnosis, and Enrollment Procedures. Our process evaluation identified challenges that included the following: (1) Identifying students from the afterschool program who achieved a low screening yield (91/420 students) and recruiting via the EMR to identify that elevated BMI did not align with efforts to reduce stigma and demedicalize the program for youths not already in the afterschool program. (2) Inadequate B'N Fit staff training limited opportunities to organizing training sessions; per diem youth leader staff had time committed to other activities. (3) The questionnaire was perceived as lengthy and difficult for students and MMCC staff to understand and complete. In addition, offsite PI obtained weight and height assessments during afterschool hours (as SBHC staff were unavailable during this time), and telephone outreach by offsite B'N Fit staff were unsustainable protocols. (4) The lack of a formalized communication protocol between SBHC (who worked during the school day) and MMCC afterschool staff (who worked during afterschool hours) delayed students enrolling through MMCC getting into the SBHC and delayed students enrolling through the SBHC getting into MMCC.

The process evaluation was used to develop new strategies for subsequent screenings (Table 4). Stakeholder input, including the school principal, MMCC staff, onsite Educational Consultant and Physical Education Faculty, and technical assistance from the HRSA granting agency, resulted in plans for (1) screening during the school day in conjunction with the schoolwide NYC Fitnessgram (weight and height data) done by physical education teachers and (2) administering the questionnaire, which was shortened to 25 items and computerized, during health class required for all students. These strategies address the limitations of initial screenings related to ensuring reduction of stigma and demedicalizing the program, while increasing the number of youths that can be fully screened potentially reaching over 400 middle school students annually.

Conducting the screening during the school day as proposed has been approved by the IRB and is currently being initiated. A bidirectional referral system involving the SBHC and the MMCC afterschool program staff was developed to ensure that overweight or obese youths, who might not otherwise join the *B'N Fit POWER* program, were diagnosed and enrolled in both settings. Utilizing the schoolwide NYC Fitnessgram data to identify all middle school students with a BMI > the 85th percentile, the PI provided a list to the MMCC staff who focused on recruiting students enrolled in afterschool and the SBHC staff who focused on all others. As students enrolled for the afterschool program in the fall, MMCC staff spoke individually with students and their parents diagnosed with a BMI > 85th percentile about registering in both MMCC and SBHC for enrollment in *B'N Fit POWER*. The SBHC staff conducted Brief Health Assessments (BHA) (which are routine visits unique to the SBHC intended to connect students to a medical home) on students diagnosed with a BMI > 85th percentile and would similarly speak with students and their parents about enrollment in the program. A per diem program monitor was hired by the MMCC afterschool program in the fall of September 2017 to create a protocol to facilitate these bidirectional referrals and as of the writing of this protocol, 35 youths have enrolled in both the SBHC and afterschool program with 11 referred through the SBHC and 24 referred through the afterschool program.

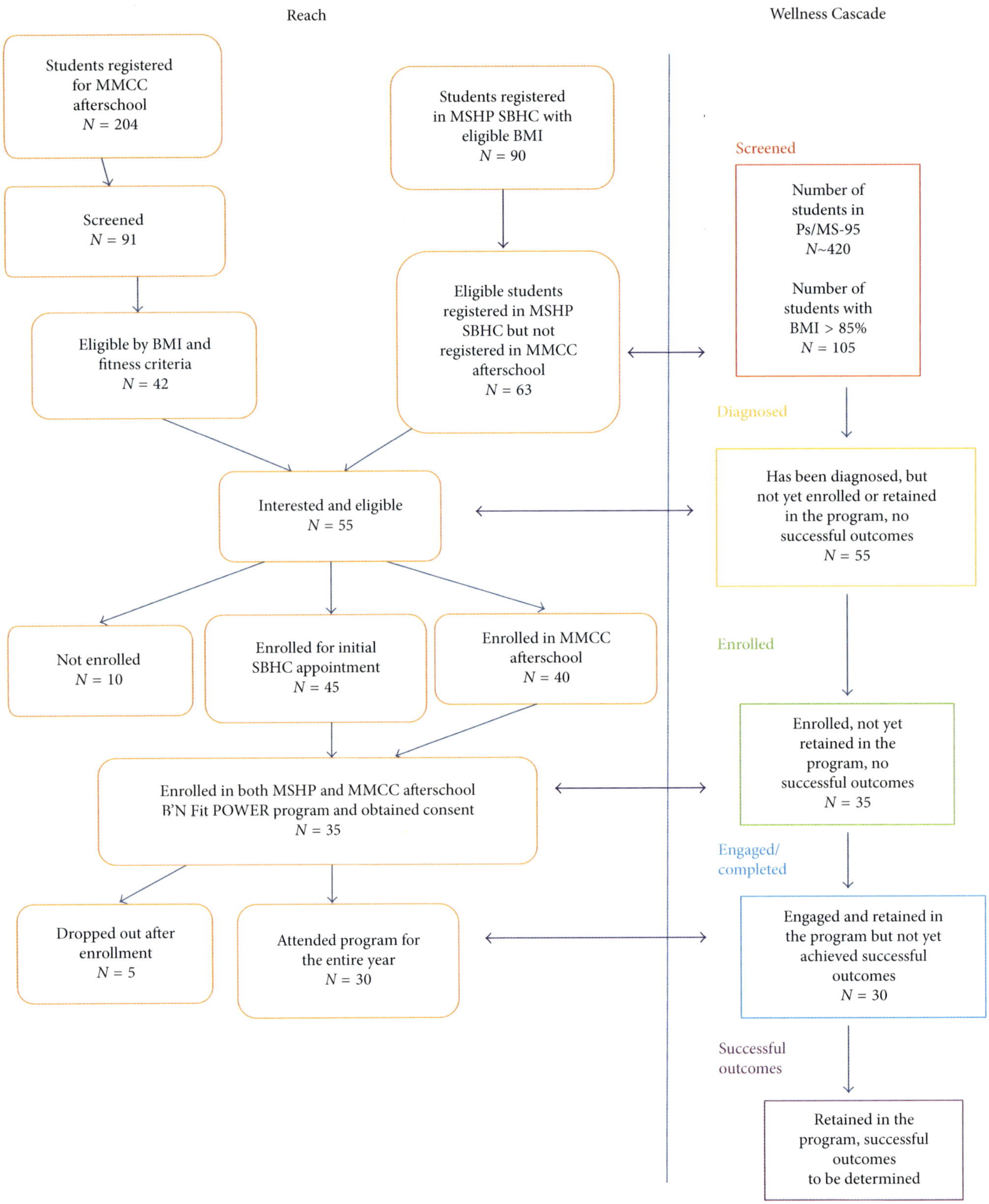

FIGURE 2: Implementation evaluation based on RE-AIM and Wellness Cascade.

3.3. Engagement in the Clinical and Afterschool Aspects of the Program. Of the 35 youths with IRB consent, 30 engaged in the program and attended elements of the program throughout the school year. To address stigma, youths in *B'N Fit POWER*, similar to the other students in the afterschool program, had the option of creating their own schedule with some minimum requirements. All students in the afterschool were assigned to leadership groups which consist of approximately 15 to 20 youths who stay together for the entire year. The structure of the MMCC afterschool program

TABLE 4: *B'N Fit POWER* integration of screening, diagnosis, and enrollment procedures.

Procedures	Existing PS-95 structure	*B'N Fit POWER* intervention at PS-95	Implementation challenges	Solutions to challenges
Screening for students with BMI ≥ 85th percentile	(i) Schoolwide NYC fitnessgram screening not routinely accessed as screening tool by MMCC or SBHC staff (ii) No routine screen by MMCC/SBHC staff	(i) Opt-out letter sent home to all students in 5th–7th grade registered in afterschool (ii) Afterschool program screening: (1) Height/weight (PI) (2) Fitnessgram (physical activity specialist) (3) *B'N Fit POWER* survey (youth leaders) (4) Healthy lifestyle handout (iii) EMR review of students in SBHC	(i) EMR identification of students with BMI > 85th percentile did not reduce stigma (ii) Low numbers screened in afterschool program (iii) Inadequate B'N Fit staff training of onsite MMCC staff (iv) Lengthy questionnaires difficult to understand and complete (v) Weight and height assessments by offsite PI unsustainable	(i) Consent letter sent to all students in school (ii) Schoolwide NYC fitnessgram data obtained by physical Education staff (iii) Access for all students (iv) B'N Fit staff training of educational consultant to train teachers to conduct questionnaire screening (v) Questionnaire shortened to 25 online items
Diagnosis	(i) No routine protocol for communicating overweight or obesity to at-risk youths (ii) SBHC BHA not always focused on screening for BMI ≥ 85th percentile	(i) Students with BMI ≥ 85th percentile recruited during routine interactions with MMCC and MSHP (ii) Emphasis was placed on explaining physical activity and health benefits of the program (iii) Telephone outreach by B'N Fit staff (iv) Distribution of flyers (v) Family information session	(i) Telephone outreach by B'N Fit staff unsustainable (ii) Low attendance at family information session	(i) NYC fitnessgram height and weight data provide shared recruitment list (ii) MMCC focus outreach on students in afterschool (iii) SBHC focus outreach on students not in afterschool
Enrollment	(i) Self-referral to SBHC (ii) Self-referral to MMCC afterschool program	(i) Self-referrals (ii) Telephone outreach (iii) Flyer distribution (iv) Information session (v) Target 85% of enrollees with BMI ≥ 85th percentile	(i) Delays in getting students enrolled in both MMCC afterschool program and SBHC related to interinstitutional communication challenges	(i) Bidirectional referrals (ii) Hired program monitor for referrals protocol implementation

BHA: Brief Health Assessment; PI: principal investigator; EMR: electronic medical record.

allowed for a seamless integration of the *B'N Fit POWER* participants into the program with other afterschool participants, particularly because there is overlap with many of the nonleadership classes and physical activity opportunities. The integration of *B'N Fit POWER* into the existing afterschool structure required no additional need to enter *B'N Fit POWER* attendance into a separate database.

3.4. Process Evaluation of Engagement in the Clinical and Afterschool Aspects of the Program. Challenges affecting implementation of a comprehensive weight management assessment in the busy SBHC and ensuring student engagement into the program included the following: (1) Lack of parental availability to obtain written consent during the school day resulted in research staff spending an unsustainable amount of time and effort to meet parents onsite and even offsite to ensure that written consents were completed. (2) Limited availability of students and families to undergo clinical assessments over the summer due to family vacations and lack of availability resulted in only 13 students undergoing their initial clinical assessments during the summer months. (3) The 60-minute initial visit was lengthy and difficult to implement during the fall school schedule during busy clinic schedule. (4) Lack of highly trained and specialized nutritionists onsite to support healthy lifestyle education placed the burden of nutrition education on the onsite medical provider, who often had little formal nutrition education and limited time to see patients. (5) While we had initially planned to do four additional follow-up visits throughout the year, the length of time it took to complete all initial visits due to high staff turnover and hospital-wide implementation of Epic in the fall requiring extensive offsite employee training (all initial visits were completed in January of 2017) made this impractical to achieve.

Table 5: *B'N Fit POWER* integration of SBHC visits and afterschool program components.

Procedures	Existing PS-95 structure	*B'N Fit POWER* intervention at PS-95	Implementation challenges	Solutions to challenges
SBHC baseline clinical assessment and follow-up visit	(i) BHA not consistently focused on screening for BMI ≥ 85th percentile (ii) No protocol for routine treatment and follow-up of youths with elevated BMI	(i) Obtain written parental consent and child assent (ii) 60-minute initial visit (iii) Patient fills out 2-page weight history, *7 Target Behavior*, and *PSC-17* questionnaires, (iv) LPN (1) Height, weight, BP (v) Medical provider: (1) Questionnaire review (2) Nutrition assessment (3) Focused PE (4) Orders labs (vi) MHP referral per routine (vii) 2nd 15-minute visit to review labs and treatment plan (viii) 4 follow-up visits to review behavior and weight goals	(i) Difficulty obtaining written parental consent (ii) Lengthy 60-minute visit difficult to implement during school schedule (iii) Lack of onsite specialized nutritionists to support healthy lifestyle education (iv) Busy clinic (v) Length of time to complete the initial visits made 4 follow-up visits impractical to achieve	(i) Obtain verbal consents from parents rather than written consent (ii) Split initial 60-minute visit into two 20-minute BHA visits: (iii) Visit 1: complete questionnaires, PE, and labs (iv) Visit 2: review lab work, and 1-page treatment plan, and target behavior education (v) Limit follow-up visits to two additional visits (vi) Completed repeat labs on those students with abnormal labs at initial visit
MMCC Afterschool Program	(i) From 3 to 6 pm daily (M-F) during year (ii) Includes DYCD mandated three hours of leadership (iii) Optional activities (iv) Routinely collect daily attendance (v) No routine curriculum for healthy lifestyle education	(i) DYCD mandated leadership includes the following: (1) *B'N Fit POWER* leadership curriculum (2) Cooking class (3) Gardening (ii) At least 5 hours of physical activity programming weekly (iii) *B'N Fit POWER* participants may sign up for any other optional activity available to the other students in the afterschool program	(i) The need for youth leader training (ii) *B'N Fit POWER* curriculum lessons were often lengthy and not well understood by youth leaders (iii) Recipes in the *B'N Fit POWER curriculum* not well accepted because ingredients not readily available in the neighborhood (iv) Busy afterschool setting	(i) Program Monitor serves as the education specialist and has reformatted and revised lesson plans to ensure clear, relatable, and relevant content (ii) Program Monitor trains youth leaders in advance of sessions (iii) Cooking specialist and WITS chefs altered recipes to better align with local community food availability

BHA: Brief Health Assessment; LPN: licensed practical nurse; MHP: mental health provider; PE: physical education; WITS: Wellness in the Schools.

The process evaluation was used to develop new strategies for subsequent clinic visits to ensure engagement into the program (Table 5). In discussions with parents and staff, the standard requirement for registering in both the SBHC and the afterschool program made the additional requirement of written research consent a barrier to completion. In an effort to streamline the consent process, in June of 2017, we obtained an amendment to the IRB to allow for verbal parental consent in combination with written child assent to facilitate study enrollment. To reduce time spent in the clinic, the initial visit was divided into two 20-minute Brief Health Assessments. The questionnaires are now being sent home and brought in completed. During the initial assessment, the history and physical exam are completed and target behaviors are identified. Labs are done during the week, and then during second 20-minute visit, the labs are discussed, comorbid conditions are reviewed, and target weight and target behaviors are discussed with 1-page treatment plan. To support healthy lifestyle education, one-page educational sheets reflecting practical approaches to making specific target behavior changes have been developed, and they increase the efficiency of providers. In consultation with MSHP staff, it was decided that each student would undergo only two additional follow-up visits, one in early winter and one in late spring. With this adjustment to the protocol, we were able to complete a first and second follow-up visit on 30 youths resulting in an 86% clinic retention rate. With the integration of the above changes, 27 students have completed their consent and baseline SBHC visit so far for the 2017/2018 school year.

The main challenges affecting the implementation of *B'N Fit POWER* into the afterschool setting included the following: (1) Lack of highly specialized and trained staff to teach the *B'N Fit POWER* comprehensive healthy lifestyle curriculum during leadership sessions and the need for youth leader training. (2) Importantly, the clinician designed *B'N Fit POWER* curriculum lessons were often lengthy and not well understood by youth leaders, who typically had a high school education and limited prior nutrition and healthy lifestyle education or experience. (3) Further, recipes contained within the *B'N Fit POWER curriculum* were also not well accepted by staff and youths because they used ingredients that were generally not readily available in the neighborhood surrounding the school. (4) Finally, the busy afterschool setting made it difficult for staff to receive training related to the curriculum and adapt recipes to better reflect cultural preferences and neighborhood grocery availability.

The process evaluation was used to develop new strategies to support student engagement into the program implementation for the 2017/2018 school year (Table 5). With much discussion and feedback from the onsite staff, an additional role for the Program Monitor, hired by MMCC, was to take on the role of serving as the MMCC education specialist to review curriculum. The curriculum has been reformatted to the lesson plan format already being used by the youth leaders; lesson plans have been edited to ensure that the content is clear, relatable, and relevant, and the Program Monitor trains youth leaders in advance of sessions to ensure that the curriculum remained relevant and engaging, and the per diem cooking specialist, who is familiar with the types of foods available in the community, has altered recipes to support the successful implementation of the recipes. We have also partnered with WITS to incorporate Department of Education alternative menu approved recipes into the cooking curriculum reinforcing concepts taught during the school day.

4. Discussion

To address health disparities in our community, we successfully engaged with a school and its onsite stakeholders and completed our first year of implementing *B'N Fit POWER*. We initiated protocols to support engagement into the school, piloted implementation of program components, and utilized our Wellness Cascade strategy to evaluate four successive steps of our program implementation corresponding to screening, diagnosis, enrollment, and engagement. While we have met a number of challenges related to the implementation process, we have developed strategies moving forward for (1) increasing the proportion of students screened from focusing on about a quarter of the middle school population to the entire middle school population; (2) ensuring that there is a mechanism for communicating with all students whose BMI > 85th percentile that there is healthy lifestyle programming available at their school and supporting linkage to care; and (3) supporting the feasibility of integrating clinical and afterschool components of the program into routine services offered at the school.

4.1. Initial Lessons Learned. The overarching lesson learned during the pilot implementation of the *B'N Fit POWER* program was that stakeholder collaboration provided the foundation for developing *B'N Fit POWER*, which included components of both successful hospital-based intensive and school-based interventions. These components included comprehensive clinical services, afterschool school program with participatory/hands on skill building student activities to teach strategies for improving dietary intake, increased physical activity, and behavioral techniques (including self-monitoring, goal setting, or coping skills) and to provide a daily dose of physical activity. *B'N Fit POWER* also included teacher training, providing a program for a duration of a year or longer, tailoring for cultural relevance, and involving parents as essential stakeholders [17, 35, 36]. The shared stakeholder responsibility facilitated delivering this content in a consistent and effective manner that ultimately results in successful implementation and sustainment of such a program. To do so, we learned how important it was for stakeholders to trust one another, the importance of giving the appropriate time and support to implement the program, particularly in our setting with few resources and limited funding, and the importance of acknowledging student stakeholder identified barriers, namely, the stigma that accompanies obesity, to program enrollment.

The B'N Fit staff has begun to earn the trust of the various stakeholders, especially with respect to "doing research" on *B'N Fit POWER* by focusing on collaborative decision-making approach [57, 58]. We learned that to gain trust we needed to consistently communicate that we valued stakeholder input and that we shared a common goal of improving the health of the students attending the school. We strove to work together as a coordinated team to accelerate the attainment of these goals during multiple stakeholder meetings in the two years leading up to the pilot intervention. Although the B'N Fit staff had extensive experience with designing, implementing, and evaluating a hospital and community-based weight management program, we acknowledged that onsite staff had more extensive experience serving large numbers of youths in their respective areas of expertise. The B'N Fit staff also joined the school-initiated School Wellness Council that meets on a monthly basis to gain a better understanding of the school health mission, current activities that promote health, and the current stakeholder strengths and resources and barriers to implementing healthy initiatives. While respecting the requirements governing the individual school, clinic, afterschool systems, and evaluation requirements, our collective priority was to ensure that the needs of the students guided our common efforts. We were thus able to streamline the screening and diagnosis protocols and align them with existing school fitness screening protocols and refine enrollment, and engagement processes by limiting time out of class to complete clinical assessments, utilize existing afterschool attendance data, and adapt the programming to be consistent with existing leadership, literacy, and STEM (science, technology, engineering, and math) requirements [59] and activities. Implementation of the PDSA evaluation cycle enabled the integration of *B'N Fit POWER* programming within the school calendar and work plans, for example, shared planning and program execution, working together to develop policies and procedures that systematized the coordination of services. Finally, support for the interprofessional team via the development of a training infrastructure facilitated more efficient use of resources and a further building of trust thereby also integrating staff engagement and empowerment into the program resulting in improved service for our target audience.

Drawing on the widely used SMART (specific, measurable, attainable, relevant or realistic, and time-bound) goal setting [60] approach enabled us to engage students and personalize setting lifestyle change goals as well as for setting program goals. We learned that careful planning was required to come up with a set number of specific annual goals for each aspect of the program and that these goals were measureable, attainable, relevant, and could be accomplished during the school year. During this process, we realized that it was imperative to consider the student's community context and stakeholder time constraints and barriers to implementation. Understanding that the Bronx is the nation's poorest urban county and least healthy county in NY State and that youths and families serviced by this program were at high risk for health disparities meant that there were high parental unemployment rates, limited financial resources, limited access to healthful foods, transportation for their children, or afterschool care for younger siblings at home. We learned that, for these youths, their families, and the staff that service these youths, minimizing the number of steps needed to engage youths in the program would support screening, diagnosis, linkage to care, and participation in the program and that the implementation of the program would need to occur over time with multiple brief actionable steps via PDSA cycles for each level of the program implementation. There is an underlying urgency to make large changes quickly to improve the health statistics in the Bronx, yet resources are sorely lacking. Applying lessons learned both from a decade of working with adolescents who are struggling to make healthy lifestyle changes and from the first year of implementing *B'N Fit POWER*, we learned that if we are a patient and focus on success with smaller goals, over time, we will empower the entire team to move forward to achieve larger goals and continue to make sustainable changes.

A final lesson learned related to acknowledging student stakeholder identified barriers, namely the stigma that accompanies obesity, to program enrollment. Our prior experience in B'N Fit with provider referrals based on BMI cutoffs resulted in youths enrolling in the B'N Fit program at the urging of their family members or provider, with a majority (70%) being in either the precontemplation or contemplation stage of change related to their interest in attending the program and making lifestyle changes; [22] most did not tell friends they attended a weight management program. While prioritizing eliminating stigma by opening enrollment to all students in the school, we acknowledged that high-risk youths may not volunteer for a popular afterschool programming expressly because they feel self-conscious, are concerned that they cannot keep up with activities and may be bullied about their physical appearance or physical limitations related to their weight, or may have other personal, familial, or social barriers to participation [61–63]. Generalized afterschool screening and open program access for all students in the afterschool program minimized stigma, as evidenced by the popularity of the program in its first year, while targeting at least 85% of the enrollees with a BMI ≥ 85th percentile. This strategy ensured adequate access to healthy lifestyle programming for high-risk youths who might not ordinarily access such a program and who would likely benefit the most from its services. Broadening the screening to include the entire school will serve to further reduce the stigma by ensuring that all students, including those not already enrolled in the existing afterschool program, undergo the same screening process. Expanding the number of students that can enroll in the afterschool *B'N Fit POWER* in the future will further increase the proportion of at risk students who have access to this program.

4.2. Limitations. Transferring the acquisition of the data from the afterschool setting to the school day setting has limitations related to the timing and accuracy of the data. Afterschool screening Fitnessgram, height and weight, and questionnaire data were obtained in April, May, and June annually, which was used for the pre- and postprogram evaluation. However, screening data are typically collected as per school protocol during physical education and health education classes from October through April. Thus, our approach for increasing the reach and efficiency for screening students does not necessarily align with a baseline and follow-up evaluation. Although the timing of the data collection conducted by the school may be viewed as a limitation, an assessment of overall school health and the impact of the interventions can be evaluated on an annual basis, and the use of this method already systematized by the school ensures sustainability of the screening process. An additional limitation relates to the use of a quasiexperimental trial to compare students receiving *B'N Fit POWER* to those students at the same school not in the program and who receive standard of care. The lack of the use of a RCT introduces selection bias, and the availability of overlapping programming activities introduces contamination thus affecting the robustness of the evaluation. Taking into consideration, however, the need for efficient use of resources and building stakeholder trust to prioritize a sustainable service for the youths, it has become clear that establishing the feasibility and acceptability of implementing the program and designing a realistic evaluation strategy is a necessary first step to designing an effectiveness trial for the program. While we conducted a process evaluation for engagement into care, we did not describe results related to actual number of students attending various components of the program as a measure of engagement and program compliance. Although attendance data were available, it was not readily accessible from the DYCD database, and the development of a protocol for accessing this data on a regular basis is necessary to track afterschool program attendance and compliance and is currently under development during the second year of the program implementation.

4.3. Next Steps. Moving forward the identification of individual stakeholders who will take on the role of all onsite training staff, implementation of quality assurance and quality control procedures, as well as the establishment of protocols to ensure collaboration among interprofessional teams will facilitate the clinical-community integration process. Utilization of tools for measuring the interprofessional collaboration and refinement of the Wellness Cascade strategy for measuring the impact of the collaboration will strengthen the integration process. Results related to engagement and completion of the program and attainment of successful outcomes will be reported in terms of the Wellness Cascade and further inform future implementation efforts.

Abbreviations

B'N Fit:	Bronx nutrition and fitness initiative for teens
CHAM:	Children's Hospital at Montefiore
StaRI:	Standards for Reporting Implementation Studies
YD:	Youth development
MSHP:	Montefiore School Health Program
SBHC:	School-Based Health Center
MMCC:	Mosholu Montefiore Community Center
WITS:	Wellness in the Schools
PIRC:	Prevention Intervention Research Center
USDA:	United States Department of Agriculture
PS/MS:	Public school/middle school
MA:	Medical Assistant
RN:	Registered Nurse
CHO:	Community Health Organizer
EMR:	Electronic Medical Record
NHLBI:	National Heart, Lung, and Blood Institute
NYC	New York City Department of Youth and
DYCD:	Community Development
PI:	Principal Investigator
HRSA:	Heath Resources and Services Administration
HbA1C:	Glycated hemoglobin test.

Acknowledgments

The study was supported by a Human Resources and Services Administration (HRSA) Healthy Tomorrows Partnership for Children Program grant (Grant no. H17MC29435) and the Life Course Methodology Core (LCMC) of the New York Regional Center for Diabetes Translation Research via a grant from the National Institute of Diabetes and Digestive and Kidney Diseases (Grant nos. DK111022-8786 and DK111022). The authors express our appreciation to our collaborators at PS/MS-95, the Mosholu Montefiore Community Center, the Montefiore School Health Program, Wellness in the Schools, the Prevention Intervention Research Center, Marni LoIacono Merves, former B'N Fit patients who served as MMCC afterschool youth leaders in the *B'N Fit POWER* program, and our students and volunteers for their innovation and commitment to the program. Most importantly, the authors thank our patients and their families for the opportunity of letting us serve them.

References

[1] C. L. Ogden, M. D. Carroll, H. G. Lawman et al., "Trends in obesity prevalence among children and adolescents in the United States, 1988–1994 through 2013-2014," *JAMA*, vol. 315, no. 21, pp. 2292–2299, 2016.

[2] A. C. Skinner and J. A. Skelton, "Prevalence and trends in obesity and severe obesity among children in the United States, 1999–2012," *JAMA Pediatrics*, vol. 168, no. 6, pp. 561–566, 2014.

[3] D. C. Seo, M. H. King, N. Kim, D. Sovinski, R. Meade, and A. M. Lederer, "Predictors for persistent overweight, deteriorated weight status, and improved weight status during 18 months in a school-based longitudinal cohort," *American Journal of Health Promotion*, vol. 30, no. 1, pp. 22–27, 2015.

[4] K. B. Watson, C. D. Harris, S. A. Carlson, J. M. Dorn, and J. E. Fulton, "Disparities in adolescents' residence in neighborhoods supportive of physical activity—United States, 2011-2012," *Morbidity and Mortality Weekly Report*, vol. 65, no. 23, pp. 598–601, 2016.

[5] D. C. Grossman, K. Bibbins-Domingo, S. J. Curry et al., "Screening for obesity in children and adolescents: US preventive services task force recommendation statement," *JAMA*, vol. 317, no. 23, p. 2417, 2017.

[6] D.-C. Seo and J. Sa, "A meta-analysis of obesity interventions among US minority children," *Journal of Adolescent Health*, vol. 46, no. 4, pp. 309–323, 2010.

[7] D. K. Wilson, "New perspectives on health disparities and obesity interventions in youth," *Journal of Pediatric Psychology*, vol. 34, no. 3, pp. 231–244, 2009.

[8] E. P. Whitlock, "Screening and interventions for childhood overweight: a summary of evidence for the US preventive services task force," *Pediatrics*, vol. 116, no. 1, pp. e125–e144, 2005.

[9] H. H. Dao, M. L. Frelut, F. Oberlin, G. Peres, P. Bourgeois, and J. Navarro, "Effects of a multidisciplinary weight loss intervention on body composition in obese adolescents," *International Journal of Obesity*, vol. 28, no. 2, pp. 290–299, 2004.

[10] L. G. Chehab, B. Pfeffer, I. Vargas, S. Chen, and M. Irigoyen, ""Energy up": a novel approach to the weight management of inner-city teens," *Journal of Adolescent Health*, vol. 40, no. 5, pp. 474–476, 2007.

[11] R. K. Evans, R. Franco, M. Stern et al., "Evaluation of a 6-month multi-disciplinary healthy weight management program targeting urban, overweight adolescents: effects on physical fitness, physical activity, and blood lipid profiles," *Pediatric Obesity*, vol. 4, no. 3, pp. 130–133, 2009.

[12] E. P. Whitlock, E. A. O'Connor, S. B. Williams, T. L. Beil, and K. W. Lutz, "Effectiveness of weight management interventions in children: a targeted systematic review for the USPSTF," *Pediatrics*, vol. 125, no. 2, pp. e396–e418, 2010.

[13] Y. Laird, S. Fawkner, P. Kelly, L. McNamee, and A. Niven, "The role of social support on physical activity behaviour in adolescent girls: a systematic review and meta-analysis,"

International Journal of Behavioral Nutrition and Physical Activity, vol. 13, no. 1, p. 79, 2016.

[14] S. J. Woolford, B. J. Sallinen, S. J. Clark, and G. L. Freed, "Results from a clinical multidisciplinary weight management program," *Clinical Pediatrics*, vol. 50, no. 3, pp. 187–191, 2011.

[15] M. Savoye, P. Nowicka, M. Shaw et al., "Long-term results of an obesity program in an ethnically diverse pediatric population," *Pediatrics*, vol. 127, no. 3, pp. 402–410, 2011.

[16] DCCT, "Lifetime benefits and costs of intensive therapy as practiced in the diabetes control and complications trial," *JAMA*, vol. 276, no. 17, pp. 1409–1415, 1996.

[17] M. J. Ickes, J. McMullen, T. Haider, and M. Sharma, "Global school-based childhood obesity interventions: a review," *International Journal of Environmental Research and Public Health*, vol. 11, no. 9, pp. 8940–8961, 2014.

[18] E. S. Belansky, N. Cutforth, E. Delong et al., "Early impact of the federally mandated local wellness policy on physical activity in rural, low-income elementary schools in Colorado," *Journal of Public Health Policy*, vol. 30, no. 1, pp. S141–S160, 2009.

[19] G. D. Foster, S. Sherman, K. E. Borradaile et al., "A policy-based school intervention to prevent overweight and obesity," *Pediatrics*, vol. 121, no. 4, pp. e794–e802, 2008.

[20] S. L. Gortmaker, K. Peterson, J. Wiecha et al., "Reducing obesity via a school-based interdisciplinary intervention among youth: planet health," *Archives of Pediatrics and Adolescent Medicine*, vol. 153, no. 4, pp. 409–418, 1999.

[21] T. N. Robinson, "Reducing children's television viewing to prevent obesity: a randomized controlled trial," *JAMA*, vol. 282, no. 16, pp. 1561–1567, 1999.

[22] J. Rieder, U. I. Khan, M. Heo et al., "Evaluation of a community-based weight management program for predominantly severely obese, difficult-to-reach, inner-city minority adolescents," *Childhood Obesity*, vol. 9, no. 4, pp. 292–304, 2013.

[23] L. R. Peralta, R. A. Jones, and A. D. Okely, "Promoting healthy lifestyles among adolescent boys: the fitness improvement and lifestyle awareness program RCT," *Preventive Medicine*, vol. 48, no. 6, pp. 537–542, 2009.

[24] D. L. Weintraub, E. C. Tirumalai, K. F. Haydel, M. Fujimoto, J. E. Fulton, and T. N. Robinson, "Team sports for overweight children: the stanford sports to prevent obesity randomized trial (SPORT)," *Archives of Pediatrics & Adolescent Medicine*, vol. 162, no. 3, pp. 232–237, 2008.

[25] D. A. Dudley, A. D. Okely, P. Pearson, and J. Peat, "Engaging adolescent girls from linguistically diverse and low income backgrounds in school sport: a pilot randomised controlled trial," *Journal of Science and Medicine in Sport*, vol. 13, no. 2, pp. 217–224, 2010.

[26] N. Eather, P. J. Morgan, and D. R. Lubans, "Improving health-related fitness in adolescents: the CrossFit Teens™ randomised controlled trial," *Journal of Sports Sciences*, vol. 34, no. 3, pp. 209–223, 2016.

[27] D. Christian, C. Todd, R. Hill et al., "Active children through incentive vouchers—evaluation (ACTIVE): a mixed-method feasibility study," *BMC Public Health*, vol. 16, no. 1, p. 890, 2016.

[28] Force C. P. S. T., *Obesity Prevention and Control: School-Based Programs*, 2017, https://www.thecommunityguide.org/sites/default/files/assets/Obesity-School-based-Programs.pdf.

[29] H. Pinnock, M. Barwick, C. R. Carpenter et al., "Standards for reporting implementation studies (StaRI) statement," *BMJ*, vol. 356, p. i6795, 2017.

[30] J. A. Hester, P. V. Stange, L. C. Seeff, J. B. Davis, and C. A. Craft, *Toward Sustainable Improvements in Population Health: Overview of Community Integration Structures and Emerging Innovations in Financing*, 2015, https://stacks.cdc.gov/view/cdc/27844.

[31] W. H. Dietz, B. Belay, D. Bradley et al., *A Model Framework that Integrates Community and Clinical Systems for the Prevention AND Management of Obesity and Other Chronic Diseases*, 2017, https://nam.edu/wp-content/uploads/2017/01/A-Model-Framework-That-Integrates-Community-and-ClinicalSystems-for-the-Prevention-and-Management-ofObesity-and-Other-Chronic-Diseases.pdf.

[32] J. L. Roth and J. Brooks-Gunn, "What exactly is a youth development program? Answers from research and practice," *Applied Developmental Science*, vol. 7, no. 2, pp. 94–111, 2003.

[33] C. McKinney, V. Bishop, K. Cabrera et al., "NuFit: nutrition and fitness CBPR program evaluation," *Journal of Prevention and Intervention in the Community*, vol. 42, no. 2, pp. 112–124, 2014.

[34] S. Stock, C. Miranda, S. Evans et al., "Healthy buddies: a novel, peer-led health promotion program for the prevention of obesity and eating disorders in children in elementary school," *Pediatrics*, vol. 120, no. 4, pp. e1059–e1068, 2007.

[35] M. Kanyamee, W. Fongkaew, J. Chotibang, P. Aree, and C. Kennedy, "An intervention study of changing eating behaviors and reducing weight in thai children aged 10–12," *Pacific Rim International Journal of Nursing Research*, vol. 17, no. 4, 2013.

[36] D. L. Katz, M. O'Connell, V. Y. Njike, M. C. Yeh, and H. Nawaz, "Strategies for the prevention and control of obesity in the school setting: systematic review and meta-analysis," *International Journal of Obesity*, vol. 32, no. 12, pp. 1780–1789, 2008.

[37] E. Jelalian, R. Mehlenbeck, E. E. Lloyd-Richardson, V. Birmaher, and R. R. Wing, "Adventure therapy' combined with cognitive-behavioral treatment for overweight adolescents," *International Journal of Obesity*, vol. 30, no. 1, pp. 31–39, 2006.

[38] P. Eskicioglu, J. Halas, M. Sénéchal et al., "Peer mentoring for type 2 diabetes prevention in first nations children," *Pediatrics*, vol. 133, no. 6, pp. e1624–e1631, 2014.

[39] M. Story, "School-based approaches for preventing and treating obesity," *International Journal of Obesity and Related Metabolic Disorders*, vol. 23, no. 2, pp. 43–51, 1999.

[40] Foundation R. W. J, *Health Outcomes: Overall Rank*, 2017, http://www.countyhealthrankings.org/app/new-york/2017/rankings/bronx/county/outcomes/overall/snapshot.

[41] J. R. Egger, K. F. Bartley, L. Benson, D. Bellino, and B. Kerker, "Childhood obesity is a serious concern in New York City: higher levels of fitness associated with better academic performance," *NYC Vital Signs*, vol. 8, no. 1, pp. 1–4, 2009.

[42] Public School 95 Sheila Mencher in Bronx, New York, 2017, http://public-schools.startclass.com/l/61172/Public-School-95-Sheila-Mencher-in-Bronx-New-York.

[43] R. da Costa Nunez, M. Adams, A. Gleason, and S. Harris, "Failures and solutions: New Yorkers' views on homelessness," in *Proceedings from an ICPH Public Opinion Poll*, New York, NY, USA, 2011.

[44] K. Atkiss, M. Moyer, M. Desai, and M. Roland, "Positive youth development: an integration of the developmental assets theory and the socio-ecological model," *American Journal of Health Education*, vol. 42, no. 3, pp. 171–180, 2011.

[45] *Education, N. Y. C. D. O. NYC Fitnessgram*, http://schools.nyc.gov/Academics/Wellness/WhatWeOffer/NycFitnessgram/Learn+About+NYC+FITNESSGRAM.htm.

[46] S. E. Barlow, "Expert committee recommendations regarding the prevention, assessment, and treatment of child and adolescent overweight and obesity: summary report," *Pediatrics*, vol. 120, no. 4, pp. S164–S192, 2007.

[47] *Service U. S. D. A. F. A. N. MyPlate*, 2017, https://www.fns.usda.gov/tn/myplate.
[48] Institute N. I. H. N. H. L. A. B., *How Much Sleep is Enough?*, 2017, https://www.nhlbi.nih.gov/health/health-topics/topics/sdd/howmuch.
[49] R. E. Glasgow, T. M. Vogt, and S. M. Boles, "Evaluating the public health impact of health promotion interventions: the RE-AIM framework," *American Journal of Public Health*, vol. 89, no. 9, pp. 1322–1327, 1999.
[50] T. McGoey, Z. Root, M. W. Bruner, and B. Law, "Evaluation of physical activity interventions in children via the reach, efficacy/effectiveness, adoption, implementation, and maintenance (RE-AIM) framework: a systematic review of randomized and non-randomized trials," *Preventive Medicine*, vol. 82, pp. 8–19, 2016.
[51] R. S. Kessler, E. P. Purcell, R. E. Glasgow, L. M. Klesges, R. M. Benkeser, and C. J. Peek, "What does it mean to "employ" the RE-AIM model," *Evaluation & the Health Professions*, vol. 36, no. 1, pp. 44–66, 2013.
[52] B. Gaglio, J. A. Shoup, and R. E. Glasgow, "The RE-AIM framework: a systematic review of use over time," *American Journal of Public Health*, vol. 103, no. 6, pp. e38–e46, 2013.
[53] M. J. Mugavero, K. R. Amico, T. Horn, and M. A. Thompson, "The state of engagement in HIV care in the United States: from cascade to continuum to control," *Clinical Infectious Diseases*, vol. 57, no. 8, pp. 1164–1171, 2013.
[54] E. A. O'Connor, C. V. Evans, B. U. Burda, E. S. Walsh, M. Eder, and P. Lozano, "Screening for obesity and intervention for weight management in children and adolescents: evidence report and systematic review for the US preventive services task force," *JAMA*, vol. 317, no. 23, p. 2427, 2017.
[55] Epic, 2017, http://www.Epic.com/software.
[56] Plan-Do-Study-Act (PDSA) Cycle, 2017, https://innovations.ahrq.gov/qualitytools/plan-do-study-act-pdsa-cycle.
[57] S. A. Kaplan, N. S. Calman, M. Golub, J. H. Davis, C. Ruddock, and J. Billings, "Racial and ethnic disparities in health: a view from the South Bronx," *Journal of Health Care for the Poor and Underserved*, vol. 17, no. 1, pp. 116–127, 2006.
[58] M. D. McKee, L. F. O'Sullivan, and C. M. Weber, "Perspectives on confidential care for adolescent girls," *Annals of Family Medicine*, vol. 4, no. 6, pp. 519–526, 2006.
[59] Education N. Y. C. D. O. STEM, 2017, http://schools.nyc.gov/Academics/STEM/default.htm.
[60] G. T. Doran, "There's a S.M.A.R.T. way to write management's goals and objectives," *Management Review*, vol. 70, no. 11, pp. 35-36, 1981.
[61] R. Cason-Wilkerson, S. Goldberg, K. Albright, M. Allison, and M. Haemer, "Factors influencing healthy lifestyle changes: a qualitative look at low-income families engaged in treatment for overweight children," *Childhood Obesity*, vol. 11, no. 2, pp. 170–176, 2015.
[62] B. J. Sallinen, S. Schaffer, and S. J. Woolford, "In their own words: learning from families attending a multidisciplinary pediatric weight management program at the YMCA," *Childhood Obesity*, vol. 9, no. 3, pp. 200–207, 2013.
[63] R. M. Puhl, J. L. Peterson, and J. Luedicke, "Weight-based victimization: bullying experiences of weight loss treatment-seeking youth," *Pediatrics*, vol. 131, no. 1, pp. e1–e9, 2013.

18

Impact of Sleeve Gastrectomy on Psychiatric Medication Use and Symptoms

Scott V. Monte,[1] Kristen M. Russo,[1] Esra Mustafa,[1] and Joseph A. Caruana[2]

[1]*University at Buffalo School of Pharmacy and Pharmaceutical Sciences, 213 Kapoor Hall, Buffalo, NY 14214, USA*
[2]*Synergy Bariatrics, A Department of ECMC, University at Buffalo School of Medicine, Buffalo, NY 14214, USA*

Correspondence should be addressed to Scott V. Monte; svmonte@buffalo.edu

Academic Editor: Aron Weller

Background. Sleeve gastrectomy (SG) has become the primary bariatric surgery procedure in the U.S. Over 50% of people presenting for surgery have psychiatric diagnoses. The study purpose was to evaluate change in anxiety and depression symptoms and medication use after SG. *Methods.* Subjects completing SG with a diagnosis of anxiety and/or depression treated with medication were retrospectively identified from the electronic medical record (EMR) of Synergy Bariatrics, a department of the Erie County Medical Center. Phone outreach was made to complete seven-point global impression of change scale classifying symptom improvement or worsening in the 3- to 6-month postoperative period. Improvement or worsening was defined as either all reported symptoms improving or worsening or ≥1 improving or worsening while remaining unchanged. If ≥1 symptom improved and worsened, it was classified as mixed. No change required the same profile before and after surgery. Medication, dose, and changes were identified by EMR, verified during interview and classified as no change, discontinued, decreased, or increased. *Results.* 59 subjects completed the interview. 21 subjects were diagnosed with anxiety. 13 (62%) had no change in therapy and 5 (24%) decreased. Symptoms improved in 12 (57%), worsened in 3 (14%), and mixed in 5 (24%). When symptoms improved, the same dose was present in 7/12 (58%) and dose decreased in 3 (25%). 51 subjects were diagnosed with depression. 32 (63%) had no change in therapy, 11 (21%) discontinued, and 4 (8%) decreased. Symptoms improved in 34 (67%), mixed in 10 (20%), worsened in 4 (8%), and unchanged in 3 (6%). When symptoms improved, the same regimen and dose was present in 21/34 cases (62%) and discontinued in 9 (26%). *Conclusion.* Anxiety symptoms improved in >50% of subjects at predominantly the same or reduced dosage. Depression symptoms improved in 67% and commonly without therapy change. These data suggest evidence that patients undergoing SG while on medication for anxiety or depression may have early symptom improvement on the same or lessened dosage.

1. Introduction

The National Institutes of Health estimates that 36% of adults in the United States are obese [1]. Bariatric surgery procedures Roux-en-Y gastric bypass (RYGB) and Sleeve gastrectomy (SG) are well-established interventions for weight loss [2]. RYGB was the most common procedure performed until 2014 when SG increased to >50% of cases [3]. One advantage of SG in comparison with RYGB is thought to be lessened concern for altered medication absorption given that only a portion of the stomach is removed and the transition to the small intestine remains continuous. This is of particular importance to people using medication therapy for depression and anxiety.

People presenting for bariatric surgery are diagnosed with depression in 36% of cases and anxiety in 11% [4]. Cunningham et al. found that less than half of people remain on the same antidepressant regimen after RYGB. In approximately 40% of those cases, an increase or switch in antidepressant was required. Only 15% decreased or discontinued therapy [5]. These data are consistent with reports of reduced absorption of selective serotonin reuptake inhibitors (SSRIs) and tricyclic antidepressants after RYGB [6]. Antianxiety medication use and absorption is not widely studied after RYGB. Prescription fill data suggest an increased use of antianxiety, sedative, and hypnotic medications following RYGB [4]. In comparison with RYGB, considerably less is known about depression and anxiety symptoms and medication use after SG. Mack et al. identified improvement in depression and stress symptoms in the 48-month period after SG [7]. However, there are no antidepressant or antianxiety medication absorption and efficacy studies after SG [8]. No studies have characterized or evaluated the overlap of change in depression or anxiety symptoms and change in medication use after RYGB or SG.

The objectives of this study were to characterize depression and anxiety symptom change; characterize antidepressant and antianxiety medication use change; and identify predictors of symptom improvement or worsening after SG.

2. Materials and Methods

Subjects with a diagnosis of depression, anxiety, or both treated with antidepressant or antianxiety medication at the time of SG surgery were identified from medical records of Synergy Bariatrics, a department of the Erie County Medical Center (Buffalo, NY) in 2016. Study investigators contacted patients by phone, and following informed consent, they were interviewed to determine change in depression and anxiety symptoms and medication use in the 3- to 6-month period after surgery. At the time of the interview study, investigators reviewed the medical chart to verify medication names, doses, and changes in therapy with the subject. Subjects were excluded if they became pregnant or experienced rehospitalization related to surgery, reoperation, or had another major surgery in the 3- to 6-month evaluation period.

A hard copy of the seven-point patient global impression of change scale (PGIC) was used to conduct and document subject survey responses (see Supplementary Appendix 1). The Patient Global Impression of Change (PGIC) is a self-report measure that reflects a patient's belief about the efficacy of treatment. PGIC is a seven-point scale that depicts a patient's rating of overall improvement [9]. Depression symptoms evaluated included feeling down or hopeless, little interest or pleasure in doing things, trouble falling asleep, sleeping too much, feeling tired or having little energy, trouble concentrating, overeating, self-dislike, and suicidal thoughts. Anxiety symptoms evaluated were anxious mood, feeling tense, feeling restless, crying easily, trouble falling asleep, trouble concentrating, little interest or pleasure in doing things, feeling tired or having little energy, and being afraid of the dark, strangers, being alone, or crowds. Investigators assessed both depression and anxiety symptoms in patients with both diagnoses. Patients with both diagnoses were treated with medications that are commonly used to treat both depression and anxiety. Symptom changes were designated as very much worse, much worse, minimally worse, minimally improved, much improved, very much improved, and those having no change versus baseline. Symptom improvement was defined as either all symptoms improving or at least one symptom improving while the remaining were unchanged. The same criteria were applied for symptom worsening. A mixed profile was noted if at least one symptom improved and worsened. No change required the same profile before and after.

Medication use was categorized as unchanged, increased, decreased, discontinued, or a switch in medication class. Increase in medication use was defined as either an increase in medication dose or frequency. The same criteria were applied for decrease in medication use.

The medical record review supplemented the interview to gather patient demographics, body mass index (BMI), excess body weight, ideal body weight, percentage of body weight lost and psychiatric diagnoses, medications, and doses. All data were maintained in a Microsoft Excel file on the internal servers of the medical practice. Data are presented descriptively and in the tabular form for change in depression and anxiety symptoms, change in medication use, and combined symptom change and medication use. Simple logistic regression was used to identify associations between independent variables and symptom improvement. Independent variables included age, gender, height, ideal body weight, weight, and excess body weight at the time of surgery, and excess body weight and percentage of excess body weight loss after surgery, death in the family, marriage or divorce, pregnancy, new or lost job, emergency room visit or hospitalization unrelated to surgery, transfer addictions of new or increased alcohol or tobacco use, prescription or recreational drug abuse, and eating disorders. Transfer addiction, after bariatric surgery, occurs when individuals trade compulsive eating for other compulsive behaviors. Other behaviors or substances may substitute for eating.

The protocol for the study was approved by the State University of New York at Buffalo Institutional Review Board.

3. Results and Discussion

Fifty-nine subjects completed interview: 38 with depression, eight with anxiety, and 13 with depression and anxiety. Subject characteristics are shown in Table 1.

3.1. Depression. Change in depression symptoms and medication use for 51 subjects are shown in Table 2. Depression symptoms improved in 34/51 (67%) subjects in the 3–6 months following SG.

Age, gender, height, ideal body weight, weight and excess body weight at the time of surgery, and percentage of excess body weight loss after surgery were not significantly associated with symptom change after SG ($p > 0.1$ for all). Death in the family, marriage, divorce, new job, lost job, and transfer addiction were also not significantly associated with symptom change. Medication use changes (no change in medication, medication increase, medication decrease, medication discontinuation, or switch in medication class) were not significantly associated with symptom change after SG. In cases where symptoms improved, 32 (94%) occurred in circumstances where medications were discontinued,

Table 1: Subject characteristics ($n = 59$).

Patient demographics ($n = 59$)	
Age	51 ± 13 years
Gender	51 females (86%)
Height	165 ± 8 cm
Weight	129 ± 28 kg
BMI	46.9 ± 8.2 kg/m^2
Ideal body weight	58 ± 9 kg
Excess body weight	71 ± 25 kg
Medication classes	No. of patients
SSRI	39 (66%)
SNRI	17 (29%)
Benzodiazepine	13 (22%)
Anticonvulsant	8 (14%)
Atypical antipsychotic	4 (7%)
Bupropion	4 (7%)
Antihistamine	1 (2%)
Trazodone	1 (2%)

BMI = body mass index; SSRI = selective serotonin reuptake inhibitor; SNRI = serotonin norepinephrine reuptake inhibitor.

Table 2: Change in depression symptoms compared to change in medication use ($n = 51$).

	Change in depression symptoms	
Symptom change	Number of patients ($n = 51$)	Percentage of patients
Unchanged	3	6%
Improved	34	67%
Worsened	4	8%
Mixed	10	19%
	Change in medication use	
Medication change	Number of patients ($n = 51$)	Percentage of patients
Unchanged	32	63%
Increased	2	4%
Decreased	4	8%
Discontinued	11	21%
Switch class	2	4%

Change in symptoms vs. change in medication use					
Symptom change	Med unchanged	Med increased	Med decreased	Med discontinued	Switch med class
Unchanged	2 (4%)	0 (0%)	1 (2%)	0 (0%)	0 (0%)
Improved	21 (41%)	1 (2%)	2 (4%)	9 (17%)	1 (2%)
Worsened	1 (2%)	1 (2%)	0 (0%)	1 (2%)	1 (2%)
Mixed	8 (16%)	0 (0%)	1 (2%)	1 (2%)	0 (0%)

decreased, or unchanged. Symptoms worsened in four (8%), were unchanged in three (6%), and were mixed in 10 (20%).

3.2. Anxiety. Change in anxiety symptoms and medication use for 21 subjects are shown in Table 3. Anxiety symptoms improved in 12/21 (57%) subjects. Gender, height, ideal body weight, weight and excess body weight at the time of surgery, and percentage of excess body weight loss after surgery were not significantly associated with symptom change after SG ($p > 0.1$ for all). Increased age was predictive of symptom improvement ($p = 0.041$). Death in the family, marriage, divorce, new job, and transfer addiction were not significantly associated with symptom change. No patients lost job. Medication use changes (no change, medication increase, medication decrease, or medication discontinuation) were not significantly associated with symptom change after SG. No patients changed medication class. In cases where symptoms improved, 11 (92%) occurred in circumstances where medications were discontinued, decreased, or unchanged. Symptoms worsened in three (14%), were unchanged in one (5%), and were mixed in five (24%).

This study is the first to characterize depression and anxiety symptom change and antidepressant and antianxiety medication use change and evaluate predictors of symptom improvement or worsening after SG. We have shown that a high percentage of patients experience improvement in their depression (67%) and anxiety (57%) symptoms after SG. Intuitive factors expected to be predictive of symptom improvement such as excess body weight at the time of surgery and percentage of excess body weight lost after surgery were not significantly associated with depression or

TABLE 3: Change in anxiety symptoms compared to change in medication use ($n = 21$).

Symptom change	Change in anxiety symptoms Number of patients ($n = 21$)	Percentage of patients
Unchanged	1	5%
Improved	12	57%
Worsened	3	14%
Mixed	5	24%

Medication change	Change in medication use Number of patients ($n = 21$)	Percentage of patients
Unchanged	13	62%
Increased	2	9%
Decreased	5	24%
Discontinued	1	5%
Switch class	0	0%

Symptom change	Med unchanged	Med increased	Med decreased	Med discontinued	Switch med class
	Change in symptoms vs. change in medication use				
Unchanged	0 (0%)	0 (0%)	1 (5%)	0 (0%)	0 (0%)
Improved	7 (33%)	1 (5%)	3 (14%)	1 (5%)	0 (0%)
Worsened	2 (9%)	1 (5%)	0 (0%)	0 (0%)	0 (0%)
Mixed	4 (19%)	0 (0%)	1 (5%)	0 (0%)	0 (0%)

anxiety symptom improvement. In fact, age was the only predictor of symptom improvement and observed in only the anxiety group. Strikingly, 94% and 92% of depression and anxiety subjects experienced symptom improvement while at the same time discontinuing, decreasing, or not changing their medication, dose, or formulation. Taken together with the lack of other independent predictors for symptom improvement, these data may suggest that SG has an independent effect on depression and anxiety. This finding would be consistent with the known effect of SG to reduce inflammatory cytokines such as interleukin-6 and C-reactive protein that are heightened in depression and anxiety [10, 11].

Antidepressant and antianxiety medication change should be anticipated in the first 3–6 months after SG. The antidepressant regimen was altered in 37% of cases. The majority discontinued or decreased medication, but four subjects (19%) required a dose increase or class switch. Antianxiety data were similar to depression in that the regimen was altered in 38% of cases and the majority discontinued or decreased medication. Two subjects required dose increase (9%). These cases where medication was increased or class switched leave open the possibility of antianxiety or antidepressant absorption being compromised in a minority of people after SG.

These data are informative to bariatric surgery providers evaluating and preparing approximately 33% people with depression and 10% with anxiety presenting for bariatric surgery but should be interpreted in the context of the following limitations. First, the sample size is small in 59 subjects. This is a retrospective study with no control group for comparison. Secondly, the evaluation period of 3–6 months after surgery affords no insight into sustainability of symptom improvement. This study examines only the preliminary stages of mental and emotional adjustment to SG and weight loss and provides no opportunity for long-term follow-up. Thirdly, antidepressant use was predominantly SSRI (66%) and serotonin norepinephrine reuptake inhibitor (29%) and antianxiety use was predominantly benzodiazepine (22%). Lastly, the investigators did not inquire about alternative explanations for symptom improvement such as initial weight loss or sense of relief due to a successful surgery.

4. Conclusion

Depression and anxiety symptoms improved in a majority of cases after SG. Antidepressant and antianxiety medication regimens were altered in approximately one-third of cases but were primarily reflected by dose decrease or discontinuation. Approximately 10–20% of cases were dose increases or class switches leaving open the possibility of compromised absorption. In depression and anxiety cases where symptoms improved, the medications were decreased or discontinued in over 90%. In the noted absence of clinical and medication factors predicting symptom improvement, these data may suggest an independent effect of SG on depression.

Disclosure

This manuscript was presented as a poster prior to publication in this journal.

References

[1] NIDDK, *Overweight & Obesity Statistics*, NIDDK, Bethesda, MD, USA, 2012.

[2] ASMBS, *Bariatric Surgery Procedures*, ASMBS, Gainesville, FL, USA, 2017.

[3] ASMBS, *Estimate of Bariatric Surgery Numbers, 2011–2015*, ASMBS, Gainesville, FL, USA, 2016.

[4] S. D. I. J. Hatoum, R. Blackstone, T. D. Hunter et al., "Clinical factors associated with remission of obesity-related comorbidities after bariatric Surgery," *JAMA Surgery*, vol. 151, no. 2, p. 130, 2016.

[5] J. L. Cunningham, C. C. Merrell, M. Sarr et al., "Investigation of antidepressant medication usage after bariatric Surgery," *Obesity Surgery*, vol. 22, no. 4, pp. 530–535, 2012.

[6] M. Geraldo, D. Feder, F. L. Affonso Fonseca, and M. R. de Fatima Veiga Gouveia, "The use of drugs in patients who have undergone bariatric surgery," *International Journal of General Medicine*, vol. 2014, pp. 219–224, 2014.

[7] I. Mack, S. Ölschläger, H. Sauer et al., "Does laparoscopic sleeve gastrectomy improve depression, stress and eating behaviour? A 4-year follow-up Study," *Obesity Surgery*, vol. 26, no. 12, pp. 2967–2973, 2016.

[8] J. P. Yska, S. van der Linde, V. V. Tapper et al., "Influence of bariatric surgery on the use and pharmacokinetics of some major drug classes," *Obesity Surgery*, vol. 23, no. 6, pp. 819–825, 2013.

[9] W. Guy, *ECDEU Assessment Manual for Psychopharmacology, DHEW Publication No. ADM 76–338*, US Government Printing Office, Washington, DC, USA, 1976.

[10] A. Mallipedhi, S. L. Prior, J. D. Barry, S. Caplin, J. N. Baxter, and J. W. Stephens, "Changes in inflammatory markers after sleeve gastrectomy in patients with impaired glucose homeostasis and type 2 diabetes," *Surgery for Obesity and Related Diseases*, vol. 10, no. 6, pp. 1123–1128, 2014.

[11] A. H. Miller, E. Haroon, C. L. Raison, and J. C. Felger, *Cytokine Targets in the Brain: Impact on Neurotransmitters and Neurocircuits*, U.S. NLM, Bethesda, MD, USA, 2013.

19

Dyslipidemia and Fatty Liver Disease in Overweight and Obese Children

Asma Deeb, [1] **Salima Attia**, [1] **Samia Mahmoud**, [2] **Ghada Elhaj**, [3] **and Abubaker Elfatih** [4]

[1] *Pediatric Endocrinology Department, Mafraq Hospital, P.O. Box 2951, Abu Dhabi, UAE*
[2] *Pediatric Clinic, Police Health Services, Abu Dhabi, UAE*
[3] *Primary Health Care Center, BaniYas, Abu Dhabi, UAE*
[4] *Biochemistry Department, Shaikh Khalifa Medical City, Abu Dhabi, UAE*

Correspondence should be addressed to Asma Deeb; adeeb@seha.ae

Academic Editor: R. Prager

Introduction. Obesity is a worldwide concern. It is associated with morbidity such as dyslipidemia and liver disease. Childhood obesity has dramatically increased, particularly in the Gulf region. We aim to assess the prevalence of dyslipidemia and fatty liver disease (FLD) in overweight and obese children and analyze the association between different anthropometric measures with dyslipidemia and fatty liver disease. *Methods.* A descriptive, cross-sectional study conducted on children referred with obesity. BMI percentiles were plotted and standardized waist circumference (WC) was generated. Family history of metabolic syndrome was recorded. Fasting lipid, liver transaminases, and ultrasound scans (US) for those with elevated enzymes were performed. Descriptive statistics were used for quantitative parameters. *Results.* 216 participants were recruited. Mean $\pm$ SD age was 10.58 $\pm$ 2.996 years. 55.3% had dyslipidemia; 11.7% had high cholesterol, 28.6% high triglyceride, 32.7% high LDL, and 18.0% low HDL. 51 (84%) had either elevated transaminases. All had liver US, and 43 had FLD. WC was strongly associated with dyslipidemia and FLD ($P = 0.04$ and 0.003). *Conclusion.* Dyslipidemia is common in overweight, obese children. FLD is prevalent in those with elevated liver transaminases. WC is an easy tool that can be utilized to screen for dyslipidemia and FLD in overweight and obese children.

1. Introduction

Obesity is an increasing health concern worldwide. It is strongly linked to morbidity and mortality through its associated health risks. Childhood obesity has dramatically increased to reach an epidemic proportion particularly in the Gulf area [1]. Sedentary life style led to emergence of obesity and the metabolic syndrome at a much younger age compared to the past which has been particularly pronounced in the Gulf area [2]. In a study by Freedman et al., 70% of obese or overweight children have at least one clinical cardiovascular risk factor; dyslipidemia, high blood pressure, or insulin resistance [3]. With the increasing prevalence of obesity, various forms of comorbidities are seen in children including dyslipidemia [4] and nonalcoholic fatty liver disease (NAFLD) [5]. Liver disease and dyslipidemia are major comorbidities for obesity at a young age [6, 7].

NAFLD is one of the most common causes of chronic liver disease associated with obesity worldwide. In 2016, NAFLD accounted for 20%–30% prevalence in Western countries and 5%–18% in Asia. The overall incidence of NAFLD in children has reached approximately 10% of which, 17% are teenagers and 40%–70% among obese children [8]. Childhood NAFLD may occur in young children. In those, the disease is usually asymptomatic with the diagnosis frequently made upon abdominal imaging [9].

Various surrogate markers have been used for dyslipidemia and fatty liver disease. Alanine aminotransferase (ALT) enzyme is known to reflect NAFLD and is used as the basis of performing liver biopsy when NAFLD is suspected [10].

Abnormalities in lipid metabolism in youth have shown an increased incidence around the world and are strongly associated with cardiovascular disease. High level of cholesterol has been reported among children and adolescents in the United States [11]. Similarly, 32% of children aged 11.4 ± 0.97 years old studied were found to have dyslipidemia in Chile [12].

Body mass index (BMI) and waist circumference (WC) are the most commonly used anthropometric measures to predict metabolic disorders related to childhood obesity [13]. As body fat distribution plays an important role in obesity-related comorbidities, WC is a commonly used parameter. In European boys and girls, Savva et al. established that WC has a better prediction for BP, HDL, and LDL than BMI [14].

While international data on dyslipidemia and nonalcoholic fatty liver disease (NAFLD) in obese children are abundant, there is paucity of studies in this field in the Arab countries and the Middle Eastern region where childhood obesity is common.

The aim of the study is to assess the prevalence of dyslipidemia and fatty liver disease in overweight and obese children. We also aim to analyze the association between various anthropometric measures and dyslipidemia and NAFLD.

2. Methods

This is a descriptive, observational, cross-sectional study conducted on children and adolescents referred for obesity management. The study is undertaken at the Paediatric Endocrinology Clinic, Mafraq Hospital, Abu Dhabi, United Arab Emirates. Overweight and obese children and adolescents referred for obesity are invited to participate in the study. Fulfilling the following criteria was ensured prior to enrolment of participants.

2.1. Inclusion and Exclusion Criteria. Patients referred to the Paediatric Endocrinology Clinic for obesity, having BMI above the 85th percentile and agreed to participate in the study were considered eligible. Children already diagnosed with diabetes or other hormonal disorders or those who are on long-term use of corticosteroids or antiepilepsy medication are considered unsuitable for the study.

2.2. Study Procedure. Patients who fulfilled the above criteria were invited to enroll in the study. Those who agreed to participate signed an assent form, and parents/guardians signed a consent form. The study was explained to participants, and they were given a study information sheet. The study is approved by the Mafraq Hospital Research and Ethics Committee.

Demographic variables including gender, age, height, weight, BMI, and waist circumference were taken. BMI was calculated as weight in kg/height^2 in meters. SDS for weight, height, and BMI were calculated. BMI percentile above the 85th and 95th were used to define overweight and obese, respectively [15]. Waist circumference was taken at the midway point between the anterior superior iliac spine and the lower rib cage and is measured by 2 study members (AD and SA). Standardized scores for waist circumference were generated based on Jackson et al. for WC percentile in Kuwaiti children and adolescents [16]. Blood pressure was taken using appropriate cuff size for age and recorded as percentile for age and sex. Detailed family history of obesity, dyslipidemia, heart disease, and diabetes in first-degree relative was taken.

Fasting blood sample was obtained from participants for lipid profile (total cholesterol, LDL, HDL, and triglyceride) and liver transaminases: alanine aminotransferase (ALT) and aspartate aminotransferase (AST). Dyslipidemia was diagnosed if any of the lipid profile parameters are found to be abnormal as follows: total cholesterol (TC) ≥ 5.2 mmol, triglyceride (TG) > 1.5 mmol, low density lipoprotein (LDL) > 2.84 mmol, or high density lipoprotein (HDL) < 0.9 mmol. Those who had elevated liver enzyme had a liver ultrasound scan (US).

2.3. Laboratory Methods. Serum ALT and AST measurement was performed on the Roche/Hitachi Cobas c702 analyzer (Roche Diagnostics GmbH, Sandhofer Strasse 116, D-68305 Mannheim) to an IFCC standardized assay that was optimized for performance and stability without pyridoxal phosphate activation. The assay has an analytical Measuring range of 5–700 IU/L, a lower detection limit (analytical sensitivity) of 5 IU/L, a within run CV (%) of 3.1% at an ALT and AST of 21.5 U/L, and a between run CV (%) of 0.6% at an ALT of 546 U/L.

Total serum total cholesterol (TC) measurement was performed on the Roche/Hitachi Cobas c702 analyzer (Roche Diagnostics GmbH, Sandhofer Strasse 116, D-68305 Mannheim) with an enzymatic, colorimetric assay. The assay has an analytical measurement range of TC 0.1–20.7 mmol/L (3.86800 mg/dL), a lower detection limit of 0.1 mmol/L (3.86 mg/dL), and a within run CV (%) of 0.6% at a TC of 2.72 mmol/L and a between run CV of 0.6% at TC of 17.9 mmol/L.

Serum lipoprotein density-cholesterol measurement was performed with the Plus- 3rd generation lipoprotein-cholesterol assay on the Roche/Hitachi Cobas c702 analyzer (Roche Diagnostics GmbH, Sandhofer Strasse 116, D-68305 Mannheim). The assay was a direct homogeneous enzymatic colorimetric enzymatic assay.

Serum Triglycerides were measured by an enzymatic colorimetric assay based on the Wahlefeld method using a lipoprotein lipase performed on the Roche/Hitachi Cobas c702 analyzer (Roche Diagnostics GmbH, Sandhofer Strasse 116, D-68305 Mannheim). The assay has an analytical measurement range of 0.1–10.0 mmol/L (8.85–885 mg/dL) and a lower limit of measurement of 0.1 mmol/L, a within run CV of 0.9 (%) at a TRIGL of 1.32 mmol/L, and a between run CV (%) of 0.60% at a TRIGL of 9.21 mmol/L.

2.4. Statistical Methods. Data were examined graphically and numerically. Descriptive statistics were used for quantitative parameters such as mean, standard deviation, minimum, maximum, and median. Frequency and percentages are used for qualitative parameters. Bivariate logistic regressions were used to examine the relationship between variables.

Table 1: Sample characteristics.

	Frequency (%)	Mean (SD)
Demographics		
Gender (male)	121 (56.0)	
Age		10.58 (2.996)
Physical exam		
Height-for-age		1.1950 ± 0.44
Weight-for-age		2.30 ± 0.704
WC-for-age		2.31 ± 1.058
WC ≥ 90th percentile	173 (89.6)	
Overweight	16 (7.0)	
Obese	200 (93.0)	
SBP-for-age		1.10 ± 1.014
DBP-for-age		0.55 ± 0.812
Acanthosis nigricans	138 (63.9)	
Family history		
Obesity	172 (80.0)	
Hyperlipidemia	117 (55.5)	
Heart disease	88 (40.7)	
Diabetes	170 (79.4)	

Statistical difference is considered significant if P value is found to be ≤0.5. Statistical analysis was performed using IBM SPSS software version 22.

3. Results

216 patients were enrolled in the study (121, 56% males). The overall age of the sample ranged between 4 and 19 years. Mean ± SD age was 10.58 ± 2.97 years. Standardized mean ± SD for height was 1.12 ± 0.44, while that for weight was 2.30 ± 0.70. 201 (93.0%) of the children were obese with a BMI ≥ 95th percentile while 15 (7.0%) were overweight.

On physical examination, a total of 138 (63.9%) of patients had acanthosis nigricans. The standardized mean ± SD for waist circumference was 2.31 ± 1.058 cm. 173 patients (89.6%) had a WC ≥ 90th percentile. The standardized mean ± SD for systolic blood pressure was 1.10 ± 1.014 mmHg while that for diastolic blood pressure was 0.55 ± 0.812 mmHg (Table 1).

3.1. Dyslipidemia. Among the total sample, 55.3% of patients had dyslipidemia. 11.7% patients had high cholesterol, 28.6% had high triglyceride, 32.7% had high LDL, and 18.0% had low HDL. Waist circumference was significantly associated with having dyslipidemia. With every unit increase (1 cm), the odds of having dyslipidemia significantly increases by 1.020 (OR = 1.020, 95% CI (1.001, 1.039), $P = 0.041$). Moreover, the odds of having dyslipidemia for patients with a waist circumference above the 90th percentile is significantly 2.760 times the odds of having dyslipidemia for patients below the 90th percentile (OR = 2.760, 95% CI (1.001, 7.615), $P = 0.05$). As for standardized waist circumference (z-scores), every increase of 1 SD, the odds of having dyslipidemia significantly increases by 1.530 (OR = 1.530, 95% CI (1.120, 2.091), $P = 0.008$) (Figure 1)

No significant associations with dyslipidemia were identified with age, gender, puberty stage, weight (absolute values), weight (z-scores), height (absolute value), height (z-scores), systolic, or diastolic blood pressure.

3.2. Elevated Liver Enzymes. Of the total 216 subjects, 210 had liver enzymes checked. 51 patients (24.3%) had either elevated AST or ALT or both (14.6% had high AST and 19.8% had high ALT).

A relationship between elevated liver enzymes with each of the following respective variables was found: age, weight (absolute value), and waist circumference. As age increases by 1 year, the odds of having elevated liver enzymes significantly increased by 1.142 (OR = 1.142, 95% CI (1.021, 1.278), $P = 0.020$). Also, as weight (absolute value) increases by 1 kg, the odds of having elevated liver enzymes significantly increased by 1.013 (OR = 1.042, 95% CI (1.000, 1.025), $P = 0.042$). Lastly, with every unit increase in waist circumference (1 cm), the odds of having elevated liver enzymes increase by 1.021. This finding is determined with a borderline significance (OR = 1.021, 95% CI (1.000, 1.043), P value = 0.052).

Gender, height (absolute value), puberty stage, height (z-scores), weight (z-scores), waist circumference (>90th percentile), waist circumference (z-scores), systolic pressure, and diastolic pressure were not significantly associated with elevated liver enzymes (Figure 2).

3.3. Fatty Liver Disease. 51 patients had high ALT or AST or both. All 51 patients had liver US. Of those, 43 had fatty liver (84%). Liver transaminases were lower in the 8 patients who did not have fatty liver. NAFLD was significantly associated with age, height (absolute value), weight (absolute value), weight (z-scores), waist circumference (absolute values), and waist circumference (z-scores) (Figure 3). As age increases by 1 year, the odds of having fatty liver significantly increase by 1.253 (OR = 1.253, 95% CI (1.072, 1.464), $P = 0.005$). As height (absolute value) increases by 1 cm, the odds of having fatty liver significantly increase by 1.032 (OR = 1.032, 95% CI (1.003, 1.062), $P = 0.030$). Moreover, as weight (absolute value) increases by 1 kg, the odds of having fatty liver significantly increase by 1.029 (OR = 1.029, 95% CI (1.013, 1.045), $P < 0.001$). Similarly, weight (z-scores) is also significantly associated with fatty liver (OR = 1.892, 95% CI (1.018, 3.518), P value = 0.044). As for waist circumference, both absolute value and z-scores are significantly associated with having fatty liver (OR = 1.044, 95% CI (1.015, 1.073), $P = 0.003$; OR = 1.534, 95% CI (1.023, 2.301), $P = 0.038$). Puberty staging showed a significant association with having a fatty liver with an OR of 3.35 ($P = 0.002$) (Figure 3). The following variables were not significantly associated with having NAFLD: gender, height (z-scores), and systolic and diastolic blood pressure.

4. Discussion

Multiple studies have shown that obesity is one of the most important risk factors of metabolic disorders in children [15]. It was shown that 70% of obese or overweight children have at least one clinical cardiovascular risk factor, 52% of them have at least two risk factors, and 12% have three or more risk factors [3].

Researchers reported that 45.8% of the overweight children showed abnormal lipid profile. 10% of the children

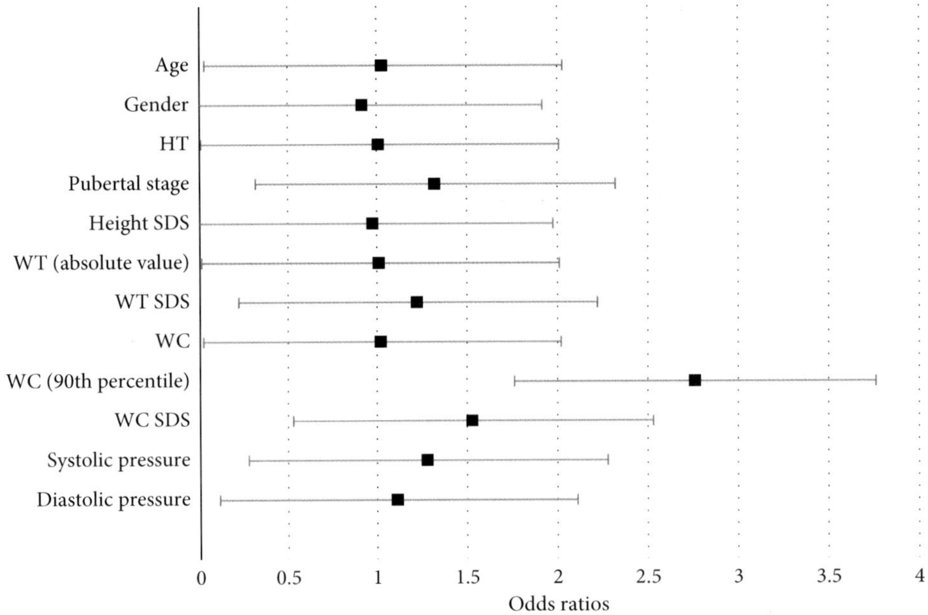

FIGURE 1: Bivariate logistic regressions between predictor variables and dyslipidemia.

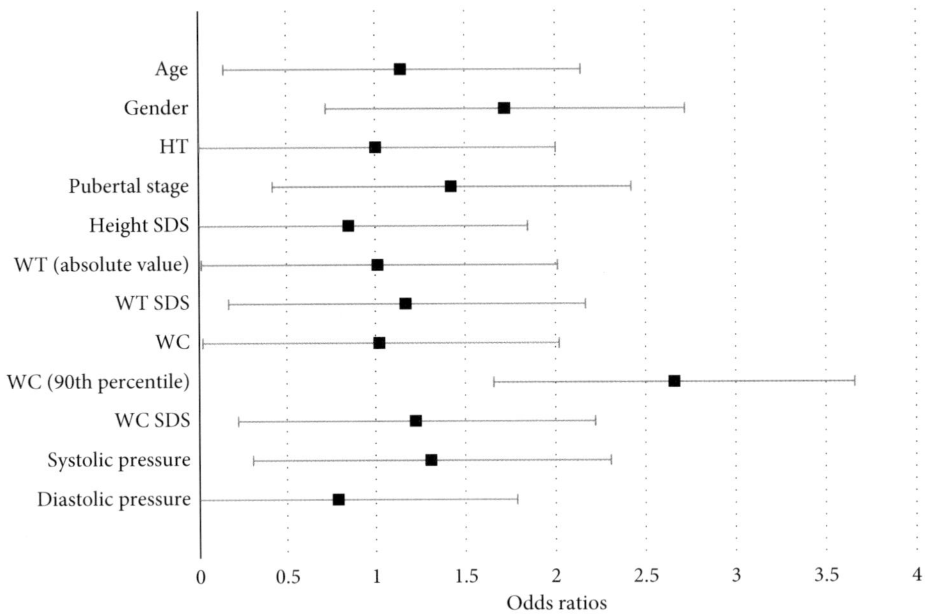

FIGURE 2: Bivariate logistic regressions between predictor variables and having elevated liver enzymes.

had high LDL levels, while 15% had increased LDL and TG with a higher prevalence in boys [17]. The results from our study revealed that, 32.7% of patients had high LDL, 18.0% had low HDL, and 28.6% of patients had high TG. Non-HDL cholesterol is a better indicator for persistent dyslipidemia and atherosclerosis in children and adults [18]. However, we were not able to run this analyte in our local lab.

In obese children, BMI has better practical utility in identifying dyslipidemia among school-aged children with obesity compared with other anthropometric measures [19]. While BMI is a useful marker for overall obesity, WC, waist-to-height ratio, and waist-to-hip ratio are more useful indices for defining abdominal obesity with WC showing the strongest relationship [20]. The International Diabetes Federation defined WC as one of the risk criteria for metabolic disorders in children [21]. In Guangzhou, China, BMI correctly identified 77% of the total dyslipidemic disorders in obese children, which was higher than that by waist hip ratio (WHR) (70.8%) ($P < 0.05$) [19]. In our study, results showed that dyslipidemia is significantly related to WC. This was in agreement with a study by Janssen et al. who reported that youths with high WC had high TG [22] and with another group of researchers who showed that the absolute WC had the strongest correlation with low HDL [13].

The probability of NAFLD increases with high WC. Studies showed that NAFLD is associated with larger WC [23]. Unlike

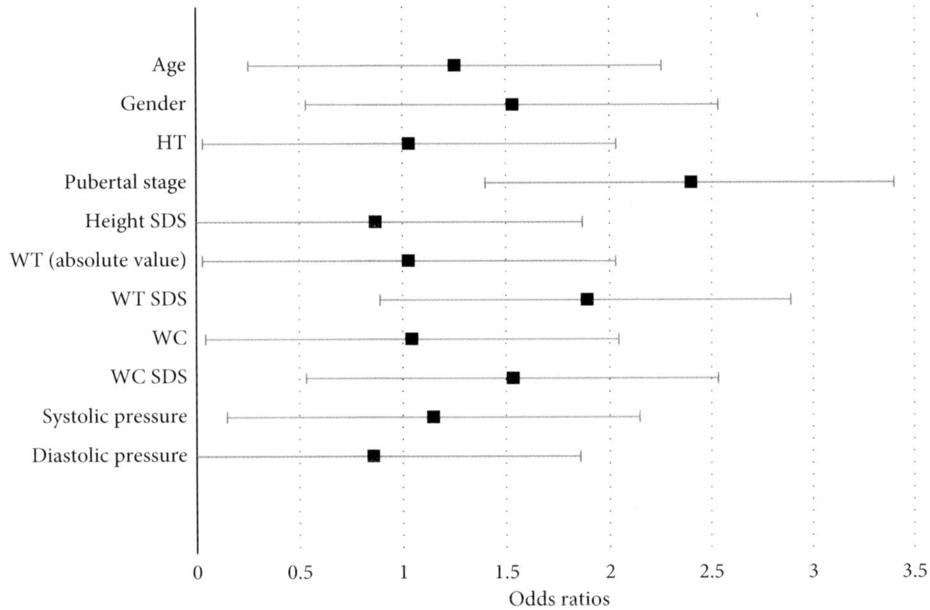

FIGURE 3: Bivariate logistic regressions between predictor variables and having fatty liver disease.

gender, pubertal status, and blood pressure, age and weight were directly proportional with dyslipidemia and NAFLD.

Elevated liver enzyme (ALT) has been considered as an indicator for NAFLD in obese children and its elevation is considered as an indication for biopsy [10]. However, in recent practice guidelines, it was highlighted that significant histological abnormalities of NAFLD, including advanced fibrosis can be seen in children with normal or mildly elevated ALT levels. Accordingly, use of ALT alone may underestimate the extent of liver injury [24].

It is stated that liver US is a predictor of NAFLD [25]. In our sample, 84% of those who had elevated liver enzymes had features of NAFLD on liver US. Patients who had normal liver US had less elevation of liver enzymes compared to those who were shown to have NAFLD on scans. While liver enzymes are used to predict presence of NAFLD, their level was not shown to correlate with the histological grade of steatosis [9].

Findings from our study have also revealed various associations of demographic and antropometric measures. Dyslipidemia is shown to be significantly associated with WC. Elevated liver enzymes appear to be seen with increased age and waist circumference. We have seen an increased liver enzyme correlating with absolute weight but not weight SDS which might reflect an association with body mass rather than age-adjusted weight.

NAFLD is more prevalent in subjects with a higher WC and is directly proportional to age, weight, and height. We did not find any gender difference in relation to the frequency of the comorbidity. Puberty status did not appear to have an impact on predisposition to comorbidities either.

History of patient's family serves as an important predictor for the various comorbidities. Parental obesity could be considered as a key factor in the development of obesity due to genetic factors and family food choices [26]. In our sample, 80% of children had family history of obesity, 79% diabetes, and 55.5% had history of hyperlipidemia. This indicates the importance of genetics and geographical variations when studying the epidemiology of obesity and their comorbidities.

Study limitation is that it represents a single center in the UAE. Involving multiple centers throughout the country will give a more comprehensive data on these obesity comorbidities.

5. Conclusion

Dyslipidemia is seen frequently in overweight and obese children and is significantly related to WC. Similarly, there is a strong association between WC and NAFLD. This study provides an insight on the higher frequency of dyslipidemia and NAFLD in children and adolescent in our region where obesity is prevalent. The findings that emerged can be utilized to help further understanding of epidemiological gap related to obesity in children in the region. WC is an easy tool that can be utilized to screen for dyslipidemia in overweight and obese children and adolescents in community setting. Efforts need to be intensified towards addressing prevention strategies and raising awareness on obesity complications among youths.

Acknowledgments

The authors acknowledge the support provided by AstraZeneca to undertake the study.

References

[1] M. Malik and A. Bakir, "Prevalence of overweight and obesity among children in the United Arab Emirates," *Obesity Reviews*, vol. 8, no. 1, pp. 15–20, 2006.

[2] D. Robinson, "Killing me sweetly," *Arabian Business-Health*, vol. 6, pp. 48–53, 2005.

[3] D. S. Freedman, Z. Mei, S. R. Srinivasan, G. S. Berenson, and W. H. Dietz, "Cardiovascular risk factors and excess adiposity among overweight children and adolescents: the Bogalusa Heart Study," *Journal of Pediatrics*, vol. 150, no. 1, pp. 12–17, 2007.

[4] S. Cook and R. E. Kavey, "Dyslipidemia and pediatric obesity," *Pediatric Clinics of North America*, vol. 58, no. 6, pp. 1363–1373, 2011.

[5] N. M. El-Koofy, G. M. Anwar, M. S. El-Raziky et al., "The association of metabolic syndrome, insulin resistance and non-alcoholic fatty liver disease in overweight/obese children," *Saudi Journal of Gastroenterology*, vol. 18, no. 1, pp. 44–49, 2012.

[6] S. Blüher, C. Meigen, R. Gausche et al., "Age-specific stabilization in obesity prevalence in German children: a cross-sectional study from 1999 to 2008," *International Journal of Pediatric Obesity*, vol. 6, no. 2, pp. 199–206, 2011.

[7] A. M. G. Cali and S. Caprio, "Obesity in children and adolescents," *Journal of Clinical Endocrinology and Metabolism*, vol. 93, no. 11, pp. s31–s33, 2008.

[8] A. M. Clemente, C. Mandato, M. Poeta, and P. Vajro, "Pediatric non-alcoholic fatty liver disease: recent solutions, unresolved issues, and future research directions," *World Journal of Gastroenterology*, vol. 22, no. 36, pp. 8078–8093, 2016.

[9] A. Shannon, N. Alkhouri, C. Carter-Kent et al., "Ultrasonographic quantitative estimation of hepatic steatosis in children with NAFLD," *Journal of Pediatric Gastroenterology and Nutrition*, vol. 53, no. 2, pp. 190–195, 2011.

[10] J. B. Schwimmer, C. Behling, R. Newbury et al., "Histopathology of pediatric nonalcoholic fatty liver disease," *Hepatology*, vol. 42, no. 3, pp. 641–649, 2005.

[11] D. Nquyen, B. Kit, and M. Carroll, "Abnormal cholesterol among children and adolescents in the United States, 2011-2014," *NCHS Data Brief*, vol. 228, pp. 1–8, 2015.

[12] S. Barja Yanez, P. Arnaiz Gómez, L. Villarroel Del Pino et al., "Dyslipidemia in school age Chilean children: prevalence and associated factors," *Nutrición Hospitalaria*, vol. 31, no. 5, pp. 2079–2087, 2015.

[13] S. Blüher, E. Molz, S. Wiegand et al., "Body mass index, waist circumference, and waist-to-height ratio as predictors of cardiometabolic risk in childhood obesity depending on pubertal development," *Journal of Clinical Endocrinology and Metabolism*, vol. 98, no. 8, pp. 3384–3393, 2013.

[14] S. C. Savva, M. Tornaritis, M. E. Savva et al., "Waist circumference and waist-to-height ratio are better predictors of cardiovascular disease risk factors in children than body mass index," *International Journal of Obesity*, vol. 24, no. 11, pp. 1453–1458, 2000.

[15] Centers for Disease Control and Prevention (CDC), *National Center for Health Statistics (NCHS). National Health and Nutrition Examination Survey Data*, U.S. Department of Health and Human Services, Hyattsville, MD, USA, http://www.cdc.gov/growthcharts/.

[16] R. T. Jackson, N. Al Hamad, P. Prakash, and M. Al Somaie, "Waist circumference percentiles for Kuwaiti children and adolescents," *Public Health Nutrition*, vol. 14, no. 1, pp. 70–76, 2011.

[17] U. Korsten-Reck, K. Kromeyer-Hauschild, K. Korsten, M. W. Baumstark, H. H. Dickhuth, and A. Berg, "Frequency of secondary dyslipidemia in obese children," *Vascular Health and Risk Management*, vol. 4, no. 5, pp. 1089–1094, 2008.

[18] Expert Panel on Integrated Guidelines for Cardiovascular Health and Risk Reduction in Children and Adolescents, "Expert panel on integrated guidelines for cardiovascular health and risk reduction in children and adolescents: summary report," *Pediatrics*, vol. 128, no. 5, pp. S213–S256, 2011.

[19] Y. Zhu, Z. Shao, J. Jing et al., "Body mass index is better than other anthropometric indices for identifying dyslipidemia in Chinese children with obesity," *PLoS One*, vol. 11, no. 3, Article ID e0149392, 2016.

[20] T. V. Barreira, S. T. Broyles, A. K. Gupta, and P. T. Katzmarzyk, "Relationship of anthropometric indices to abdominal and total body fat in youth: sex and race differences," *Obesity*, vol. 22, no. 5, pp. 1345–1350, 2014.

[21] P. Zimmet, G. Alberti, F. Kaufman et al., "The metabolic syndrome in children and adolescents," *The Lancet*, vol. 369, no. 9579, pp. 2059–2061, 2007.

[22] I. Janssen, P. T. Katzmarzyk, S. R. Srinivasan et al., "Combined influence of body mass index and waist circumference on coronary artery disease risk factors among children and adolescents," *Pediatrics*, vol. 115, no. 6, pp. 1623–1630, 2005.

[23] T. Trasher and M. Abelmalek, "Non-alcoholic fatty liver disease Non-alcoholic fatty liver disease," *North Carolina Medical Journal*, vol. 50, pp. 1–5, 2016.

[24] N. Chalasani, Z. Younossi, J. E. Lavine et al., "The diagnosis and management of nonalcoholic fatty liver disease: practice guidance from the American Association for the Study of Liver Diseases," *Hepatology*, vol. 67, no. 1, pp. 328–357, 2018.

[25] P. Vajro, S. Lenta, P. Socha, A. Dhawan, P. McKiernan, and U. Baumann, "Diagnosis of nonalcoholic fatty liver disease in children and adolescents: position paper of the ESPGHAN Hepatology Committee," *Journal of Pediatric Gastroenterology and Nutrition*, vol. 54, no. 5, pp. 700–713, 2012.

[26] J. J. Reilly, J. Armstrong, A. R. Dorosty et al., "Early life risk factors for obesity in childhood: cohort study," *BMJ*, vol. 330, no. 7504, p. 1357, 2005.

20

Trial Characteristics and Appropriateness of Statistical Methods Applied for Design and Analysis of Randomized School-Based Studies Addressing Weight-Related Issues

Moonseong Heo,[1] Singh R. Nair,[2] Judith Wylie-Rosett,[1] Myles S. Faith,[3] Angelo Pietrobelli,[4,5] Nancy R. Glassman,[6] Sarah N. Martin,[1] Stephanie Dickinson,[7] and David B. Allison[7]

[1]*Department of Epidemiology and Population Health, Albert Einstein College of Medicine, Bronx, NY, USA*
[2]*Department of Anesthesiology, Montefiore Medical Center, Bronx, NY, USA*
[3]*Department of Counseling, School, and Educational Psychology, Graduate School of Education, University at Buffalo-SUNY, Buffalo, NY, USA*
[4]*Department of Pediatrics, University of Verona, Verona, Italy*
[5]*Pennington Biomedical Research Center, Baton Rouge, LA, USA*
[6]*D. Samuel Gottesman Library, Albert Einstein College of Medicine, Bronx, NY, USA*
[7]*Department of Epidemiology and Biostatistics, School of Public Health, Indiana University-Bloomington, Bloomington, IN, USA*

Correspondence should be addressed to Moonseong Heo; moonseong.heo@einstein.yu.edu

Academic Editor: Chris I. Ardern

Objective. To evaluate whether clustering effects, often quantified by the intracluster correlation coefficient (ICC), were appropriately accounted for in design and analysis of school-based trials. *Methods.* We searched PubMed and extracted variables concerning study characteristics, power analysis, ICC use for power analysis, applied statistical models, and the report of the ICC estimated from the observed data. *Results.* $N = 263$ papers were identified, and $N = 121$ papers were included for evaluation. Overall, only a minority (21.5%) of studies incorporated ICC values for power analysis, fewer studies (8.3%) reported the estimated ICC, and 68.6% of studies applied appropriate multilevel models. A greater proportion of studies applied the appropriate models during the past five years (2013–2017) compared to the prior years (74.1% versus 63.5%, $p = 0.176$). Significantly associated with application of appropriate models were a larger number of schools ($p = 0.030$), a larger sample size ($p = 0.002$), longer follow-up ($p = 0.014$), and randomization at a cluster level ($p < 0.001$) and so were studies that incorporated the ICC into power analysis ($p = 0.016$) and reported the estimated ICC ($p = 0.030$). *Conclusion.* Although application of appropriate models has increased over the years, consideration of clustering effects in power analysis has been inadequate, as has report of estimated ICC. To increase rigor, future school-based trials should address these issues at both the design and analysis stages.

1. Introduction

Pediatric and adolescent obesity is a global concern as the range of its health consequence includes cardiovascular diseases, diabetes, poor quality of life, disability, mental health problems, and even adulthood mortality [1–5]. Despite this concern, the prevalence of pediatric and adolescent obesity has not decreased in the United States (US) or globally over the past several decades [6, 7]. In addition, financial and care burdens for preventing and treating pediatric obesity are substantial at both the individual or family level and societal or governmental level [8]. As such, countless trials have been conducted over the world to address pediatric and adolescent obesity and prevention, treatment, or diet guidelines based on evidence collected from the findings of those trials have been published [9, 10].

Many opine that schools represent "key settings" or "ideal settings" for obesity prevention or intervention, and numerous school-based studies have been conducted worldwide [11, 12]. The scope of interventions in school-based trials is broad ranging from education to health behaviors focusing on nutrition and physical activities [13–15]. However, the appropriate evaluation of intervention effectiveness critically hinges on proper trial design and statistical analysis of school-based trial data. Importantly, the data from school-based trials naturally form multiple levels of hierarchy. For example, when students are to be followed up multiple times for outcome measurements during the course of a study, repeatedly measured outcomes are nested within students who are in turn nested within schools. This hierarchical nature forms a three-level data structure so that clustering effects, also known as design effects, of outcome data at the school and student levels should be taken into account not only at the design stage but also at the analysis stage.

The critical issue is that required sample sizes are likely to be underestimated if such clustering effects are not taken into account [16–20]. This is especially so when the interventions are assigned at the highest level of data hierarchy. Likewise, the standard errors of estimated intervention effects at the analytic stage are smaller than what it should be and so are p values, likely increasing the type I error rate [21]. Anecdotally, errors in neglecting such clustering seem not uncommon [22].

The primary aim of this review is to evaluate statistical methods applied to published school-based randomized trials addressing weight issues. The evaluation is focused on assessing appropriateness of power analysis and applied statistical methods as to whether clustering effects often represented by correlations of subject outcomes within schools, which is also known as the intracluster (or intraclass) correlation coefficient (ICC) [23], are properly accounted for in the design and analysis of school-based trials. Specifically, we aim to examine (1) whether study characteristics are different between the past five years (2013–2017) and the prior years (1995–2012), that is, between pre- and postera of the updated, extended CONSORT statement for cluster randomized trials published in the year 2012 [24] and (2) whether appropriateness of statistical methods is associated with study characteristics.

2. Methods

2.1. Search Strategy. We searched PubMed for papers meeting the following inclusion criteria:

(i) Published in journals indexed in PubMed
(ii) From the PubMed inception year
(iii) Randomized school-based trials
(iv) Written in English
(v) Outcomes involving weight-related issues
(vi) Subjects of age younger than 25 years that include young adults.

To this end, we applied a Boolean algebraic combination of MeSH (*Me*dical *S*ubject *H*eadings) as follows: ("Body Weight"[MeSH] OR "Body Mass Index"[MeSH]) AND "Schools"[MeSH] AND (Randomized Controlled Trial[ptyp] AND English[lang] AND ("adolescent"[MeSH Terms] OR "child"[MeSH Terms:noexp] OR "child, preschool"[MeSH Terms] OR "young adult"[MeSH Terms])). With this search strategy, we identified a total of 263 papers as of December 8, 2017, and the earliest publication year was 1995.

2.2. Exclusion Criteria. We retrieved full texts of all of those papers, and two authors (MH and SN) applied the following exclusion criteria for the review:

(i) Protocol paper.
(ii) Not a randomized study.
(iii) Not a school-based intervention.
(iv) Analysis of subjects of age beyond the range.
(v) Outcome is not related to weight issues.
(vi) Baseline or subgroup analysis of a parent study.
(vii) Single-school trials.

When the two raters' ratings were not concordant due to unclear descriptions in the text regarding study design parameters or analytic methods, the rating was resolved by consensus between them.

2.3. Extracted Variables and Classifications. We extracted the following study characteristic variables from the included studies: the publication year (past 5 years (2013–2017) versus the prior years (1995–2012)); number of schools; analytic sample sizes of individuals, which are the size of the completers at the final follow-up when available; randomization level (cluster versus individual); length of follow-up in months (<12 versus ≥ 12 months); number of repeated measurements including baseline (2 versus >2); location of the trial (the US versus others); and types of schools (preschool, elementary/primary, middle, and high school, and college).

As per the randomization level, the "cluster" classification category includes any higher level units in which all subjects received the identical interventions or treatments. Therefore, the cluster unit could be schools, classes, health centers, communities, camps, and so on. Nevertheless, we extracted the number of involved schools, instead of the number of the various randomized cluster units, for the number of schools variable. If randomization occurred at the individual/student level within schools or other cluster units, we classified the randomization level for such trials as "individual." When multiple types of schools are involved in a trial, we classified such cases into the school type of the lowest level. For instance, if a trial involved preschool and primary schools, then this case was classified as "preschool" for the school type.

With respect to the presence of power analysis and appropriateness of applied statistical methods, we extracted the report of power analysis (yes versus no); consideration of the intracluster correlation coefficient (ICC) for power analysis (yes versus no); primary statistical analysis models (multilevel versus no); and the report of the ICC estimated from statistical analysis (yes versus no). If the description of power analysis or sample size determination referred to a protocol paper and was not provided in the text to an evaluable extent, we classified such cases as no report of power analysis. As the terminologies of statistical models are not standardized across the papers, we classified the following models as "multilevel" models in which a "clustering" effect at some level of the data hierarchy had presumably been taken into account in the analysis: generalized mixed-effects model, mixed-effects model, linear mixed-effects model, multilevel mixed-effects model, hierarchical models, random-intercept models, mixed models, logistic mixed-effects models, generalized estimating equation models, and the likes. We consider the application of those multilevel analyses appropriate. Other models that do not take the clustering effects into account were classified as "no" multilevel model: for example, paired t-test, chi-square test, analysis of variance (ANOVA), analysis of covariance (ANCOVA), linear or logistic regression models, and repeated-measures AN(C)OVA at the individual level.

2.4. Statistical Analysis. Descriptive statistics are provided in terms of frequency, percentages, median, and the first (Q1) and the third (Q3) quartiles. There were three missing values for the number of schools, and studies with those missing values were excluded from analyses involving the number of schools. The follow-up length and number of measurements are analyzed as both continuous and dichotomized variables. Comparisons of study characteristics, the presence of power analysis, and appropriateness of statistical methods between the publication years 2013–2017 versus 1995–2012 are made using Wilcoxon rank-sum tests or Fisher exact tests. The same sets of these tests are also applied to testing associations of study characteristics and the presence of power analysis with application of appropriate multilevel analysis. Statistical significance is declared at $p < 0.05$ (two-tailed). SAS v9.4 was used for all analyses.

3. Results

3.1. Reasons for Exclusion. The application of the exclusion criteria resulted in 121 papers (Supplementary Materials (available here)) with 1995 as the earliest publication year after exclusion of 142 papers. The reasons for exclusions are displayed in Table 1. Although it is possible that a study was excluded for multiple reasons, the most common reason was due to single-school trials (34.5%) followed by protocol papers (25.4%).

Table 1: Reasons for exclusion.

Reasons	N	%
Single-school trial	49	34.5
Protocol paper	36	25.4
Baseline or subgroup analysis of a parent study	27	19.0
Not a randomized trial	18	12.7
Students of age beyond the age range	7	4.9
Not a school-based trial	5	3.5
Total	142	

Note. Although it is possible that studies could be excluded for multiple reasons, we classified the reasons in a mutually exclusive manner.

3.2. Study Characteristics between the Past Five Years and the Prior Years. Detailed results are presented in Table 2. There were 63 (52%) and 58 (48%) studies included for analysis between the years 2013–2017 versus 1995–2012, respectively. None of the listed study characteristics, except the school type, significantly differ between those time frames. We note that the initial extended CONSORT guideline statement for cluster randomized trials was published in the year 2004 [25], but we did not further categorize years into three time frames including those before 2005 due to a relatively small number of included studies during that time period ($N = 19$ or 7.3%). Overall, the vast majority of studies randomized interventions at a cluster level (89.3%), and the analytic sample size is relatively large with a median of 620 students. The majority (58.9%) of studies had only two measurements: one at baseline or before intervention and the other at the end of the trial/follow-up or after intervention. Most (57.0%) of the studies were conducted outside the US, and more so for the past five years compared to the prior years (63.8% versus 50.8%, $p = 0.198$). The number of countries outside the US was 30 from all continents; one study involved six European countries. The primary/elementary schools most often served as experimental settings (68.6%); however, those schools were significantly less utilized during the past 5 years compared to the prior years (56.9% versus 79.4%, $p = 0.010$). Perhaps for this reason, the distributions of overall types of schools are significantly different between years ($p = 0.038$).

3.3. Power Analysis, ICC, and Multilevel Models between the Past Five Years and the Prior Years. Results from the comparisons of power analysis and application of multilevel models between years are presented in Table 3. A minority (43.0%) of the studies reported power analysis adequately in the text, and the proportion was not significantly different between the past five years and the prior years (48.3% versus 38.1%, $p = 0.258$). However, most studies applied multilevel analytic methods (68.6%), and the proportion was greater for the past five years (74.1% versus 63.5%, $p = 0.176$). About one-fifth of studies (21.5%) took the ICC into consideration for power analysis, and the past five years did not see a significant increase in this proportion. A smaller number of studies (8.3%) reported ICCs estimated from the statistical analysis of trial data, and the proportions decreased, though not significantly, during the past five years.

3.4. Association between Multilevel Analysis and Study Characteristics. As presented in Table 4, a majority of study characteristics are associated with the application of appropriate multilevel statistical models. Specifically, a larger number of schools ($p = 0.030$), a larger size of the analytic sample ($p = 0.002$), longer follow-up ($p = 0.014$), and randomization at a cluster level ($p < 0.001$) were all significantly associated with the application of appropriate models. The location of trials was not significantly associated with the appropriateness ($p = 1.000$). The studies with appropriate multilevel models were more likely to have incorporated the ICC into power analysis ($p = 0.016$) and reported the ICC

Table 2: Study characteristics by study years: median (Q1, Q3), N (%).

Study characteristics	All years (N = 121)	1995–2012 (N = 63)	2013–2017 (N = 58)	p value
Number of schools*	13 (7, 28)	14 (8, 31)	12 (6, 20)	0.434
Analytic sample size	620 (340, 1182)	670 (407, 1295)	610 (310, 1083)	0.269
Follow-up length in months	12 (6, 24)	12 (6, 24)	12 (5, 20)	0.078
Number of repeated measurements	2 (2, 3)	2 (2, 3)	2 (2, 3)	0.098
Randomization at a cluster level	108 (89.3%)	57 (90.5%)	51 (87.9%)	0.772
Follow-up ≥1 year	68 (56.2%)	38 (60.3%)	30 (51.7%)	0.365
Two measurements including baseline	70 (57.9%)	32 (50.8%)	38 (65.5%)	0.140
Trials conducted outside the US	69 (57.0%)	32 (50.8%)	37 (63.8%)	0.198
School type				0.038
Preschool	11 (9.1%)	3 (4.8%)	8 (13.8%)	
Primary/elementary school	83 (68.6%)	50 (79.4%)	33 (56.9%)	
Middle school	20 (16.5%)	7 (11.1%)	13 (22.4%)	
High school	5 (4.1%)	3 (4.8%)	2 (3.5%)	
College	2 (1.7%)	0 (0.0%)	2 (3.5%)	

*N = 3 is missing.

Table 3: Power analysis and statistical methods by study years: N (%).

Power analysis statistical methods	All years (N = 121)	1995–2012 (N = 63)	2013–2017 (N = 58)	p value
Power analysis conducted and reported	52 (43.0%)	24 (38.1%)	28 (48.3%)	0.258
ICC taken into account for power analysis	26 (21.5%)	13 (20.6%)	13 (22.4%)	0.828
Multilevel analysis performed	83 (68.6%)	40 (63.5%)	43 (74.1%)	0.176
ICC estimated from the analysis reported	10 (8.3%)	7 (11.1%)	3 (5.2%)	0.327

Table 4: Association between multilevel analysis and study characteristics and power analysis: median (Q1, Q3), N (%).

Study characteristics	Multilevel analysis		p value
	Yes (N = 83)	No (N = 38)	
Number of schools*	16 (8, 32)	10 (6, 18)	0.030
Analytic sample size	816 (432, 1323)	472 (181, 869)	0.002
Follow-up length in months	12 (6, 24)	7 (4, 18)	0.014
Number of measurements	2 (2, 3)	2 (2, 3)	0.558
Randomization at a cluster level	82 (98.8%)	26 (68.4%)	<0.001
Follow-up ≥1 year	52 (62.7%)	16 (42.1%)	0.048
Two measurements including baseline	47 (56.6%)	23 (60.5%)	0.843
Trials conducted outside the US	47 (56.6%)	22 (57.9%)	1.000
Power analysis and ICC			
Power analysis conducted and reported	39 (47.0%)	13 (34.2%)	0.236
ICC taken into account for power analysis	23 (27.7%)	3 (7.9%)	0.016
ICC estimated from the analysis reported	10 (12.1%)	0 (0.0%)	0.030

*N = 3 is missing.

from the analysis of trial data ($p = 0.030$). As should be the case, no studies with non-multilevel models reported ICC estimates. However, even among studies with multilevel models, only a minority (12.1%) reported ICC estimates.

4. Discussion

The primary finding of this review is that the proportion of studies which failed to apply multilevel models to analyzing school-based data appears to be relatively high at 31.4%. In addition, even if multilevel models were applied, specification of levels of clustering effects was rarely described (data not shown). For instance, clustering effects of only the highest-level units of data hierarchy seem to have been taken into account, ignoring additional potential clustering effects of lower-levels units. Taken together, significance of findings based on p values from those studies might have possibly been falsely declared especially when the p values are close to 0.05. Furthermore, less than half of all studies reported power analysis, and approximately one-fifth of all studies, or equivalently about half of the studies that reported power analysis, took the ICC into consideration for power analysis. Therefore, it is likely that a majority of studies might have been underpowered implying that even if the study findings are significant, one cannot rule out the possibility of type I error.

The magnitudes of ICC for power analysis were mostly low, and rationales for such a hypothesized ICC are seldom clearly described. The dearth of rationale might have been due to the lack of information regarding ICC estimates, published or not, pertinent to their studies. This is reflected on the very low proportion of studies (8.3%) that reported ICCs estimated from their data analysis. To this end, the reporting of the ICC estimated from data analysis would be critical for designing future studies with adequate sample sizes. Even if the ICC appears to be very small, it needs to be accounted for power analysis. For example, when the number of students is as small as 30 for each school, the number of required schools with ICC = 0.01 increases by 29% for the same power, compared to when ICC = 0, regardless of hypothesized effect sizes. Therefore, the impact of a small ICC on the sample size could be substantial.

Detailed design characteristics are often referred to protocol papers published earlier, and adequacy of power analysis was not evaluable in the text of outcome papers. Classification of such outcome papers as no report of power analysis might have underestimated the proportion of studies with power analysis because the protocol papers might have properly reported power analysis. However, we surmise that it is fairly rare for a school-based study to be conducted exactly as planned or designed in the protocol papers as school environments are dynamic and changes may alter aspects of the design or analysis plans including sample size determinations/power analysis, statistical methods, and outcome parameters. If outcomes papers do not clearly delineate these aspects, it may be unclear to know whether the power analysis in the earlier protocol paper would be appropriate for the applied statistical methods for the analysis of trial outcomes. We believe that this issue would be a research topic worthy to investigate. After all, the following key design elements should be reported in the outcome analysis papers: target power, significance level, hypothesized effect sizes and ICCs and their rationales, the number of clusters, the number of levels, anticipated attrition rates, and the planned sample size of the subjects. This description can enable readers to effectively and clearly evaluate whether the study has been analyzed as designed, not being forced to compare with detailed elements described in the protocol papers.

Many trials are excluded from evaluation due to the utilization of single schools. These studies are mostly college-based trials likely because multicollege trials may be difficult to conduct compared to the other types of schools. Nonetheless, it is not possible to take the clustering effect into account not only for power analysis but also for statistical analysis, nor is it possible to estimate ICCs from data analysis from single-school/cluster studies. Although it could bring up an issue as to what extent clustering effects should be considered in general, this limitation should be addressed in regard to limited generalizability or transportability of the findings from single-school trials. Identical or similar findings from replicate studies in other school settings would validate the findings.

Our findings also have implications for doctoral programs training future obesity researchers, particularly those conducting school-based interventions. The programs include but are not limited to health, clinical, and school psychology subspecialties. Researchers should ensure that the most rigorous and appropriate methodologies, including issues related to clustering addressed in this study, are included as part of the core curriculum. In this way, students learn early in their careers the practice of reporting such information. To this point, the American Psychological Association (APA) recently released two APA Publications and Communications Board Task Force reports addressing standards for reporting study results. Separate reports were made for quantitative studies [26], as well as qualitative, meta-analytic, and mixed-methods research [27].

Although our review is confined to school-based trials, the findings may be applicable to other cluster randomized trials using different settings and different types of interventions and treatments in other research areas [28–31]. Collectively, therefore, it would be ideal for reports of cluster randomized trials in general to adhere to the aforementioned 2012 updated CONSORT guideline [24] for both outcome and protocol papers. This guideline proposes all the design and analysis elements that should be reported in a standardized manner on manuscripts based on cluster randomized trials. If reports are standardized, it will be beneficial for researchers not only to plan or design school-based trials or other cluster randomized trials but also to more efficiently conduct systematic reviews and meta-analyses with greater statistical power and clearer transparencies.

4.1. Limitations. There are limitations that should be counted when interpreting results from this review. First, the search strategy was rather incomprehensive including only PubMed papers, and the keywords for search may be coarse. Therefore, studies that would have been eligible and added to our evaluations might not have been captured, and the scopes of potentially missing studies are unknown. As is the case for review papers in general, subjective ratings may not be completely avoided even if efforts are placed in minimizing misclassification errors. For instance, we did not evaluate whether potential confounding factors were appropriately controlled for in the data analysis. This evaluation might rely more on subjective judgments with substantial knowledge on the research topics under study and also might be difficult to reach a consensus. Lastly, again, the proportion of the studies with the reported power analysis might have been underestimated because studies that referred detailed power analysis to a protocol paper without a minimum level of description in the text were counted as papers with no report of power analysis.

5. Conclusions

In conclusion, the extent of the application of multilevel models to analyzing school-based trials appears to have so far been inadequate. Key elements such as the hypothesized ICC for power analysis or sample size determinations and the reported ICC estimated from data analyses of school-based trials are missing for a majority of studies. Future school-based trials should specifically address these issues at both design and analysis stages, preferably adhering to the extended CONSORT guideline to increase rigor and reproducibility of experimental settings and study findings. Clinical implications drawn based on the outcomes from school-based trials with rigorously well-performed design, conduct, and analysis would be the most useful to advance knowledge for preventing and treating pediatric and adolescent obesity epidemic.

Disclosure

The opinions expressed are those of the authors and not necessarily of the NIH or any other organization.

Funding

This study was in part supported by R01DK097096, P30DK111022, UL1 TR001073, R25DK099080, and R25HL124208.

References

[1] A. Must, P. F. Jacques, G. E. Dallal, C. J. Bajema, and W. H. Dietz, "Long-term morbidity and mortality of overweight adolescents: a follow-up of the Harvard Growth Study of 1922 to 1935," *New England Journal of Medicine*, vol. 327, no. 19, pp. 1350–1355, 1992.

[2] A. Must, J. Spadano, E. H. Coakley, A. E. Field, G. Colditz, and W. H. Dietz, "The disease burden associated with overweight and obesity," *JAMA*, vol. 282, no. 16, pp. 1523–1529, 1999.

[3] A. Must and R. S. Strauss, "Risks and consequences of childhood and adolescent obesity," *International Journal of Obesity*, vol. 23, pp. S2–S11, 1999.

[4] G. Twig, G. Yaniv, H. Levine et al., "Body-mass index in 2.3 million adolescents and cardiovascular death in adulthood," *New England Journal of Medicine*, vol. 374, no. 25, pp. 2430–2440, 2016.

[5] A. W. Harrist, T. M. Swindle, L. Hubbs-Tait, G. L. Topham, L. H. Shriver, and M. C. Page, "The social and emotional lives of overweight, obese, and severely obese children," *Child Development*, vol. 87, no. 5, pp. 1564–1580, 2016.

[6] C. L. Ogden, M. D. Carroll, H. G. Lawman et al., "Trends in obesity prevalence among children and adolescents in the United States, 1988-1994 through 2013-2014," *JAMA*, vol. 315, no. 21, pp. 2292–2299, 2016.

[7] M. Ng, T. Fleming, M. Robinson et al., "Global, regional, and national prevalence of overweight and obesity in children and adults during 1980-2013: a systematic analysis for the Global Burden of Disease Study 2013," *The Lancet*, vol. 384, no. 9945, pp. 766–781, 2014.

[8] D. Yach, D. Stuckler, and K. D. Brownell, "Epidemiologic and economic consequences of the global epidemics of obesity and diabetes," *Nature Medicine*, vol. 12, no. 1, pp. 62–66, 2006.

[9] S. E. Barlow, "Expert committee recommendations regarding the prevention, assessment, and treatment of child and adolescent overweight and obesity: summary report," *Pediatrics*, vol. 120, no. 4, pp. S164–S192, 2007.

[10] U.S. Department of Health and Human Services and U.S. Department of Agriculture, 2015–2020 Dietary Guidelines for Americans, HHS and USDA, Washington, DC, USA, 8th edition, December 2015, http://health.gov/dietaryguidelines/2015/guidelines/.

[11] J. Clarke, B. Fletcher, E. Lancashire, M. Pallan, and P. Adab, "The views of stakeholders on the role of the primary school in preventing childhood obesity: a qualitative systematic review," *Obesity Reviews*, vol. 14, no. 12, pp. 975–988, 2013.

[12] M. Story, M. S. Nanney, and M. B. Schwartz, "Schools and obesity prevention: creating school environments and policies to promote healthy eating and physical activity," *Milbank Quarterly*, vol. 87, no. 1, pp. 71–100, 2009.

[13] T. Baranowski, L. Adams, J. Baranowski et al., "A school-based intervention for diabetes risk reduction," *New England Journal of Medicine*, vol. 363, no. 5, pp. 443–453, 2010.

[14] D. L. Katz, M. O'Connell, V. Y. Njike, M. C. Yeh, and H. Nawaz, "Strategies for the prevention and control of obesity in the school setting: systematic review and meta-analysis," *International Journal of Obesity*, vol. 32, no. 12, pp. 1780–1789, 2008.

[15] T. Brown and C. Summerbell, "Systematic review of school-based interventions that focus on changing dietary intake and physical activity levels to prevent childhood obesity: an update to the obesity guidance produced by the National Institute for Health and Clinical Excellence," *Obesity Reviews*, vol. 10, no. 1, pp. 110–141, 2009.

[16] M. J. Fazzari, M. Y. Kim, and M. Heo, "Sample size determination for three-level randomized clinical trials with randomization at the first or second level," *Journal of Biopharmaceutical Statistics*, vol. 24, no. 3, pp. 579–599, 2014.

[17] A. W. Brown, P. Li, M. M. Bohan Brown et al., "Best (but oft-forgotten) practices: designing, analyzing, and reporting cluster randomized controlled trials," *American Journal of Clinical Nutrition*, vol. 102, no. 2, pp. 241–248, 2015.

[18] B. J. George, T. M. Beasley, A. W. Brown et al., "Common scientific and statistical errors in obesity research," *Obesity*, vol. 24, no. 4, pp. 781–790, 2016.

[19] A. Donner and N. Klar, "Pitfalls of and controversies in cluster randomization trials," *American Journal of Public Health*, vol. 94, no. 3, pp. 416–422, 2004.

[20] A. Donner and N. Klar, *Design and Analysis of Cluster Randomization Trials in Health Research*, Arnold, London, UK, 2000.

[21] D. Cousineau and L. Laurencelle, "A correction factor for the impact of cluster randomized sampling and its applications," *Psychological Methods*, vol. 21, no. 1, pp. 121–135, 2016.

[22] P. Li, A. W. Brown, J. M. Oakes, and D. B. Allison, "Comment on "school-based obesity prevention intervention in Chilean children: effective in controlling, but not reducing obesity"," *Journal of Obesity*, vol. 2015, Article ID 183528, 2 pages, 2015.

[23] M. K. Campbell, P. M. Fayers, and J. M. Grimshaw, "Determinants of the intracluster correlation coefficient in cluster randomized trials: the case of implementation research," *Clinical Trials*, vol. 2, no. 2, pp. 99–107, 2005.

[24] M. K. Campbell, G. Piaggio, D. R. Elbourne, and D. G. Altman, "Consort 2010 statement: extension to cluster randomised trials," *BMJ*, vol. 345, no. 1, p. e5661, 2012.

[25] M. K. Campbell, D. R. Elbourne, and D. G. Altman, "CONSORT statement: extension to cluster randomised trials," *BMJ*, vol. 328, no. 7441, pp. 702–708, 2004.

[26] M. Appelbaum, H. Cooper, R. B. Kline, E. Mayo-Wilson, A. M. Nezu, and S. M. Rao, "Journal article reporting standards for quantitative research in psychology: The APA Publications and Communications Board task force report," *American Psychologist*, vol. 73, no. 1, pp. 3–25, 2018.

[27] H. M. Levitt, M. Bamberg, J. W. Creswell, D. M. Frost, R. Josselson, and C. Suarez-Orozco, "Journal article reporting standards for qualitative primary, qualitative meta-analytic, and mixed methods research in psychology: The APA Publications and Communications Board task force report," *American Psychologist*, vol. 73, no. 1, pp. 26–46, 2018.

[28] N. M. Ivers, M. Taljaard, S. Dixon et al., "Impact of CONSORT extension for cluster randomised trials on quality of reporting and study methodology: review of random sample of 300 trials, 2000-8," *BMJ*, vol. 343, no. 1, p. d5886, 2011.

[29] P. S. Fleming, D. Koletsi, A. Polychronopoulou, T. Eliades, and N. Pandis, "Are clustering effects accounted for in statistical analysis in leading dental specialty journals?," *Journal of Dentistry*, vol. 41, no. 3, pp. 265–270, 2013.

[30] S. Dell-Kuster, R. A. Droeser, J. Schafer et al., "Systematic review and simulation study of ignoring clustered data in surgical trials," *British Journal of Surgery*, vol. 105, no. 3, pp. 182–191, 2018.

[31] H. Oltean and J. J. Gagnier, "Use of clustering analysis in randomized controlled trials in orthopaedic surgery," *BMC Medical Research Methodology*, vol. 15, no. 1, p. 17, 2015.

21

Adipose Tissue-Secreted Factors Alter Bladder Cancer Cell Migration

Nisha Hariharan,[1] Keith A. Ashcraft,[2] Robert S. Svatek,[2] Carolina B. Livi,[1] Desiree Wilson,[1] Dharam Kaushik,[2] Robin J. Leach,[1,2] and Teresa L. Johnson-Pais[2]

[1]*Department of Cell Systems and Anatomy, University of Texas Health Science Center, San Antonio, TX 78229, USA*
[2]*Department of Urology, University of Texas Health Science Center, San Antonio, TX 78229, USA*

Correspondence should be addressed to Teresa L. Johnson-Pais; paist@uthscsa.edu

Academic Editor: Sayed S. Hoseini

Background. Obesity is associated with an increased risk of bladder cancer recurrence. This study investigated the role of adipose tissue in bladder cancer progression. *Methods.* Gene expression profiling was performed on adipose tissues collected from normal weight ($n = 5$), overweight ($n = 11$), and obese ($n = 10$) patients with invasive bladder cancer, and adipose stromal cells (ASCs) were obtained from two normal weight, two overweight, and two obese patients. Conditioned media (CM) was characterized and evaluated for its effects on the proliferation, migration, and invasive potential of T24 bladder cancer cells. *Results.* Expression profiling demonstrated depot-specific or body mass index-specific differences. Increased T24 cell migration was observed using CM harvested from all ASCs. ASC CM from an obese patient significantly increased T24 cell migration and invasion compared to ASC CM collected from normal weight and overweight patients. We identified abundant expression of CXCL1, PAI1, IL6, CX3CL1, and CCL2 in all CM. Exogenous treatment of T24 cells with PAI1, IL6, and CXCL1 enhanced migration. Depletion of CXCL1, PAI1, and IL6 in an obese patient ASC CM abrogated T24 migration. *Conclusion.* Factors secreted by adipose tissue influence the migration of bladder tumor cells and could play an active role in tumor progression.

1. Introduction

An estimated 79,000 urinary bladder cancer cases will be newly diagnosed and are expected to result in 16,870 deaths in the United States in 2017 [1]. Bladder cancer is the fourth most common cancer among American men and the eighth most common cause of cancer deaths [1, 2]. The bladder is surrounded by visceral adipose tissue, and bladder cancer staging is based on involvement of perivesical fat. Tumors with extravesical invasion of the tumor into the perivesical fat (pathologic stage T3) are highly predisposed to lymph node involvement and distant metastasis [3, 4]. Obesity appears to play an important role in the development of bladder cancer. An epidemiological study of 1,719 incident bladder cancer cases demonstrated that obese individuals had a 28% increased risk for bladder cancer compared to normal weight individuals [5]. Obesity has been shown to be associated with worse cancer-specific outcomes in bladder cancer patients in a large multi-institutional cohort. In patients with body mass index (BMI) > 30 kg/m^2, there was a 67% increased risk of cancer recurrence and a 43% increased risk of cancer-specific mortality [6]. In addition, a meta-analysis of 14 prospective cohort studies showed a positive association between bladder cancer and obesity and a potential association between BMI and bladder cancer risk with the risk increasing by 3.1% for each 5 kg/m^2 increase [7].

Several studies have reported a positive association of obesity severity with adverse outcomes in many cancer types [8–10]. Studies of obesity and prostate cancer revealed that the periprostatic adipose tissue secretes high levels of interleukin-6 (IL6), compared to subcutaneous adipose tissue, which modulates cancer aggressiveness [11, 12]. Subcutaneous and visceral adipose depots show differential patterns of gene expression in obese patients with and without endometrial cancer [13]. Adipose tissue is heterogeneous, and the stromal vascular fraction that is enriched for the adipose stromal cells (ASCs) is a potent source of numerous cytokines and chemokines [14]. The altered expression of the various secreted factors from the adipose tissue in the overweight and obese states has been observed to have mitogenic effects in numerous cancers [15–21].

Here, we sought to gain an understanding of the role of adipose tissue in bladder cancer and to determine whether bladder tumors are affected by the dysfunctional adipose tissue in the obese state. We characterized the gene expression profiles of adipose tissue collected from various patients across a spectrum of BMI. In addition, we observed that secreted factors from bladder cancer patients' adipose tissue influence the proliferation and migratory and invasive capacity of human bladder cancer cells.

2. Materials and Methods

2.1. Patient Recruitment and Tissue Procurement. All adipose tissue samples were obtained through a bladder cancer repository maintained in the Department of Urology that has full institutional review board (IRB) approval at the University of Texas Health Science Center at San Antonio. Fresh adipose tissue samples were provided without identifiers The research protocol for this study was assessed by the IRB and determined to be nonhuman research (protocol number: HSC20130350N). Adipose tissue was obtained from 26 male patients who were undergoing radical cystectomy for locally advanced bladder cancer. Adipose tissue was collected from the fat surrounding the urinary bladder and subcutaneous tissue. Care was taken to extract fat surrounding the bladder and when tumor was present, immediately adjacent to the tumor site. This method was the same for all patients/samples. When no bladder tumor was present, fat was removed from the scarred area (resection site) which corresponded to where the tumor was before transurethral resection. An assessment for the presence of contaminating tumor cells in the whole fat surrounding the bladder was not performed. The patients were stratified into three BMI groups according to the World Health Organization standards: normal weight ($n = 5$, BMI < 25 kg/m^2), overweight ($n = 11$, BMI $= 25$–29.9 kg/m^2), and obese ($n = 10$, BMI ≥ 30 kg/m^2).

2.2. Adipose Tissue Explant Conditioned Media. Specimens (0.5–2.0 g) of the bladder and subcutaneous adipose tissue, when available, and based on the quantity of available tissues were placed in primary whole adipose tissue explant cultures using a modified protocol adapted from Thalmann et al. [22]. Adipose tissue (500 mg) was incubated as an explant overnight in the serum-free Dulbecco's modified Eagle's–Ham's F-12 medium (DMEM/F12) (1 : 1 v/v) (Corning, Manassas, VA) supplemented with 1% penicillin-streptomycin and antimycotic agent. The explant cultures were maintained at 37°C in a 5% CO_2 atmosphere for 48 hours. The explant culture media was subsequently collected, centrifuged, and frozen at −80°C as whole adipose tissue explant conditioned media (FCM).

2.3. Isolation of Adipose Stromal Cells (ASCs) and Preparation of ASC CM. Bladder and subcutaneous adipose tissue (1-2 g) from normal weight ($n = 2$), overweight ($n = 2$), and obese patients ($n = 2$), from whom there was sufficient tissue available, was digested with Blendzyme (Roche, Indianapolis, IN) to release the individual cell components, placed in a shaker rotating at 75 rpm for 60 minutes, filtered with 100-micron mesh, and plated on 60 mm tissue culture dishes [23]. The ASCs were expanded in DMEM/F12 with 10% fetal bovine serum (FBS). To prepare ASC conditioned media (ASC CM), 7.5×10^4 ASCs seeded in DMEM/F12 media supplemented with 2% FBS and 1% penicillin and amphotericin-B in 35 mm dishes were allowed to adhere and then washed with phosphate-buffered saline (PBS) and switched to serum-free DMEM/F12 media supplemented with 1% penicillin and amphotericin-B. After 48 hours, ASC CM was collected and stored at −80°C.

2.4. Morphology and Flow Cytometry Analysis of Patient-Derived ASCs. ASC cultures from early passages (1–6 population doublings) were harvested and resuspended in DMEM/F12 with 2% FBS. The cells were then centrifuged and suspended in cold PBS at a concentration of 10^6 cells/100 μl. Cell aliquots were stained with monoclonal mouse anti-human antibodies against the following antigens: CD44-peridinin-chlorophyll-protein/cyanin 5.5, CD90-phycoerthyrin (PE), PE/Cy7-CD105, CD73-fluorescein isothiocyanate, CD34-Alexa Fluor 647, CD45-Pacific Blue (PB), CD11b-PB, and CD31-PB (BioLegend, San Diego, CA) for 30 minutes in the absence of light at 4°C. The cells that were stained with a single antibody coupled with a fluorescent dye were acquired for compensation purposes. After incubation, the cells were washed and resuspended in cold PBS. Flow cytometry was performed using a Becton Dickinson LSR II. A gate was set to include only the viable propidium iodide-negative cells. The number of cells staining positive for a given cell surface marker was determined by the percentage of cells present within an established gate. A minimum of 10,000 events were counted for each analysis.

2.5. Adipogenic Differentiation of Patient ASCs. Adipogenic differentiation of ASCs was performed as previously described [24]. Subcutaneous and bladder-associated ASCs plated in the growth media were cultured until confluence in a 35 mm dish. The medium was removed, and the cells were incubated with or without the adipogenic differentiation medium consisting of the DMEM/F12 medium supplemented with 10% FBS with the addition of 1 μM dexamethasone (Sigma-Aldrich, St. Louis, MO), 10 μg/ml recombinant human insulin, and 0.5 mM 1-methyl-3-isobutyl xanthine (IBMX) (Sigma-Aldrich) for three days. This medium was replaced every three days with the same medium without IBMX for the adipogenic differentiation maintenance period. After 15 days of differentiation, stromal and adipogenic cells were fixed in 1% paraformaldehyde in PBS and stained using the lipid stain Oil Red O.

2.6. Gene Expression. Total RNA was isolated from adipose specimens of approximately 100 mg in weight. The frozen patient adipose tissue was homogenized in the QIAzol lysis reagent (Qiagen, Valencia, CA), and the ASCs were disrupted using a Mini-Beadbeater-16 cell disrupter (BioSpec, Bartlesville, OK). Once homogenized, chloroform was added and the homogenate was centrifuged to separate the aqueous phase from the organic phase. The aqueous phase, containing the RNA, was transferred to a new tube and processed with the RNeasy lipid tissue mini kit (Qiagen) for the whole adipose tissue and RNeasy mini kit (Qiagen) for the ASCs, according to the manufacturer's instructions. RNA quantity was assessed using a NanoDrop spectrophotometer (Thermo Fisher Scientific, Waltham, MA), and RNA integrity and purity were assessed using the Agilent 2100 Bioanalyzer (Agilent Technologies, Santa Clara, CA). For cRNA probe labeling, 500 ng of total RNA was used in the Illumina TotalPrep RNA Amplification protocol to create the cRNA probe (Thermo Fisher Scientific, Waltham, MA). The hybridization cocktail containing the labeled cRNA probes was hybridized to the Human HT-12v4 Whole-Genome Expression BeadChip microarray (Illumina, San Diego, CA). The arrays were subsequently processed and imaged using the Illumina iScan, according to the manufacturer's protocol. GenomeStudio software (Illumina) was used for background correction, data normalization, and filtering. Data analysis was performed using GeneSpring 12.6 (Agilent Technologies). Gene function and network enrichments for selected genes were performed using Pathway Architect. The threshold set for significantly dysregulated genes was a p value < 0.05 and a twofold or higher change. The moderated T-test was used to compare gene expression changes between groups, and a $p < 0.05$ was considered statistically significant. A candidate gene prioritization analysis was performed on the identified gene transcripts based on functional annotations using the ToppGene Suite [25].

2.7. Measurement of Protein Levels. Potential protumor factors in the conditioned medium obtained from whole fat explants (FCM) from different anatomical sites from six of the 26 patients for whom there was sufficient tissue available (normal, $n = 1$; overweight, $n = 2$; obese, $n = 3$) and from patient ASC cultures (ASC CM) (normal, $n = 2$; overweight, $n = 2$; obese, $n = 2$) were screened for 41 secreted cytokines/growth factors and six adipokines using the MILLIPLEX MAP 41-plex Human Cytokine/Chemokine Panel and the Human Adipokine Panel 1 (Billerica, MA), which were evaluated using FLEXMAP 3D™ (Luminex, Austin, TX).

2.8. Cell Lines and Culture Conditions. The human transitional cell carcinoma cell line T24 was purchased from ATCC and cultured as recommended in McCoy's 5A media supplemented with 10% FBS, 1% penicillin-streptomycin, and antimycotic agent. The cell line was authenticated using short tandem repeat DNA fingerprinting by the University of Texas MD Anderson Cancer Center Characterized Cell Line Core, NCI # CA016672. Cell viability was determined using trypan blue dye exclusion.

2.9. Cell Proliferation. Approximately 2×10^3 T24 cells were plated in triplicate in a 96-well flat-bottomed cell culture plate, and each well was treated with (1) whole fat conditioned media (FCM), (2) media only (negative control), or (3) ASC CM. After 24 hours in culture, cell proliferation was assessed using the CellTiter 96 AQ MTS (3-(4,5-dimethylthiazol-2-yl)-5-(3-carboxymethoxyphenyl)-2-(4-sulfophenyl)-2H-tetrazolium) assay (Thermo Fisher Scientific) following the manufacturer's protocol.

2.10. Cell Migration Using the Transwell System. T24 cells (2×10^5 cells) were plated in duplicate on the top of 8-micron Transwell inserts (BD Biosciences, San Jose, CA) and exposed to serum-free media (SFM) (negative control), whole fat explant FCM (diluted 1 : 6 in SFM), or ASC CM (diluted 1 : 6 in SFM) in the lower chamber. FCM and ASC CM were diluted 1 : 6 to demonstrate that the effects were not nonspecific effects of high levels of protein present in the CM. The positive control consisted of the complete culture medium as the chemoattractant. The cells were allowed to transmigrate across the porous membrane at 37°C in a 5% CO_2 incubator. After the cells were incubated for 18 hours, the inserts were removed, and tumor cells on the upper membrane were detached with a sterile cotton swab. Inserts were stained with the Hema-3 staining system (Thermo Fisher Scientific). Pictures of the migrated cells were taken in five random microscopic fields per insert with 150x magnification using a Nikon Eclipse Ti bright-field microscope, and the average number of migrated cells/fields was determined by counting.

2.11. Cell Invasion Assay Using Matrigel. Cell invasion was assayed using a reconstituted extracellular matrix membrane (Matrigel; BD Biosciences, San Jose, CA). T24 cells (1.8×10^5 cells) were seeded in duplicate in the upper well of Transwell chambers precoated with 20 μg Matrigel. The media tested in the lower chamber was (1) explant CM (diluted 1 : 6 in SFM), (2) ASC CM (diluted 1 : 6 in SFM), or (3) SFM (negative control). The positive control included the complete culture medium in the lower well. The cells were incubated for 21 hours at 37°C in a 5% CO_2 incubator. Following incubation, noninvading cells on the top of the upper chamber were removed using a sterile cotton swab, and the cells that invaded through the Matrigel were stained with the Hema-3 staining system (Fisher Scientific). The invading cells were counted in five random microscopic fields per insert with 150x magnification using a Nikon Eclipse Ti bright-field microscope.

2.12. Stimulatory Effect of Selected Secreted Factors on Bladder Cancer Cell Migration. To test whether the cytokines identified in the conditioned media mediated the bladder cancer cell migration, media containing the following selected recombinant factors: interleukin-8 (IL8) at 10 ng/ml, chemokine (C-X-C motif) ligand 1 (CXCL1) at 10 ng/ml, plasminogen activator inhibitor 1 (PAI1) at 40 nM, interleukin-6 (IL6) at 5 ng/ml, fractalkine (CX3CL1) at 10 ng/ml, and monocyte chemoattractant protein 1 (CCL2) at 1 ng/ml, was placed in the lower well of a Transwell system. The concentration of the factors was determined from the quantities detected in the CM. T24 cells (2×10^5 cells) were plated in duplicate on the top of 8-micron Transwell inserts, and cell migration was assayed as described above. In addition, the activity of the IL6, PAI1, and CXCL1 was also individually blocked by the addition of the respective neutralizing antibody in the lower chamber. The IL6 and CXCL1 antibodies were obtained from R&D Systems (Minneapolis, MN), and the PAI1 antibody was obtained from EMD Millipore (Billerica, MA).

2.13. Depletion of Secreted Factors in Patient ASC CM. ASC CM from an obese patient was depleted of IL6, PAI1, and CXCL1 by incubation with neutralizing antibodies against the three factors (described above) at 4°C overnight with constant rotation. The antibodies were removed by adding 20 μl/ml Protein-G agarose beads (GE Healthcare Life Sciences, Pittsburg, PA) and incubating for four hours with rotation. CM containing the agarose beads was spun at 260 ×g for three minutes, and the supernatant was collected for use in the migration assay [26]. The positive control ASC CM was not incubated with the neutralizing antibodies but were treated with the Protein-G agarose beads. T24 cells (1.8×10^5 cells) were plated in duplicate on the top of 8-micron Transwell inserts (BD Biosciences), and the CM (depleted and control) was added in the lower wells. The cells were allowed to migrate for 21 hours. The Transwell inserts (BD Biosciences) were subsequently stained with the Hema-3 staining system to detect the migrated cells (Thermo Fisher Scientific). The migrated cells were counted in five random microscopic fields per insert with 150x magnification using a Nikon Eclipse Ti bright-field microscope.

2.14. Statistical Analysis. One-way ANOVA tests followed by multiple comparison testings were performed using the GraphPad Prism software, version 5.00 (GraphPad Software, San Diego, CA; www.graphpad.com) to determine statistically significant differences between groups. Differences were considered significant if $p \leq 0.05$.

3. Results

A total of 26 male bladder cancer patients who had invasive bladder cancer provided adipose tissue for analysis (patient demographics in Supplementary Table 1 in Supplementary Material available online). The patients were between 56 and 85 years of age. Approximately 70% of the patients were current or former smokers, 31% of them had previously received bacillus Calmette–Guérin (BCG) treatment, and 31% of them received treatment with neoadjuvant chemotherapy. At the time of cystectomy, downstaging of the tumor was observed in most of the patients and is a common occurrence in patients who receive neoadjuvant chemotherapy. Thus, the patients can have less than T2 disease at cystectomy, including T0-T1. The patient BMI range for each category was normal (19.21–24.86), overweight (25.07–29.97), and obese (30.08–41.91) Results were not stratified based on smoking, BCG therapy, or chemotherapy treatment.

Whole-genome gene expression was performed using RNA isolated from visceral adipose tissue surrounding the bladder from normal weight ($n = 5$), overweight ($n = 11$), and obese ($n = 10$) men with bladder cancer. A summary of the relationship between the differentially expressed genes in adipose tissue is presented as a Venn diagram in Figure 1(a). The analysis demonstrated that when comparing the gene expression profiles from obese versus normal weight men, 252 gene transcripts were found to be differentially expressed ($p < 0.05$ at a minimum of twofold differential expression). A candidate gene prioritization analysis was performed on the 252 gene transcripts based on functional annotations using the ToppGene Suite [25]. The top biological process in which these genes are involved in is secretion, with a total of 28 genes or 11% of the genes. Two hundred and two significant gene transcripts were found to be at least twofold differentially regulated ($p < 0.05$) when comparing the gene expression patterns between the adipose tissue surrounding the bladder of normal weight men and overweight men. A candidate gene prioritization performed on these 202 gene transcripts based on functional annotations using the ToppGene Suite revealed immune response, defense response, inflammatory response, regulation of the immune system process, and leukocyte activation as the top biological processes. Interestingly, the molecular functional annotation identified that the cytokine-cytokine receptor interaction pathway involved 12 of the differentially expressed genes. Comparison of gene expression patterns of bladder adipose tissue between obese and overweight men identified 161 genes that were at least twofold differentially regulated ($p < 0.05$). Candidate gene prioritization of the 161 genes using ToppGene revealed regulation of secretion, locomotion, regulation of the apoptotic process, regulation of the programmed cell death, and regulation of secretion by cells as the top biological processes.

To understand how adipose tissue contributes to paracrine signaling in bladder cancer, FCM from whole fat explants was assayed for their ability to affect the migration and invasion potential of T24 human bladder cancer cells. FCM from matched bladder and subcutaneous adipose tissue from three patients had a variable effect on T24 migration (Figure 1(b)). FCM also did not stimulate the invasive capability of T24 cells (Figure 1(c)). Since we observed a large variability in the migration of T24 cells when exposed to FCM across the different specimens, and because adipose tissue is a mixture of different cell types with the possibility that contaminating tumor cells may have been present in the whole fat, we chose to purify and expand the ASC population from the whole bladder fat and subcutaneous fat for further analysis.

To characterize the cells isolated as ASCs, selected ASC cultures were analyzed for the expression of common stem cell surface markers using flow cytometry. The subcutaneous and bladder ASCs tested positive for the cell surface markers CD73, CD44, CD90, CD105, and CD34 and negative for CD45, CD11b, and CD31 (data not shown). The cultured ASCs show similar cell surface markers as those of

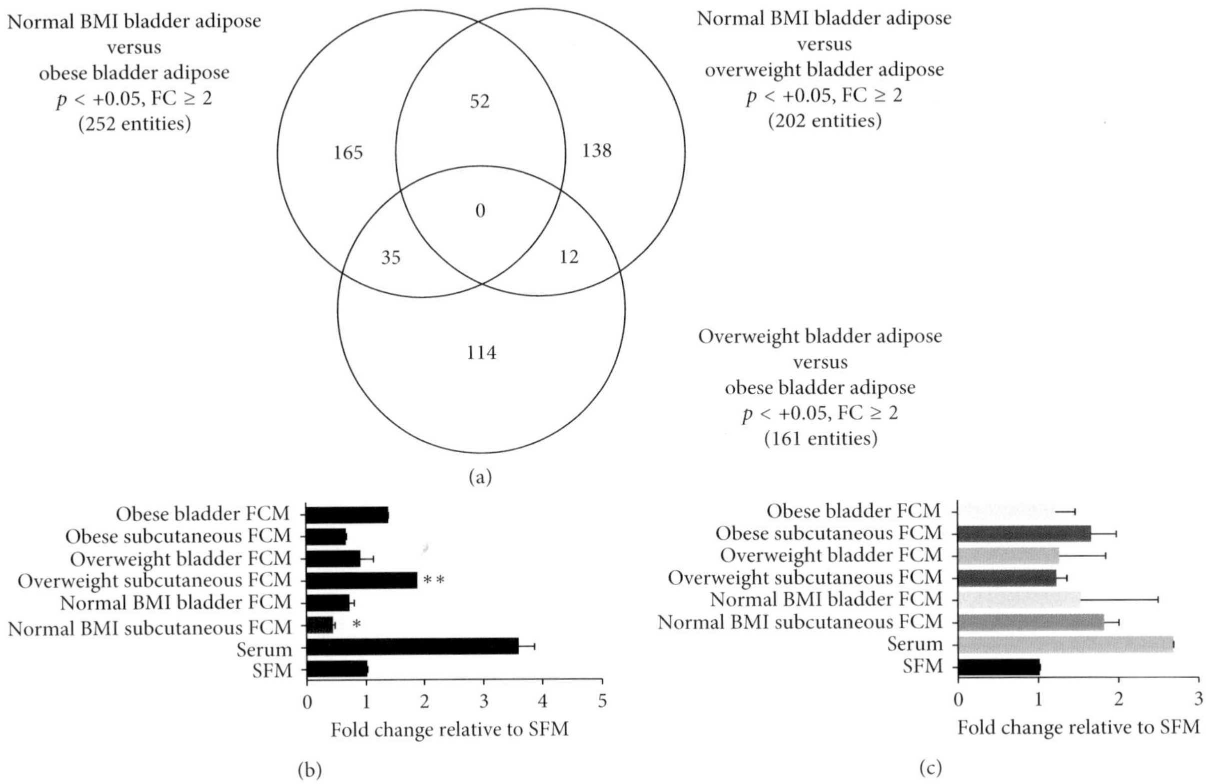

FIGURE 1: Gene expression profiling of bladder adipose tissue and effects of the influence of explant CM on T24 cancer cell behavior. (a) A Venn diagram representative of gene transcripts differentially regulated in the patient bladder fat between the groups: normal BMI versus obese, normal BMI versus overweight, and overweight versus obese. (b) Adipose whole explant CM from a normal weight patient, an overweight patient, and an obese patient was placed in the bottom of a Boyden chamber, and T24 cells were placed in the upper chamber. Serum-free media (SFM) was used as a control. Migrated cells were stained and counted. $^{*}p<0.05$ and $^{**}p<0.01$ are statistically significant. (c) Fat CM harvested from a normal weight patient, an overweight patient, and an obese bladder cancer patient was placed in the bottom of a Transwell invasion chamber, and T24 cells were placed in the upper chamber. Serum-free media (SFM) was used as a control. Invasive cells were stained and counted. $^{*}p<0.05$ and $^{**}p<0.01$ are statistically significant.

mesenchymal stem cells. Furthermore, ASC cultures treated with adipogenic differentiation media were able to undergo adipogenic differentiation, which was demonstrated by the staining of fat droplets using Oil Red O (Figures 2(a) and 2(b)). Gene expression analysis was performed using ASCs isolated from matched bladder and subcutaneous adipose tissue from two normal weight and two obese patients. The gene expression patterns of the ASC cluster based on both fat site and BMI status (Figure 2(c)). Bladder ASCs have a unique expression signature compared to subcutaneous ASCs. Comparison of gene expression profiles between ASCs derived from the subcutaneous and bladder depots in an obese patient revealed 15,394 differentially expressed transcripts with 7,615 transcripts that were at least twofold upregulated in the bladder depot showing a stratification based on BMI as well.

Conditioned media was prepared from ASC cultures derived from bladder and subcutaneous adipose tissue from a normal weight patient, an overweight patient, and an obese patient, and this media was able to induce migration of T24 cells (Figure 3(a)). Also, the ASC CM showed a greater effect in inducing T24 cell migration than what was previously observed with the explant CM (Figure 1(b)). Interestingly, the ASC CM (from both subcutaneous and bladder adipose tissue) obtained from an obese patient was able to cause a significant increase in T24 cell migration, compared to the respective depot-specific ASC CM obtained from a normal weight patient (Figure 3(a)). These results suggest that adipose stromal cells secrete factors that enhance the ability of T24 cells to migrate. Since it is difficult to control for the concentration of these factors in the explant FCM between specimens due to differences in the cellularity of the specimens, this may explain the variability in the stimulation of migration between the explant FCM and ASC CM. Only ASC CM obtained from an obese patient was also able to cause a significant increase in the invasiveness of T24 cells (Figure 3(b)). Conditioned media from whole fat or ASCs did not influence the proliferation rate of T24 cells *in vitro* (data not shown).

To determine which secreted factors may be influencing T24 behavior, the whole adipose tissue explant FCM and ASC CM were evaluated for the presence of 41 known cytokines/growth factors and six adipokines. In the adipose CM, we found that interleukin-8 (IL8), interleukin-6 (IL6), GRO1 oncogene (CXCL1), and fractalkine (CX3CL1) were present in high levels among several others (total 25 factors) detected above control SFM. The adipokine plasminogen activator inhibitor 1 (PAI1) was also present in high levels.

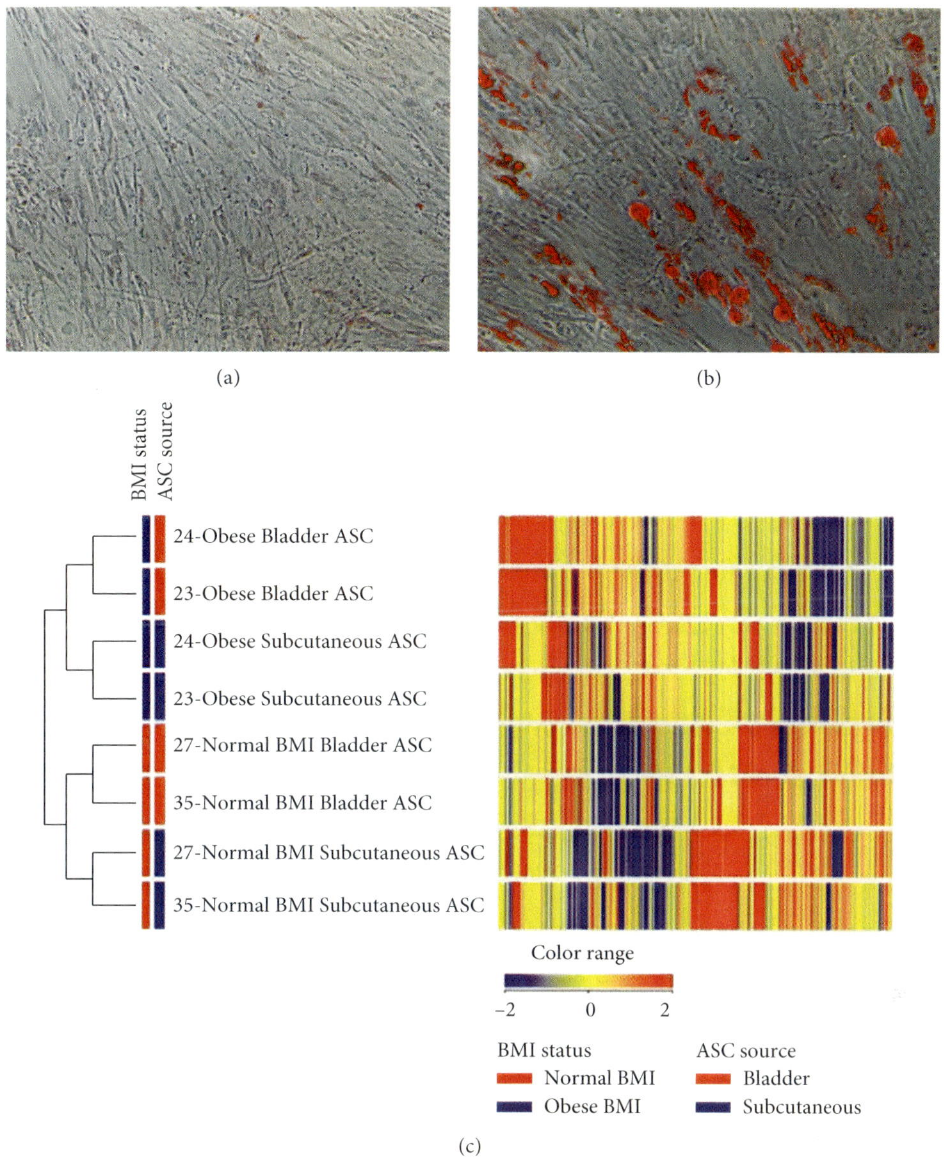

FIGURE 2: Characterization of bladder ASCs. Primary ASC cultures were allowed to grow to confluence in 6-well plates and were treated (a) without or (b) with the adipogenic differentiation medium. Adipogenic cells were stained using Oil Red O. (c) A heat map representative of differential gene expression in ASCs isolated from matched bladder and subcutaneous sites from two normal weight and two obese patients shows clustering based on the BMI status and ASC source. Transcripts are at least twofold differentially regulated ($p < 0.05$). The heat map indicates upregulation (red), downregulation (blue), and comparable levels of gene expression (yellow) and clustering based on the anatomical source of ASCs, as well as the BMI. PT = patient ID; BL = bladder; SQ = subcutaneous.

High levels of monocyte chemoattractant protein 1 (CCL2), CXCL1, IL6, IL8, and PAI1 were also found in patient ASC CM, irrespective of patient BMI. We chose to focus our investigations on the secreted factors that were detected in both the adipose CM and ASC CM. Data from studies of the bladder and other cancers implicate IL6, IL8, CXCL1, and PAI1 as factors that may play a role in the ability of the adipose CM and ASC CM to alter the migratory potential of the T24 cells [18, 27–32].

We determined whether the selected soluble factors IL8, CCL2, CX3CL1, IL6, PAI1, and CXCL1 contributed to the FCM- and ASC CM-mediated stimulation of T24 cell migration. However, exogenous treatment with CCL2, CX3CL1, and IL8 added individually did not stimulate the migration potential of T24 cells in a Transwell migration assay (data not shown). Subsequently, T24 cells were exposed to recombinant human IL6, PAI1, or CXCL1 individually placed in the lower chamber of a Transwell system. The addition of 5 ng/ml recombinant human IL6 was able to significantly enhance T24 migration in a Transwell assay, and blocking its function using a neutralizing antibody significantly reduced the migration potential (Figure 4(a)). Treatment of T24 cells with recombinant human PAI1 (40 nM, comparable to PAI1 levels found in patient ASC CM) caused a significant increase in migration (Figure 4(b)). Addition of recombinant human CXCL1 (10 ng/ml) to SFM alone was able to significantly

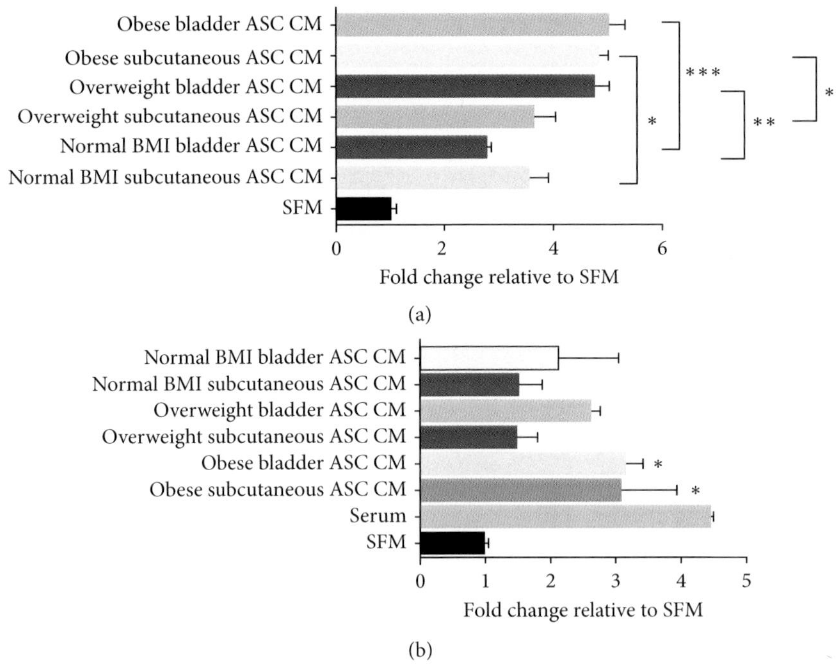

FIGURE 3: Effect of ASC CM on the migration and invasion potential of T24 cells. (a) ASC CM harvested from a normal weight patient, an overweight patient, and an obese bladder cancer patient was placed in the bottom of a Transwell invasion chamber, and T24 cells were placed in the upper chamber. Migrated cells were stained and counted. $^{*}p < 0.05$, $^{**}p < 0.01$, and $^{***}p < 0.001$ are statistically significant. (b) ASC CM harvested from a normal weight patient, an overweight patient, and an obese bladder cancer patient was placed in the bottom of a Transwell Matrigel invasion chamber, and T24 cells were placed in the upper chamber. Invasive cells were stained and counted. $^{*}p < 0.05$ is statistically significant.

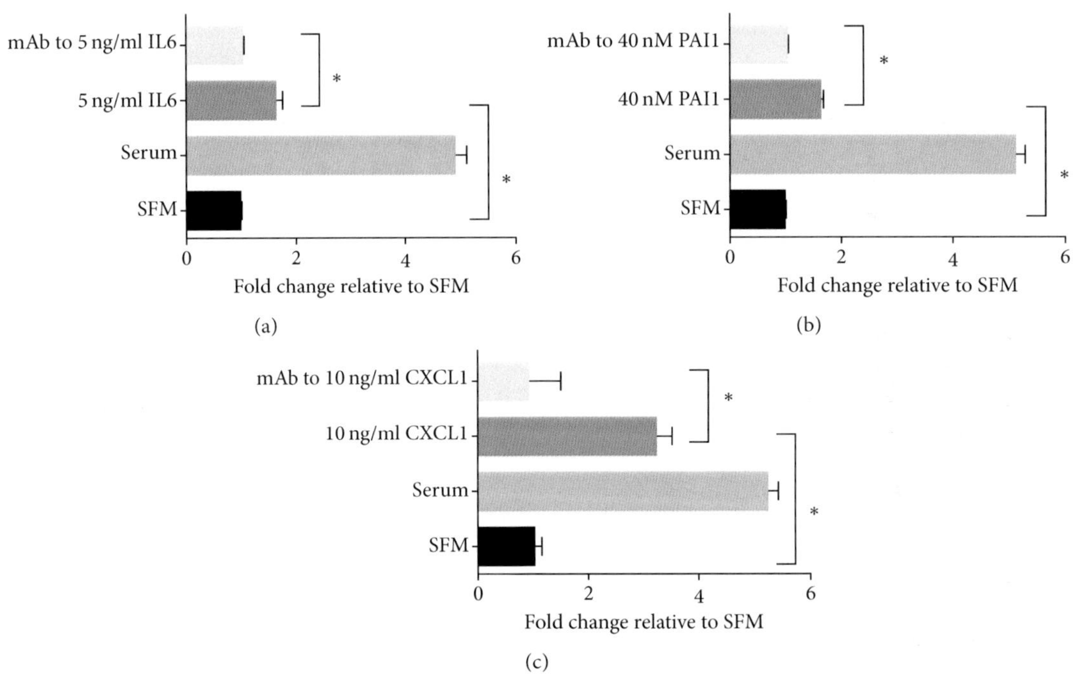

FIGURE 4: The activities of IL6, PAI1, and CXCL1 stimulate T24 migration. (a) Recombinant IL6 was added to serum-free media placed in the bottom of a Transwell chamber. Neutralizing antibody (Ab) against IL6 was added to block the activity. (b) Recombinant PAI1 was added to serum-free media placed in the bottom of a Transwell chamber. Neutralizing Ab against PAI1 was added to block the activity of PAI1. (c) Recombinant CXCL1 was added to serum-free media placed in the bottom of a Transwell chamber. Neutralizing Ab against CXCL1 was added to neutralize the CXCL1 activity. To each treatment, serum-free media (SFM) was used as a control. Migrated cells were stained and counted. $^{*}p < 0.05$ is statistically significant.

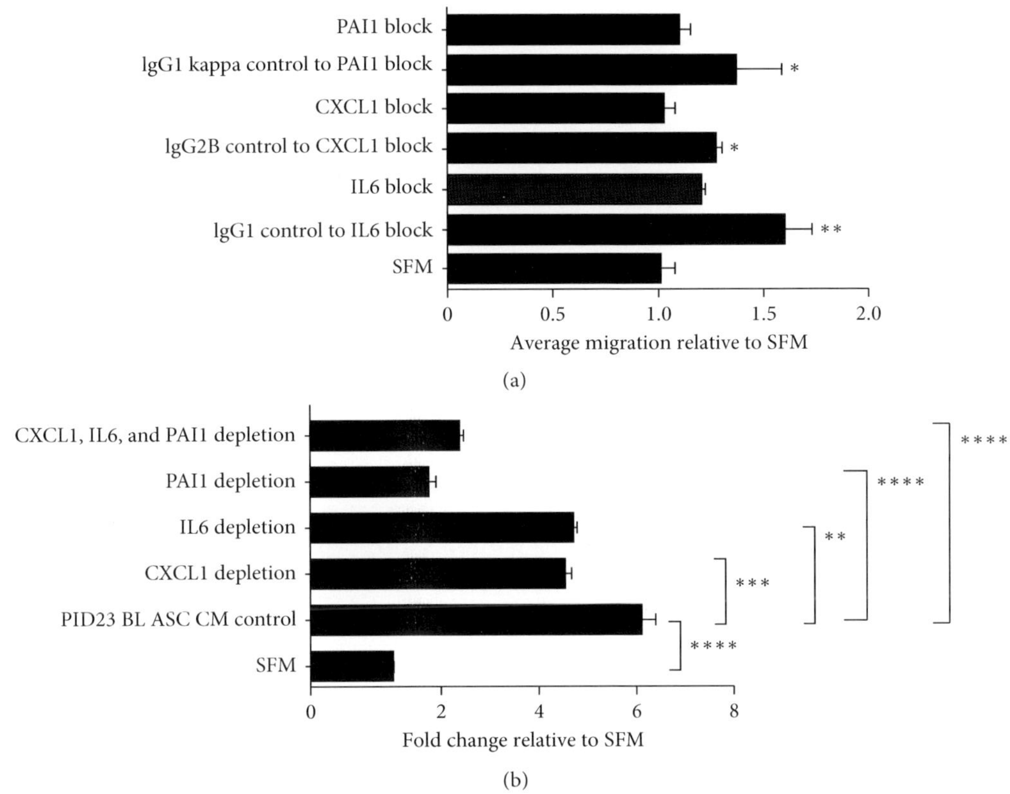

FIGURE 5: Blocking or depleting IL6, CXCL1, and PAI1 reduces migration of T24 cells. (a) Blocking the activity of exogenously added recombinant IL6, CXCL1, and PAI1 with neutralizing antibodies significantly reduces T24 migration in a Transwell assay compared to treatment with an isomeric IgG control. One-way ANOVA with uncorrected Fisher's LSD test: $^{*}p < 0.05$ and $^{**}p < 0.01$ are statistically significant. (b) Depletion of IL6, PAI1, and CXCL1 in an obese patient ASC CM was performed by treating with neutralizing antibodies. T24 migration was assessed in a Transwell system, and migrated cells were stained and counted. One-way ANOVA: $^{*}p < 0.05$, $^{**}p < 0.01$, $^{***}p < 0.001$, and $^{****}p < 0.0001$ are statistically significant.

increase the migration of T24 cells compared to the control SFM, and addition of the neutralizing antibody (10 μg/ml) to deplete the exogenous recombinant CXCL1 showed significant reduction in the migratory potential (Figure 4(c)). We then tested whether blocking the function of the selected factors IL6, PAI1, and CXCL1 using a neutralizing antibody or treatment with the appropriate isotype-matched control was able to affect T24 cell migration. Interestingly, exposure of T24 cells to recombinant IL-6, PAI-1, and CXCL1 added together in the lower chamber of the Transwell system followed by the individual addition of neutralizing antibodies to either IL6, PAI1, or CXCL1 in the lower chamber significantly abrogated the ability of the ASC CM to induce T24 migration (Figure 5(a)). In addition, neutralization of IL6, PAI1, or CXCL1 together or individually in the obese ASC CM abrogated the ASC CM-mediated stimulatory effect on T24 cell migration, indicating that each of the secreted factors contributed significantly to enhance T24 cell migration *in vitro* (Figure 5(b)).

4. Discussion

An increasing number of studies point towards a positive association between BMI and bladder cancer risk. Therefore, it is important to understand how adipose tissue exerts its effects on the bladder tumor progression. Global gene expression profiling of adipose tissue surrounding the bladder has been applied to identify genes and regulatory pathways associated with the obese/overweight state in the context of bladder cancer. The relevant biological processes found to be altered in the obese/overweight state included the pathways of secretion and inflammation-mediated cytokine signaling.

This study demonstrates that visceral adipose tissue is a potential source of secreted factors that can induce bladder cancer cell migration *in vitro*, and the ASC population is a source of factors that have the potential to impact bladder carcinogenesis. Although whole adipose tissue explants produce a surplus of cytokines in varying quantities, we focused on IL6, IL8, CXCL1, CX3CL1, CCL2, and PAI1, whose levels were found to be secreted in high levels by the whole fat. There was no site-specific or BMI-specific trend in cytokine profiles in the whole fat explant CM. Although it was not determined if there was bladder tumor cell contamination in the whole fat specimens, the subsequent analyses utilized a population of purified and characterized ASCs that exhibited the expression of cell surface markers and adipogenic differentiation potential consistent with ASCs and not bladder tumor cells. Similar to the whole adipose tissue, high levels of IL6, IL8, CXCL1, CX3CL1, CCL2, and PAI1 were present in ASC conditioned media with no site-specific or BMI-specific trend in cytokine profiles.

Exogenous treatment of T24 bladder cancer cells using recombinant human IL6, PAI1, or CXCL1 enhanced their migratory potential. Functional blocking of these three factors using neutralizing antibodies abrogated the enhanced T24 cell migration. Neutralizing the function of IL6, PAI1, and CXCL1 in an obese patient ASC CM abrogated the ASC CM-mediated stimulatory effect on T24 cell migration. We observed that blocking of IL6, PAI1, or CXCL1 alone in the obese ASC CM abrogated the ASC CM-mediated stimulatory effect on T24 cells, indicating that each of the secreted factors contributes significantly to induce cell migration. These data provide evidence that IL6, PAI1, and CXCL1 are important factors in promoting T24 cell migration.

IL6 was previously found to be secreted by ASCs, and it caused significant stimulation of MCF-7 breast cancer cell migration, while depletion of IL6 in the ASC conditioned media decreased migration and invasion [18]. CXCL1 is reported to be produced in human breast cancer cell line MDA-MB-23 supernatants, where its downregulation is involved in the protein kinase Syk-mediated suppression of cell migration [28]. Studies in other cancers show that CXCL1 expression plays a role in regulating the invasive potential of colon carcinoma cells [29]. PAI1 is known to regulate urokinase-type plasminogen activator (uPA), by blocking its interaction with substrates. PAI1 controls local proteolysis in the extracellular matrix by inhibiting uPA [30]. However, the role of PAI1 in tumor carcinogenesis is unclear. The expression of PAI1 has been found to be elevated in tissues from patients with transitional cell carcinoma of the bladder compared to healthy controls [31]. Previous studies also report that the inhibition of PAI1 expression in T24 bladder cancer xenografts resulted in inhibition of angiogenesis and apoptosis leading to reduced tumor growth [32]. It appears that CXCL1 and PAI1 secreted by adipose tissue and bladder-derived ASCs play an important role in inducing the migration of bladder cancer cells. Targeting the cytokines secreted by ASCs in the stromal compartment and the bladder cancer cells might prove to be a new effective approach for bladder cancer therapy.

Acknowledgments

This study was funded by the Sandra and Stanley Rosenburg Endowment Fund, a UT Health San Antonio Cancer Center Pilot Grant (RJL), and RP140105 CPRIT Research Training Award (Keith A. Ashcraft). Gene expression data were generated by the UT Health San Antonio Mays Cancer Center Genomics Shared Resource Facility and flow cytometry data were generated by the Flow Cytometry Shared Resource Facility, which are supported by the University of Texas Health Science Center, San Antonio, and NIH-NCI P30 CA054174 (Mays Cancer Center at University of Texas Health Science Center).

References

[1] R. L. Siegel, K. D. Miller, and A. Jemal, "Cancer statistics, 2016," *CA: A Cancer Journal for Clinicians*, vol. 66, no. 1, pp. 7–30, 2016.

[2] http://www.cancer.net/cancer-types/bladder-cancer/statistics.

[3] Y. Neuzillet, T. Lebret, V. Molinie et al., "Perivesical fat invasion in bladder cancer: implications for prognosis comparing pT2b, pT3a and pT3b stages and consequences for adjuvant chemotherapy indications," *British Journal of Urology International*, vol. 110, no. 11, pp. 1736–1741, 2012.

[4] E. Scosyrev, J. Yao, and E. Messing, "Microscopic invasion of perivesical fat by urothelial carcinoma: implications for prognosis and pathology practice," *Urology*, vol. 76, no. 4, pp. 908–913, 2010.

[5] C. Koebnick, D. Michaud, S. C. Moore et al., "Body mass index, physical activity, and bladder cancer in a large prospective study," *Cancer Epidemioloogy, Biomarkers & Prevention*, vol. 17, no. 5, pp. 1214–1221, 2008.

[6] T. F. Chromecki, E. K. Cha, H. Fajkovic et al., "Obesity is associated with worse oncological outcomes in patients treated with radical cystectomy," *British Journal of Urology International*, vol. 111, no. 2, pp. 249–255, 2012.

[7] L. Zhao, X. Tian, X. Duan, Y. Ye, M. Sun, and J. Huang, "Association of body mass index with bladder cancer risk: a dose-response meta-analysis of prospective cohort studies," *Oncotarget*, vol. 8, no. 20, pp. 33990–34000, 2017.

[8] Â. Moreira, S. S. Pereira, M. Costa et al., "Adipocyte secreted factors enhance aggressiveness of prostate carcinoma cells," *PLoS One*, vol. 10, no. 4, article e0123217, 2015.

[9] T. Mistry, J. E. Digby, K. M. Desai, and H. S. Randeva, "Obesity and prostate cancer: a role for adipokines," *European Urology*, vol. 52, no. 1, pp. 46–63, 2007.

[10] H. Wang, A. Maitra, and H. Wang, "Obesity, intrapancreatic fatty infiltration, and pancreatic cancer," *Clinical Cancer Research*, vol. 21, no. 15, pp. 3369–3371, 2015.

[11] D. S. Finley, V. S. Calvert, J. Inokuchi et al., "Periprostatic adipose tissue as a modulator of prostate cancer aggressiveness," *Journal of Urology*, vol. 182, no. 4, pp. 1621–1627, 2009.

[12] R. Ribeiro, C. Monteiro, V. Cunha et al., "Human periprostatic adipose tissue promotes prostate cancer aggressiveness in vitro," *Journal of Experimental and Clinical Cancer Research*, vol. 31, no. 1, p. 32, 2012.

[13] S. C. Modesitt, J. Y. Hsu, S. R. Chowbina, R. T. Lawrence, and K. L. Hoehn, "Not all fat is equal: differential gene expression and potential therapeutic targets in subcutaneous adipose, visceral adipose, and endometrium of obese women with and without endometrial cancer," *International Journal of Gynecological Cancer*, vol. 22, no. 5, pp. 732–741, 2012.

[14] G. R. Hajer, T. W. van Haeften, and F. L. J. Visseren, "Adipose tissue dysfunction in obesity, diabetes, and vascular diseases," *European Heart Journal*, vol. 29, no. 24, pp. 2959–2971, 2008.

[15] R. C. van Kruijsdijk, E. van der Wall, and F. L. J. Visseren, "Obesity and cancer: the role of dysfunctional adipose tissue," *Cancer Epidemiology, Biomarkers & Prevention*, vol. 18, no. 10, pp. 2569–2578, 2009.

[16] J. Park, D. M. Euhus, and P. E. Scherer, "Paracrine and endocrine effects of adipose tissue on cancer development and progression," *Endocrine Reviews*, vol. 32, no. 4, pp. 550–570, 2011.

[17] A. L. Strong, M. E. Burow, J. M. Gimble, and B. A. Bunnell, "Concise review: the obesity cancer paradigm: exploration of the interactions and crosstalk with adipose stem cells," *Stem Cells*, vol. 33, no. 2, pp. 318–326, 2015.

[18] M. Walter, S. Liang, S. Ghosh, P. J. Hornsby, and R. Li, "Interleukin 6 secreted from adipose stromal cells promotes

migration and invasion of breast cancer cells," *Oncogene*, vol. 28, no. 30, pp. 2745–2755, 2009.

[19] L. Prantl, F. Muehlberg, N. M. Navone et al., "Adipose tissue-derived stem cells promote prostate tumor growth," *The Prostate*, vol. 70, no. 15, pp. 1709–1715, 2010.

[20] V. Pistone Creydt, S. J. Fletcher, J. Giudice et al., "Human adipose tissue from normal and tumoral breast regulates the behavior of mammary epithelial cell," *Clinical and Translational Oncology*, vol. 15, no. 2, pp. 124–131, 2012.

[21] B. G. Rowan, J. M. Gimble, M. Shenq, M. Anbalagan, R. K. Jones, and T. P. Frazier, "Human adipose tissue-derived stromal/stem cells promote migration and early metastasis of triple negative breast cancer xenografts," *PLoS One*, vol. 9, no. 2, article e89595, 2014.

[22] S. Thalmann, C. E. Juge-Aubry, and C. A. Meier, "Explant cultures of white adipose tissue," *Methods in Molecular Biology*, vol. 456, pp. 195–199, 2008.

[23] A. J. Katz, A. Tholpady, S. S. Tholpady, H. Shang, and R. C. Ogle, "Cell surface and transcriptional characterization of human adipose-derived adherent stromal (hADAS) cells," *Stem Cells*, vol. 23, no. 3, pp. 412–423, 2005.

[24] K. R. Silva, S. Liechocki, J. R. Carneiro et al., "Stromal-vascular fraction content and adipose stem cell behavior are altered in morbid obese and post bariatric surgery ex-obese women," *Stem Cell Research & Therapy*, vol. 6, no. 1, p. 72, 2015.

[25] J. Chen, E. E. Bardes, B. J. Aronow, and A. G. Jegga, "ToppGene suite for gene list enrichment analysis and candidate gene prioritization," *Nucleic Acids Research*, vol. 37, pp. W305–W331, 2009.

[26] C. P. Chen, Y. Y. Chen, J. P. Huang, and Y. H. Wu, "The effect of conditioned medium derived from human placental multipotent mesenchymal stromal cells on neutrophils: possible implications for placental infection," *Molecular Human Reproduction*, vol. 20, no. 11, pp. 1117–1125, 2014.

[27] K. Inoue, J. W. Slaton, B. Y. Eve et al., "Interleukin 8 expression regulates tumorigenicity and metastases in androgen-independent prostate cancer," *Clinical Cancer Research*, vol. 6, no. 5, pp. 2104–2119, 2000.

[28] J. Li and N. Sidell, "Growth-related oncogene produced in human breast cancer cells and regulated by Syk protein-tyrosine kinase," *International Journal of Cancer*, vol. 117, no. 1, pp. 14–20, 2005.

[29] A. Li, M. L. Varney, and R. K. Singh, "Constitutive expression of growth regulated oncogene (gro) in human colon carcinoma cells with different metastatic potential and its role in regulating their metastatic phenotype," *Clinical & Experimental Metastasis*, vol. 21, no. 7, pp. 571–579, 2004.

[30] C. E. Leik, E. J. Su, P. Nambi, D. L. Crandall, and D. A. Lawrence, "Effect of pharmacologic plasminogen activator inhibitor-1 inhibition on cell motility and tumor angiogenesis," *Thrombosis and Haemostasis*, vol. 4, no. 12, pp. 2710–2715, 2006.

[31] M. Becker, T. Szarvas, M. Wittschier et al., "Prognostic impact of plasminogen activator inhibitor type 1 expression in bladder cancer," *Cancer*, vol. 116, no. 19, pp. 4502–4512, 2010.

[32] E. Gomes-Giacoia, M. Miyake, S. Goodison, and C. J. Rosser, "Targeting plasminogen activator inhibitor-1 inhibits angiogenesis and tumor growth in a human cancer xenograft model," *Molecular Cancer Therapeutics*, vol. 12, no. 12, pp. 2697–2708, 2013.

22

Identification and Characterization of Families That Are Positively Deviant for Childhood Obesity in a Latino Population

Byron A. Foster,[1,2] Christian A. Aquino,[3] Sharol Mejia,[3] Barbara J. Turner,[2,3] and Arvind Singhal[4,5]

[1]*Departments of Dermatology and Pediatrics, Oregon Health & Science University, Portland, OR, USA*
[2]*Center for Research to Advance Community Health, University of Texas Health San Antonio, San Antonio, TX, USA*
[3]*School of Medicine, University of Texas Health San Antonio, San Antonio, TX, USA*
[4]*Department of Communication, The University of Texas at El Paso, El Paso, TX, USA*
[5]*Inland University of Applied Sciences, Elverum, Norway*

Correspondence should be addressed to Byron A. Foster; fosterb@ohsu.edu

Academic Editor: R. Prager

Background. Childhood obesity is a complex public health challenge that requires innovative, sustainable solutions. Positive deviance, inspired by the science of complexity, is an approach that examines what allows certain individuals to succeed despite being predicted to fail. This study is aimed at identifying and defining positive deviants for early childhood obesity. *Methods.* This case control study used medical record data to identify Latino children aged 2–5 and classify them using their longitudinal weight change. Parents of children with trajectories toward a healthy weight from an obese weight (cases) and parents of children with stable obese weight trajectories over time (controls) were recruited. Mixed-methods analyses were used including a semi-structured interview and quantitative surveys evaluating diet, physical activity, sleep, feeding practices, and self-efficacy. Qualitative description was applied to the qualitative data; quantitative data were analyzed using descriptive statistics and logistic regression modeling. *Results.* Of eligible Latino children identified from the overall data set ($n = 1,621$), 257 (16%) had trajectories toward a healthy weight, and among these, 21 positively deviant cases completed the study with 23 matched controls. Positive deviant families were characterized by lower education, higher self-efficacy, and a more Mexican cultural orientation. Findings suggest that effective engagement of other caregivers and creating healthy food environments were important determinants of healthy weight outcomes. *Conclusions.* Positive deviants (cases) were distinct from controls in several parenting strategies such as creating healthy food environments and engaging caregivers. They had higher self-efficacy despite lower education. There were fewer differences in diet and physical activity than expected.

1. Introduction

As early childhood obesity strongly predicts adolescent and adult weight [1], effective interventions directed at this age group are needed to reduce lifetime risk of diabetes and cardiovascular disease. Low-income Latino children are at highest risk for obesity among racial-ethnic groups [2] and experience significant healthcare access disparities [3]. Prior interventions have demonstrated mixed results in Latino, preschool-aged children. Well-designed, theory-based interventions showed no effect on adiposity in Head Start [4, 5] or community settings [6]. However, other studies using either a home-based intervention targeting healthier routines [7] or a parenting skills intervention on nutrition have shown more promising results [8]. These mixed results highlight the need for further community-based research. Approaches that identify what is already working in low-income Latino families can inform the development of interventions for the larger community.

Positive deviance is an approach to solve complex problems such as childhood obesity that asks, theoretically, what is working in the community, particularly among the most disadvantaged ones [9, 10]. By identifying individuals who have found a way to achieve a desirable outcome in spite of adversity, and discovering their uncommon and replicable practices, the positive deviance approach presents an innovative, inside-out approach to solve complex problems [11–13]. In other words, there may be families at high risk for continued obesity who have successfully achieved a healthy weight and have used existing assets and resources to do so. Identifying their behaviors may yield lessons applicable for the rest of the community.

Applications of positive deviance theory to childhood malnutrition are well established [14, 15]; however, applications to address childhood obesity are very limited. Of the few studies published, their limitations include examination of cross-sectional data on weight [16] or the lack of control groups [17]. The current study addresses these limitations by identifying subjects through a longitudinal analysis of children's weight, and employing a case-control design, coupled with mixed-methods analysis to define positive deviants' characteristics and behaviors. We examined both known associations with obesity (feeding behaviors, physical activity, sleep, and screen time) along with a semistructured interview to elicit potentially novel behaviors.

2. Methods

2.1. Overall Design. This study identified children as positive deviants (cases) who had been obese and then were able to reduce their adiposity to a healthier weight. Children who remained persistently obese served as controls. Parents of the children classified as cases and controls were recruited to participate in this mixed-methods study that included a semistructured interview and a questionnaire on their lifestyles, eating habits, and physical activity.

2.2. Study Participants and Growth Trajectory Analysis. Medical record data from a large, safety-net healthcare provider in San Antonio, TX, were used to identify the weight trajectories. We focused on the most recent data from 2013 to 2015 (49,860 children) to examine weight-based trajectories and to minimize recall bias in our parental interviews. A data analyst with the health system pulled the growth chart data from the medical records using an HIPAA waiver obtained for this study.

Children were included in the growth trajectory analysis if they were obese (≥95th percentile for body mass index (BMI) per CDC guidelines) during 2–5 years, had at least three height and weight measurements over more than one year to determine a BMI z-score trajectory, were of Latino ethnicity, and lived in a San Antonio zip code.

A latent class linear mixed model with a linear link function and a diagonal variance-covariance structure was used to classify each child into a distinct group based on their BMI z-score trajectory [18]. Due to high variability in the BMI z-scores over time, a median filter (Tukey's Running Median Smoothing [19]) was used to reduce noise in the data. The variables used to model the repeated BMI z-scores were sex and age. Sex was treated as a fixed effect, while age varied by subjects (random effect) who entered the study at different times. The mean posterior probabilities of class membership were used to assess the classification accuracy, which in turn determined the number of classes allowed in the model.

2.3. Recruitment. After classification of children by weight trajectory, their parents were recruited to participate as either cases (positive deviants) or controls (Figure 1). Potential positive deviants had a negative BMI z-score trajectory over time (from an obese toward a healthy weight), were of Latino ethnicity, and with public insurance (based on their medical record). Controls had either a flat or an increasing BMI z-score trajectory by the latent class modeling and were matched by ethnicity and insurance status. Growth trajectory classes were visually confirmed on growth charts prior to recruitment. The sample size was determined by the qualitative data until thematic saturation was reached.

A letter, in English and Spanish, outlined the purpose and design of the study and was sent to all of the potential positive deviants. An option allowing recipients to return a postcard opting out of further communication was provided. An HIPAA waiver was obtained as part of the research protocol to do this. We recruited controls from the larger population of controls. A research assistant conducted follow-up phone calls with potential participants to determine if they met the eligibility criteria. Children were excluded from participation as either a case or a control if they had a diagnosis of intellectual disability or developmental delay, a seizure disorder, diabetes, cerebral palsy, a genetic problem, or if they were taking medication for attention deficit/hyperactivity disorder (these medications affect growth trajectories and physical activity).

2.4. Study Visit and Measures. Parents participated in a semistructured interview in either English or Spanish, followed by a quantitative assessment at either a clinical research center, a local library, or their home. All of the quantitative measures described below have been validated in Spanish except for the Comprehensive Feeding Practices Questionnaire [20]. Quantitative data were collected on REDCap [21].

2.5. Semistructured Interview. The semistructured interview was designed to elicit parents' opinions about the health of their child, including any changes purposely adopted or attempted related to their child and their child's health. Questions were grouped into general health and perceptions of health, feeding practices, physical activities, changes in weight, food purchasing and preparation, parent modeling, family rules and interactions, neighborhood and community resources, and school.

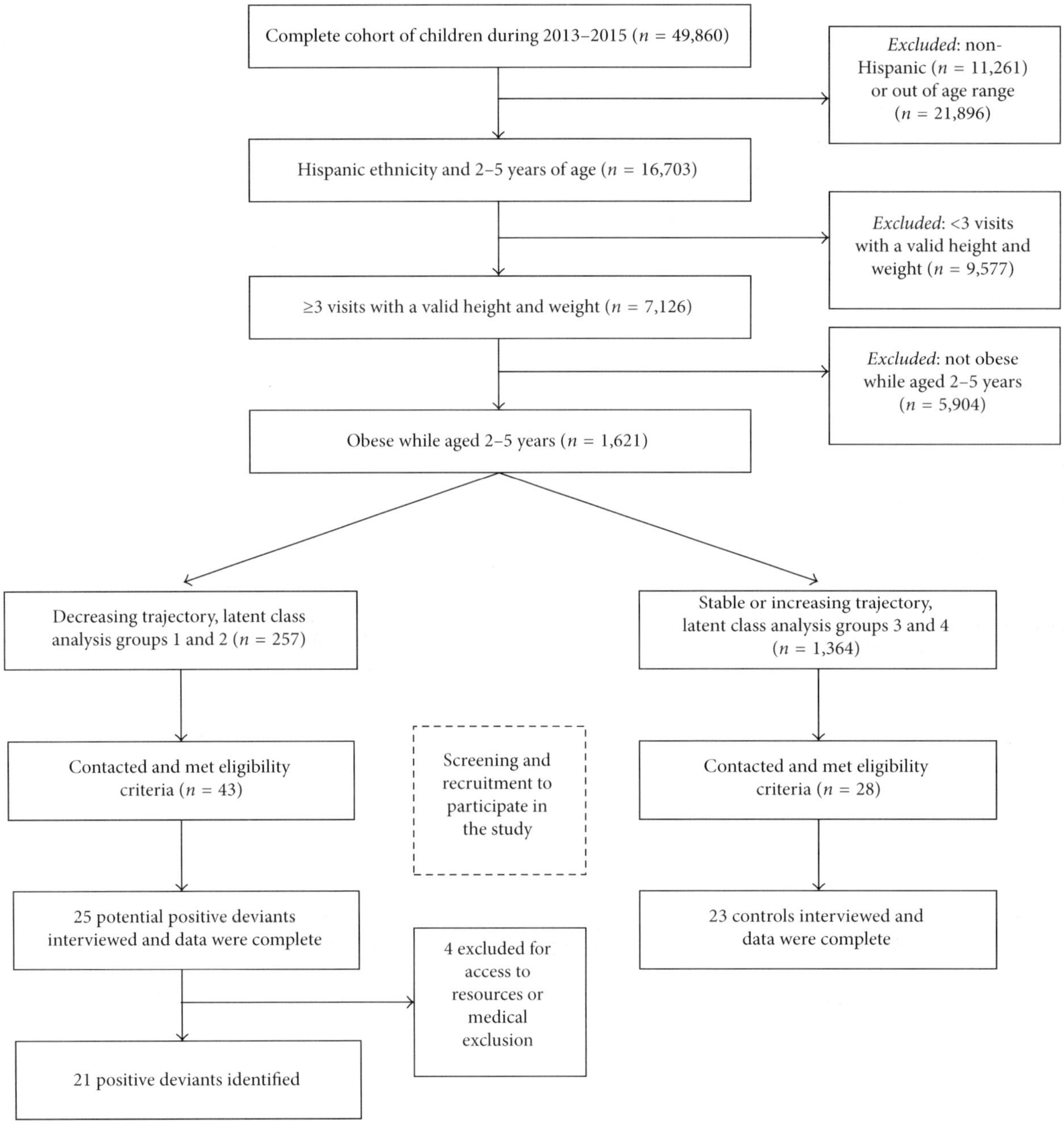

FIGURE 1: Identification of cases (positive deviants) and controls from a large, healthcare data set using inclusion and exclusion criteria as well as latent class trajectories.

2.6. Demographics. The structure of the Behavioral Risk Factor Surveillance System Questionnaire [22] was used to gather demographic characteristics including parental sex, height, weight, race/ethnicity, household size, income, employment, and education.

2.7. Food Frequency Questionnaire. The Block Kids Food Screener (BKFS), developed by NutritionQuest (Berkeley, CA, USA) [23], was administered to parents to assess their child's dietary intake of nutrients and food groups.

2.8. Feeding Practices. The Comprehensive Feeding Practices Questionnaire (CFPQ) [20] consisting of 49 questions and 12 Likert subscales was administered. Parents self-reported the frequency and degree of agreement/disagreement with described practices and behaviors.

2.9. Screen Time, Sleep, and Outside Play. Participating parents were queried on their child's screen time using questions from the National Survey of Early Childhood Health [24]. Previously validated questions about their sleep habits [25] and outside play [26] were asked.

2.10. Food Security. To explore the relationship between food insecurity and obesity among low-income families, we asked questions to parents to assess their level of food insecurity using the US Department of Agriculture's (USDA) questions [27].

2.11. Self-Efficacy. To explore potential relationships between self-efficacy and effective weight maintenance, parents also completed the General Self-Efficacy Scale [28].

2.12. Acculturation. To gauge the differential diversity of acculturation among Latino children in San Antonio, the Acculturation Rating Scale for Mexican Americans-II (ARSMA-II) was administered [29]. This included two subscales on the degree of Anglo and/or Mexican Orientation and three subscales that examined the degree of marginalization.

2.13. Data Analysis

2.13.1. Qualitative. Each semistructured interview was recorded and professionally transcribed in either English or Spanish, and all Spanish interviews were translated to English (Verbal Ink, Los Angeles, USA). Dedoose software was employed to facilitate the collaborative coding process. Each semistructured interview was coded independently by two authors using qualitative description, and differences were resolved through discussion. Qualitative description was used as the analytic method to stay "close" to data and be pragmatic. The purpose of qualitative coding was to capture events and experiences through rich descriptions and not to generate theory from data or serve a deep interpretive function [30, 31].

2.13.2. Quantitative. Descriptive statistics were used to compare the groups by demographic characteristics and their responses to the administered surveys using SPSS 23.0 (IBM, USA). Logistic regression was performed to assess the strongest predictors of positive deviance status (dependent variable) with factors significant on bivariate analysis at $p \leq 0.10$ included in the forward, stepwise regression analyses, using a probability of Wald statistics for variable elimination.

2.14. Ethics and Incentives. This study was approved by the Institutional Review Board of the University of Texas Health Science Center at San Antonio. The Bexar County Translational Advisory Board provided input at all stages of the study. All parents provided written informed consent to participate and received a $50 stipend for their participation.

3. Results

3.1. Identification of Positive Deviants. Of the 49,860 children in the data set from 2013 to 2015, there were 16,703 who were both Latino and 2–5 years of age (Figure 1). Of these, 57% (9,577) were excluded for reason of not having 3 or more visits spread over at least 12 months in order to assess a weight trajectory. Finally, 23% (1,621) of that sample was found to be obese (≥95th BMI percentile for age and sex) during the period and thus eligible for inclusion. From the latent class analysis, 16% (257) of children had a decreasing trajectory over time for their BMI *z*-score (groups 1 or 2) and 84% (1,364) had a stable or increasing trajectory (groups 3 or 4). Of the 257 children with a decreasing trajectory, we were able to contact and screen 43 children who were potentially positive deviants with 25 completing the study visit. Of the 1,364 controls, we screened them for eligibility on a rolling basis as we contacted them, with 23 controls completing the study, matched on ethnicity and insurance. The difference in the recruitment rate can be explained pragmatically: if a control needs to reschedule a visit, we moved onto the next control on the list. However, for positive deviants, given the limited number, we kept attempting to reschedule though that proved futile.

Since the screening did not fully evaluate the degree of access to resources (a core component to determine positive deviance), we reviewed the educational level and income data of the enrolled (potentially positively deviant) participants. Of the positive deviants interviewed, three had access to extra resources (either having a high income or being a medical provider) and one was identified as starting a medication for attention deficit disorder (something not identified at the time of screening). These participants were excluded from the final analysis.

3.2. Demographic Characteristics of Participants. The mean age of children enrolled was 71 months (SD = 15), 22/44 (50%) families reported an income of less than 25,000 USD per year, and 37/44 (84%) were on public insurance (Table 1). About half (24/44) of family members chose to complete the interview and surveys in English and the rest in Spanish. Six subjects reported having private insurance during the interview whose medical record had identified them as having public insurance. The positive deviants had a lower level of education than the controls, with most (69%) having less than a high school education compared with 39% of controls ($p = 0.02$). As expected, the BMI *z*-score was lower at the time of enrollment in the positive deviance group compared with the controls ($p < 0.001$) (Table 1).

3.3. Feeding Practices. Using the Comprehensive Feeding Practices Questionnaire, positive deviants reported a higher level of agreement with practices related to restricting their child's diet to limit less healthy foods and sweets on a Likert scale from 1 to 5, with a mean score of 4.1 (SD = 1.0) versus a mean of 3.5 (SD = 1.0) for controls ($p = 0.06$, *t*-test). There were no differences in the subscales of modeling, food as reward, encouraging balance and variety, the food environment, and restriction for weight control (Table 2).

3.4. Dietary Intake. After screening the food frequency data for quality, 43 children had valid food frequency data. Overall, the two groups were similar in their dietary intake overall with no major differences in nutrient or food group estimates at $p < 0.05$ (Table 2). The only observed difference at the $p < 0.10$ level between positive deviants and controls was lower mean amounts of total protein ($p = 0.09$).

Table 1: Baseline demographic characteristics of study children and parents.

	Controls (n = 23)	Positive deviants (n = 21)	All (n = 44)	p value
Child age (months), mean (SD)[1]	71 (18)	69 (12)	71 (15)	0.75
Child sex (female), n (%)[2]	10 (44%)	10 (48%)	20 (46%)	0.51
Child BMI percentile, median (IQR)[3]	98.8 (96.9–99.3)	93.2 (82.8–96.5)	96.8 (91.6–99.2)	<0.01
Child BMI z-score, mean (SD)[1]	2.17 (0.60)	1.50 (0.72)	1.82 (0.74)	<0.01
Parental age (years), mean (SD)[1]	34 (7)	37 (11)	35 (9)	0.37
Interviewed parent sex (female), n (%)[2]	23 (100%)	20 (95%)	43 (98%)	0.48
Parent BMI, mean (SD)[1]	33 (7)	30 (7)	32 (7)	0.21
Preferred language (English), n (%)[2]	13 (57%)	11 (52%)	24 (55%)	1.0
Hispanic, n (%)[2]	23 (100%)	21 (100%)	44 (100%)	1.0
Household size, median (IQR)[3]	5 (4–6)	4 (3–5)	4 (3–5)	0.13
Income, n (%)[2]				0.47
Less than $25,000	11 (48%)	11 (52%)	22 (50%)	
Less than $50,000	6 (26%)	7 (33%)	13 (30%)	
$50,000 or more	5 (22%)	1 (5%)	6 (14%)	
Not known/not sure	1 (4%)	2 (10%)	3 (7%)	
Marital status, n (%)[2]				0.18
Married	14 (61%)	8 (38%)	22 (50%)	
Divorced/separated	1 (4%)	4 (19%)	5 (11%)	
Never married/member of an unmarried couple	8 (35%)	9 (43%)	17 (39%)	
Education level, n (%)[2]				0.02
Less than high school	9 (39%)	14 (67%)	23 (52%)	
High school diploma or equivalent	3 (13%)	5 (24%)	8 (18%)	
Any college or college graduate	11 (48%)	2 (10%)	13 (30%)	
Insurance, n (%)[2]				0.67
Private	4 (17%)	2 (10%)	6 (14%)	
Public	19 (83%)	18 (86%)	37 (84%)	
None	0	1 (5%)	1 (2%)	

[1]t-test; [2]chi-squared test; [3]Mann–Whitney test.

3.5. Physical Activity, Sleep, and Screen Time. Positive deviants reported higher outside physical activity time per week (p = 0.09). There were no significant differences in reported screen time (data not shown) or sleep patterns between the groups (Table 2).

3.6. Self-Efficacy, Acculturation, and Food Security. Overall, a trend of higher overall self-efficacy was observed in the positive deviant group compared with controls (p = 0.10) (Table 2). There were no differences in the three subscales of self-efficacy (initiative, effort, or persistence).

There was a different distribution of acculturation levels between the positive deviants and controls (p = 0.01) (Table 2), with positive deviants having more of a Mexican orientation. There were no major differences seen in the marginalization subscales (data not shown).

Only 59% of the families had high food security (Table 2). There were no differences by group on food security status as assessed by the USDA measure.

3.7. Multivariable Analysis. For variables associated with being a positive deviant at $p < 0.10$ in the bivariate analysis, we examined the data for potential interactions between significant variables. Across all parents, self-efficacy was positively associated with education and Pearson's correlation coefficient (r) = 0.39 ($p < 0.01$). However, when examining positive deviants and controls separately, this association was only found to be true for controls with r = 0.60 ($p < 0.01$). For positive deviants, there was no significant correlation between general self-efficacy assessed with the GSES and education (r = 0.17; p = 0.46).

Given that education was associated with being a positive deviant and in an unexpected direction, we further examined the subset of parents with low education (less than high school) for differences between positive deviants and controls. Only looking at those with less than a high school education, there was a difference in self-efficacy between positive deviants (mean GSES initiative scale = 4.2 (SD = 0.7)) and controls (mean GSES initiative scale = 3.3 (SD = 1.3); p = 0.04).

Stepwise logistic regression model building for prediction of positive deviance status yielded a final model with variables for self-efficacy and education level with an overall classification accuracy of 74% and a Nagelkerke's R^2 of 0.37. The continuous variable self-efficacy had an estimated OR of 5.0 (95% CI: 1.2–21.2; p = 0.03). The education level less than high school compared with college or more had an estimated OR of 20.1 (95% CI: 2.7–149.6; p = 0.003) and high school compared with college or more had an estimated OR of 17.0 (95% CI: 1.8–163.7; p = 0.01).

3.8. Qualitative Analysis. There were five different thematic foci that emerged from the qualitative data analysis that distinguished positive deviants (Table 3). First, positive deviants created a healthy food environment. They did not favor having unhealthy foods in the house and purposely took healthy foods out of the house with them on outings in

TABLE 2: Parent-reported general self-efficacy, acculturation, food security, child physical activity, child sleep habits, and child dietary patterns between positive deviants and controls.

	Controls ($n = 23$)	Positive deviants ($n = 21$)	All ($n = 44$)	p value
General self-efficacy, mean (SD)				
Overall score	4.24 (0.67)	4.41 (0.48)	4.32 (0.59)	0.10
Initiative score	3.95 (1.04)	4.43 (0.69)	4.18 (0.91)	0.17
Effort score	4.41 (1.07)	4.37 (0.65)	4.39 (0.89)	0.12
Persistence score	4.38 (0.71)	4.43 (0.75)	4.40 (0.72)	0.92
Acculturation levels, n (%)				0.01
Very Mexican oriented	8 (35%)	5 (25%)	13 (30%)	
Mexican oriented to approximately balanced bicultural	5 (22%)	9 (45%)	14 (33%)	
Slightly Anglo oriented bicultural	10 (44%)	2 (10%)	12 (28%)	
Strongly Anglo oriented	0	4 (20%)	4 (9%)	
Food security, n (%)				0.43
High food security	11 (48%)	15 (71%)	26 (59%)	
Marginal food security	6 (26%)	2 (10%)	8 (18%)	
Low food security	5 (22%)	3 (14%)	8 (18%)	
Physical activity				
Days playing outside, mean (SD)	5.2 (1.9)	6.1 (1.7)	5.6 (1.8)	0.11
Time playing outside per day (minutes), mean (SD)	81 (45)	106 (74)	93 (61)	0.18
Active play time (hours per week), mean (SD)	7.2 (5.4)	11.1 (9.3)	9.1 (7.7)	0.09
Sleep				
Sleep (hours per day), mean (SD)	9.9 (1.7)	10.0 (1.0)	10.0 (1.4)	0.90
Child naps (yes), n (%)	7 (30%)	8 (38%)	15 (34%)	0.75
Dietary patterns (estimates shown as mean (SD) intake per day)				
Fruit, including fruit juice (cups)	1.4 (0.7)	1.5 (0.9)	1.4 (0.8)	0.50
Vegetables (cups)	0.6 (0.4)	0.5 (0.3)	0.6 (0.4)	0.84
Potatoes, including French fries (cups)	0.2 (0.2)	0.2 (0.2)	0.2 (0.1)	0.60
Whole grains (ounces)	0.5 (0.3)	0.3 (0.3)	0.4 (0.3)	0.11
Saturated fat (grams)	16.1 (7.3)	13.5 (5.7)	15.0 (6.7)	0.23
Meat, poultry, and fish (ounces)	2.4 (1.5)	1.8 (1.4)	2.1 (1.5)	0.24
Dairy (cups)	1.5 (0.8)	1.4 (0.5)	1.5 (0.7)	0.44
Legumes (cups)	0.2 (0.3)	0.1 (0.1)	0.2 (0.2)	0.55
Sugar added to foods/drink (tsp)	4.9 (2.2)	5.8 (5.2)	5.3 (3.7)	0.47
Energy intake (kcal)	1141 (447)	992 (336)	1080 (407)	0.27
Protein (grams)	51 (22)	40 (15)	47 (20)	0.09
Fat (grams)	46 (20)	38 (17)	43 (19)	0.21
Carbohydrate (grams)	134 (49)	127 (42)	131 (46)	0.61
Fiber (grams)	12 (6)	10 (3)	11 (5)	0.41
Sugars occurring in foods, juice (grams)	65 (25)	72 (28)	68 (26)	0.43
Energy from sugary beverages (kcal)	25 (25)	40 (77)	31 (52)	0.38
Sugary beverages (servings)	0.2 (0.2)	0.2 (0.3)	0.2 (0.2)	0.77
CFPQ scales				
Environment (parents make healthy food available in the home)	4.3 (0.6)	4.2 (0.8)	4.2 (0.7)	0.83
Restriction for health (parents control the child's food intake to limit unhealthy foods)	3.5 (1.0)	4.1 (1.0)	3.8 (1.0)	0.06
Parents use food as reward	2.3 (0.9)	2.1 (0.8)	2.2 (0.9)	0.34
Modeling (parents demonstrate healthy eating)	4.2 (1.0)	4.4 (0.9)	4.3 (0.9)	0.60
Encourage balance and variety	4.3 (0.6)	4.6 (0.6)	4.4 (0.6)	0.18
Restriction for weight control (parents control intake to influence weight)	3.1 (0.9)	2.9 (1.0)	3.0 (1.0)	0.63

kcal = kilocalories; SD = standard deviation.

order to have a healthy option available. Second, positive deviants displayed message consistency: they believed that their child knew what foods they could or could not eat for snacks. Third, positive deviants expressed greater self-efficacy in making changes, for instance, being proactive to overcome their child's picky eating habits in contrast to let it be an ongoing challenge (picky eating was more common in controls). Fourth, positive deviants made incremental changes; for instance, they were more likely to reduce unhealthy snacks rather than trying to

Table 3: Representative quotes for each of the five themes identified from the qualitative description analysis alongside representative quotes from controls where appropriate.

Positive deviants	Controls
1. Creating healthy food environments	
"... why am I going to have this at the house and her being tempting in eating it. I'd rather not have it and this way whenever she opens the refrigerator well she's not going to be tempted." PD13	"They can't just freely go out, open up a bag of chips. They'll say, 'Mom, can I open up these Doritos?' Then, I'll look to see what I have to make sure... and I'll be like, 'All right, well, just get a little bit.'" C1
"That's why I always make sure that they have them in the fridge, because I'd rather them eat as much fruit as they want than have to worry about giving them junk.... they're at the bottom of the fridge drawer. He just opens it." PD5	"...but he likes to steal candy. He'll come in the middle of the night. He'll go in the refrigerator, take the yogurts. He'll take the sweet bread we leave out at night on the table." C12
"When we leave from here, I take a container with fruit for her. Sometimes–she really likes eating celery sticks. I take some celery for her." PD14	"...he's really disciplined, he'll tell me. 'Mommy, can I grab this?' 'Yes.' And potato chips, we do buy potato chips, but I don't let them eat an entire bag." C50
2. Message consistency related to snacks	
"She really knows not to eat junk food, which she can't eat it because we don't have it. When she goes over to her cousins, she doesn't eat there. She knows." PD28	"I noticed that the kids eat dinner over there and I cook dinner of here. There's like a free for all kind of. Yeah, there's was structure for them but it was like if the girls were hungry you know we're going to eat this, we're going to eat that. Just whatever they wanted." C4
"Every Sunday we go out for walks with our bikes and he walks with us, for about two hours." PD2	
3. Confidence in making changes	
"I don't drink soda anymore either, so me and her... It was just something I wanted to do... it hasn't been hard at all." PD23	"I would I like for her to eat veggies, but she doesn't... Yeah, she doesn't like them." C6
"...Just the food part. We're still having challenges on that. Hopefully, we can overcome that and just look for ideas. I'm always on Pinterest. I look at ideas of other parents because I'm pretty sure I'm not the only one that has picky eaters." PD2	"I stay away from certain foods, but I don't... I guess, I do. I stay away from the foods that I know that my doctor would say no to. As far as portions, I've gotten smaller, but that's about it." C8
4. Making incremental changes	
"Go out with them to play. Also before we hardly went out–and if we do not go out at least we do something for a while in the yard, we do activities, run or play or bicycle or so." PD15	"He always wanted the Debbie cakes and ice cream, he was always stuck on peanut butter and jelly and then I changed it." C5
"She would eat like bag of chips too... It's rare now. It's maybe once or twice, she'll eat it during the week." PD23	
5. Engaging the entire family	
"Well, I mean, I figure we're all eating the same thing, because if I make changes with one–then one is going to say, "Why are you guys eating that and the rest are not?" So, everyone is the same. We all eat the same thing." PD12	"I'm not drinking no more soda, so she doesn't drink soda no more... She just drinks when she's with my mom or sister, like I said, or her dad." C9
"I already prohibited him from bringing her candy. I told him, 'You can bring her things that she can eat, but healthy things. Fruit–bring her fruit, any kind of fruit you want to. She loves fruit, apples, grapes.' I did struggle for a while to get him used to it, but it's been a long time since he's brought her that." PD14	"Yeah, because he'll go and he'll ask my grandpa, "Can I have this?" My grandpa will give it to him, even though I've already told my son no. My grandpa doesn't know that so it just depends." C13

eliminate them completely, or were more likely to gradually increase time spent on physical activity rather than abruptly introduce a new rigorous physical activity. Finally, positive deviants successfully engaged the whole family in implementing changes, including engaging the grandparents, and also found opportunities for the whole family to be engaged in a collective physical activity.

What were the notable similarities across groups? Both positive deviants and controls tended to implement rules and limits for the entire family rather than for the individual child. Fathers tended to be more lenient when it came to eating practices in both groups. Controls often described the challenge of other lenient caregivers (fathers and grandparents) feeding their child whatever they wanted, whereas positive deviants largely described this as a challenge they overcame. There were no differences noted in eating together as a family (commonly described), perceptions of good and bad foods, using food as a reward, dealing with food insecurity, grocery shopping, food preparation, serving size, utilization of nutritional assistance, or eating out. The qualitative descriptions of physical activity were remarkably similar between positive deviants and controls in types of activity, frequency, and degree of parent involvement. No differences in the qualitative data were seen in descriptions of use of community resources, food security, health perceptions, parent modeling, or motivations (family members with diabetes being the most common).

Parents were specifically asked about goals or metrics they set related to their children's health and weight. There were no differences in the description of the goal between the groups. The most common goals were age-appropriate clothing sizes, less bullying at school, decreased weight (total body weight), and specific changes in diet patterns (e.g., less-fried foods). Notably, only positive deviants mentioned using doctor visits to track weight.

4. Discussion

This study is novel in utilizing a large healthcare data set to screen growth charts for potential positive deviants and including a set of controls. Furthermore, an in-depth, mixed-methods approach was employed to compare groups. Five primary qualitative themes distinguished positive deviants from the controls. Self-efficacy was identified as a quantitative predictor of positive deviance, despite the positive deviants having a lower level of educational achievement.

The creation of a healthy food environment emerged as a difference between positive deviants and controls in the qualitative data. Notably, there was no difference in parental self-rating of their creation of a healthy food environment on the CFPQ subscale with an overall mean of 4.2 (SD = 0.7) (p = 0.83), perhaps a function of the social desirability bias. Although an association between the home food environment and early childhood obesity has been known [32], only recently have interventions specifically targeted home food environments. An intervention done in a relatively affluent, white population showed a significant reduction in adiposity [33], while an intervention done in a primarily Latino population showed no effect on the home food environment [34]. Family-based interventions that emphasize changes to the home environment have been effective in older age groups [35, 36].

Household-wide rule changes and message consistency were noted in another positive deviance investigation into childhood obesity [17]. In the current study, controls also attempted to implement household-wide rule changes, whereas consistency was in the domain of positive deviants. In the controls, there were multiple examples of parents reporting making household-wide changes to rules and then later describing the different exceptions to those rules. It is notable that the few interventions shown to be effective in this demographic have targeted household routines or emphasized consistency [7, 8].

We identified more restriction related to unhealthy foods but not restriction related to weight status among positive deviants. Restrictive feeding has been hypothesized to contribute to later obesity via the proposed sequelae of overconsumption of restricted, more palatable foods when the restrictions are relaxed [37], although longitudinal data have not confirmed that association [38]. The relationship between restrictive feedings may be in response to weight status [39], and interactions exist between the parenting style, child temperament, and restrictive feeding [40].

Successful engagement of other care providers was unique to positive deviants. Grandparents represented a common care provider, particularly for Latino families [41]. In this study, both grandparents and fathers were described as being more indulgent overall, consistent with prior findings [42]. The key difference in positive deviants was the mother's described ability to effectively change or reign in their indulgent behavior. Although this finding is unique to this study, one of the few other studies using this approach identified a similar construct of social support in positive deviants [43].

Self-efficacy emerged as a predictor of positive deviance in the quantitative data—a finding reinforced in the qualitative descriptions. This finding is consistent with previous studies: interventions designed to facilitate greater self-efficacy (i.e., motivational interviewing) are effective [44, 45]. The qualitative data suggested greater self-efficacy specific to picky eating in positive deviants. Recent longitudinal data on picky eating in early childhood and subsequent weight status have not shown a consistent relationship, although these studies were not done in a Latino population [46, 47]. A recent study in a low-income, mixed race, preschool population found no association between picky eating and obesity but did find an association with healthy eating patterns and picky eating [48]. The picky eating noted among controls in the current study was a significant source of frustration and may also reflect lower general self-efficacy.

The finding of lower education associated with positive deviance status was unexpected. The qualitative data seemed to indicate a pattern of positive deviants listening more to what the doctor told them about their child's weight status compared with controls who more often described the doctor's opinion as incorrect. Lower education has been associated with lower preference for shared decision-making and more paternalistic communication [49], and lower education has been associated with higher vaccine adherence [50]. This finding combined with high general self-efficacy may have contributed to the difference for the positive deviants. Remarkably, the GSES score for positive deviants with less than a high school education was similar to that of the controls with a college education.

We observed a significant association of positive deviance with a slight Mexican orientation on the acculturation scales. Among adults, it has been observed that lower acculturation to the dominant culture in the United States is associated with a healthier lifestyle [51]. However, in contrast to the adult data and our findings, prior studies in children have found an association between obesity and lower acculturation [52–54]. More recent adult data suggest that the observed association may be related to time in the United States and the community context rather than acculturation per se [55].

We observed a lower reported intake of protein among positive deviants compared with controls. In adult studies of dietary interventions for obesity, the data suggest that higher protein intake correlates with greater weight loss [56, 57]. However, our finding is consistent with cohort studies in early childhood examining macronutrient intake [58–60].

In general, positive deviance studies are well positioned to identify novel strategies to address complex problems by using qualitative methods to elicit previously unidentified themes. Notably, most of the studies applying positive deviance to malnutrition [15] are designed to apply findings directly to the community with a very short time between eliciting findings and implementation of the intervention. In contrast, the few studies using the positive deviance approach in obesity [16, 43, 61] have a longer time interval between eliciting findings and intervention in the community.

The vast majority of projects in the field of malnutrition pair up positive deviance with the hearth method of community engagement, teaching the local community about how they can use the findings from their own community in a community health effort. The work on obesity in the United States has been more research-focused. In this context, positive deviance may still provide insight into how to tailor interventions to the population and which components of an intervention are most relevant. Additionally, incorporating findings common across studies such as household-wide implementation of rules may prove to be beneficial.

4.1. Limitations. This study was not powered to detect a difference around the quantitative measures of physical activity, diet, sleep, or other factors. The fact that no major differences emerged in these categories could be either due to a lack of power, potentially social desirability bias in answering the questionnaires driving both responses upwards, or that no differences existed at the time of assessment. Also, parents' reported physical activity and total caloric intake do approximate recommendations in both groups, which may limit the external validity. Using the significance cutoff of $p \leq 0.10$ allowed for identification of possible differences and use of the qualitative data to correlate across data types. However, this increases the possibility of type 1 error. Other limitations include the cross-sectional nature of the collected data and the potential for recall bias as the changes in behaviors or parenting were across time in growth chart trajectories. This study did not investigate data on other siblings' growth trajectories, or the parents' weight changes over the same period. The control group was matched by ethnicity and insurance status; the addition of neighborhood matching could have improved the matching process and controlled for other community-level changes. Although children of 2–5 years were eligible, using the weight trajectory definition of three or more measurements over a one-year period plus the time to conduct the analysis and do recruitment biased the sample toward an older population as seen by the mean age of five years.

5. Conclusion

Using electronic medical records to identify families of children successful in losing their weight identified several behavioral strategies that positively deviant parents employed, for instance, creating healthier food environments, providing consistent messages, effective engagement of caregivers and family members, and a proclivity to encourage incremental changes.

Disclosure

The NIH had no role in the study design, the collection, analysis, and interpretation of data, the writing of the report, or the decision to submit the paper for publication.

Acknowledgments

This study was funded by the National Institutes of Health to BAF with Grant no. K23DK109199.

References

[1] Z. J. Ward, M. W. Long, S. C. Resch, C. M. Giles, A. L. Cradock, and S. L. Gortmaker, "Simulation of growth trajectories of childhood obesity into adulthood," *New England Journal of Medicine*, vol. 377, no. 22, pp. 2145–2153, 2017.

[2] C. L. Ogden, M. D. Carroll, C. D. Fryar, and K. M. Flegal, "Prevalence of obesity among adults and youth: United States, 2011-2014," *NCHS Data Brief*, no. 219, pp. 1–8, 2015.

[3] G. Flores and L. R. Vega, "Barriers to health care access for Latino children: a review," *Family Medicine*, vol. 30, no. 3, pp. 196–205, 1998.

[4] S. M. Davis, O. B. Myers, T. H. Cruz et al., "CHILE: outcomes of a group randomized controlled trial of an intervention to prevent obesity in preschool Hispanic and American Indian children," *Preventive Medicine*, vol. 89, pp. 162–168, 2016.

[5] M. L. Fitzgibbon, M. R. Stolley, L. Schiffer, L. Van Horn, K. KauferChristoffel, and A. Dyer, "Hip-Hop to Health Jr. for Latino preschool children," *Obesity*, vol. 14, no. 9, pp. 1616–1625, 2006.

[6] N. F. Butte, D. M. Hoelscher, S. E. Barlow et al., "Efficacy of a community-versus primary care-centered program for childhood obesity: TX CORD RCT," *Obesity*, vol. 25, no. 9, pp. 1584–1593, 2017.

[7] J. Haines, J. McDonald, A. O'Brien et al., "Healthy habits, happy homes: randomized trial to improve household routines for obesity prevention among preschool-aged children," *JAMA Pediatrics*, vol. 167, no. 11, pp. 1072–1079, 2013.

[8] W. Slusser, F. Frankel, K. Robison, H. Fischer, W. G. Cumberland, and C. Neumann, "Pediatric overweight prevention through a parent training program for 2–4 year old Latino children," *Childhood Obesity*, vol. 8, no. 1, pp. 52–59, 2012.

[9] A. Singhal, "Communicating what works! Applying the positive deviance approach in health communication," *Health Communication*, vol. 25, no. 6-7, pp. 605-606, 2010.
[10] A. Singhal, J. Sternin, and L. Dura, "Combating malnutrition in the land of a thousand rice fields: positive deviance grows roots in Vietnam," *Positive Deviance wisdom series*, vol. 1, pp. 1–8, 2009.
[11] A. Singhal and K. Greiner, "Using the positive deviance approach to reduce MRSA at the Veterans Administration Healthcare System in Pittsburgh," in *Leading Change in Healthcare: Transforming Organizations Using Complexity, Positive Psychology, and Relationship Centered-Care*, A. Suchman, D. Sluyter, and P. Williamson, Eds., pp. 177–209, Radcliffe Publishing, New York, NY, USA, 2011.
[12] D. R. Marsh, D. G. Schroeder, K. A. Dearden, J. Sternin, and M. Sternin, "The power of positive deviance," *BMJ*, vol. 329, no. 7475, pp. 1177–1179, 2004.
[13] M. Zeitlin, "Nutritional resilience in a hostile environment: positive deviance in child nutrition," *Nutrition Reviews*, vol. 49, no. 9, pp. 259–268, 1991.
[14] D. R. Marsh, H. Pachón, D. G. Schroeder et al., "Design of a prospective, randomized evaluation of an integrated nutrition program in rural Vietnam," *Food and Nutrition Bulletin*, vol. 23, no. 4, pp. 36–47, 2002.
[15] J. Costa Machado, R. Minardi Mitre Cotta, and L. Saraiva da Silva, "The positive deviance approach to change nutrition behavior: a systematic review," *Revista Panamericana de Salud Pública*, vol. 36, no. 2, pp. 134–140, 2014.
[16] B. A. Foster, J. Farragher, P. Parker, and D. E. Hale, "A positive deviance approach to early childhood obesity: cross-sectional characterization of positive outliers," *Childhood Obesity*, vol. 11, no. 3, pp. 281–288, 2015.
[17] M. Sharifi, G. Marshall, R. Goldman et al., "Exploring innovative approaches and patient-centered outcomes from positive outliers in childhood obesity," *Academic Pediatrics*, vol. 14, no. 6, pp. 646–655, 2014.
[18] C. Proust-Lima, V. Philipps, A. Diakite, and B. Liquet, *LCMM: Estimation of Latent Class Mixed Models, Joint Latent Class Mixed Models and Mixed Models for Curvilinear Outcomes*, 2013.
[19] J. W. Tukey, *Exploratory Data Analysis*, Addison-Wesley Pub. Co., Boston, MA, USA, 1977.
[20] D. Musher-Eizenman and S. Holub, "Comprehensive feeding practices questionnaire: validation of a new measure of parental feeding practices," *Journal of Pediatric Psychology*, vol. 32, no. 8, pp. 960–972, 2007.
[21] P. A. Harris, R. Taylor, R. Thielke, J. Payne, N. Gonzalez, and J. G. Conde, "Research electronic data capture (REDCap)–a metadata-driven methodology and workflow process for providing translational research informatics support," *Journal of Biomedical Informaticszfvac*, vol. 42, no. 2, pp. 377–381, 2009.
[22] CDC, *Behavioral Risk Factor Surveillance System Questionnaire*, CDC, Atlanta, GA, USA, 2009.
[23] O. Garcia-Dominic, R. P. Treviño, R. M. Echon et al., "Improving quality of Food Frequency Questionnaire response in low-income Mexican American children," *Health Promotion Practice*, vol. 13, no. 6, pp. 763–771, 2012.
[24] S. J. Blumberg, N. Halfon, and L. M. Olson, "The National Survey of Early Childhood Health," *Pediatrics*, vol. 113, no. 6, pp. 1899–1906, 2004.
[25] I. Iglowstein, O. G. Jenni, L. Molinari, and R. H. Largo, "Sleep duration from infancy to adolescence: reference values and generational trends," *Pediatrics*, vol. 111, no. 2, pp. 302–307, 2003.
[26] T. Remmers, S. ML. Broeren, C. M. Renders, R. A. Hirasing, A. van Grieken, and H. Raat, "A longitudinal study of children's outside play using family environment and perceived physical environment as predictors," *International Journal of Behavioral Nutrition and Physical Activity*, vol. 11, no. 1, p. 76, 2014.
[27] USDA, *U.S. Household Food Security Survey Module*, USDA, Washington, DC, USA, 2012.
[28] R. J. Bosscher and J. H. Smit, "Confirmatory factor analysis of the general self-efficacy scale," *Behaviour Research and Therapy*, vol. 36, no. 3, pp. 339–343, 1998.
[29] I. Cuellar, B. Arnold, and R. Maldonado, "Acculturation Rating Scale for Mexican Americans-II: a revision of the original ARSMA scale," *Hispanic Journal of Behavioral Sciences*, vol. 17, no. 3, pp. 275–304, 1995.
[30] S. Sullivan-Bolyai, C. Bova, and D. Harper, "Developing and refining interventions in persons with health disparities: the use of qualitative description," *Nursing Outlook*, vol. 53, no. 3, pp. 127–133, 2005.
[31] M. A. Neergaard, F. Olesen, R. S. Andersen, and J. Sondergaard, "Qualitative description-the poor cousin of health research?," *BMC Medical Research Methodology*, vol. 9, no. 1, p. 52, 2009.
[32] S. M. P. L. Gerards and S. P. J. Kremers, "The role of food parenting skills and the home food environment in children's weight gain and obesity," *Current Obesity Reports*, vol. 4, no. 1, pp. 30–36, 2015.
[33] L. J. Stark, L. M. Clifford, E. K. Towner et al., "A pilot randomized controlled trial of a behavioral family-based intervention with and without home visits to decrease obesity in preschoolers," *Journal of Pediatric Psychology*, vol. 39, no. 9, pp. 1001–1012, 2014.
[34] R. E. Boles, L. Yun, S. J. Hambidge, and A. Davidson, "Influencing the home food and activity environment of families of preschool children receiving home-based treatment for obesity," *Clinical Pediatrics*, vol. 54, no. 14, pp. 1387–1390, 2015.
[35] L. H. Epstein, A. Valoski, R. R. Wing, and J. McCurley, "Ten-year outcomes of behavioral family-based treatment for childhood obesity," *Health Psychology*, vol. 13, no. 5, pp. 373–383, 1994.
[36] B. H. Wrotniak, L. H. Epstein, R. A. Paluch, and J. N. Roemmich, "Parent weight change as a predictor of child weight change in family-based behavioral obesity treatment," *Archives of Pediatrics and Adolescent Medicine*, vol. 158, no. 4, p. 342, 2004.
[37] L. L. Birch and J. O. Fisher, "Mothers' child-feeding practices influence daughters' eating and weight," *American Journal of Clinical Nutrition*, vol. 71, no. 5, pp. 1054–1061, 2000.
[38] K. W. Bauer, J. Haines, A. L. Miller et al., "Maternal restrictive feeding and eating in the absence of hunger among toddlers: a cohort study," *International Journal of Behavioral Nutrition and Physical Activity*, vol. 14, no. 1, p. 172, 2017.
[39] K. E. Rhee, S. M. Coleman, D. P. Appugliese et al., "Maternal feeding practices become more controlling after and not before excessive rates of weight gain," *Obesity*, vol. 17, no. 9, pp. 1724–1729, 2009.
[40] N. Shloim, L. R. Edelson, N. Martin, and M. M. Hetherington, "Parenting styles, feeding styles, feeding practices, and weight status in 4-12 year-old children: a systematic review of the literature," *Frontiers in Psychology*, vol. 6, p. 1849, 2015.
[41] E. R. Pulgarón, A. M. Patiño-Fernández, J. Sanchez, A. Carrillo, and A. M. Delamater, "Hispanic children and the obesity

epidemic: exploring the role of abuelas," *Families, Systems, and Health*, vol. 31, no. 3, pp. 274–279, 2013.

[42] N. Z. Mena, K. Gorman, K. Dickin, G. Greene, and A. Tovar, "Contextual and cultural influences on parental feeding practices and involvement in child care centers among Hispanic parents," *Childhood Obesity*, vol. 11, no. 4, pp. 347–354, 2015.

[43] M. Sharifi, G. Marshall, R. Marshall et al., "Accelerating progress in reducing childhood obesity disparities: exploring best practices of positive outliers," *Journal of Health Care for the Poor and Underserved*, vol. 24, no. 2, pp. 193–199, 2013.

[44] M. Borrello, G. Pietrabissa, M. Ceccarini, G. M. Manzoni, and G. Castelnuovo, "Motivational interviewing in childhood obesity treatment," *Frontiers in Psychology*, vol. 6, p. 1732, 2015.

[45] K. Resnicow, F. McMaster, A. Bocian et al., "Motivational interviewing and dietary counseling for obesity in primary care: an RCT," *Pediatrics*, vol. 135, no. 4, pp. 649–657, 2015.

[46] J. F. Rohde, M. N. Händel, M. Stougaard et al., "Relationship between pickiness and subsequent development in body mass index and diet intake in obesity prone normal weight preschool children," *PLoS One*, vol. 12, no. 3, Article ID e0172772, 2017.

[47] E. E. Antoniou, A. Roefs, S. P. J. Kremers et al., "Picky eating and child weight status development: a longitudinal study," *Journal of Human Nutrition and Dietetics*, vol. 29, no. 3, pp. 298–307, 2016.

[48] C. L. Brown, E. M. Perrin, K. E. Peterson et al., "Association of picky eating with weight status and dietary quality among low-income preschoolers," *Academic Pediatrics*, vol. 18, no. 3, pp. 334–341, 2017.

[49] A. Schneider, T. Körner, M. Mehring, M. Wensing, G. Elwyn, and J. Szecsenyi, "Impact of age, health locus of control and psychological co-morbidity on patients' preferences for shared decision making in general practice," *Patient Education and Counseling*, vol. 61, no. 2, pp. 292–298, 2006.

[50] D. A. Salmon, L. H. Moulton, S. B. Omer, M. P. DeHart, S. Stokley, and N. A. Halsey, "Factors associated with refusal of childhood vaccines among parents of school-aged children: a case-control study," *Archives of Pediatrics and Adolescent Medicine*, vol. 159, no. 5, pp. 470–476, 2005.

[51] R. Pérez-Escamilla, "Acculturation, nutrition, and health disparities in Latinos," *American Journal of Clinical Nutrition*, vol. 93, no. 5, pp. 1163–1167, 2011.

[52] C. Lind, G. G. Mirchandani, B. C. Castrucci, N. Chávez, A. Handler, and D. M. Hoelscher, "The effects of acculturation on healthy lifestyle characteristics among Hispanic fourth-grade children in Texas public schools, 2004-2005," *Journal of School Health*, vol. 82, no. 4, pp. 166–174, 2012.

[53] J. P. Moreno, E. Vaughan, D. Hernandez, R. T. Cameron, J. P. Foreyt, and C. A. Johnston, "The impact of acculturation level on weight status and weight outcomes in Hispanic children," *Journal of Racial and Ethnic Health Disparities*, vol. 3, no. 4, pp. 582–589, 2016.

[54] M. Fialkowski, R. Ettienne, R. Rivera et al., "Ethnicity and acculturation: do they predict weight status in a longitudinal study among Asian, Hispanic, and non-Hispanic White early adolescent females?," *Adolescent Health, Medicine and Therapeutics*, vol. 6, p. 1, 2015.

[55] C. R. Isasi, G. X. Ayala, D. Sotres-Alvarez et al., "Is acculturation related to obesity in Hispanic/Latino adults? Results from the Hispanic Community Health Study/Study of Latinos," *Journal of Obesity*, vol. 2015, Article ID 186276, 8 pages, 2015.

[56] T. P. Wycherley, L. J. Moran, P. M. Clifton, M. Noakes, and G. D. Brinkworth, "Effects of energy-restricted high-protein, low-fat compared with standard-protein, low-fat diets: a meta-analysis of randomized controlled trials," *American Journal of Clinical Nutrition*, vol. 96, no. 6, pp. 1281–1298, 2012.

[57] O. Ajala, P. English, and J. Pinkney, "Systematic review and meta-analysis of different dietary approaches to the management of type 2 diabetes," *American Journal of Clinical Nutrition*, vol. 97, no. 3, pp. 505–516, 2013.

[58] T. Voortman, K. VE. Braun, J. C. Kiefte-de Jong, V. WV. Jaddoe, O. H. Franco, and E. H. van den Hooven, "Protein intake in early childhood and body composition at the age of 6 years: the Generation R Study," *International Journal of Obesity*, vol. 40, no. 6, pp. 1018–1025, 2016.

[59] A. Beyerlein, U. M. Uusitalo, S. M. Virtanen et al., "Intake of energy and protein is associated with overweight risk at age 5.5 years: results from the prospective TEDDY study," *Obesity*, vol. 25, no. 8, pp. 1435–1441, 2017.

[60] L. Pimpin, S. Jebb, L. Johnson, J. Wardle, and G. L. Ambrosini, "Dietary protein intake is associated with body mass index and weight up to 5 y of age in a prospective cohort of twins1,2," *American Journal of Clinical Nutrition*, vol. 103, no. 2, pp. 389–397, 2016.

[61] H. L. Stuckey, J. Boan, J. L. Kraschnewski, M. Miller-Day, E. B. Lehman, and C. N. Sciamanna, "Using positive deviance for determining successful weight-control practices," *Qualitative Health Research*, vol. 21, no. 4, pp. 563–579, 2011.

23

Determinants of Walking among Middle-Aged and Older Overweight and Obese Adults: Sociodemographic, Health, and Built Environmental Factors

Samuel N. Forjuoh,[1,2] Marcia G. Ory,[2] Jaewoong Won,[3] Samuel D. Towne Jr.,[2] Suojin Wang,[4] and Chanam Lee[3]

[1] *Department of Family & Community Medicine, Baylor Scott & White Health, College of Medicine, Texas A&M Health Science Center, Temple, TX, USA*
[2] *Department of Health Promotion & Community Health Sciences, School of Public Health, Texas A&M University, College Station, TX, USA*
[3] *Department of Landscape Architecture & Urban Planning, College of Architecture, Texas A&M University, College Station, TX, USA*
[4] *Department of Statistics, College of Science, Texas A&M University, College Station, TX, USA*

Correspondence should be addressed to Samuel N. Forjuoh; samuel.forjuoh@bswhealth.org

Academic Editor: Eliot Brinton

Background. This study examined the association between selected sociodemographic, health, and built environmental factors and walking behaviors of middle-aged and older overweight/obese adults. *Methods.* Subjective data were obtained from surveys administered to community-dwelling overweight/obese adults aged ≥50 years residing in four Texas cities from October 2013 to June 2014, along with objective data on neighborhood walkability (Walk Score™). Multivariate logistic regression identified factors predicting the odds of walking the recommended ≥150 minutes per week for any purpose. *Results.* Of 253 participants, the majority were non-Hispanic white (81.8%), married (74.5%), and male (53.4%) and reported an annual income of ≥$50,000 (65.5%). Approximately, half were employed (49.6%) or had at least a college degree (51.6%). Walking the recommended ≥150 minutes per week for any purpose (n = 57, 22.5%) was significantly associated with having at least a college degree (OR = 5.55, 95% CI = 1.79–17.25), having no difficulty walking a quarter of a mile (OR = 5.18, 95% CI = 1.30–20.83), and being unemployed (OR = 3.25, 95% CI = 1.18–8.93) as well as perceived presence of sidewalks/protected walkways (OR = 3.56, 95% CI = 1.10–11.50) and perceived absence of distracted drivers in the neighborhood (OR = 4.08, 95% CI = 1.47–11.36). *Conclusion.* Addressing neighborhood conditions related to distracted drivers and pedestrian infrastructure may promote walking among middle-aged and older overweight/obese individuals.

1. Introduction

The global public health burden of obesity is well established as is the influence of physical activity on the health and well-being of individuals who are overweight or obese [1, 2]. In the United States, obesity is a major public health problem for all ages, but particularly for middle-aged and older adults who do not seem to engage in adequate physical activity. This is a timely issue given projections that those aged 65 years or older are expected to nearly double between 2012 and 2050 [3]. In fact, obesity is higher among middle-aged and older adults than among their younger counterparts [4]. Approximately two-thirds of the adult population in the United States is overweight and nearly one-third is obese [4, 5], yet most do not get adequate physical activity [6].

The federal 2008 Physical Activity Guidelines for Americans recommend adults to avoid inactivity and have at least 150 minutes of moderate-intensive aerobic activity weekly and muscle-strengthening activities on two or more days every week. For older adults who cannot do 150 minutes of moderate-intensive aerobic activity due to chronic conditions, the recommendation is for them to be physically active as their abilities and conditions allow [7]. However, most middle-aged and older adults do not meet this guideline. In 2014, the percentage of adults aged 45–54 years and 55–64 years who met the federal 2008 Physical Activity Guidelines for Americans for both aerobic activity and muscle-strengthening exercise was 19.3% and 16.1%, respectively, compared to 25.1% and 31.1% for those aged 25–44 years and 18–24 years, respectively. The corresponding rates for those aged 65–74 years and 75 years or older were 14.4% and 7.9%, respectively [8]. Physical activity in old age is particularly important for disease prevention, health maintenance, quality of life, overall independence, and fall prevention [7, 9, 10]. Preventing or delaying chronic diseases is a salient issue as nearly nine in 10 older adults have at least one chronic condition, with nearly three in four having at least two chronic conditions [11]. Thus, identifying factors that may lessen the burden of chronic disease as individuals age is especially timely with this rapidly aging population [3].

Although there are numerous ways to be physically active, walking is one of the most popular and frequently recommended forms of physical activity, especially for middle-aged and older adults who may have difficulty with certain forms of rigorous physical activity and in line with the current recommendation of ≥150 minutes of exercise per week (as opposed to specifying 30 minutes of moderate-intensity exercise five days per week) for older adults [12, 13]. In fact, walking or jogging was rated the highest among older adults' favorite activities in a large nationally representative sample of older adults [14].

Walking is important for preventing obesity as well as promoting better health and reducing healthcare costs for those who are already obese [15, 16]. Cognizant of the physical activity guidelines by the physicians in our setting [17], walking was cited as the most common activity recommended by family physicians for their obese patients, along with bicycling and swimming [18]. Regular physical activity such as walking can prevent or ameliorate the effects of many chronic conditions that afflict middle-aged and older adults, lower their quality of life, and contribute to the leading causes of death. Therefore, promoting walking as a form of physical activity in middle-aged and older adults can directly benefit them through improved quality of life and reduced burden of chronic conditions. This is especially true for middle-aged and older adults who are overweight or obese.

While prior studies have uncovered predictors of walking among older adults, including the barriers and motivators [19, 20], less is known about the predictors of walking among middle-aged and older adults who are overweight or obese. The predictors for the latter population could be different given the added morbidity or chronic medical condition to their aging condition. In an exploratory study, Lee et al. [21] addressed barriers and motivators to walking among overweight and obese adults, but the sample included all adults aged 18 years or older and the focus was on age variations in barriers or motivators with little mention of health predictors of walking among this population. They, however, concluded that overweight and obese adults may experience considerable modifiable environmental barriers to walking.

This study examined factors associated with the walking behaviors of middle-aged and older overweight and obese adults, focusing on the influence of selected sociodemographic, health, and built environmental factors. In line with the behavioral-environment health model [21], it is important to understand which multilevel factors are most correlated with reported walking as a form of physical activity. Additionally important is having both subjective and objective measures of the built environment.

2. Methods

2.1. Study Design, Setting, and Participants. A cross-sectional survey was conducted from October 2013 to June 2014 in a large university-affiliated, integrated multispecialty healthcare system associated with a 220,000-member Health Maintenance Organization in four central Texas cities (Temple, Killeen, College Station, and Bryan). These cities included peri-urban environments where urban and rural features coexist within cities, which can exhibit diverse neighborhood contexts with a range of street and development patterns from car-dependent to fairly walkable environments. The survey used a standardized, online, and paper questionnaire that included open-ended and multiple choice questions. Study participants were community-dwelling overweight or obese adults aged ≥50 years residing in one of the four cities and seen by a family physician in a primary care clinic in the previous three years who reported some level of walking as a form of physical activity. Objective data were also collected using Walk Score to capture walkability (i.e., accessibility to destinations) of the survey respondent's residential neighborhood. The study protocol was reviewed and approved by the Institutional Review Boards of Baylor Scott & White Health and the Texas A&M University.

2.2. Recruitment Procedure and Data Collection. Details of the research methods, including the procedures for recruitment and data collection, have been published elsewhere [19, 22, 23]. In brief, participants were recruited via electronic medical records (EMRs) that were utilized to conduct initial patient screening by age and geographic residence. Primary care providers were then provided with a list generated from the EMRs to identify potentially eligible patients from a sampling list, from which 7,543 recruitment letters were sent out. The sample was restricted to those who (a) had no difficulty reading, writing, and speaking English; (b) were not terminally ill; and (c) did not live in a nursing home or assisted-living community. In order to ensure patients' capability of walking as a form of physical activity, screening questions on the ability to walk in their neighborhood without major difficulty or for a quarter of a mile (approximately 2-3 city blocks) or for about 5–10 minutes were included at the front of the survey instrument.

The link to the online survey was sent to participants who opted for the online version (69.5%) via provided email addresses, while paper surveys were mailed to those who opted for the paper version (30.5%) to their provided addresses. Designed to take approximately 20 minutes to complete, the survey included questions on sociodemographic, health, and built environmental factors potentially related to walking. Previously validated or tested instruments including the Behavioral Risk Factor Surveillance System developed by the Centers for Disease Control and Prevention [24], Starting-The-Conversation developed by the University of North Carolina Prevention Partners [25], the International Physical Activity Questionnaire [26], and the Neighborhood Environment Walkability Scale [27] informed the survey. Each participant was offered a $10 gift card at the completion of the survey.

2.3. Study Measures. The primary study outcome measure was walking the recommended ≥150 minutes per week for any purpose. This measure of walking behavior was obtained by combining two survey items that estimated walking days for any purpose in a typical week and walking minutes for any purpose in each day. The outcome variable was dichotomized into (a) walking ≥150 minutes per week for any purpose (as a proxy for meeting the federal 2008 Physical Activity Guidelines for Americans) and (b) walking <150 minutes per week for any purpose (as a proxy for not meeting the guidelines for physical activity).

We used Walk Score as one of our predictor variables to measure walkability of each participant's residential environment [28–30]. Walk Score is calculated based on an accessibility-based measure to various walkable destinations from home, providing an objective and disaggregated estimate of walkability around each participant's residence. Walk Score can be used to categorize areas that are walkable (Walk Score ≥ 50) versus those that are car-dependent (Walk Score < 50) [28]. Neighborhood perception, captured from the survey, was conceptualized with several questions related to the built environments that focused on (1) neighborhood safety from traffic, for example, "There is so much traffic along nearby streets that it makes it difficult or unpleasant to walk in my neighborhood"; (2) neighborhood safety from crime, for example, "My neighborhood streets are well lit at night"; (3) neighborhood safety from physical injury risks, for example, "There are many broken sidewalks in my neighborhood"; (4) behavioral factors in neighborhood safety, for example, "There are many distracted drivers in my neighborhood (e.g., on the cell phone while driving)"; (5) social aspects of the neighborhood, for example, "People in my neighborhood know each other"; and (6) attractiveness of the neighborhood, for example, "There are many attractive buildings, homes or gardens to see in my neighborhood."

Other predictor variables were also captured from the survey and included anthropometric (i.e., being overweight or obese), social interaction (e.g., someone to walk with, dog in household), and demographic characteristics (e.g., age, gender, education) as well as health (e.g., difficulty walking for a quarter of a mile and health condition) variables.

2.4. Statistical Analyses. Descriptive statistics were used to characterize participants' anthropometric and sociodemographic data as well as their health conditions, walking, and built environmental behaviors. Pearson chi-square tests were then used to assess differences between participants who reported walking versus not walking the recommended ≥150 minutes per week. Finally, multivariate logistic regression was used to predict walking the recommended ≥150 minutes per week for any purpose using the selected sociodemographic, health, and built environmental factors. Those variables that showed statistical significance in the bivariate tests and were clinically sensible and plausible were added to the multivariate model. Adjusted odds ratios and 95% confidence limits of the final multivariate model are reported. All analyses were conducted in 2016 using Stata 13 (StataCorp, College Station, TX). Statistical significance was set at the $P < 0.05$ level.

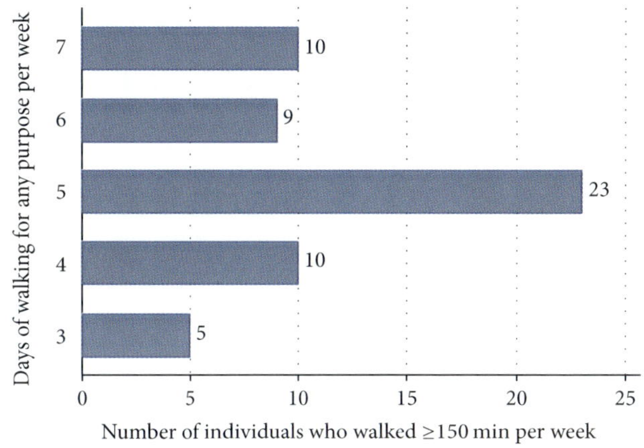

FIGURE 1: Number of days of walking for any purpose by middle-aged and older overweight and obese individuals who walked ≥150 minutes per week.

3. Results

3.1. Survey Response and Walking Behaviors. Of the 496 patients who participated in the survey (adjusted response rate, 6.8%), 102 participants were excluded for not meeting the study eligibility criteria (e.g., did not live in our study areas, lived in assisted facilities, and aged <50 years) or screening criteria (e.g., did not walk) or completing the survey. Of the remaining 394 participants, 141 were excluded for not being overweight or obese. Analyses for this study were therefore based on the remaining 253 participants who were overweight or obese adults, of whom 57 (22.5%) reported walking the recommended ≥150 minutes per week for any purpose.

Of the 57 who reported walking the recommended ≥150 minutes per week for any purpose, most (40.4%, $n = 23$) reported walking 5 days per week, 17.5% ($n = 10$) reported walking 7 days per week, and another 17.5% ($n = 10$) reported walking 4 days per week, while 15.8% ($n = 9$) reported walking 6 days per week and 8.8% ($n = 5$) reported walking 3 days per week (Figure 1). The most popularly used places for walking were the neighborhood streets, green places with water features, and malls or shopping centers (Figure 2).

3.2. Anthropometric, Demographic, and Health Characteristics. Of the total sample who were overweight or obese adults

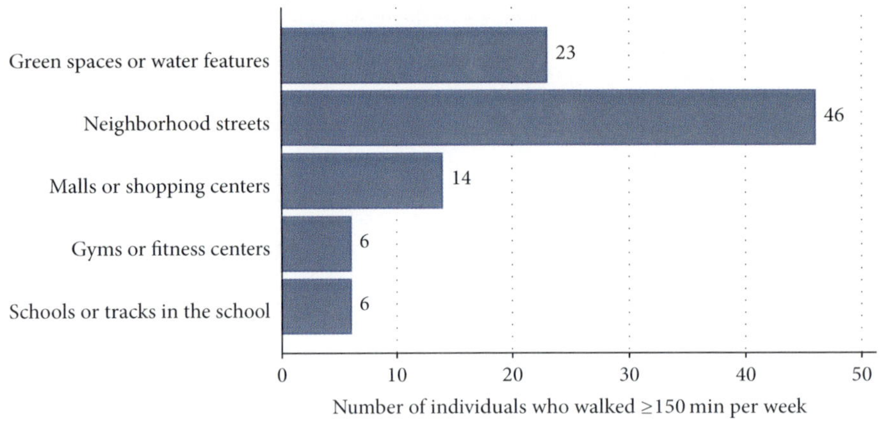

FIGURE 2: Places for walking for any purpose by middle-aged and older overweight and obese individuals who walked ≥150 minutes per week.

(n = 253), the majority were overweight (55.7%), non-Hispanic white (81.8%), married (74.5%), and male (53.4%) and reported an annual household income of ≥$50,000 (65.4%). Approximately, half were aged ≥65 years (48.2%), employed (49.6%), or had at least a college degree (51.6%). They were generally healthy, with 51.0% reporting very good to excellent health and 35.6% reporting good health. Overall, 23.8% reported having a little or some difficulty walking for a quarter of a mile. Nearly half of them reported receiving a primary care provider recommendation to be more physically active (Table 1).

3.3. Social Support and Built Environmental Characteristics. Table 2 summarizes the bivariate social support and built environmental characteristics of the overweight or obese participants. Few respondents reported having caregiving responsibilities for elders (15.1%), while a substantial number reported having a dog in the household (41.9%), and almost half of them reported having someone to walk with (49.0%). The vast majority (91.3%) resided in less walkable or car-dependent areas (Walk Score < 50) than walkable areas (Walk Score ≥ 50). The mean and median Walk Scores were 20.4 and 17.0, respectively, with a range from 0 to 72. However, no significant differences were seen between those who walked the recommended ≥150 minutes per week for any purpose and those who did not in terms of these social support variables.

Of the built environmental factors related to neighborhood safety from traffic, one showed a significant difference between those overweight or obese adults who walked the recommended ≥150 minutes per week for any purpose and those who did not. Among those overweight or obese adults who walked the recommended ≥150 minutes per week for any purpose, significantly more participants strongly agreed/agreed that there are crosswalks and pedestrian signals to help walkers cross busy streets in the neighborhood than those who strongly disagreed/disagreed (26.4% versus 18.2%, P = 0.01). Similarly, one variable among the built environmental factors related to neighborhood safety from physical injury risk showed a significant difference between the two groups. Significantly more overweight or obese participants strongly agreed/agreed that they were worried about falling when walking in the neighborhood than those who strongly disagreed/disagreed (25.4% versus 11.4%, P = 0.045). None of the other built environmental variables related to neighborhood safety from crime and behavioral risk factors showed statistically significant differences.

3.4. Factors Associated with Walking the Recommended ≥150 Minutes per Week for any Purpose among Overweight or Obese Adults in Multivariate Model. The strongest determinants of overweight or obese participants walking the recommended ≥150 minutes per week for any purpose in a multivariate model (Table 3) were related to respondent's educational levels and favorable neighborhood perceptions. Compared to those with a high school diploma or some college, participants with a college degree or higher were more than five times as likely to walk the recommended ≥150 minutes per week for any purpose (OR = 5.55, 95% CI = 1.79–17.25). Walking the recommended ≥150 minutes per week for any purpose was significantly associated with participants who strongly disagreed/disagreed that there were many distracted drivers (e.g., on the cell phone while driving) in their neighborhood (OR = 4.08, 95% CI = 1.47–11.36) and those who strongly agreed/agreed that there are sidewalks or protected walkways (e.g., walking trails) in their neighborhood (OR = 3.56, 95% CI = 1.10–11.50). Those employed were significantly less likely to walk the recommended ≥150 minutes per week compared to those unemployed (OR = 0.31, 95% CI = 0.11–0.85) as were those who reported some difficulty walking for a quarter of a mile (OR = 0.19, 95% CI = 0.05–0.77).

Nearly threefold more participants strongly disagreed/disagreed that drivers do not yield to pedestrians or bicyclists in the neighborhood than those who strongly agreed/agreed, meaning that most felt that drivers do yield. The disagreement with "Drivers do not yield to pedestrians or bicyclists in my neighborhood" predicted a borderline association with extra walking (P = 0.087). As would be expected, there was a positive relationship between extra walking and having a dog in the household, although the trend was also only borderline in strength (P = 0.098). Being overweight or obese and health condition as well as other social interaction

TABLE 1: Anthropometric, demographic, and health characteristics of study participants.

Variable	Total participants (N = 253)		Walked ≥150 min per week for any purpose (n = 57)		Walked <150 min per week for any purpose (n = 196)		P value
	FREQ[a]	%	FREQ[a]	%[b]	FREQ[a]	%[b]	
Weight status							0.94
Overweight	141	55.7	32	22.7	109	77.3	
Obese	112	44.3	25	22.3	87	77.7	
Age group (years)							0.65
50–64	131	51.8	28	21.4	103	78.6	
≥65	122	48.2	29	23.8	93	76.2	
Gender							0.63
Male	135	53.4	32	23.7	103	76.3	
Female	118	46.6	25	21.2	93	78.8	
Race/ethnicity							0.53
Other	46	18.2	12	26.1	34	73.9	
Non-Hispanic white	206	81.8	45	21.8	161	78.2	
Marital status							0.22
Divorced/widowed	64	25.5	11	17.2	53	82.8	
Married/living with a partner	187	74.5	46	24.6	182	75.4	
Education							**0.012**[*]
High school or some college	118	48.4	18	15.2	100	84.8	
College graduate or graduate	126	51.6	36	28.6	90	71.4	
Employment							0.198
Not employed	126	50.4	33	26.2	93	73.8	
Employed	124	49.6	24	19.3	100	80.7	
Annual household income							0.070
<\$50,000	85	34.6	14	16.5	71	83.5	
≥\$50,000	161	65.4	43	26.7	118	73.3	
Difficulty walking for a quarter of a mile							**0.002**[**]
Not at all difficult	192	76.2	52	27.1	140	72.9	
Only a little/somewhat	60	23.8	5	8.3	55	91.7	
Health condition							0.37
Poor to fair	34	13.4	5	14.7	29	85.3	
Good	90	35.6	19	21.1	71	78.9	
Very good to excellent	129	51.0	33	25.6	96	74.4	
Received PCP recommendation to be more physically active							0.177
No	130	51.8	34	26.1	96	73.9	
Yes	121	48.2	23	19.0	98	81.0	

Boldface indicates statistical significance ($^{*}P < 0.05$; $^{**}P < 0.01$). [a]May not add to total due to missing data. [b]Row %. PCP = primary care provider.

factors such as having someone to walk with and care-giver responsibilities for elders as well as Walk Score were not significantly associated with the odds of walking the recommended ≥150 minutes per week for any purpose among overweight or obese adults.

Counter-intuitively, walking the recommended ≥150 minutes per week for any purpose was significantly associated with participants who strongly agreed/agreed that most drivers exceeded the posted speed limits while driving, strongly disagreed/disagreed that walkers and bikers on the streets can be easily seen, and strongly agreed/agreed that there is so much traffic along nearby streets (Table 3).

4. Discussion

In this cross-sectional study of community-dwelling overweight and obese adults aged 50 years or older in central Texas, 22.5% reported walking the recommended ≥150

Table 2: Social and built environmental characteristics of study participants' neighborhood.

Variable	Total participants (N = 253)		Walked ≥150 min per week for any purpose (n = 57)		Walked <150 min per week for any purpose (n = 196)		P value
	FREQ[a]	%	FREQ[a]	%[b]	FREQ[a]	%[b]	
Someone to walk with							0.75
No	129	51.0	28	21.7	101	78.3	
Yes	124	49.0	29	23.4	95	76.6	
Have caregiving responsibilities for elders							0.80
No	214	84.9	49	22.9	165	77.1	
Yes	38	15.1	8	21.0	30	79.0	
Dog in household							0.21
No	147	58.1	29	19.7	118	80.3	
Yes	106	41.9	28	26.4	78	73.6	
Walk Score (WS)							0.61
WS < 50 (less walkable)	231	91.3	53	22.9	178	77.1	
WS ≥ 50 (walkable)	22	8.7	4	18.2	18	81.8	
†There is so much traffic along nearby streets that it makes it difficult to walk							0.35
Strongly agree/agree	73	28.7	19	26.4	53	73.6	
Strongly disagree/disagree	181	71.3	37	20.9	140	79.1	
†Most drivers exceed the posted speed limits while driving in my neighborhood							0.94
Strongly agree/agree	120	47.8	27	22.5	93	77.5	
Strongly disagree/disagree	131	52.2	30	22.9	101	77.1	
†There are sidewalks or protected walkways (e.g., trails) in my neighborhood							0.12
Strongly disagree/disagree	110	44.0	20	18.2	90	81.8	
Strongly agree/agree	140	56.0	37	26.4	103	73.6	
†There are crosswalks and pedestrian signals to help walkers cross busy streets							**0.01***
Strongly disagree/disagree	163	65.5	28	17.2	135	82.8	
Strongly agree/agree	86	34.5	27	31.4	59	68.6	
‡My neighborhood streets are well lit at night							0.44
Strongly disagree/disagree	109	43.1	22	20.2	87	79.8	
Strongly agree/agree	144	56.9	35	24.3	109	75.7	
‡Walkers and bikers on the streets can be easily seen by people from their homes							0.98
Strongly disagree/disagree	162	65.3	36	22.2	126	77.8	
Strongly agree/agree	86	34.7	19	22.1	67	77.9	
‡I see and speak to other people when I am walking in my neighborhood							0.07
Strongly disagree/disagree	42	16.7	5	11.9	37	88.1	
Strongly agree/agree	210	83.3	52	24.8	158	75.2	

Table 2: Continued.

Variable	Total participants ($N = 253$)		Walked ≥150 min per week for any purpose ($n = 57$)		Walked <150 min per week for any purpose ($n = 196$)		P value
	FREQ[a]	%	FREQ[a]	%[b]	FREQ[a]	%[b]	
[¥]There are many broken sidewalks in my neighborhood							0.57
Strongly agree/agree	63	25.2	16	25.4	47	74.6	
Strongly disagree/disagree	187	74.8	41	21.9	146	78.1	
[¥]I am worried about falling when I walk in my neighborhood							**0.045**[*]
Strongly agree/agree	205	82.3	52	25.4	153	74.6	
Strongly disagree/disagree	44	17.7	5	11.4	39	88.6	
[¥]My neighbors could be counted on to help in case of need							0.16
Strongly disagree/disagree	42	16.7	6	14.3	36	85.7	
Strongly agree/agree	210	83.3	51	24.3	159	75.7	
[$]There are many distracted drivers in my neighborhood (e.g., on phone while driving)							0.199
Strongly agree/agree	156	61.7	31	19.9	125	80.1	
Strongly disagree/disagree	97	38.3	26	26.8	71	73.2	
[$]Drivers do not yield to pedestrians or bicyclists in my neighborhood							0.26
Strongly agree/agree	83	33.6	15	18.1	68	81.9	
Strongly disagree/disagree	164	66.6	40	24.4	124	75.6	
[$]There is drug dealing in my neighborhood							0.43
Strongly agree/agree	211	85.8	49	23.2	162	76.8	
Strongly disagree/disagree	35	14.2	6	17.1	29	82.7	

Boldface indicates statistical significance ([*] $P < 0.05$). [a]May not add to total due to missing data. [a]Row %. [†]Traffic safety. [‡]Crime safety. [¥]Physical injury risk safety. [$]Behavioral risk safety.

TABLE 3: Adjusted ORs and 95% CI of walking the recommended ≥150 minutes per week for any purpose.

Variable	OR	95% CI	*P* value
Education			
High school or some college	1.00	—	
College graduate or graduate school	5.55	1.79–17.25	**0.003****
Difficulty walking for a quarter of a mile			
Not at all difficult	1.00	—	
Only a little or somewhat difficult	0.19	0.05–0.77	**0.020***
There are many distracted drivers in the neighborhood			
Strongly agree/agree	1.00	—	
Strongly disagree/disagree	4.08	1.47–11.36	**0.007****
There are sidewalks or protected walkways in neighborhood			
Strongly disagree/disagree	1.00	—	
Strongly agree/agree	3.56	1.10–11.50	**0.034***
Drivers do not yield to pedestrians or bicyclists			
Strongly agree/agree	1.00	—	
Strongly disagree/disagree	2.67	0.87–8.22	0.087
¶Most drivers exceed the posted speed limits while driving			
Strongly disagree/disagree	1.00		
Strongly agree/agree	2.85	1.10–7.41	**0.031***
¶Walkers and bikers on the streets can be easily seen			
Strongly agree/agree	1.00		
Strongly disagree/disagree	4.00	1.17–13.70	**0.027***
¶There is so much traffic along nearby streets			
Strongly disagree/disagree	1.00		
Strongly agree/agree	4.33	1.47–12.66	**0.008****
Employment			
Not employed	1.00	—	
Employed	0.31	0.11–0.85	**0.022***
Annual household income			
<$50,000	1.00	—	
≥$50,000	1.55	0.47–5.20	0.474
Age group (years)			
50–64	1.00	—	
≥65	0.87	0.30–2.51	0.791
Race/ethnicity			
Other	1.00	—	
Non-Hispanic white	0.35	0.10–1.21	0.096
Marital status			
Divorced, widowed, separated, or never married	1.00	—	
Married or living with a partner	0.73	0.20–2.63	0.625
Gender			
Male	1.00	—	
Female	0.78	0.30–2.06	0.621
Weight status			
Overweight	1.00	—	
Obese	1.30	0.52–3.26	0.570

TABLE 3: Continued.

Variable	OR	95% CI	P value
Health condition			
Poor to fair	1.00	—	
Good	3.13	0.47–20.67	0.237
Very good to excellent	6.87	0.96–49.33	0.055
Someone to walk with			
No	1.00	—	
Yes	0.51	0.19–1.38	0.183
Dog in household			
No	1.00	—	
Yes	2.07	0.87–4.90	0.098
Has caregiving responsibilities for elders			
No	1.00	—	
Yes	0.64	0.17–2.33	0.495
Walk Score			
Less walkable	1.00	—	
Walkable	1.71	0.40–7.27	0.467

$N = 209$. Likelihood Ratio Chi^2 = 53.33 ($P = 0.014$). Pseudo $R^2 = 0.245$. Boldface indicates statistical significance ($^*P < 0.05$; $^{**}P < 0.01$). ¶Counter-intuitive association.

minutes per week for any purpose and three personal variables, including having at least a college degree, not having any difficulty walking for a quarter of a mile, and not being employed, were identified as significant personal level determinants of walking the recommended ≥150 minutes per week for any purpose after controlling for other covariates. Unfortunately, no comparable state or national data on the percentage of overweight and obese adults in a comparable age group who walked ≥150 minutes per week could be found.

From the neighborhood built environmental variables, strong disagreement with the perception that there are many distracted drivers (e.g., on the cell phone while driving) in one's neighborhood was found to be positively associated with walking the recommended ≥150 minutes per week for any purpose. Further, strong agreement that there are sidewalks or protected walkways (e.g., trails) in one's neighborhood was found to be associated with the increased odd of walking ≥150 minutes per week for any purpose. Thus, the relative importance of having sidewalks and protected walkways in one's neighborhood for walking can serve as a target for environmental interventions that focus on either maintaining or building such structures. It is also possible that those who walk more are more likely to know the pedestrian infrastructure in the neighborhood, such as sidewalks and walkways. Therefore, programs and campaigns to increase awareness of pedestrian infrastructure available in the neighborhood, as well as policies aimed to reduce distracted drivers, may also require further attention as components of future walking intervention programs. To the best of our knowledge, this is the first study to assess determinants of walking among a population of overweight and obese middle-aged and older adults. However, these factors are the same as found for older adults of all weight status, including normal weight [19].

Features in the built environment may be more favorable for certain segments of the population such as those who are more educated, less healthy, unemployed, or retired [31]. In the current study, walking the recommended ≥150 minutes per week for any purpose was found to be associated with individuals with at least a college degree and those unemployed possibly including those who are retired. Higher education can enhance an individual's knowledge about health promotion, including the need for more physical activity such as walking [32, 33] even for those who may be overweight or obese as found in this study. Thus, those seeking to promote physical activity campaigns and other interventions can use the results of this study to set targets and to tailor marketing materials. Similarly, physicians seeking to encourage patients to be more active may also use this information to target and tailor encouragement for physical activity to particularly at-risk patients (e.g., those with lower educational levels). Also, being unemployed or retired may be associated with the needed time to engage in more physical activity such as walking [34].

Safety from traffic and behavioral risks such as that found in this study, along with safety from crime and injury risks, are among the foremost factors for promoting walking [35]. Exposure of middle-aged or older adults to increased risks of being hit by a distracted driver due to lack of sidewalks or protected walkways may deter them from walking. In fact, older adults bear disproportionately high rates of fatality from traffic crashes, accounting for 18% of all pedestrian deaths, although they account for only 13% of the total population [36]. Neighborhoods without distracted drivers and with ample safety features such as sidewalks or protected walkways will definitely promote walking even among middle-aged and older overweight and obese adults.

Despite the fact that the majority of the participants in this study resided in less walkable areas, one in five reported walking the recommended ≥150 minutes per week for any purpose. This finding is encouraging and may imply that enhancing the walkability of the neighborhood will make more individuals walk in their neighborhood. Prior studies have shown associations between higher neighborhood walkability and decreased prevalence of overweight and obesity, possibly via increased physical activity such as walking [37, 38].

Several seemingly counter-intuitive associations were found with walking the recommended ≥150 minutes per week for any purpose. These included strong agreement that most drivers exceeded the posted speed limits while driving and that there was so much traffic along nearby streets making it difficult or unpleasant to walk in one's neighborhood as well as strong disagreement that walkers and bikers on the neighborhood streets can be easily seen by people from their homes and were rather unusual. However, these findings are likely due to the increased awareness of or sensitivity to those neighborhood conditions influencing pedestrians among those who walk more. For example, those who walk a lot (meeting the recommended ≥150 minutes) are more likely to witness and consider inadequate driver behaviors, lack of visual surveillance, and heavy traffic to be problematic. The observation of so much traffic can be balanced with some observed positive, albeit insignificant, driver behavior of yielding to pedestrians or bicyclists. This observation may indicate that heavy traffic is associated with neighborhood walking, but safe driving behaviors should be encouraged. Although designing the roadway to reduce traffic is very important, driver behavior towards pedestrians may be more important for promoting neighborhood walking.

Our study had some limitations that must be taken into consideration in the interpretation of the findings. First, the limitation of our study to the selected four sites reduces the generalizability of the findings as was the exclusion of non-English speaking subjects which may have missed others, particularly Hispanics, who are a large subset with documented overweight and obesity problems. Second, our study had a very low response rate, further impacting the generalizability of study findings. However, this is typical of studies that depend on EMRs for subject recruitment [21, 39], and the actual refusal rate once a patient was identified was rather very low (0.15%, 11 out of 7,543). Further, our intent was to explore the associations between different correlates and walking behaviors in an understudied population rather than to conduct a larger more national epidemiological study. Third, the survey item for walking behavior we used was "how many days in a typical week do you walk in your neighborhood." We did not thoroughly define respondents' neighborhood boundary, and the definition might have been different across respondents. Finally, the cross-sectional design of the study precludes determination of causality.

5. Conclusions

In conclusion, we found that neighborhood perceptions and built environmental characteristics appear to be important determinants of the walking behaviors of middle-aged and older overweight and obese individuals as presented previously [40] and to be presented in an upcoming conference [41]. Enhancing the neighborhood environments, especially those related to pedestrian walkways, driver behaviors, visual surveillance, and traffic conditions, has the potential to promote walking among these individuals as well as the general population. Such enhancement may include providing walking trails and beautiful neighborhoods conducive for walking. However, these neighborhood environment enhancements ought to take cognizance of the needs of middle-aged and older individuals who may be overweight or obese.

Disclosure

This paper was presented, in part, at the 5th World Conference on Controversies & Consensus in Diabetes, Obesity, and Hypertension, Istanbul, Turkey, Nov. 5–7, 2015.

Acknowledgments

The authors thank Vanessa Hoelscher for study coordination and Phyllis Davis for secretarial duties. The study was supported by Baylor Scott & White Health Institutional Research Fund (no. 120803).

References

[1] Y. C. Wang, K. McPherson, T. Marsh, S. L. Gortmaker, and M. Brown, "Health and economic burden of the projected obesity trends in the USA and the UK," *The Lancet*, vol. 378, no. 9793, pp. 815–825, 2011.

[2] J. M. Jakicic, B. H. Marcus, K. I. Gallagher, M. Napolitano, and W. Lang, "Effect of exercise duration and intensity on weight loss in overweight, sedentary women: a randomized trial," *Journal of the American Medical Association*, vol. 290, no. 10, pp. 1323–1330, 2003.

[3] J. M. Ortman, V. A. Velkoff, and H. Hogan, *An aging nation: the older population in the United States*, US Census Bureau, Washington, DC, USA, 2014.

[4] C. L. Ogden, M. D. Carroll, B. K. Kit, and K. M. Flegal, "Prevalence of childhood and adult obesity in the United States, 2011-2012," *The Journal of the American Medical Association*, vol. 311, no. 8, pp. 806–814, 2014.

[5] K. M. Flegal, D. Carroll, B. K. Kit, and C. L. Ogden, "Prevalence of obesity and trends in the distribution of body mass index among US adults, 1999–2010," *Journal of the American Medical Association*, vol. 307, no. 5, pp. 491–497, 2012.

[6] Centers for Disease Control and Prevention, "One in five adults meet overall physical activity guidelines, 2016," http://www.cdc.gov/media/releases/2013/p0502-physical-activity.htm.

[7] U.S. Department of Health and Human Services, *2008 Physical Activity Guidelines for Americans*, U.S. Department of Health and Human Services, Washington, DC, USA, 2008.

[8] National Center for Health Statistics, *Health, United States, 2015: With Special Feature on Racial and Ethnic Health Disparities*, Hyattsville, MD, USA, 2016.

[9] W. Chodzko-Zajko, *ACSM's Exercise for Older Adults*, Lippincott Williams & Wilkins, 2013.

[10] B. Elsawy and K. E. Higgins, "Physical activity guidelines for older adults," *American Family Physician*, vol. 81, no. 1, pp. 55–59, 2010.

[11] G. Anderson, *Chronic Care: Making The Case for Ongoing Care*, Robert Wood Johnson Foundation, Princeton, NJ, USA, 2010.

[12] K. E. Mobily, "Walking among older adults," *World Leisure Journal*, vol. 56, no. 2, pp. 130–140, 2014.

[13] "Exercise Recommendations for Older Adults, 2016," http://www.todaysgeriatricmedicine.com/news/ex_092210_03.shtml.

[14] S. L. Szanton, R. K. Walker, L. Roberts et al., "Older adults' favorite activities are resoundingly active: findings from the NHATS study," *Geriatric Nursing*, vol. 36, no. 2, pp. 131–135, 2015.

[15] I.-M. Lee and D. M. Buchner, "The importance of walking to public health," *Medicine and Science in Sports and Exercise*, vol. 40, no. 7, pp. S512–S518, 2008.

[16] M. E. Nelson and S. C. Folta, "Further evidence for the benefits of walking," *American Journal of Clinical Nutrition*, vol. 89, no. 1, pp. 15-16, 2009.

[17] Y. Hong, M. G. Ory, C. Lee, S. Wang, J. Pulczinski, and S. N. Forjuoh, "Walking and neighborhood environments for obese and overweight patients: perspectives from family physicians," *Family Medicine*, vol. 44, no. 5, pp. 336–341, 2012.

[18] S. N. Forjuoh, C. Lee, S. Wang, Y. Hong, and M. G. Ory, "Family physicians? perception on environmental influences in promoting physical activity in their obese patients," *Open Journal of Preventive Medicine*, vol. 02, no. 04, pp. 423–428, 2012.

[19] M. G. Ory, S. D. Towne, J. Won, S. N. Forjuoh, and C. Lee, "Social and environmental predictors of walking among older adults," *BMC Geriatrics*, vol. 16, no. 1, article no. 155, 2016.

[20] J. Van Cauwenberg, P. Clarys, I. De Bourdeaudhuij et al., "Physical environmental factors related to walking and cycling in older adults: the Belgian aging studies," *BMC Public Health*, vol. 12, no. 1, article no. 142, 2012.

[21] C. Lee, M. G. Ory, J. Yoon, and S. N. Forjuoh, "Neighborhood walking among overweight and obese adults: age variations in barriers and motivators," *Journal of Community Health*, vol. 38, no. 1, pp. 12–22, 2013.

[22] S. D. Towne, J. Won, S. Lee et al., "Using walk score™ and neighborhood perceptions to assess walking among middle-aged and older adults," *Journal of Community Health*, vol. 41, no. 5, pp. 977–988, 2016.

[23] S. N. Forjuoh, C. Lee, J. Won, S. D. Towne, S. Wang, and M. G. Ory, "Correlates of receiving a recommendation for more physical activity from a primary care provider," *American Journal of Preventive Medicine*, vol. 52, no. 2, pp. 207–214, 2016.

[24] Centers for Disease Control and Prevention, *Behavioral Risk Factor Surveillance System survey data*, Department of Health and Human Services, Centers for Disease Control and Prevention, Atlanta, Ga, 2009.

[25] A. E. Paxton, L. A. Strycker, D. J. Toobert, A. S. Ammerman, and R. E. Glasgow, "Starting the conversation: performance of a brief dietary assessment and intervention tool for health professionals," *American Journal of Preventive Medicine*, vol. 40, no. 1, pp. 67–71, 2011.

[26] The International Physical Activity Questionnaire, "Short Last 7 Days Self-Administered Format, 2002," http://www.ipaq.ki.se.

[27] E. Cerin, B. E. Saelens, J. F. Sallis, and L. D. Frank, "Neighborhood environment walkability scale: Validity and development of a short form," *Medicine and Science in Sports and Exercise*, vol. 38, no. 9, pp. 1682–1691, 2006.

[28] Walk Score™, "Walk score methodology, 2016," https://www.walkscore.com/methodology.shtml.

[29] D. T. Duncan, J. Aldstadt, J. Whalen, S. J. Melly, and S. L. Gortmaker, "Validation of Walk Score® for estimating neighborhood walkability: an analysis of four US metropolitan areas," *International Journal of Environmental Research and Public Health*, vol. 8, no. 11, pp. 4160–4179, 2011.

[30] L. J. Carr, S. I. Dunsiger, and B. H. Marcus, "Walk Score™ as a global estimate of neighborhood walkability," *American Journal of Preventive Medicine*, vol. 39, no. 5, pp. 460–463, 2010.

[31] A. Forsyth, R. C. Brownson, and K. Day, "The built environment, walking, and physical activity: is the environment more important to some people than others?" *Transportation Research Part D: Transport and Environment*, vol. 14, no. 1, pp. 42–49, 2009.

[32] A. K. Van Der Bij, M. G. H. Laurant, and M. Wensing, "Effectiveness of physical activity interventions for older adults—a review," *American Journal of Preventive Medicine*, vol. 22, no. 2, pp. 120–133, 2002.

[33] C. L. Craig, R. C. Brownson, S. E. Cragg, and A. L. Dunn, "Exploring the effect of the environment on physical activity: a study examining walking to work," *The American Journal of Preventive Medicine*, vol. 23, no. 2, pp. 36–43, 2002.

[34] S. Chung, M. E. Domino, S. C. Stearns, and B. M. Popkin, "Retirement and physical activity: analyses by occupation and wealth," *American Journal of Preventive Medicine*, vol. 36, no. 5, pp. 422–428, 2009.

[35] J. Won, C. Lee, S. N. Forjuoh, and M. G. Ory, "Neighborhood safety factors associated with older adults' health-related outcomes: a systematic literature review," *Social Science and Medicine*, vol. 165, pp. 177–186, 2016.

[36] National Highway Traffic Safety Administration, *Traffic Safety Facts 2009*, Department of Transportation, Washington, DC, USA, 2009.

[37] M. Chiu, B. R. Shah, L. C. Maclagan, M.-R. Rezai, P. C. Austin, and J. V. Tu, "Walk score® and the prevalence of utilitarian walking and obesity among Ontario adults: a cross-sectional study," *Health Reports*, vol. 26, no. 7, pp. 3–10, 2015.

[38] M. I. Creatore, R. H. Glazier, and Moineddetal, "Association of neighborhood walkability with change in overweight, obesity, and diabetes," *Journal of the American Medical Association*, vol. 315, no. 20, pp. 2211–2220, 2016.

[39] J. Murphy, M. Schwerin, J. Eyerman, and J. Kennet, "Barriers to survey participation among older adults in the national survey on drug use and health: The importance of establishing trust," *Survey Practice*, vol. 1, no. 2, 2008.

[40] S. N. Forjuoh, M. G. Ory, J. W. Won, S. Towne, S. J. Wang, and C. Lee, "Socio-environmental correlates of walking among overweight and obese older adults in an integrated healthcare system," in *Proceedings of the 5th World Conference on Controversies & Consensus in Diabetes, Obesity, and Hypertension*, Istanbul, Turkey, Nov 5–7, 2015.

[41] S. N. Forjuoh, M. G. Ory, J. W. Won, S. Towne, S. J. Wang, and C. Lee, "Determinants of walking among middle-aged and older overweight and obese adults: Demographic, health, and socio-environmental factors," in *Proceedings of the 19th International Conference on Obesity*, Singapore, Singapore, Jul 4-5, 2017.

"Culture Is So Interspersed": Child-Minders' and Health Workers' Perceptions of Childhood Obesity

Roger Figueroa,[1] Jaclyn Saltzman,[2] Jessica Jarick Metcalfe,[2] and Angela Wiley[3]

[1] *University of Illinois at Urbana-Champaign, 905 South Goodwin Ave., 230 Bevier Hall MC-180, Urbana, IL 61801, USA*
[2] *University of Illinois at Urbana-Champaign, 904 W. Nevada St., #1014, MC-081, Urbana, IL 61801, USA*
[3] *University of Illinois at Urbana-Champaign, 904 W. Nevada St., #2004, MC-081, Urbana, IL 61801, USA*

Correspondence should be addressed to Roger Figueroa; rfiguer2@illinois.edu

Academic Editor: Sharon Herring

Introduction. Forty-one million children globally are overweight or obese, with most rapid rate increases among low- and middle-income nations. Child-minders and health workers play a crucial role in obesity prevention efforts, but their perceptions of childhood obesity in low- and middle-income countries are poorly understood. This study aims to (1) explore child-minders and health workers' perceptions of the causes, consequences, potential strategies, and barriers for childhood obesity prevention and intervention in Cape Town, South Africa and (2) to provisionally test the fit of a socioecological framework to explain these perceptions. *Methods.* Twenty-one interviews were recorded, transcribed, and analyzed through analytic induction. *Results.* Participants identified multilevel factors and contexts, as well as potential consequences and priorities of interest in addressing childhood obesity. An adapted childhood obesity perceptions model was generated, which introduces an overarching cultural dimension embedded across levels of the socioecological framework. *Conclusions.* Culture plays a pivotal role in explaining obesogenic outcomes, and the results of this study demonstrate the need for further research investigating how obesity perceptions are shaped by cultural frames (e.g., social, political, and historical). Understanding the causes, consequences, and potential interventions to address obesity through a cultural lens is critical for promoting health in low- and middle-income nations.

1. Introduction

The World Health Organization reports that nearly 41 million children globally are overweight or obese, with the most rapid increases in overweight and obesity rates reported in low- and middle-income nations [1]. As low-income countries shift to participate more in the global economy, obesity and malnutrition emerge as simultaneous health burdens [2]. Low- and middle-income countries such as South Africa have a high rate of childhood obesity across all economic levels and age groups [3], with rural youth affected most by underweight and urban youth affected most by overweight [4]. It is important to note that South Africa has been recently classified as an upper-middle income country but has a significant number of low-income settings within its borders, due in part to the 23.9% unemployment rate [5].

Childhood obesity is a particularly challenging phenomenon because it predicts obesity in adulthood, as well as cardiovascular and metabolic disease, but is resistant to treatment in the majority of cases [6–8]. South Africa has the highest obesity rates in Africa [3, 9, 10]. Rates of obesity and overweight among South African children are increasing at a similar pace as developed countries in prior decades at 13.5% [11], suggesting further research on implementing successful interventions to address this issue is needed.

Given the country's complicated history embedded in its cultural, economic, and political landscapes, it is imperative that researchers and policymakers avoid overgeneralizing Westernized views and data when designing interventions for childhood obesity in South Africa. Specifically, the effects of Apartheid-era policies and current unemployment and homelessness rates [12, 13] may reduce the effectiveness of intervention and prevention programs that were developed in high-income nations with different economic, health, and education infrastructure. It is also important to highlight South Africa's racial and cultural make-up, including Native

Africans, European descendants (whites), and coloured (predominantly mixed race descendants from East and Central Africa) as well as Asian descendants [14]. Baseline data on South African perceptions related to childhood obesity are needed to underpin effective intervention in this multifaceted context.

Risk for childhood obesity cannot be traced to one specific factor but is rather the result of numerous interacting contributors across levels of influence, as previously proposed in the Six C's Model [15]. Bronfenbrenner's ecological model provides grounding for this transdisciplinary framework that explores risk and protective factors for childhood obesity, at the cellular, child, clan, community, country, and cultural levels (Figure 1). The Six C's Model of childhood obesity presents a framework for considering these contributing factors across concentric levels of influence [15]. Harrison and colleagues summarized the literature on biological (cell), psychological/behavioral (child), social and familial (clan), economic and political (community and country), and cultural predictors of childhood obesity in the United States in order to create the Six C's Model. The Six C's Model, like other socioecological approaches, conceptualizes the individual as embedded within the context of development over time and poses that factors within the concentric contexts are bidirectionally influential [15]. For example, a factor within the community sphere (e.g., school lunch availability and nutritional quality) is affected by the national economy (country sphere) and in turn has the potential to affect family finances (clan), child eating behavior (child), and ultimate adiposity (cell). However, the model's generalizability across cultures has not yet been explored. For the purposes of this study, culture can be defined as a system of shared and learned patterns of thoughts consisting not only of practical information about the world but also of values, attitudes, and beliefs [16].

Culturally rich accounts are important because—depending on a country's historical, political, social, and economic context—fat (or obesity) serves as a cultural indicator of such disparate characteristics as benevolence, greed, wealth, success, power, and failure [17]. Simply put, culture shapes how individuals perceive obesity [18, 19]. These and other interacting contributors across socioecological levels play a crucial role in how individuals may perceive obesity.

It is important to examine *perceptions* about childhood obesity using a theoretical framework as a first step toward addressing multiple factors contributing to childhood obesity. Understanding how members of the public perceive the causes of obesity promotes discussion of relevance to public health practitioners. Specifically, theory-based research on obesity perceptions will allow researchers to identify whether key figures in South African obesity prevention efforts will view obesity according to the relatively well-accepted social constructions of the phenomenon (e.g., obesity as "epidemic," socially acceptable discrimination of obese individuals) [20]. The job of public health and medical professionals is to provide an avenue to healthful behavior, sensitive to public perceptions of what it means to be obese. However, given that obesity is a health issue complicated by social stigma that varies from culture to culture, it is critical that practitioners are aware of how obesity is perceived. To be obese is not simply to be perceived as being fat, or not thin, or not fitting some societally proscribed standard of beauty. To be obese is to have a ratio of weight for height that is strongly correlated with increased risk for cardiovascular disease, stroke, diabetes, or arthritis in joints [21]. To be obese is to be told to lose weight or suffer the consequences described above [22], but then to be given no viable long-term options for the prescribed weight loss [23]. Thus, culturally informed examination of perceptions of obesity is critical in order for researchers and practitioners to identify promising avenues for prevention and intervention.

Understanding patient perceptions about obesity and its consequences may give providers opportunities to prescribe health behavior change to their patients in a sensitive manner (e.g., taking into account patients readiness to engage in healthy habits for health versus lose weight). Using objective indicators—such as cholesterol levels, blood pressure, or oxygen uptake—to discuss obesity-related health problems may be a more fruitful path to behavior change than focusing on weight loss alone [24]. Importantly, it is clear that shaming patients into weight loss is not an effective method to change nutrition and physical activity behaviors [25]. In order to change health behaviors at the individual and family levels, researchers must first identify how relevant stakeholders perceive obesity in specific communities and cultures, before prevention and intervention efforts can be developed or addressed.

Child-minders (called child care providers in some contexts) and health workers are important components of the community sphere in the Six C's Model, because they provide valuable health information to patients, clients, and community members. Both groups have access to children and their parents and provide support for children's health and well-being. Community-based prevention tools can be effectively implemented in their places of work including schools, hospitals, early childhood education programs, and through the media [3, 26]. A study exploring perceptions about risk factors for obesity among low-income Latinos in Texas found parents, caregivers, and health workers as important players in preventing obesity among children [27]. Health workers are central to the prevention and treatment of childhood obesity; parents, schools, and society in general consistently turn to providers regarding weight-related health [28]. Given this and considering the limited time spent during medical training on nutrition and physical activity [29], clinicians are prime targets for intervention [30].

While child-minders and health workers are important agents in the health ecology of children, little research has tested the fit of novel theories to their perceptions about the causes and consequences of childhood obesity. Even less work has explored this among care providers in low- and middle-income countries. Being able to explore the current perceptions of these professionals using a sound theoretical framework would allow for identification of areas for further intervention and involvement of stakeholders in addressing childhood obesity.

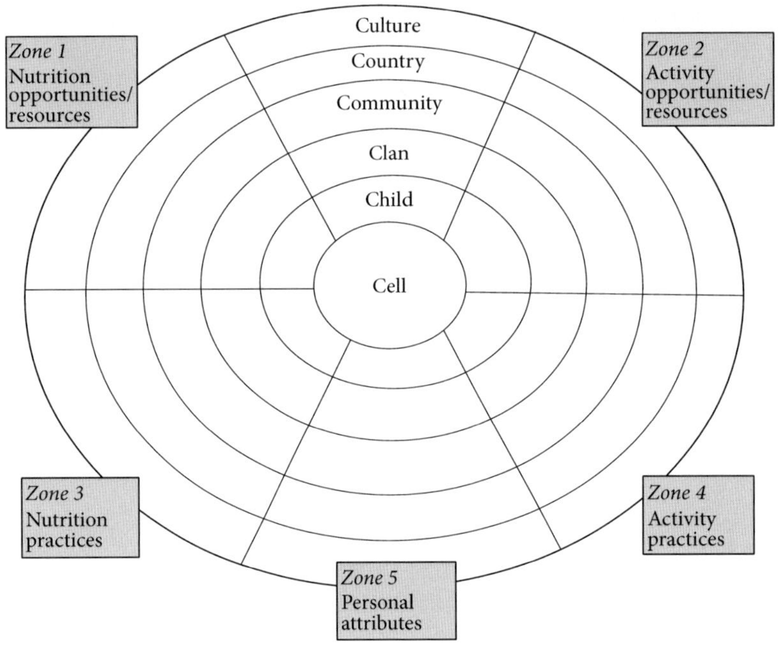

FIGURE 1: The Six C's Ecological Developmental Model of contributors to overweight and obesity in childhood [15].

This study uses an existing socioecological framework to explore the current perceptions of childhood obesity among a purposive sample of child-minders and health workers in Cape Town, South Africa. Our first aim (Aim 1) is to qualitatively explore perceived causes and consequences of, as well as the perceived strategies for and barriers to, addressing childhood obesity among health workers and child-minders in Cape Town, South Africa. Our second aim (Aim 2) is to examine whether the perceptions and understandings of childhood obesity among child-minders and health workers can be organized according to a preexisting socioecological model of childhood obesity (Figure 1). Focusing on these objectives using a qualitative approach will support further initiatives in testing the relationship between the theoretical fit of actual and perceived factors associated with childhood obesity in low- and middle-income countries.

2. Materials and Methods

Recently, there has been a call for more qualitative work focused on obesity that allows for more detailed and nuanced insights about obesity [31]. More specifically, Perez and Ball [31] have found that, of current publications focused on obesity, qualitative studies only account for approximately 1% of the total studies. This study aims to reduce this gap in the literature by qualitatively examining perceptions of obesity among South Africans.

2.1. Research Design. Semistructured in-depth interviews were conducted between January and June 2014 in Cape Town, South Africa. We used an adapted obesity perceptions interview protocol [27] with questions organized by levels and constructs of a transdisciplinary (TD) conceptual framework (Six C's) to explore participants' perceptions of the multiple levels of influence on children's obesity risk (see the following list). In this study, the target population was child-minders and health workers. The research ethics board at the University of Illinois at Urbana-Champaign approved this study (IRB Reference number: 14411).

Adapted Semistructured Facilitation Protocol for Conducting Interviews [27]

(1) Introductory Remarks

(1a) Introductions

(1b) Consent forms

(1c) Ground rules: timing, reinforcement of no right or wrong answers, confidentiality.

(1d) Audio-recording initiation (if applicable)

(2) Exploration of childhood obesity perceptions

In general, what would you say are the main causes to "overweight or obesity" in children?

Probing questions:

What consequences are you most concern about?

How concerned are you about childhood obesity in your community? Why?

What roles do the following play in child obesity? If possible, please expand as to why.

(2a) What is the role of a child or an individual in childhood obesity?

(2b) What are the roles of family and friends in childhood obesity?

TABLE 1: Key characteristics of study sites in Cape Town, South Africa.

	Khayelitsha	Rondebosch	Heideveld
Region	Western Cape, CT	Western Cape, CT	Western Cape, CT
Size of study area	10,000/km^2	2,300/km^2	9,600/km^2
Population of study area	391,749	14,591	17,388
Race/Ethnicity & Language information within region*	*Race:* Black African (98.6%), Coloured (0.6%); *Language:* Xhosa (90.5%), English (3.2%)	*Race:* White (62.7%), Black African (16.5%), Coloured (9.6%), Indian/Asian (6.1%); *Language:* English (84.3%), Afrikaans (7.6%), Other (8.1%)	*Race:* Black African (5.3%), Coloured (92.3%); *Language:* Afrikaans (63.1%), English (34.4%)
Number of interviewees	12	1	8
Recruitment Strategy		Purposeful; Snowball Sampling	

*These data were not collected among participants. Source: [42–44].

(2c) What are the roles of parents in childhood obesity?

(2d) What are the roles of grandparents in childhood obesity?

(2e) What are the roles of childcare providers (child-minders) in childhood obesity?

(2f) What are the roles of health Provider in childhood obesity?

(2g) What is the role of the community (e.g., schools, environment) in child obesity?

(2h) What is the role of the government in childhood obesity?

(2i) What is the role of media in childhood obesity?

(2j) What is the role of culture in childhood obesity?

Probing questions:

How and why they play a role in child obesity?

(3) In your opinion, what would be helpful for the community you work with to prevent childhood obesity?

(3a) Are there any potential solutions?

(3b) Are there any intervention strategies to address childhood obesity?

(3c) Would you name any major barriers to such?

(4) Concluding remarks

Would participant like to add anything else to this discussion?

(4a) No further comments conclude the interview.

(4b) Thank participants very much for being part of this research study!

(4c) Participants receive incentive valued in $10 as an appreciation token for their time.

2.2. Recruitment and Data Collection. Following IRB approval, participants were recruited using a purposive sampling technique (i.e., snowball sampling) [32]. Under the purposive sampling assumptions participants were screened to reflect the following inclusion criteria: (1) willing to do interviews in English, unless they had communicated prior to the face-to-face meeting that they would like to bring a translator on site, (2) over 21 years of age, and (3) currently employed as a health worker or child-minder in the Cape Town area. Project collaborators provided a preestablished list of potential study sites. These sites were contacted using e-mail notifications and face-to-face visits with a recruitment letter describing study criteria. As recruitment of participants who met criteria proceeded, snowball sampling was used to allow participants to identify more participants with similar characteristics (i.e., other known child-minders and health workers) to contribute rich information to this study. This population was of interest to us because they serve as health information outlets [27] and might be key players in the prevention of child obesity [33–37]. Each participant gave written, informed consent prior to participating in the present study. Initially, sample size requirements were informed by Creswell [38, 39], in which is suggested that a sample size between 20 and 30 participants would lead to theoretical saturation. In addition, Francis and colleagues [40] have found that theory-based interview studies including health workers would reach theory-based saturation between interviews 13 and 17. These findings are fairly consistent with Guest and colleagues [41], who reported that the first 12 interviews produced 97% of the main codes in their results.

2.3. Participants. There were twenty-one (21) participants in this study. Initially, 13 participants were recruited in January 2014 in Cape Town, South Africa, in the communities of Khayelitsha and Rondebosch. A second round of interviews with 8 new participants took place in May and June 2014 in the community of Heideveld (see Table 1). Interviews took approximately 30 minutes on average. Participants completed a demographic questionnaire, which included questions regarding age, gender, income, years living in South Africa and Cape Town, and language. They self-reported their occupation and education. Individual interviews were conducted by the first author and were audio-recorded (n = 16). Participants also had the option to opt out of the audio portion of the interview (n = 5) by typing their answers to the interview protocol independently and emailing them to the first author. Participants' remuneration for their time was valued at $10 USD (approximately 150 ZAR). With the exception of one interview, all interviews were conducted in English. A translator was on site to assist in an interview with a child-minder who preferred to communicate in Xhosa.

2.4. Data Analysis. Interviews were transcribed verbatim by a professional transcription agency and checked for accuracy by the first author. Using an analytic induction approach, the first author coded the first round of interviews (data collected in January 2014) in the first phase of analysis. Analytic induction is a technique that formulates a set of preliminary hypotheses from analyzing a small number of cases. These are tested and reformulated with the remainder of the available data. It tests a limited number of hypotheses with all available data, in an effort to understand the larger phenomena [45–47]. We formulated preliminary hypotheses for each ecological level of the Six C's Model [15] to test the fit of participants' perceptions about causes and consequences of childhood obesity. We also formulated preliminary hypotheses for each of the open questions about potential solutions and barriers to addressing childhood obesity.

The first author initiated analysis of the data by reading each transcript while identifying general themes (open coding), then coding each transcript line-by-line. Codes were compared and used to form core categories to represent the data. After analyzing the first portion of the data, the research team moved ahead to test the resulting hypotheses. Diagrams were created to illustrate themes and interrelationships between cases, categories, and/or processes [45]. When relevant, "negative cases" that did not fit the emerging hypotheses were analyzed to either revise or add new dimensions to the analysis [47]. Analyses continued until all cases were analyzed. The final interpretation of the data tested a conceptual framework where results were systematically reported in relation to categories derived from data that addressed the research questions [45, 46].

Two coauthors, formally trained in qualitative methodologies, independently coded a subset of cases following the first author's coding system. More specifically, they engaged in initial (line-by-line) and intermediate coding. Then, the research team met to develop a merged coding template. All investigators in the research team were knowledgeable about the Six C's ecological framework and its application and took into account these sensitizing concepts while analyzing the data. Consensus about a final version of this codebook was agreed upon and coding issues, if any, were resolved during the analysis stage via consensus within the research team [48]. During the intermediate coding stage, coauthors independently coded a subset of transcripts; categories that

TABLE 2: Frequency of demographic characteristics, (n = 21).

Category	Average/frequency
Age*	38.45
Gender	
Male	5
Female	16
Occupation	
Health worker	8
Child-minder	13
Years in Cape Town*	
5 or less	2
6–10	1
11–15	1
16–20	4
20 or more	12
Years in South Africa*	
5 or less	—
6–10	—
11–15	2
16–20	—
20 or more	18
Education*	
Some high school	7
Matriculation	2
Technical college	2
University degree	6
Graduate degree	3
Did not respond	2
Income* (in ZAR)	
Less than 10.000	8
10.000 to 15.000	2
25.000 to 30.000	1
30.000 to 35.000	1
35.000 or more	8
Primary Language*	
Afrikaans	3
Xhosa	5
English	11
Swahili	1

*One participant opted to not complete the demographic questionnaire.

emerged were compared with those identified by the first author. Finally, all investigators triangulated the findings at all stages of data analysis and summarized analyses with a systematic report of the findings and a conceptual framework that represented the most salient concepts in the data from all cases [48].

3. Results

3.1. Sample Characteristics. In total, five men and sixteen women represented our sample (see Table 2). All men in our sample had occupations in the health field, while child-minders were all women. The average age in our sample was

38.45 years. The majority of participants had lived in South Africa for more than 20 years, with more than half residing in the city of Cape Town. There were no noticeable differences between child-minders and health workers in regard to the length of time they had lived in South Africa. In South Africa, the poverty line as of March 2011 was between 5,316 ZAR ($360 USD) and 7,440 ZAR ($504 USD) annually [49]. This is significantly lower than in the US, where the poverty line is $11,000 a year per person [50], equal to about 150,000 ZAR. Our sample of child-minders reported annual income levels close to the South African poverty line (less than 10,000 ZAR), whereas a majority of health workers reported earning more than 35,000 ZAR annually. In terms of education, child-minders on average had less than a college degree, whereas health workers had at least a college degree. Education varied considerably among participants: most had some high school ($n = 7$), with fewer indicating matriculation ($n = 2$), technical college attendance ($n = 1$), attainment of a university degree ($n = 6$), graduate school attendance ($n = 3$), and unknown ($n = 2$). Participants were all fluent in English with the exception of one, but their primary languages were Swahili ($n = 1$), Afrikaans ($n = 3$), Xhosa ($n = 5$), and English ($n = 11$). Given the inherent socioeconomic differences between child-minders and health workers in this sample, we chose not to further stratify by income or education in our analyses, in order to preserve our focus on participants' perspectives and beliefs as child-minders and health workers, rather than their status.

3.2. Aim 1: Evaluating Obesity Perceptions of Child-Minders and Health Workers

3.2.1. Comparisons between Child-Minders and Health Workers. Participants were asked about factors at every level of the Six C's model (Figure 1), and whether they perceived these factors to be associated with childhood obesity outcomes. Findings from the in-depth interviews revealed an array factors associated with obesity: contributing factors to childhood obesity, consequences of childhood obesity, contexts in which contributing factors affect childhood obesity outcomes, and priorities regarding childhood obesity prevention and treatment.

A close examination of the data indicated that there were both differences and similarities between child-minders and health workers in the way they discussed childhood obesity. Child-minders were more likely to mention peer influences on eating behaviors than health workers, likely because they observe children interacting while eating on a daily basis. Health workers were more likely to emphasize nutritional issues common in the South African population (like missing breakfast or nutritional deficits), whereas child-minders focused on more individualized issues contributing to childhood obesity (like overeating and lack of physical activity). Education was mentioned more frequently by health workers, who claimed that many South Africans (children especially) are not well educated about healthy eating and the consequences of childhood obesity. Both groups attended to issues of access and affordability, emphasizing the prevailing effect of socioeconomic situation (SES) on eating and physical activity.

These findings suggest that child-minders were more likely to identify influences at the child (i.e., overeating, physical activity) and community levels (i.e., peer-relationships), whereas health workers were more likely to emphasize influences at the country level (i.e., education, nutritional deficits). Almost all participants noted that healthy foods are usually more expensive and that poorer individuals are more likely to live in dangerous neighborhoods where it is not safe to let children play outside. Strikingly, both child-minders and health workers noted prevailing cultural trends that encouraged obesity among South Africans, for example, the pattern that often obesity is not viewed as problematic but instead is associated with wealth and power.

3.2.2. Combined Participants' Perceptions. Overall, participants were knowledgeable and aware of a range of factors contributing to obesity including biological, behavioral, familial, and environmental influences. Two key themes emerged that were related to biological contributing factors: genetics and malnutrition. In addition, behavioral factors attributed to childhood obesity that emerged in our data were diet and physical activity. In regard to familial factors attributed to childhood obesity, participants gave specific examples of the role of parents, grandparents, and even siblings. Two other key themes emerged regarding environmental factors affecting childhood obesity outcomes: lack of access to healthy foods and limited opportunities for physical activity. With regard to consequences of childhood obesity, participants expressed concern about increased healthcare costs because of high obesity rates, comorbidities, and mortality, as well as increased likelihood of developing noncommunicable diseases such as heart disease, type 2 diabetes, cancer, hypertension, cholesterol, stroke, osteoarthritis, liver, and gallbladder disease.

The interview protocol explored contexts where contributing factors might affect childhood obesity outcomes including schools, community, health facilities, food environments (e.g., fast foods, food deserts), and government. Lastly, priorities for preventing childhood obesity emerged as participants talked about education, physical activity, and safe environments. See the emergent themes and example excerpts in Table 3.

3.3. Aim 2: Assessing the Fit of the Six C's Model for Child-Minders and Health Workers' Combined Perceptions of Childhood Obesity Causes and Consequences. The multitude of factors that emerged from the in-depth interviews are displayed in Table 4, organized according to the original Six C's theoretical model (Figure 1). Overall, participants identified causal factors and consequences of childhood obesity at each level of the ecology proposed by the Six C's Model, as well as strategies for and barriers to childhood obesity prevention. Participants were able to readily provide examples that support the general fit of the Six C's Model of childhood obesity. However, "culture" was not identified as a concentric sphere but rather was described as a driving influence embedded and infused

TABLE 3: Thematic content of participants' perceptions.

Themes	Example excerpts
Perceived biological contributing factors	"Some of them they are fat because of they were born with a fat family." "Other factors contributing to obesity include genetic factors and high rates of stunting in children who later become obese." "But maybe, assuming there is a gene that causes you to want to be, like, you know. But if that same gene were a cancer gene, then you would make a plan to avoid it." "But when it's a fat gene, like it could possibly that easy, then you're just like: well, my mother was fat. I'm just gonna [inaudible] weigh more. So it's the same concept. Because once they overeat, there are many other problems. It is going to break you down and it's going to be a lot sooner than cancer was going to."
Perceived behavioral contributing factors	"One is when they are finished to eat the food, there is no exercise. That's what they do, is eat the food, after that they do sleeping, so its going to gain the weight faster because there is no activity." "Of course this sometimes contributes to obesity and also if you don't watch a child, he's going to eat and eat and eat." "One is [fat] when they are finished to eat the food, there is no exercise. That's what they do is eat the food, after that [what] they do [is] sleeping so it's [the child] going to gain the weight faster because there is no activity."
Perceived familial contributing factors	"I think it's the way that parents feed their children. They overfeed them." "If my grandmother's fat, I'm fat, oh well, we're just a fat family." "They come across psychological things where they emotionally eat. Mother are, 'Oh, you're crying, I'll give you chocolate, I'll give you food.'"
Perceived environmental contributing factors	"Obviously the crime and that kind of thing does play a role because all the mother ensures that the child is safe while she's at work, so she encourages the child to stay at home because it's safer in the house than on the outside of the house." "Most of the time in low socioeconomic systems... They only have minimal to feed the children, so it's usually the high carb things that sort of fill them up very quickly... So they just feed them what they can afford and it's usually the high carb things that make you pick up very quick weight."
Perceived cultural contributing factors	"That's very hard to talk about. Culture is so interspersed. You can't distinguish anymore what was cultural and what was choice. It might not have been the choice of people, just to eat mealie-meal and all that stuff. Part of your culture was to have lots of meat and lots of veggies." "We have many different cultures. Here in South Africa, we've got many people, living their own ways. We've got Muslims, as well. I think our culture doesn't care about what the children eat. They like the children to be big, in order for people to see that this child's family, they come from a very well–off family, and they are fed all the time, which is not good. It is really not good." "... I said black culture, like myself, so I was born in an age that a man has to get married to a person heavy, not the slim. (Unclear) And whenever you're sick, your wife can head back to bring to the hospital, and if there is any problem, she can... When you're obese, you got power. People don't think there's power in someone that's slim."
Perceived consequences	"Consequences I am concerned about? ALL of them! Diet and level of physical activity affects every aspect of one's body- so this list could actually be much longer... Coronary heart disease, Type 2 diabetes, cancers (endometrial, breast, and colon), hypertension (high blood pressure), high total cholesterol, stroke, liver and gallbladder disease, and osteoarthritis (a degeneration of cartilage and its underlying bone within a joint)." "The children you will see they not like, you know children they will always feeling tired, you will see them tired and the children, they get sick. Most of the time that will cause a heart attack and that will cause as well diabetes because diabetes also is caused by obesity. When you eat not good food you will gain a lot of weight and that will cause diabetes."
Perceived contextual contributing factors	"It also encourages the children to eat more and more, because we've got some of the shops where they sell that goods, and then you try to control the nutrition for a child at home but when she or he is at school they can eat everything that has been sold." "The unfortunate thing is, the way we prepare the food is not ok. Steamed, and cooked and boiled in water. Soup is food for poor people. That is something in colored communities, whereas we know that soup is a great way of getting nutrition. But for the longest time, soup wasn't associated with health. It was associated with poverty." "It's unsafe to play in the park."

Table 3: Continued.

Themes	Example excerpts
Perceived priorities regarding childhood obesity prevention/treatment	"Insufficient attention is given to teaching school children about healthy diets and lifestyle. Not enough physical activity is promoted or engaged in at schools." "In some communities, there aren't even sidewalks, so how can you tell mothers to go for a walk to take the children for a walk? How can you walk to the park when you're likely to be assaulted or raped?"

Table 4: Factors affecting childhood obesity by the Six C's spheres.

Codes	Cell[a]	Child	Clan	Community	Country	Culture
Causes	Heredity	(i) Eating habits (ii) Food preferences (iii) Sedentarism (iv) Screen time (v) Skipping meals (vi) "Happiness"	(i) Force feeding (ii) Parenting styles (and Grandparents) (iii) Spoiling children	(i) Child-minders' feeding styles (ii) Lack of play infrastructure (iii) Access to junk food (iv) Lack of role models	(i) Socio economic status (ii) Media advertising (iii) Food availability and affordability (iv) Food packaging (v) Geographic location	(i) Cultural foods (ii) Traditional practices (iii) Food preparation (iv) Political (Historical)
Consequences	Cancer	(i) Gaining weight (ii) Health risks (iii) Negative body image (iv) Weight stigma (v) Eating disorders (vi) Stress (vii) Delayed development (viii) Tiredness (ix) Low self-esteem (x) Laziness (xi) Suicide	(i) Happiness (ii) Strict parental routines (iii) Lack of participation in sports (iv) Bullying	(i) Healthcare sector profit (ii) Scholastic performance	(i) Childhood obesity incidence (ii) Malnutrition (iii) Population outcomes	(i) Protective factor of HIV stigma (ii) Cultural beliefs about weight and diet
Strategies	—	(i) Limiting feeding (ii) Monitoring weight status (iii) Increasing knowledge (iv) Playing, dancing, exercising (v) Weight loss (vi) Increasing F & V consumption (vii) Limiting screen time (viii) Snack variety	(i) Cooking (ii) Workshops (iii) Family mealtimes (iv) Breastfeeding (v) Serving sizes (vi) Love & Hope (vii) Role modeling (viii) Social support (ix) Reward systems (x) Home visits by dietitians	(i) Health counseling (ii) Health education (iii) Community gardening (iii) Building fitness facilities (iv) Meal routines at childcare (v) Healthcare stakeholders' meetings (vi) Support groups	(i) Dietary guidelines (ii) Subsidizing food products/supplements (iii) Fortified food offering (iv) Food stamps (v) Gardening (vi) Built environment (vii) Media-related (viii) Food production (ix) Access to media outlets (x) Collaborations across sectors	(i) Walkability (ii) Access to nature (iii) Traditional dances
Barriers		(i) Emotional eating (ii) Palatable/desirable foods	(i) "Clean your plate" (ii) Family structure (iii) Lack of quality time	(i) Living conditions (ii) Lack of neighborhood safety (iii) Time constraints (iv) Lack of training (v) People's attitudes	(i) Lack of options (ii) Funding (iii) Soil contaminants (iv) Food insecurity	(i) Myths about women/black culture (ii) "Big," "Fat" as healthy, endearing

[a]There were no questions exploring perceptions about the cell-level contribution to childhood obesity prevention.

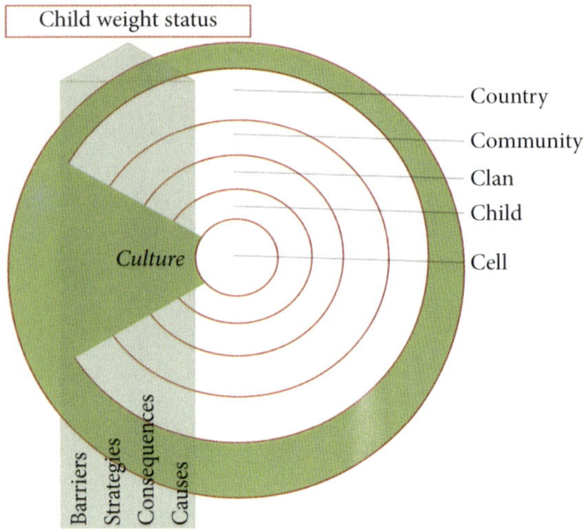

FIGURE 2: Six C's of childhood obesity perceptions among child-minders and health workers in South Africa.

within each of the other spheres (Figure 2). Therefore, we will propose an adaptation of the original Six C's Model based on our data later in this manuscript. First, we will briefly discuss the causal factors, consequences, strategies, and barriers that child-minders and health workers perceived as influencing childhood obesity, at each level of the original Six C's model (Table 4). Then, we will discuss how culture influences and is infused within each sphere according to our revised model.

At the cell level, hereditary and biological factors, such as genetic predisposition, were perceived as causal factors of childhood obesity. One participant saw cancer as related to obesity, noting, "obesity leads to so many other problems including cancer." Participants did not discuss strategies for prevention or barriers to such efforts in relation to cell-level characteristics.

At the child level, many factors were discussed as contributing to childhood obesity, including eating habits, food preferences, sedentary habits, screen time, skipping meals, and "happiness." Consequences at the child level included health risks, negative body image, weight stigma, eating disorders, stress, delayed development, fatigue, low self-esteem, laziness, and suicide. Some general strategies to address obesity at the child level included limiting feeding, monitoring weight status, increasing knowledge, promoting physical activity (playing, dancing, and exercising), weight loss, increasing fruit and vegetable consumption, limiting screen time, and providing snack variety. Barriers at the child level included emotional eating and highly desirable or palatable foods.

At the clan level, force-feeding, grandparents, parenting styles, and "spoiling" children were identified as potential causes of childhood obesity. Interestingly, both happiness and bullying were identified as consequences, in addition to more reactionary consequences, such as strict parent routines and lack of participation in sports. Many strategies were identified for prevention, including concrete ideas such as promoting breastfeeding and home visits by dieticians, and more abstract thoughts such as promoting love and hope. Barriers included family-norms around cleaning one's plate, and lack of quality time.

At the community level, child-minder feeding styles, lack of playground infrastructure, and access to junk foods were identified as causes of childhood obesity. Consequences at this level were more limited and focused on profits for healthcare and scholastic performance in the local communities. In contrast, many concrete strategies that utilized community resources were identified, including gardening programs, health education, and stakeholder's meetings. Finally, barriers to change included poor living conditions, safety, time constraints, attitudes towards obesity, and lack of training.

At the country level, socioeconomic status, media, and food availability were identified as top causes of childhood obesity, whereas consequences included malnutrition and population health outcomes over time. Strategies focused on government-based initiatives (i.e., revising dietary guidelines, providing subsidies, and food stamps), as well as private-sector initiatives (i.e., fortifying foods, increasing healthy food production, and promoting positive media outreach around health behaviors). However, providers identified funding as a prime barrier to government and industry involvement at the national level.

Finally, although our codes are listed under the cultural level in Table 4, it is important to note that the cultural causes, consequences, strategies, and barriers related to childhood obesity were consistently linked to factors at other levels, and participants resisted parsing culture out from other factors. Indeed, when asked how a child's culture plays a role in childhood obesity, one child-minder said: "That's very hard to talk about. Culture is so interspersed. You can't distinguish anymore what was cultural and what was choice. It might not have been the choice of people, just to eat mealie-meal and all that stuff. Part of your culture was to have lots of meat and lots of veggies."

As in other ecological models, culture is presented in the original Six C's Model as a distal sphere in which other contexts are embedded. In an interesting preliminary finding of this study, the data suggest that cultural influences are present within multiple levels of the child's ecology, interacting with other factors more proximally. We therefore propose that "culture" is a global theme or core category in our adapted model. This core category, "culture is so interspersed," emerged with the greatest explanatory power in regard to the main phenomenon (i.e., childhood obesity) because (1) it is intertwined with multiple ecological spheres (child, clan, community, and country) (2) and it links central structural categories (i.e., perceived causal factors, consequences, strategies, and barriers) that were identified in the data.

When asked about culture, participants used many words and phrases interchangeably, such as "black culture" or "in South Africa" or "in Cape Town" or "in the Western Cape" or "African culture". The embedded nature of culture across ecological contexts is apparent in the common references to its prevalent and complex nature, for example, as follows.

3.4. Excerpt 1: Jennifer (Pseudonym)

```
1 Interviewer (I): "How does children's
2 culture play a role in childhood
3 obesity?"
4 Jennifer (J): "That's very hard to
5 talk about. Culture is so
6 interspersed. You can't distinguish
7 anymore what was cultural and what was
8 choice. It might not have been the
9 choice of people, just to eat mealie-
10 meal and all that stuff. Part of your
11 culture was to have lots of meat and
12 lots of veggies."
13 J: "I really believe that, because
14 when I go to [inaudible], to events
15 there, it's lots of veggies on my
16 plate. The unfortunate thing is, the
17 way we prepare the food is not okay."
```

3.5. Excerpt 2: Matthew (Pseudonym)

```
1 Interviewer (I): "And then lastly, the
2 culture... [inaudible] How it plays a
3 role?"
4 Matthew (M): "...A culture is to eat
5 like this. We have a specific kind of
6 function, and with that function, we
7 have this particular - we have many
8 functions, cultural functions, as we
9 call it, and those functions are very
10 much associated with food. And not
11 good food. It's overly - it's not bad
12 food, but it's cultural food."
```

Overall, participants noted how multiple cultures that are embedded within South African society are implicated in eating behaviors. Participants gave examples about the role of "their" culture and black culture specifically in obesity, often in a positive light. Some discussed how healthy habits (i.e., physical activity) may or may not be afforded by one's culturally influenced environment. For example, one individual noted, "I think the culture can help the children. Our culture, we can go to the mountain to fetch the wood, so I walk every day. It can make you lose weight if you are overweight." Given the prevalence of this "culture" theme and its interrelationship with other ecological levels, we represent culture in our adapted model as a central influence that intersects with other ecological levels (Figure 2).

4. Discussion

In sum, participants articulated the multiple contributors to and consequences of obesity as well as potential strategies for and barriers to obesity prevention within South Africa, according to an ecological framework. Culture seems to play a critical role in shaping these perceptions, but also in addressing childhood obesity in this context. This study contributes much needed qualitative data focused on childhood obesity [31] and assesses multiple levels of influence. The aims of this study were to (a) qualitatively explore the perceived causes and consequences of, as well as the potential strategies for and barriers to, addressing childhood obesity among health workers and child-minders in Cape Town, South Africa, and (b) provisionally test the fit of a socioecological theory (the Six C's Model) to explain child-minders' and health workers' perceptions about childhood obesity in South Africa.

As hypothesized, each level of the Six C's Model was validated in the responses of study respondents. In this sense, our model is generally consistent with other scholars' conceptualization of the socioecological factors that influence childhood obesity [15]. Participants were able to articulate an array of multilevel factors and contexts that contribute to obesity outcomes, as well as potential consequences of childhood obesity, and priorities of interest in addressing childhood obesity. This pattern is consistent with previous research targeting perceptions of obesity in ethnic minorities in the United States [27] in which participants were able to identify multiple obesogenic factors affecting their community.

Socioecological models may be particularly useful for understanding childhood obesity in understudied (and underresourced) populations. These models are also powerful for focusing research on different levels of the framework. For example, Kime [51] addresses the socioecological factors at the family level as related to obesity, whereas Sano and colleagues' work [52] explored socioecological factors associated with food insecurity among Latino immigrants via qualitative methods, focusing on the community sphere. The current study supports the importance of examining the specific constellations of contributors and barriers perceived at each ecological level by specific populations. Such an approach could help tailor childhood obesity interventions for greater efficacy in at-risk populations.

Unlike the Six C's Model, in our data, "culture" emerged as a core category embedded within each of the other spheres instead of being the outermost level of the model. Our adapted model of childhood obesity perceptions introduces a cross-cutting cultural dimension in which participants perceive cultural elements to interact in a variety of ways with other factors at varying levels. Though there were a variety of factors, consequences, strategies, and barriers reported at each level of the Six C's Model, many of these factors were described as being culturally influenced. Participants reported different cultural elements related to childhood obesity, such as the role of South African and black culture on the perception of body weight and body image and behavioral habits such as physical activity and eating habits, as well as noting bidirectional effects between culture and other factors at multiple levels of socioecological influence.

These findings support the notion that obesity might be a "culture-bound syndrome." Ritenbaugh [53] was one of the first scholars to articulate the centrality of culture in shaping obesity. The emergent core category in our study ("culture is so interspersed") illustrates the embedded relationship of culture throughout other socioecological factors that affect individual and child weight outcomes. There are various possible constellations and interrelationships between these socioecological factors of interest (e.g., causal factors, consequences, strategies, and barriers) and child weight outcomes. These complex relationships, including potential mediators and moderators, are wound into the cultural milieu. Ritenbaugh's [53] "culture bound perspective" highlights four important features of obesity: it cannot be understood apart from its specific cultural or subcultural context; its etiology summarizes and symbolizes core meanings and behavioral norms; its diagnosis relies on culture-specific technology and ideology; and successful treatment is accomplished by participants embedded within the surrounding culture. Given these key features of childhood obesity, it is not surprising that each aspect was present in our data. Ritenbaugh emphasizes each culture's uniqueness, as well as their particular genetic and environmental pools. If obesity can be understood as a culturally bound syndrome, it is important to acknowledge the implications for obesity related research moving forward.

In an important example, Shugart [17] has argued that culture plays a pivotal role in explaining obesogenic outcomes, but not without having sociopolitical implications. For example, if an individual's culture is the main explanatory factor in predicting their own obesity outcomes, then the onus is on the individual to make behavioral changes contrary to their cultural upbringing. This finding needs to be taken into account carefully to prevent negative consequences when addressing obesity.

In Iran, for instance, researchers have found that the causes of childhood obesity are perceived to relate to macrolevel policy influences, the school environment, sociocultural factors, and family and individual behavioral factors, all acting in combination [54]. A key emergent theme in this study was the pervasive influence of the Iranian government's policies on children's food intake and physical activity, in which the political and sociocultural context does not encourage girls and women to participate in active lifestyles [54]. This example emphasizes the point that each culture is unique and needs to be understood within its own context and circumstances.

One significant shortcoming of previous "culture-bound syndrome" research is that it has focused on cultural/popular media images, body shapes, and women weight standards, with little focus on the public health implications of obesity. This study aims to close that gap, promoting translational obesity-related research that aims to improve the health and well-being of individuals, by showcasing the perceptions of individuals working directly with those affected by childhood obesity. Such an orientation provides an opportunity to address health rather than appearance or normative values [28]. Ultimately, we seek to make a contribution beyond just advancing the field of health promotion, by bridging public health and social justice.

This study adds to the scarce qualitative literature that aims to understanding and addressing childhood obesity. Additionally, our interview protocol for assessing obesity perceptions within ecological contexts might be a tool for those interested in exploring childhood obesity and related issues in diverse communities. It could be used also as a resource for initiating dialogue so that perceived contributing factors are understood within their appropriate context. Finally, it could also aid in assessing the cultural background of an individual who intends to engage in health behavior modifications because culture is crucial in order for these efforts to be effective [55].

4.1. Study Limitations. There are various limitations that future studies must address. Firstly, there were notable differences between child-minders and health workers: particularly gender, income, and community characteristics. In future studies, it would be ideal to recruit participants in these groups with similar characteristics. Due to constraints during the data collection process, it was difficult to conduct face-to-face interviews with all participants. To allow us to recruit more participants and gather more data, some participants were permitted to respond to the interview questions via e-mail responses. The data are limited in that there may be some variations in responses across these data collection modalities. Lastly, most participants were low- to middle-income. We do observe some variability in the income levels of participants; however, only one participant was from a high-income community (Rondebosch). Additionally, there were noticeable differences in income between child-minders and health workers. This may limit the generalizability of the results in this study. Future studies may cast a wider net to allow comparative analyses.

4.2. Implications. The implications of this research shed light on areas that could aid child-minders and health workers in childhood obesity prevention efforts. Previous research indicates that preventative health strategies that incorporate the views of target participants have improved likelihood of success [56]. Health workers and child-minders are important stakeholders, who are familiar with the culture in which their clients live and have important roles relevant for health promotion. They can provide a range of perspectives that can help to identify priorities and directions in planning culturally relevant childhood obesity interventions [57].

Understanding the causes, consequences of and potential solutions to obesity through these and other individuals' cultural lenses could inform tailored, culturally sensitive, and effective intervention programs promoting child health. Working with these professionals in South Africa would require clear communication that attends to cultural norms regarding weight and health behavior.

Our data indicated that South African care providers do not perceive that genetic factors play a central role in childhood obesity, even though these are critically associated with the phenomena in the Six C's Model. Further exploration of perceptions about these various hereditary traits and genetic predispositions is warranted. According to Swinburn and colleagues [58] "the genetic background loads the gun, but the environment pulls the trigger." Future work should help us better understand how to educate the public about the nuances of genetics and its role in obesity, including emphasizing that acknowledging the role genetics plays does not diminish the involvement of other socioecological factors in the obesity problem (e.g., health behaviors, environmental factors). This research could aid social scientists in bridging the gap in the public eye between genetic research and these other behavioral, social, and environmental factors associated with obesity.

Most importantly, our findings suggest that the role of culture should be taken into account carefully, since culture is both interspersed and widely varied in South Africa. To address the potential challenges of targeting this and other culturally rich populations, researchers and practitioners need to be sensitive to participants' ethnic identities and culture and avoid altering behavior that is closely attached to cultural beliefs. Rather, it would be ideal to add elements to behavioral interventions that leverage culturally rooted strengths in targeted populations. For example, many families perceive mealtimes as times of joy and connection. While eating healthfully is important, severe food restrictions and prohibitions might well be perceived as punishment and be culturally unacceptable. A potential alternative could be modifying environmental features to coexist with cultural practices and encourage positive reinforcement of health behaviors.

5. Conclusion

The findings outlined in this study emphasize the pervasive influence of culture on individual, biological, behavioral, familial, and environmental factors that influence childhood obesity. Future studies and obesity prevention efforts should investigate and attend to the key role that culture plays in shaping individual health behaviors. Culturally tailored approaches with key community stakeholders in multiple sectors may be crucial to develop effective strategies addressing childhood obesity prevention efforts.

Competing Interests

The authors declare that there is no conflict of interests regarding the publication of this paper.

Acknowledgments

The research team wants to acknowledge the following individuals for their outstanding logistical support: Jan Brooks, Dr. Ruopeng An, Jessica Dickson, Sarai Coba, Sedick Pandit, Oliver Hagan, Andrew Ndwanya, and the participants in this study. This research was supported by the training grant "Illinois Transdisciplinary Obesity Prevention Program (I-TOPP)" funded by the National Institute of Food and Agriculture, US Department of Agriculture, under Award no. 2011-67001-30101.

References

[1] World Health Organization (WHO), *Report of the Commission on Ending Childhood Obesity*, Ending Childhood Obesity Commission, Geneva, Switzerland, 2016.

[2] Food and Agriculture Organization of the United Nations (FAO), *Obesity in Developing Countries: Causes and Implications*, 2015, http://www.fao.org/docrep/003/y0600m/y0600m05.htm.

[3] H. S. Kruger, T. Puoane, M. Senekal, and M.-T. Van Der Merwe, "Obesity in South Africa: challenges for government and health professionals," *Public Health Nutrition*, vol. 8, no. 5, pp. 491–500, 2005.

[4] M. A. Monyeki, A. Awotidebe, G. L. Strydom, J. H. de Ridder, R. L. Mamabolo, and H. C. Kemper, "The challenges of underweight and overweight in South African children: are we winning or losing the battle? A systematic review," *International Journal of Environmental Research and Public Health*, vol. 12, no. 2, pp. 1156–1173, 2015.

[5] The World Bank, *South Africa Economic Update: Promoting Domestic Competition between Firms Could Help Spur Growth, Reduce Poverty*, 2016, http://www.worldbank.org/en/country/southafrica/publication/south-africa-economic-update-promoting-faster-growth-poverty-alleviation-through-competition.

[6] Y. Wang and T. Lobstein, "Worldwide trends in childhood overweight and obesity," *International Journal of Pediatric Obesity*, vol. 1, no. 1, pp. 11–25, 2006.

[7] G. P. August, S. Caprio, I. Fennoy et al., "Prevention and treatment of pediatric obesity: an endocrine society clinical practice guideline based on expert opinion," *Journal of Clinical Endocrinology and Metabolism*, vol. 93, no. 12, pp. 4576–4599, 2008.

[8] P. W. Franks, R. L. Hanson, W. C. Knowler, M. L. Sievers, P. H. Bennett, and H. C. Looker, "Childhood obesity, other cardiovascular risk factors, and premature death," *New England Journal of Medicine*, vol. 362, no. 6, pp. 485–493, 2010.

[9] J. H. Goedecke, C. L. Jennings, and E. V. Lambert, "Obesity in South Africa," in *Chronic Diseases of Lifestyle in South Africa, 2005*, K. Steyn, J. Fourie, and N. Temple, Eds., pp. 65–79, 1995.

[10] M.-T. Van Der Merwe and M. S. Pepper, "Obesity in South Africa," *Obesity Reviews*, vol. 7, no. 4, pp. 315–322, 2006.

[11] Z. Mchiza and E. Maunder, "Fighting childhood obesity," *South African Journal of Clinical Nutrition*, vol. 26, no. 3, pp. 100–102, 2013.

[12] H. Coovadia, R. Jewkes, P. Barron, D. Sanders, and D. McIntyre, "The health and health system of South Africa: historical roots of current public health challenges," *The Lancet*, vol. 374, no. 9692, pp. 817–834, 2009.

[13] Statistics South Africa, *City of Cape Town*, 2011, http://www.statssa.gov.za/?page_id=1021&id=city-of-cape-town-municipality.

[14] H. A. Strydom, "Minority rights issues in post-apartheid South Africa," *Loyola of Los Angeles International and Comparative Law Journal*, vol. 19, pp. 873–914, 1996.

[15] K. Harrison, K. K. Bost, B. A. McBride et al., "Toward a developmental conceptualization of contributors to overweight and obesity in childhood: the six-cs model," *Child Development Perspectives*, vol. 5, no. 1, pp. 50–58, 2011.

[16] J. W. Carey, "Linking qualitative and quantitative methods: integrating cultural factors into public health," *Qualitative Health Research*, vol. 3, no. 3, pp. 298–318, 1993.

[17] H. A. Shugart, "Weight of tradition: culture as a rationale for obesity in contemporary U.S. news coverage," *Obesity Reviews*, vol. 14, no. 9, pp. 736–744, 2013.

[18] A. A. Agne, R. Daubert, M. L. Munoz, I. Scarinci, and A. L. Cherrington, "The cultural context of obesity: exploring perceptions of obesity and weight loss among Latina immigrants," *Journal of Immigrant and Minority Health*, vol. 14, no. 6, pp. 1063–1070, 2012.

[19] M. Davidson and K. A. Knafl, "Dimensional analysis of the concept of obesity," *Journal of Advanced Nursing*, vol. 54, no. 3, pp. 342–350, 2006.

[20] R. M. Puhl and C. A. Heuer, "Obesity stigma: important considerations for public health," *American Journal of Public Health*, vol. 100, no. 6, pp. 1019–1028, 2010.

[21] World Health Organization (WHO), "What are the health consequences of being overweight?" 2013, http://www.who.int/features/qa/49/en/.

[22] M. L. Loureiro and R. M. Nayga Jr., "Obesity, weight loss, and physician's advice," *Social Science and Medicine*, vol. 62, no. 10, pp. 2458–2468, 2006.

[23] L. Montesi, M. E. Ghoch, L. Brodosi, S. Calugi, G. Marchesini, and R. D. Grave, "Long-term weight loss maintenance˜for obesity: a multidisciplinary approach," *Diabetes, Metabolic Syndrome and Obesity: Targets and Therapy*, vol. 9, pp. 37–46, 2016.

[24] M. Harris, "The role of primary health care in preventing the onset of chronic disease, with a particular focus on the lifestyle risk factors of obesity, tobacco and alcohol," in *Canberra: National Preventative Health Taskforce*, pp. 1–21, National Preventative Health Taskforce, Canberra, Australia, 2008.

[25] S. N. Bleich, W. L. Bennett, K. A. Gudzune, and L. A. Cooper, "Impact of physician BMI on obesity care and beliefs," *Obesity*, vol. 20, no. 5, pp. 999–1005, 2012.

[26] Center for Disease Control and Prevention (CDC), "Community Efforts," 2015 http://www.cdc.gov/obesity/strategies/community.html.

[27] R. Figueroa, E. Sosa, A. Cordova, S. Wilmoth, M. He, and S. Wu, "Health communication and obesity prevention in hispanic communities: a qualitative exploration of media's roles," *Journal of Research in Obesity*, vol. 2014, Article ID 722324, 18 pages, 2014.

[28] N. Stettler, "Comment: the global epidemic of childhood obesity: is there a role for the paediatrician?" *Obesity Reviews, Supplement*, vol. 5, supplement 1, pp. 1–3, 2004.

[29] American College of Sports Medicine (ACSM), *All Medical Students and Physicians Need Training in Nutrition and Physical Activity to Help Combat America's Obesity Epidemic*, 2014, http://www.acsm.org/about-acsm/media-room/news-releases/2014/06/24/all-medical-students-and-physicians-need-training-in-nutrition-and-physical-activity-to-help-combat-america-s-obesity-epidemic.

[30] Center for Disease Control and Prevention (CDC), *Health Equity Resource Toolkit for State Practitioners Addressing Obesity Disparities*, 2015, https://www.cdc.gov/obesity/downloads/CDCHealthEquityObesityToolkit508.pdf.

[31] A. Perez and G. D. Ball, "Are we overlooking the qualitative 'look' of obesity?" *Nutrition & Diabetes*, vol. 5, no. 7, article no. e174, 2015.

[32] M. Q. Patton, *Qualitative Evaluation and Research Methods*, Sage Publications, Newbury Park, Calif, USA, 2nd edition, 1990.

[33] B. Fees, S. Trost, M. Bopp, and D. A. Dzewaltowski, "Physical activity programming in family child care homes: providers' perceptions of practices and barriers," *Journal of Nutrition Education and Behavior*, vol. 41, no. 4, pp. 268–273, 2009.

[34] K. R. Hesketh, E. M. F. van Sluijs, R. E. Blaine, E. M. Taveras, M. W. Gillman, and S. E. B. Neelon, "Assessing care providers' perceptions and beliefs about physical activity in infants and toddlers: baseline findings from the Baby NAP SACC study," *BMC Public Health*, vol. 15, no. 1, article 100, 2015.

[35] L. A. King, J. H. M. Loss, R. L. Wilkenfeld, D. L. Pagnini, M. L. Booth, and S. L. Booth, "Australian GPs' perceptions about child and adolescent overweight and obesity: the weight of opinion study," *British Journal of General Practice*, vol. 57, no. 535, pp. 124–129, 2007.

[36] N. Larson, D. S. Ward, S. B. Neelon, and M. Story, "What role can child-care settings play in obesity prevention? a review of the evidence and call for research efforts," *Journal of the American Dietetic Association*, vol. 111, no. 9, pp. 1343–1362, 2011.

[37] P. Tucker, M. M. van Zandvoort, S. M. Burke, and J. D. Irwin, "Physical activity at daycare: childcare providers' perspectives for improvements," *Journal of Early Childhood Research*, vol. 9, no. 3, pp. 207–219, 2011.

[38] J. W. Creswell, *Qualitative Inquiry and Research Method: Choosing among Five Approaches*, Sage, Thousand Oaks, Calif, USA, 2nd edition, 2007.

[39] J. W. Creswell, *Qualitative Inquiry and Research Design: Choosing among Five Approaches*, Sage, Thousand Oaks, Calif, USA, 2013.

[40] J. J. Francis, M. Johnston, C. Robertson et al., "What is an adequate sample size? Operationalising data saturation for theory-based interview studies," *Psychology and Health*, vol. 25, no. 10, pp. 1229–1245, 2010.

[41] G. Guest, A. Bunce, and L. Johnson, "How many interviews are enough? An experiment with data saturation and variability," *Field Methods*, vol. 18, pp. 59–82, 2006.

[42] Statistics South Africa, *Census: Heideveld*, 2011, http://census2011.adrianfrith.com/place/199029022.

[43] Statistics South Africa, *Census: Khayelitsha*, 2011, http://census2011.adrianfrith.com/place/199038.

[44] Statistics South Africa, *Census: Rondebosch*, 2011, http://census2011.adrianfrith.com/place/199041030.

[45] B. G. Glaser and A. L. Strauss, "The constant comparative method of qualitative analysis," *Social Problems*, vol. 12, no. 4, pp. 436–445, 1968.

[46] V. Minichiello, R. Aroni, E. Timewell, and L. Alexander, *In-Depth Interviewing: Principles, Techniques, Analysis*, Longman, Sydney, Australia, 2nd edition, 1995.

[47] H. R. Bernard and G. W. Ryan, *Analyzing Qualitative Data: Systematic Approaches*, Sage Publications, 2009.

[48] M. Q. Patton, *How to Use Qualitative Methods in Evaluation*, Sage Publications, London, UK, 1987.

[49] Statistics South Africa, *Poverty Trends in South Africa: An Examination of Absolute Poverty between 2006 and 2011*, 2014, http://www.statssa.gov.za/publications/Report-03-10-06/Report-03-10-06March2014.pdf.

[50] U. S. Department of Health and Human Services (USDHHS), *2015 Poverty Guidelines*, 2016, https://aspe.hhs.gov/2015-poverty-guidelines#threshholds.

[51] N. Kime, "Children's eating behaviours: the importance of the family setting," *Area*, vol. 40, no. 3, pp. 315–322, 2008.

[52] Y. Sano, S. Garasky, K. A. Greder, C. C. Cook, and D. E. Browder, "Understanding food insecurity among latino immigrant families in rural America," *Journal of Family and Economic Issues*, vol. 32, no. 1, pp. 111–123, 2011.

[53] C. Ritenbaugh, "Obesity as a culture-bound syndrome," *Culture, Medicine and Psychiatry*, vol. 6, no. 4, pp. 347–361, 1982.

[54] B. Mohammadpour-Ahranjani, M. J. Pallan, A. Rashidi, and P. Adab, "Contributors to childhood obesity in Iran: the views of parents and school staff," *Public Health*, vol. 128, no. 1, pp. 83–90, 2014.

[55] F. Douglas, J. Clark, L. Craig, J. Campbell, and G. McNeill, "'It's a balance of just getting things right': mothers' views about pre-school childhood obesity and obesity prevention in Scotland," *BMC Public Health*, vol. 14, no. 1, article 1009, 2014.

[56] K. Hesketh, E. Waters, J. Green, L. Salmon, and J. Williams, "Healthy eating, activity and obesity prevention: a qualitative study of parent and child perceptions in Australia," *Health Promotion International*, vol. 20, no. 1, pp. 19–26, 2005.

[57] A. Smibert, R. Abbott, D. Macdonald, A. Hogan, and G. Leong, "School, community, and family working together to address childhood obesity: perceptions from the KOALA lifestyle intervention study," *European Physical Education Review*, vol. 16, no. 2, pp. 155–170, 2010.

[58] B. A. Swinburn, G. Sacks, K. D. Hall et al., "The global obesity pandemic: shaped by global drivers and local environments," *The Lancet*, vol. 378, no. 9793, pp. 804–814, 2011.

The First Step of Health Policy-Making for Lifestyle Modifications at Middle Age: Problem Identification in 40- to 60-Year-Old Population

Simin Mouodi,[1] Seyed Reza Hosseini,[1] Reza Ghadimi,[2] Ali Bijani,[1] Robert Graham Cumming,[3] Hassan Ashrafian Amiri,[1] Fatemeh Bayani,[1] and Shima Sum[1]

[1] *Social Determinants of Health Research Center, Health Research Institute, Babol University of Medical Sciences, Babol, Iran*
[2] *Health Research Institute, Babol University of Medical Sciences, Babol, Iran*
[3] *School of Public Health, University of Sydney, Sydney, NSW, Australia*

Correspondence should be addressed to Seyed Reza Hosseini; hosseinirezaseyed@gmail.com

Academic Editor: David H. St-Pierre

Background. The purpose of this study was to determine the current situation of lifestyle behaviors and related outcomes, as the first step to make proper local health policies for improvement of health lifestyle behaviors. *Materials and Methods.* This analytic research has been conducted as a cross-sectional study on the middle-aged (40–60 years old) population of Amirkola, Northern Iran. The Persian translation of the Health-Promoting Lifestyle Profile II questionnaire and the International Physical Activity Questionnaire were used for data collection. Also, anthropometric variables, blood pressure, fasting blood sugar, and serum lipids profile were examined. *Results.* Three hundred one individuals have been enrolled in the study. Results showed that 10.6% of the participants had unhealthy lifestyle behaviors in the subdomain of spiritual growth; 46.8% in the subdomain of health responsibility; and 48.2% in the subdomains of stress management, physical activity, and nutrition; men had more physical activity than women ($p < 0.001$). Totally, 189 persons (63.9%) had serum cholesterol greater than or equal to 200 mg/dL; seventy-five individuals (25%) had high blood pressure. One hundred twenty-six persons (81.8%) of women and 103 (70.1%) of men were overweight or obese. *Conclusions.* Health lifestyle behaviors in 40- to 60-year-old population need a proper intervention to improve the current situation.

1. Introduction

The increasing prevalence of noncommunicable diseases (NCDs), especially cardiovascular diseases, diabetes, cancer, and chronic respiratory disorders, has driven health policy-makers to implement effective programs for prevention and control of these diseases, worldwide [1–3]. These major NCDs share four behavioral risk factors which represent one's lifestyle, namely, tobacco use, unhealthy diet, physical inactivity, and harmful use of alcohol [4]. As lifestyles become more sedentary and diets change more rapidly than ever, these diseases are becoming more common and are striking at a younger age [5]. Recently, greater efforts have been made to best encourage people to have an active living and healthier lifestyle, including making better nutritional patterns and physical activity (PA) choices [6–13]. The World Health Organization (WHO) advocates to all countries, either developed or developing, to make sustainable policies for fighting NCDs, as the most important health threats [1]. The WHO reported that NCDs kill 16 million people each year before their 70th birthdays [1]. Unhealthy diet and lack of physical activity are leading global risks to health [14]. Globally, 1 in 4 adults is not active enough [15]. Worldwide obesity has more than doubled since 1980; in 2014, more than 1.9 billion adults, 18 years and older, were overweight; of these, over 600 million were obese. Thirty-nine percent of adults aged 18 years and above were overweight in 2014, and 13% were obese [16].

Recent studies predicted that disability-adjusted life years related to cardiovascular diseases would be increased more than twofold in 2025 compared with 2005 in Iranian adults aged ≥30 years [17]. The Isfahan Cohort Study conducted in the central part of Iran showed that the incidence rates for almost all cardiovascular diseases were high in adults aged 35 years and above [18]. According to the third national surveillance of risk factors of non-communicable diseases in Iranian adults (aged 15–64 years), the prevalence of diabetes, hypertension, obesity, central obesity, hypertriglyceridemia, and hypercholesterolemia was reported to be 8.7%, 26.6%, 22.3%, 53.6%, 36.4%, and 42.9%, respectively [19]; furthermore, the prevalence of low physical activity was estimated to be 44.8%, and the odds of lower physical activity in the women were three times greater than those in men [20]. The survey of Tehran Lipid and Glucose Study in adult population (aged 30–74 years) over 6 years of follow-up suggested that current situation of non-communicable disease risk factors needs a proper lifestyle intervention regarding changes in nutritional habits and increased physical activity for primary prevention of cardiovascular diseases in Iranian adults [21, 22].

Considering the importance of novel, local, cost-effective, and culturally acceptable interventions to change sedentary lifestyle [23–26] and due to limited published articles related to the adults' lifestyle behaviors in the northern region of Iran, this study aimed to evaluate the current situation of health-promoting lifestyle profile, physical activity, anthropometric variables, and the profile of plasma lipids and glucose in the middle-aged population of Northern Iran, near Caspian Sea. The results can be used as the first step of policy-making to implement proper interventions [12, 27] for lifestyle modifications in this region.

2. Materials and Methods

This analytic research has been conducted as a cross-sectional study on the middle-aged (40–60 years old) population of Amirkola, Northern Iran. Sample size was determined based on data from the previous studies by considering $p = 0.5$ and $d = 0.06$ for a sample comprising 267 individuals [28]; in addition, taking a possible loss to follow-up into account, a safety margin of 10–15% was used [29]. Considering that the entire population of this area is covered by the family physician program, we used various methods to invite and recruit middle-aged population, including (1) informing local health care workers and family physicians; (2) public announcements by local health volunteers (nonemployed women who have voluntary co-operation with health centers); (3) distribution of public notices in households, public gathering places, mosques, banks, post offices, local markets, and stores; and (4) selecting the research center in the central part of the city, close to the local health centers, in the access of people of the region and keeping this center active at various times of the morning and evening on Saturdays to Thursdays each week in order to be responsive to the clients. At first, the volunteers who referred to the research center have been checked for exclusion criteria; then, they were divided into 4 groups according to their sex and age (male and female; in the age groups of 40–49 and 50–60 years); at the same time, using the information available about households which were associated with the health centers of the region, the researchers called the households which had at least one person in the age group of 40–60 years and invited them to participate in the study. Simple random sampling was used to select these households. Sampling continued until each of the four groups had nearly the same number of participants. Women in the pregnancy or breast-feeding period, the persons who could not read and write (and could not read the written informed consent form of the study), and those who were undergoing specific nutrition regimens, prescribed by a physician, have been excluded.

The Persian translation of the Health-Promoting Lifestyle Profile II (HPLP-II) questionnaire was used to investigate participants' lifestyles. This questionnaire includes 52 questions in six lifestyle subscales (spiritual growth with "11 questions," health responsibility "13 questions," interpersonal relations "8 questions," stress management "6 items," physical activity "7 questions," and nutritional habits "7 questions"). Each question has a four-point response scale to determine the frequency of that behavior, ranging from 1–4: "1" representing "never" and "4" representing "routinely." An average of ≥2.50 was considered to be a positive response in each question [30]; therefore, considering the number of questions in each subdomain, the cutoff point for health behaviors related to spiritual growth was considered as 27.5, health responsibility as 32.5, interpersonal relations as 20, stress management as 15, physical activity, and nutritional habits as 17.5. The HPLP-II instrument has been translated in different languages [31, 32]; validity and reliability of its Iranian version have been confirmed in previous studies [33, 34].

We used the International Physical Activity Questionnaire (IPAQ) to assess physical activity (PA) of the participants. Validity and reliability of its Iranian version have been confirmed in the year 2012 [35]. This questionnaire includes four parts ((1) activities at work; (2) housework, gardening, and caring for family; (3) PA in transportation; and (4) recreation, sport, and leisure time) and asks about the intensity and time a person spent being physically active in the last 7 days. For each domain, participants recorded the number of days and time spent each day undertaking vigorous- and moderate-intensity activities separately along with the time spent walking. Vigorous physical activities are defined as activities that take hard physical effort and make a person breathe much harder than normal such as lifting heavy things, digging, heavy construction work, or climbing stairs, and moderate activities are defined as activities that take moderate physical effort and make them breathe somewhat harder than normal such as carrying light loads. These values (vigorous activity, moderate activity, and walking) were used to calculate the PA levels, as specified in the official IPAQ instruction manual. Each type of activity was weighted by its energy requirements as MET (metabolic equivalent of task). By multiplying MET value of particular activity (3.3 METs for walking, 4.0 METs for moderate PA, and 8.0 METs for vigorous PA), total MET minutes per week was calculated. Vigorous and moderate activities were defined as those lasting for at least 10 minutes continuously [35]. Questions related to time spent sitting on a weekday or weekend were excluded from analysis. Study population was classified into the levels of PA according to MET minutes/week: "minimally active" for individuals who achieved a minimum of at least 600 MET minutes/week, "highly active" for those who had a minimum of at least 1500 MET minutes per week, and "inactive" persons for those who had not met the above two categories [36].

Other data which were collected included age, gender, education level, occupation, marital status, living region (urban or rural), and history of comorbid physical or mental disorders. Also, weight and height, blood pressure, fasting blood sugar, and serum lipids profile were examined. Body mass index (BMI) was calculated as weight (in kilograms)/height^2 (in meters).

Other anthropometric measures which have been assessed included body fat percentage and waist and buttock circumferences. These variables have been measured with a tape. Also, waist-to-hip ratio (WHR) and waist-to-height ratio (WHtR) [37, 38] have been calculated.

Waist circumference was measured around the midpoint between the lower margin of the last palpable rib and the top of the iliac crest, and buttock measurement was taken at the maximum circumference over the buttocks. All measurements were taken once over light clothing, and values were recorded in centimeters.

Body fat percentage was measured by using the hand-to-foot bioelectrical impedance analysis technique with a digital body fat calculator (BF511 model; Omron company). This technique has been reported as a simple, quick, and non-invasive method which can give reliable measurements of body composition with minimal intra- and interobserver variability; the results are available immediately and reproducible with <1% error on repeated measurements [39].

Blood pressure was measured with the participant in the sitting position, using a digital sphygmomanometer (Omron M6 brand), and the average of two times blood pressure measurement ≥140/90 mmHg was defined as hypertension. Early morning venous blood samples (5 mL) were collected after fasting for at least 12 hours to assess fasting blood sugar (FBS), total cholesterol, high-density lipoprotein (HDL) cholesterol, low-density lipoprotein (LDL) cholesterol, and triglyceride (TG) levels; these values were measured using Pars Azmoon kits via the autoanalyzer respons®910 DiaSys system. All of the laboratory tests have been conducted in a particular laboratory which had undertaken external quality control.

According to the National Cholesterol Education Program Adult Treatment Panel III Report [37], cutoff points for fasting blood glucose, total serum cholesterol, triglyceride, and LDL levels have been considered less than 126, 200, 150, and 100 mg/dL, respectively. The HDL cholesterol cutoff point was considered less than 40 mg/dL in men and less than 50 mg/dL in women. Also, serum TG levels in the range of 150–199 were classified as borderline-high TG, 200–499 as high TG, and >500 mg/dL as very high TG categories.

Data analysis was performed by SPSS 17 package; the chi-square test, Fisher's exact test, and *t*-test were used for data analysis with a significance level of $p < 0.05$. The Kolmogorov–Smirnov test was used to evaluate the normal distribution of quantitative data.

All of the participants signed a written informed consent form. They have been assured that their information would be kept confidential. This research has been approved by the Ethics Committee of Babol University of Medical Sciences as registration code Mubabol.Rec.1394.45.

3. Results

Three hundred one individuals have been enrolled in this study. The mean age of the participants was 49.67 ± 5.42 (range of 40–60 years); 154 persons (51.2%) were female with the mean age of 49.0 ± 5.13 years, and 147 (48.8%) were male with the mean age of 50.4 ± 5.64. Basic characteristics of the participants divided into the two age groups are presented in Table 1. This table shows that these two age groups had no significant difference in their baseline characteristics ($p > 0.05$), except in their occupation ($p = 0.047$).

Lifestyle behaviors according to the HPLP-II questionnaire are presented in Table 2. Thirty-two participants (10.6%) in the subdomain of spiritual growth, 141 participants (46.8%) in the subdomain of health responsibility, 145 participants (48.2%) in the subdomain of interpersonal relations, and 145 participants (48.2%) in the subdomains of stress management, physical activity, and nutrition had scores less than average. There was no significant difference between the two age groups about distribution of the average score of lifestyle behaviors except in the nutrition subscale ($p = 0.033$); the age group of 50–60 years had higher scores in this subscale. Men and women had no significant difference in the total score and subdomains of lifestyle behavior ($p > 0.05$) except in the subdomain of health responsibility ($p < 0.001$); in this subscale, women had higher scores.

Distribution of PA in two sexes divided into the two age groups is presented in Table 3. Totally, 24 women (15.6%) and 1 man (0.7%) were inactive, 36 women (23.4%) and 13 men (8.8%) were minimally active, and 94 women (61.0%) and 133 men (90.5%) were highly active according to MET min/week. A significant statistical difference was observed between two sexes about their physical activity ($p < 0.001$); men had more physical activity than women.

Anthropometric measures, blood pressure, fasting blood sugar, and serum lipids profile of the participants divided into two age groups are presented in Table 4. This table shows that these two age groups have significant differences in height, waist circumference, WHR, WHtR, and systolic blood pressure ($p < 0.05$). We found significant differences in mean systolic blood pressure, BMI, body fat percentage, waist and buttock circumferences, WHR, WHtR, fasting blood glucose, and TG and HDL serum levels between male and female persons ($p < 0.05$). Mean systolic blood pressure and waist circumference, WHR, WTR, fasting blood glucose, and TG serum level were higher in men; BMI, body fat percentage, buttock circumference, WHtR, and HDL were higher in women.

Table 1: Basic descriptive characteristics of the participants.

Variables	Age groups 40–49 years (N = 145), n (%)	50–60 years (N = 156), n (%)	Total (N = 301), n (%)	p value
Education level				
Less than diploma	88 (60.7)	89 (57.1)	177 (58.8)	
Diploma	37 (25.5)	50 (32.1)	87 (28.9)	0.408
Higher than diploma	20 (13.8)	17 (10.9)	37 (12.3)	
Occupation				
Shopkeepers	7 (4.8)	5 (3.2)	12 (4.0)	
Housewives	72 (49.7)	63 (40.4)	135 (44.9)	
Employees	18 (12.4)	31 (19.9)	49 (16.3)	0.047
Others	48 (33.1)	57 (36.5)	105 (34.9)	
Marital status				
Married	140 (96.6)	146 (93.6)	286 (95.0)	0.066
Single, divorced, or widowed	5 (3.4)	10 (6.4)	15 (5.0)	
Living region				
Urban	142 (97.9)	150 (96.2)	292 (97.0)	0.288
Rural	3 (2.1)	6 (3.8)	9 (3.0)	
Past medical history of physical disorders				
No	118 (81.4)	117 (75.0)	235 (78.1)	0.181
Yes	27 (18.6)	39 (25.0)	66 (21.9)	
Past medical history of mental disorders				
No	142 (97.9)	146 (93.6)	288 (95.7)	0.064
Yes	3 (2.1)	10 (6.4)	13 (4.3)	

Table 2: Distribution of the average score of lifestyle behaviors according to the HPLP-II questionnaire.

Lifestyle subdomains	Mean score of lifestyle subdomains in two age groups 40–49 years (N = 145)	50–60 years (N = 156)	Total mean ± SD (min–max)	p value
Spiritual growth	33.81 ± 5.31	33.81 ± 4.98	33.81 ± 5.13 (16–44)	0.999
Health responsibility	34.11 ± 7.38	32.70 ± 7.34	33.38 ± 7.38 (16–51)	0.097
Interpersonal relations	23.87 ± 4.57	23.76 ± 4.00	23.81 ± 4.27 (10–32)	0.820
Stress management	13.76 ± 3.07	13.59 ± 2.88	13.67 ± 2.97 (7–22)	0.622
Physical activity	12.99 ± 4.67	13.03 ± 4.84	13.01 ± 4.75 (7–28)	0.934
Nutrition	20.12 ± 3.32	20.63 ± 3.04	20.38 ± 3.18 (11–28)	0.165
Total score	138.65 ± 19.80	137.51 ± 18.63	138.06 ± 19.18 (88–191)	0.609

Table 3: Distribution of physical activity in men and women within age groups of 40–49 and 50–60 years.

IPAQ parameters	Mean ± SD of IPAQ parameters in the two age groups (MET min/week)					
	40–49 years			50–60 years		
	Female (N = 79)	Male (N = 66)	p value	Female (N = 75)	Male (N = 81)	p value
Walking	755.9 ± 974.5	4033.3 ± 40.39.2	<0.001	924.9 ± 834.4	2901.4 ± 3145.8	<0.001
Moderate activity	1889.1 ± 2112.9	2850.3 ± 3383.1	0.039	1782.4 ± 2602.0	4395.3 ± 5650.7	<0.001
Vigorous activity	209.1 ± 1008.2	992.1 ± 2397.2	0.009	336.5 ± 2026.0	1514.6 ± 3470.2	<0.001
Total physical activity	2854.1 ± 3143.0	7875.7 ± 5625.9	<0.001	3043.8 ± 3503.0	8811.3 ± 7550.6	<0.001

In this research, we found 19 individuals (6.4%) with FBS greater than or equal to 126 mg/dL: 5 (3.3%) of women and 14 (9.7%) of men; 189 persons (63.9%) with serum cholesterol greater than or equal to 200 mg/dL: 93 (61.6%) of women and 96 (66.2%) of men; 58 persons (19.6%) with borderline-high TG, 79 persons (26.7%) with high TG; and 6 persons (2.0%) with very high TG levels. One hundred thirteen (74.3%) of women and 126 (86.9%) of men had normal HDL levels (p = 0.006), and 85 persons (28.6%) had LDL cholesterol less than or equal to 100 mg/dL. Fifty-one subjects (17.0%) had systolic blood pressure greater than or equal to 140 mmHg, 55 persons (18.3%) had diastolic blood pressure greater than or equal to 90 mmHg, and totally 75 individuals (25%) had high blood pressure.

Relative distribution of body mass index categories in two sexes is presented in Figure 1. Nobody has BMI less than 18.5 kg/m^2 in this study. One hundred twenty-six persons

Table 4: Anthropometric variables, blood pressure, fasting blood sugar, and serum lipids profile of the participants.

Variables	Age groups 40–49 years (N = 145)	Age groups 50–60 years (N = 156)	Total mean ± SD (min–max)	p value
BMI (kg/m^2)	28.2 ± 4.6	28.3 ± 4.2	28.3 ± 4.4 (19.2–46.5)	0.773
Body fat percentage	32.3 ± 9.3	30.9 ± 11.2	31.6 ± 10.3 (5.1–52.2)	0.240
Waist circumference (cm)	93.4 ± 10.4	95.7 ± 8.7	94.6 ± 9.6 (70.0–123.0)	0.032
Buttock circumference (cm)	108.0 ± 8.8	107.1 ± 8.7	107.6 ± 8.7 (88.5–138.0)	0.372
WHR	0.86 ± 0.07	0.89 ± 0.06	0.88 ± 0.07 (0.71–1.09)	<0.001
WHtR	0.56 ± 0.06	0.58 ± 0.06	0.57 ± 0.60 (0.42–0.76)	0.001
Systolic blood pressure (mmHg)	121.2 ± 15.4	128.4 ± 16.9	124.9 ± 16.6 (88–186)	<0.001
Diastolic blood pressure (mmHg)	80.0 ± 9.9	81.1 ± 10.5	80.6 ± 10.3 (47–122)	0.347
FBS (md/dL)	95.5 ± 25.9	100.8 ± 34.5	98.3 ± 30.8 (60–330)	0.139
Total cholesterol (mg/dL)	212.0 ± 48.0	219.8 ± 44.9	216.1 ± 46.5 (115–457)	0.149
TG (mg/dL)	186.3 ± 138.9	162.7 ± 92.3	173.9 ± 117.0 (37–1108)	0.084
HDL (mg/dL)	55.9 ± 15.7	58.4 ± 14.1	57.2 ± 14.9 (21–117)	0.149
LDL (mg/dL)	113.2 ± 30.0	119.1 ± 26.9	116.3 ± 28.6 (47–233)	0.075

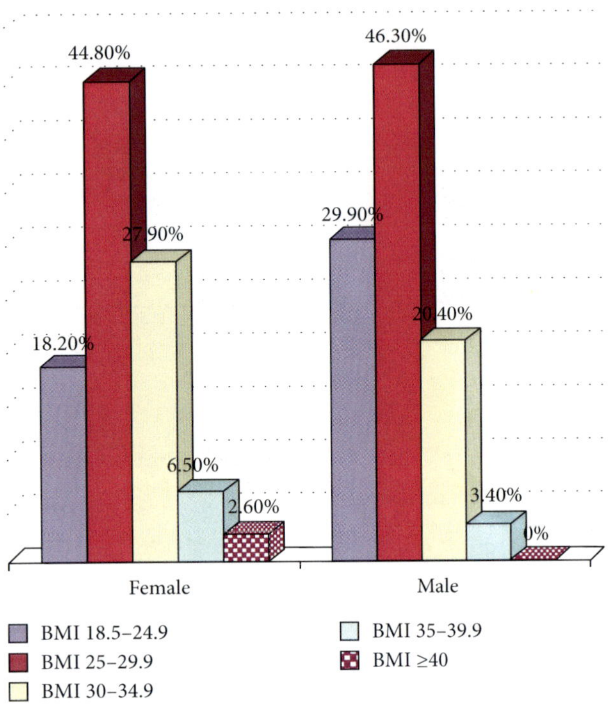

Figure 1: Body mass index distribution in two sexes.

(81.8%) of women and 103 (70.1%) of men were overweight or obese.

4. Discussion

We found that 10.6% of 40- to 60-year-old adults had unhealthy lifestyle behaviors in the subdomain of spiritual growth; 46.8% in the subdomain of health responsibility; and 48.2% in the subdomains of stress management, physical activity, and nutrition. This finding shows that interventional approaches for improvement of health-promoting behaviors in this region should primarily focus on stress management skills, physical activity, and healthy nutrition program. In the research performed by Enjezab et al. in Yazd, the central part of Iran, in which 483 middle-aged women were assessed, spiritual growth and physical activity subdomains had the highest and the lowest scores, respectively [40]; the research done by Mirghafourvand et al. in Tabriz, the northwest part of Iran, in which 322 infertile couples were examined, showed that the highest mean score was for the nutrition subscale and the lowest was for physical activity and health responsibility subscales in both men and women [41]; in another research conducted by Mirghafourvand et al., women in reproductive age scored highest in interpersonal relations and lowest in physical activity [42]. In the research carried out by Kim et al. in the United Arab Emirates which evaluated health-promoting lifestyle behaviors among Arabs and Koreans, spiritual growth and interpersonal relations had the highest scores; Arabs scored low on physical activity, and Koreans scored low on health responsibility [43]. These differences in health lifestyle behaviors can be related to ethnic characteristics, cultural variations, and the properties of the population under study which can have impact on the results.

In our study, the 50- to 60-year-old participants had higher scores in the nutrition subscale of the HPLP-II questionnaire; also, women had higher scores in the subdomain of health responsibility. These results show that we should pay more attention to dietary patterns of young adults and should implement interventional plans to encourage men to improve their health care. Okubo et al. reported in their study that older people tended to pay more attention to their diets than younger adults [44]. Vlassoff reported that gender is an important factor which can influence the determinants and consequences of health and illness. He suggested the involvement of both men and women in health education and interventions for promotion of health lifestyles [45], and Bertakis et al. reported that women had a significantly higher number of visits to their primary care clinic and diagnostic services than men. In their study, mean charges for primary care, specialty care, emergency treatment, and diagnostic services and annual total charges were higher for women than men [46].

In this study, nearly 16% of women were inactive and 23.4% of them were minimally active, and men had more physical activity than women. The World Health Organization recommends that adults aged 18–64 should do at least 150 minutes of moderate-intensity aerobic PA or do at least 75 minutes of vigorous-intensity PA throughout the week or an equivalent combination of moderate- and vigorous-intensity activity. This organization advices that, for additional health benefits, adults should increase their moderate-intensity PA to 300 minutes per week or engage in 150 minutes of vigorous-intensity aerobic PA per week [47]; therefore, considering the results, we should implement interventional programs to improve PA in 40- to 60-year-old population, especially for women. In the research done by Asgari et al. in Iran, 32.5% of study population aged 15–64 years did exercise at least 10 minutes in their free time [48], and in the research performed by Jurakić et al., conducted on 1032 Croatians aged 15 years and above, the lowest physical activity was found in the 15–24 age group (42.7 MET hours/week) and the highest in the 55–64 age group (72.0 MET hours/week); they reported that the majority of participants (74%) reached the level of at least 30 minutes of moderate physical activity 5 days a week, which is considered as the lowest level of physical activity for achieving health benefits [49]. In a systematic review conducted to explore the PA patterns among South Asian adults, the overall prevalence of inactivity was reported as follows: India 18.5%–88.4%, Pakistan 60.1%, and Sri Lanka 11.0%–31.8% [50]. In the research of Anjana et al. which was conducted among individuals aged ≥20 years in four regions of India, similar to the results of our study, men were significantly more active than women [51]. Yates et al. evaluated differences in levels of PA between white and South Asian populations in Leicestershire, UK. They showed that South Asian participants self-reported less moderate-intensity to vigorous-intensity PA (30 versus 51 min/day) and walking (11 versus 17 min/day) [52]. Considering a wide variation in the prevalence of physical inactivity within and between countries [50], these differences in the results can be justifiable.

Mean systolic blood pressure, waist circumference, WHR, WTR, fasting blood glucose, and TG serum level were higher in men; BMI, body fat percentage, buttock circumference, WHtR, and HDL were higher in women. In this research, 6.4% of the participants had FBS ≥126 mg/dL; 63.9% had serum cholesterol ≥200 mg/dL; and 19.6% had borderline-high TG, 26.7% high TG, and 2.0% had very high TG levels. Nine percent of study population had HDL <40 mg/dL, and nearly 29% had LDL ≤100 mg/dL. Almost twenty-five percent of the persons had blood pressure ≥140/90 mmHg. Seventy-six percent of 40- to 60-year-old adults were overweight or obese (BMI ≥ 25).

In the research of Asgari et al. in Iran, 7.7% were diabetics and 25.2% were hypertensive at the age of 25–64 years. Obesity, overweight, and hypercholesterolemia were 14.8, 28.6, and 15.1, respectively, at the age of 15–64 years [48]. In the research of Bakhshi et al. in Iran, 22.3% of the adults aged ≥15 years in all provinces of this country were reported obese. Among all racial/ethnic groups, the highest prevalence value was observed in Turk/Gilak/Lor/Turkmen Iranian ethnicities group (25.5%) [53]. In the research of Krishna Kumar Aryal in Nepal among 15- to 69-year-old population, 21% were overweight or obese. The prevalence of raised blood pressure and raised blood glucose including those on medication was 26% and 4%, respectively; also, almost 23% of study population had raised total cholesterol (total cholesterol ≥190 mg/dL or under current medication for raised cholesterol). The World Health Organization advices to all countries to implement proper policies to reduce modifiable risk factors for NCDs and underlying social determinants through creation of health-promoting environments [4]. We should have policy options in our region to improve health lifestyle behaviors and control the current situation of NCD-related risk factors.

The most important strength of our research was evaluation of NCD-related risk factors in a population-based sample.

We did not take into account some of the behaviors such as alcohol, tobacco, and substance abuse which we did not intend to enter in this study, and this can be considered as a limitation of this research.

5. Conclusion

Health lifestyle behaviors in 40- to 60-year-old population need a proper intervention to improve the current situation.

Acknowledgments

The financial support of the Vice Chancellor for Research and Technology of Babol University of Medical Sciences and the kind cooperation of the middle-aged population of Amirkola to participate in this project are greatly appreciated.

References

[1] M. Chan and M. R. Bloomberg, *Political Will Need to Win Fight against Noncommunicable Diseases*, World Health Organization, Geneva, Switzerland, 2016, http://www.who.int/mediacentre/commentaries/political-noncommunicable-diseases/en.

[2] G. El-Kassas and F. Ziade, “Exploration of the dietary and lifestyle behaviors and weight status and their self-perceptions among Health Sciences University students in North Lebanon,” *BioMed Research International*, vol. 2016, Article ID 9762396, 14 pages, 2016.

[3] W. C. Willett, J. P. Koplan, R. Nugent, C. Dusenbury, P. Puska, and T. A. Gaziano, “Prevention of chronic disease by means of diet and lifestyle changes,” in *Disease Control Priorities in Developing Countries*, J. G. B. D. T. Jamison, A. R. Measham, and G. Alleyne, Eds., The International Bank for Reconstruction and Development/The World Bank, Washington, DC, USA, 2nd edition, 2006.

[4] World Health Organization, *Global Action Plan for the Prevention and Control of NCDs 2013-2020*, World Health Organization, Geneva, Switzerland, 2013.

[5] C. Hancock, *Review the Benefits of Physical Activity for Health and Well-Being*, C3 Collaborating for Health, London, UK, 2012.

[6] P. Bully, A. Sánchez, E. Zabaleta-Del-Olmo, H. Pombo, and G. Grandes, “Evidence from interventions based on theoretical models for lifestyle modification (physical activity, diet, alcohol

and tobacco use) in primary care settings: a systematic review," *Preventive Medicine*, vol. 76, pp. S76–S93, 2015.

[7] Y. Ye, W. Zhong, X. Lin et al., "Association between sedentary life style and risks of metabolic syndrome and diabetes mellitus type 2," *Zhonghua Liu Xing Bing Xue Za Zhi*, vol. 35, no. 11, pp. 1235–1240, 2014, in Chinese.

[8] C. Julia, S. Péneau, V. A. Andreeva et al., "Weight-loss strategies used by the general population: how are they perceived?," *PLoS One*, vol. 9, no. 5, Article ID e97834, 2014.

[9] M. Ezzati and E. Riboli, "Behavioral and dietary risk factors for noncommunicable diseases," *New England Journal of Medicine*, vol. 369, pp. 954–964, 2013.

[10] A. S. Page and B. M. Winklhofer-Roob, "Five-minutes-to-twelve for implementation of early changes in dietary and lifestyle behaviour across Europe," *International Journal of Obesity*, vol. 35, no. 1, pp. S1–S2, 2011.

[11] G. Claire, "Obesity: effectiveness of a brief physician intervention," *Nature Reviews Endocrinology*, vol. 13, no. 1, p. 5, 2017.

[12] I. A. Macdonald and R. Atkinson, "Public health initiatives in obesity prevention: the need for evidence-based policy," *International Journal of Obesity*, vol. 35, no. 4, p. 463, 2011.

[13] T. A. Wadden, V. L. Webb, C. H. Moran, and B. A. Bailer, "Lifestyle modification for obesity: new developments in diet, physical activity, and behavior therapy," *Circulation*, vol. 125, no. 9, pp. 1157–1170, 2012.

[14] World Health Organization, *Healthy Diet. Fact Sheet No. 394*, World Health Organization, Geneva, Switzerland, 2015, http://www.who.int/mediacentre/factsheets/fs394/en.

[15] World Health Organization, *Physical Activity. Fact Sheet No. 385*, World Health Organization, Geneva, Switzerland, 2017, http://www.who.int/mediacentre/factsheets/fs385/en.

[16] World Health Organization, *Obesity and Overweight. Fact Sheet No. 311*, World Health Organization, Geneva, Switzerland, 2016, http://www.who.int/mediacentre/factsheets/fs311/en.

[17] M. Sadeghi, A. A. Haghdoost, A. Bahrampour, and M. Dehghani, "Modeling the burden of cardiovascular diseases in Iran from 2005 to 2025: the impact of demographic changes," *Iranian Journal of Public Health*, vol. 46, no. 4, pp. 506–516, 2017.

[18] M. Talaei, N. Sarrafzadegan, M. Sadeghi et al., "Incidence of cardiovascular diseases in an Iranian population: the Isfahan Cohort Study," *Archives of Iranian Medicine*, vol. 16, no. 3, pp. 138–144, 2013.

[19] A. Esteghamati, A. Meysamie, O. Khalilzadeh et al., "Third national surveillance of risk factors of non-communicable diseases (SuRFNCD-2007) in Iran: methods and results on prevalence of diabetes, hypertension, obesity, central obesity, and dyslipidemia," *BMC Public Health*, vol. 9, no. 1, p. 167, 2009.

[20] H. Fakhrzadeh, S. Djalalinia, M. Mirarefin et al., "Prevalence of physical inactivity in Iran: a systematic review," *Journal of Cardiovascular and Thoracic Research*, vol. 8, no. 3, pp. 92–97, 2016.

[21] S. Ebrahimof, F. Hosseini-Esfahani, P. Mirmiran, M. Fallah-Kezabi, and F. Azizi, "Food Patterns and Framingham Risk Score in Iranian adults: Tehran Lipid and Glucose Study: 2005–2011," *Metabolic Syndrome and Related Disorders*, vol. 16, no. 1, pp. 64–71, 2018.

[22] F. Azizi, "Tehran lipid and glucose study: a legacy for prospective community-based research," *Archives of Iranian Medicine*, vol. 17, no. 6, pp. 392-393, 2014.

[23] W. V. Brown, H. E. Bays, R. La Forge, and G. Sikand, "JCL roundtable: gender differences in risk reduction with lifestyle changes," *Journal of Clinical Lipidology*, vol. 9, no. 4, pp. 486–495, 2015.

[24] N. Mastellos, L. H. Gunn, L. M. Felix, J. Car, and A. Majeed, "Transtheoretical model stages of change for dietary and physical exercise modification in weight loss management for overweight and obese adults," *Cochrane Database of Systematic Reviews*, vol. 5, no. 2, article CD008066, 2014.

[25] M. Razavi, S. Fournier, D. S. Shepard, G. Ritter, G. K. Strickler, and W. B. Stason, "Effects of lifestyle modification programs on cardiac risk factors," *PLoS One*, vol. 9, no. 12, Article ID e114772, 2014.

[26] H. A. Tagoe and F. A. A. Dake, "Healthy lifestyle behaviour among Ghanaian adults in the phase of a health policy change," *Globalization and Health*, vol. 7, no. 1, p. 7, 2011.

[27] World Health Organization, *Module 5: Understanding Health Policy Processes*, World Health Organization, Geneva, Switzerland, 2005, http://www.who.int/hac/techguidance/tools/disrupted_sectors/adhsm_mod5_en.

[28] K. Hajian-Tilaki, "Sample size estimation in epidemiologic studies," *Caspian Journal of Internal Medicine*, vol. 2, no. 4, pp. 289–298, 2011.

[29] L. Jahangiry, D. Shojaeizadeh, A. Montazeri, M. Najafi, K. Mohammad, and M. Yaseri, "Adherence and attrition in a web-based lifestyle intervention for people with metabolic syndrome," *Iranian Journal of Public Health*, vol. 43, no. 9, pp. 1248–1258, 2014.

[30] S. Zhang, F. Tao, A. Ueda, C. Wei, and J. Fang, "The influence of health-promoting lifestyles on the quality of life of retired workers in a medium-sized city of Northeastern China," *Environmental Health and Preventive Medicine*, vol. 18, no. 6, pp. 458–465, 2013.

[31] C. N. Wei, K. Harada, K. Ueda, K. Fukumoto, K. Minamoto, and A. Ueda, "Assessment of health-promoting lifestyle profile in Japanese university students," *Environmental Health and Preventive Medicine*, vol. 17, no. 3, pp. 222–227, 2012.

[32] I. L. Mullins, T. O'Day, and T. Y. Kan, "Validation of the Health-Promoting Lifestyle Profile II for Hispanic male truck drivers in the Southwest," *Clinical Nursing Research*, vol. 22, no. 3, pp. 375–394, 2013.

[33] P. T. Tanjani, M. Azadbakht, G. Garmaroudi, R. Sahaf, and Z. Fekrizadeh, "Validity and reliability of Health Promoting Lifestyle Profile II in the Iranian elderly," *International Journal of Preventive Medicine*, vol. 7, no. 1, p. 74, 2016.

[34] I. Mohammadi Zeidi, A. Pakpour Hajiagha, and B. Mohammadi Zeidi, "Reliability and validity of Persian version of the Health-Promoting Lifestyle Profile," *Journal of Mazandaran University of Medical Sciences*, vol. 22, no. 1, pp. 103–113, 2012.

[35] M. H. Baghiani Moghaddam, F. Bakhtari Aghdam, M. Asghari Jafarabadi et al., "The Iranian version of International Physical Activity Questionnaire (IPAQ) in Iran: content and construct validity, factor structure, internal consistency and stability," *World Applied Sciences Journal*, vol. 18, no. 8, pp. 1073–1080, 2012.

[36] IPAQ Instruction Office, *Guidelines for Data Processing and Analysis of the International Physical Activity Questionnaire (IPAQ)-Short Form*, IPAQ Instruction Office, Barcelona, Spain, 2004, http://www.institutferran.org/documentos/scoring_short_ipaq_april04.

[37] National Cholesterol Education Program (NCEP) Expert Panel on Detection, Evaluation, and Treatment of High Blood

Cholesterol in Adults (Adult Treatment Panel III), "Third report of the National Cholesterol Education Program (NCEP) expert panel on detection, evaluation, and treatment of high blood cholesterol in adults (adult treatment panel III) final report," *Circulation*, vol. 106, no. 25, pp. 3143–3421, 2002.

[38] D. D. Reidpath, J. C. Cheah, F. C. Lam, S. Yasin, I. Soyiri, and P. Allotey, "Validity of self-measured waist and hip circumferences: results from a community study in Malaysia," *Nutrition Journal*, vol. 12, no. 1, p. 135, 2013.

[39] M. Dehghan and A. T. Merchant, "Is bioelectrical impedance accurate for use in large epidemiological studies?," *Nutrition Journal*, vol. 7, no. 1, p. 26, 2008.

[40] B. Enjezab, Z. Farajzadegan, F. Taleghani, A. Aflatoonian, and M. A. Morowatisharifabad, "Health promoting behaviors in a population-based sample of middle-aged women and its relevant factors in Yazd, Iran," *International Journal of Preventive Medicine*, vol. 3, no. 1, pp. S191–S198, 2012.

[41] M. Mirghafourvand, F. Sehhati, and M. Rahimi, "Health-promoting lifestyle and its demographic predictors in infertile couples referred to infertility clinic of Tabriz Al-Zahra Hospital, 2013," *Journal of Caring Sciences*, vol. 3, no. 3, pp. 175–184, 2014.

[42] M. Mirghafourvand, A. Baheiraei, S. Nedjat, E. Mohammadi, S. M. Charandabi, and R. Majdzadeh, "A population-based study of health-promoting behaviors and their predictors in Iranian women of reproductive age," *Health Promotion International*, vol. 30, no. 3, pp. 586–594, 2015.

[43] H. J. Kim, S. Choi-Kwon, H. Kim, Y. H. Park, and C. K. Koh, "Health-promoting lifestyle behaviors and psychological status among Arabs and Koreans in the United Arab Emirates," *Research in Nursing and Health*, vol. 38, no. 2, pp. 133–141, 2015.

[44] H. Okubo, S. Sasaki, K. Murakami et al., "Designing optimal food intake patterns to achieve nutritional goals for Japanese adults through the use of linear programming optimization models," *Nutrition Journal*, vol. 14, no. 1, p. 57, 2015.

[45] C. Vlassoff, "Gender differences in determinants and consequences of health and illness," *Journal of Health, Population and Nutrition*, vol. 25, no. 1, pp. 47–61, 2007.

[46] K. D. Bertakis, R. Azari, L. J. Helms, E. J. Callahan, and J. A. Robbins, "Gender differences in the utilization of health care services," *Journal of Family Practice*, vol. 49, no. 2, pp. 147–152, 2000.

[47] World Health Organization, *Global Recommendations on Physical Activity for Health*, WHO, Geneva, Switzerland, 2010, http://whqlibdoc.who.int/publications/2010/9789241599979.

[48] F. Asgari, H. Aghajani, M. Haghazali, and H. Heidarian, "Non-communicable diseases risk factors surveillance in Iran," *Iranian Journal of Public Health*, vol. 38, no. 1, pp. 119–122, 2009.

[49] D. Jurakić, Z. Pedišić, and M. Andrijašević, "Physical activity of Croatian population: cross-sectional study using International Physical Activity Questionnaire," *Croatian Medical Journal*, vol. 50, pp. 165–173, 2009.

[50] C. D. Ranasinghe, P. Ranasinghe, R. Jayawardena, and A. Misra, "Physical activity patterns among South-Asian adults: a systematic review," *International Journal of Behavioral Nutrition and Physical Activity*, vol. 10, no. 1, p. 116, 2013.

[51] R. M. Anjana, R. Pradeepa, A. K. Das et al., "Physical activity and inactivity patterns in India–results from the ICMR-INDIAB study (Phase-1) [ICMR-INDIAB-5]," *International Journal of Behavioral Nutrition and Physical Activity*, vol. 11, no. 1, p. 26, 2014.

[52] T. Yates, J. Henson, C. Edwardson, D. H. Bodicoat, M. J. Davies, and K. Khunti, "Differences in levels of physical activity between white and South Asian populations within a healthcare setting: impact of measurement type in a cross-sectional study," *BMJ Open*, vol. 5, no. 7, article e006181, 2015.

[53] E. Bakhshi, J. Koohpayehzadeh, B. Seifi et al., "Obesity and related factors in Iran: the STEPS Survey, 2011," *Iranian Red Crescent Medical Journal*, vol. 17, no. 6, article e22479, 2015.

Ethnic Differences in Risk Factors for Obesity among Adults

Liang Wang,[1] Jodi Southerland,[2] Kesheng Wang,[1] Beth A. Bailey,[3] Arsham Alamian,[1] Marc A. Stevens,[1] and Youfa Wang[4]

[1]*Department of Biostatistics and Epidemiology, College of Public Health, East Tennessee State University, Johnson City, TN, USA*
[2]*Department of Community and Behavioral Health, College of Public Health, East Tennessee State University, Johnson City, TN, USA*
[3]*Department of Family Medicine, Quillen College of Medicine, East Tennessee State University, Johnson City, TN, USA*
[4]*Fisher Institute of Health and Well-Being, Systems-Oriented Global Childhood Obesity Intervention Program, Department of Nutrition and Health Sciences, College of Health, Ball State University, Muncie, IN, USA*

Correspondence should be addressed to Liang Wang; wangl2@etsu.edu

Academic Editor: Aron Weller

Little attention has been given to differences in obesity risk factors by racial/ethnic groups. Using data from the 2011-2012 California Health Interview Survey, we examined differences in risk factors for obesity among Whites, Latinos, Asians, and African Americans among 42,935 adults (24.8% obese). Estimates were weighted to ensure an unbiased representation of the Californian population. Multiple logistic and linear regression analyses were used to examine the differences in risk factors for obesity. Large ethnic disparities were found in obesity prevalence: Whites (22.0%), Latinos (33.6%), African Americans (36.1%), and Asians (9.8%). Differences in risk factors for obesity were also observed: Whites (gender, age, physical activity, smoking, arthritis, and diabetes medicine intake), Latinos (age, arthritis, and diabetes medicine intake), Asians (age, binge drinking, arthritis, and diabetes medicine intake), and African Americans (gender, physical activity, smoking, binge drinking, and diabetes medicine intake). Females were more likely to be obese among African Americans (odds ratio (OR) = 1.43, 95% confidence interval (CI) = 1.05–1.94), but less likely among Whites (OR = 0.80, 95% CI = 0.74–0.87). Race/ethnicity should be considered in developing obesity prevention strategies.

1. Introduction

The obesity epidemic in the United States (U.S.) has become a public health crisis [1–6]. Data from the 2011-2012 U.S. national survey showed that the prevalence of adult obesity was 34.9% and varied by ethnicity (e.g., 10.8% for non-Hispanic Asians, 32.6% for non-Hispanic Whites, 42.5% for Hispanics, and 47.8% for non-Hispanic Blacks) [3]. With the exception of Asians, the prevalence of grade 2 obesity (body mass index [BMI] $\geq$ 35) and grade 3 obesity (BMI $\geq$ 40) was significantly higher among racial/ethnic minorities than in Whites, particularly among females [3]. Numerous cross-sectional and longitudinal studies have identified similar trends [4–6]. National health objectives call for the elimination of health disparities and achievement of health equity [7]. Racial/ethnic minorities currently comprise 36.3% of the U.S. population and are expected to increase to more than 50% of the total population by 2050 [8, 9]. Disproportionate increases in the prevalence of obesity have led to persistent disparities, particularly among non-Whites [6].

Among adults in California, 35.0% were overweight and 24.7% were obese in 2014 [10]. An earlier report showed racial/ethnic differences in average BMI in Californian adults for both sexes, with larger difference in females [11]. Limited studies have reported the recent prevalence of obesity among Californian adults by demographics. To date, most research in adult obesity trends has focused on differences in the prevalence of obesity by individual, socioeconomic, or neighborhood characteristics [12–15], with less attention given to differences in obesity risk factors by racial/ethnic groups.

This study aimed to examine obesity-related risk factors among four major ethnic groups (Whites, Latinos, Asians, and African Americans [AAs]) in California using data from the 2011-2012 California Health Interview Survey (CHIS). This information can be used to develop targeted obesity prevention interventions and help eliminate health disparities over time.

2. Methods

2.1. Data and Sample Selection. The CHIS is a collaborative study of the University of California, Los Angeles Center for Health Policy Research, the California Department of Health Services, and the Public Health Institute. As one of the largest health surveys in the nation, this population-based random-digit dial telephone survey has been conducted every other year in California since 2001. The survey examines public health and healthcare access issues in the state. The 2011-2012 CHIS is the sixth data collection cycle for this survey since 2001. Among the randomly selected households, one adult who was 18 years or older was then randomly selected as the respondent. Details about the sampling design and methodology can be found elsewhere [16]. Procedures for data collection and analysis were approved by the Institutional Review Boards (IRBs) at the participant universities and agencies. The current study was approved by the IRB of the authors' university.

Due to small sample sizes for Pacific Islander ($n = 73$, 0.17%), American Indian/Alaskan native ($n = 636$, 1.48%), and other single/multiple racial groups ($n = 3,065$; 7.14%), we combined them as "other." In the current study, a total of 42,935 adults were included in the analysis, including 26,376 (61.43%) Whites, 6,453 (15.03%) Latinos, 4,253 (9.91%) Asians, 2,079 (4.84%) AAs, and 3,774 (8.79%) adults classified as "other."

3. Measures

3.1. Dependent Variable. Obesity was defined as a BMI of 30 kg/m^2 or more. BMI was calculated from self-reported height and weight.

3.2. Independent Variables. Respondents' race was categorized as White, Latino, Asian, AA, and other. Gender was dichotomized to male or female. Respondents' age at the time of the interview was categorized into three levels: 18–44 years, 45–64 years, and 65 years or older. In addition, respondents were asked about employment status, for example, (i) "full-time employment (>21 hours/week)," (ii) "part-time employment (0–20 hours/week)," (iii) "employed and not at work," (iv) "unemployed and looking for work," and (v) "unemployed and not looking for work." In the present study, employment status was dichotomized to yes (i–iii) or no (iv, v). For physical activity, respondents answered "yes" or "no" to the question "Have you walked at least 10 minutes for leisure in the past 7 days?" Respondents were also asked about smoking habits. Responses included "currently smokes," "quit smoking," and "never smoked regularly." In the present study, smoking status was defined as "never," "current," or "past." Binge drinking for males was defined as those who had five or more drinks on at least one occasion in the past month while female binge drinkers were those that had four or more drinks. Frequent binge drinking was defined as engaging in binge drinking daily or weekly, monthly, or more than monthly but less than weekly in the past year. Infrequent binge drinking was defined as engaging in binge drinking once in the past year, more than once but less than monthly in the past year. For arthritis status, respondents answered "yes" or "no" to the question "Has a doctor ever told have arthritis, gout, or lupus?" With regard to diabetes medicine intake, respondents answered "yes" or "no" to the question "Are you currently taking diabetes pills to lower blood sugar?" Furthermore, serious psychological distress (SPD) was determined using the Kessler psychological distress scale (K6) [17], which comprises six questions asking how often during the past 30 days a person felt "so sad that nothing could cheer them up," "nervous," "restless," "hopeless," "worthless," or that "everything was an effort." SPD is a nonspecific measure of psychological distress that has been psychometrically validated and can detect community DSM-IV cases from noncases. Responses are scored from 0 (none of time) to 4 (all the time) and summed to produce a total score. A score of 13 or above was defined as having SPD [17].

3.3. Statistical Analysis. Estimates from the CHIS sample were weighted to ensure an unbiased representation of the Californian population. SAS PROC SURVEYLOGISTIC procedure was used to estimate odds ratios (ORs) and 95% confidence intervals (CIs) for the association between independent variables and the prevalence of obesity. SAS PROC SURVEYREG procedure was used to estimate regression coefficients and standard errors for the association between independent variables and BMI. Multiple logistic and linear regression analyses were used to examine the association between all the independent variables and obesity and BMI. Race was found to have significant interactions with gender, age, physical activity, binge drinking, and diabetes medicine intake (all P-interaction < 0.05). Multiple logistic and linear regression analyses were then used to examine the differences in risk factors for obesity and BMI in Whites, Latinos, Asians, and AAs, respectively. All analyses were performed using SAS statistical software, version 9.2 (SAS Institute, Cary, NC, USA).

4. Results

Overall, the prevalence of obesity was 24.8% among Californian adults. Compared to Whites (22.0%), Latinos (33.6%) and AAs (36.1%) had a higher prevalence of obesity while Asians had a lower prevalence (9.8%). Individuals who were male, between the ages of 45–64 years, and unemployed had a higher prevalence of obesity than their counterparts. Other risk factors for obesity included lack of physical activity, past smoking, arthritis, use of diabetes medicine, and presence of SPD (Table 1).

Figure 1 shows the prevalence of obesity by ethnicity and gender. Asian women had the lowest prevalence of obesity, whereas AA women had the highest. Gender disparity in obesity prevalence appeared to be largest in AAs. Among men, ethnic disparities in obesity prevalence were largest

TABLE 1: The prevalence (%) of obesity according to characteristics of participants, the 2011-12 CHIS (n = 42,935).

Characteristics	Sample size	Prevalence (%)	95% CI	P value*
Overall	42,935	24.8	24.2–25.4	
Race				
White	26,376	**22.0**	**21.3–22.7**	
Latino	6,453	**33.6**	**31.8–35.4**	
Asian	4,253	**9.8**	**8.2–11.4**	**<0.0001**
African American	2,079	**36.1**	**32.8–39.4**	
Other	3,774	**29.9**	**27.5–32.4**	
Gender				
Male	17,848	**25.8**	**24.9–26.6**	**<0.0001**
Female	25,087	**23.9**	**23.1–24.7**	
Age in years				
18–44	12,010	**21.8**	**20.8–22.8**	
45–64	16,810	**30.1**	**28.9–31.3**	**<0.0001**
65+	14,115	**23.1**	**22.1–24.1**	
Employment				
No	21,424	**26.3**	**25.2–27.4**	**0.0005**
Yes	21,511	**23.9**	**23.0–24.7**	
Physical activity				
No	15,823	**28.0**	**26.9–29.2**	**<0.0001**
Yes	26,763	**23.0**	**22.1–23.8**	
Smoking status				
Never	25,405	**23.3**	**22.5–24.2**	
Current	4,977	**25.2**	**23.3–27.1**	**<0.0001**
Past	12,553	**28.6**	**27.3–29.8**	
Binge drinking				
Never	32,863	24.9	24.2–25.7	
Infrequent	5,948	25.2	23.5–26.9	0.378
Frequent	4,124	23.4	21.1–25.7	
Arthritis				
No	29,760	**22.5**	**21.8–23.2**	**<0.0001**
Yes	13,175	**33.9**	**32.5–35.3**	
Diabetes medicine intake				
No	38,234	**22.7**	**22.1–23.3**	**<0.0001**
Yes	3,396	**48.6**	**45.8–51.5**	
Serious psychological distress				
No	41,199	**24.4**	**23.9–25.0**	**<0.0001**
Yes	1,515	**35.2**	**30.7–39.7**	

CHIS, California Health Interview Survey; CI, confidence interval.
* P value is calculated from χ^2 test.
Notes. Sampling weights were used in analysis. Results in bold indicate statistically significant findings.

between Latino and Asians. Among women, disparities were largest between AAs and Asians. Overall, these differences were greater among women than among men.

Multivariate regression analyses of the associations between all potential risk factors and obesity/BMI are shown in Table 2. Multiple logistic regression analyses showed that compared to Whites, Latinos (OR = 1.94, 95% CI = 1.76–2.15) and AAs (OR = 1.96, 95% CI = 1.66–2.31) had an increased likelihood of being obese while Asians (OR = 0.41, 95% CI = 0.34–0.50) had a lower likelihood of being obese. Other risk factors for obesity included being male, 45–64 years of age, unemployment, lack of physical activity, past smoking, arthritis, and diabetes medicine intake (all $P < 0.001$). Multiple linear regression analyses showed similar results for risk factors of BMI.

Table 3 shows the risk factors associated with obesity for each ethnic group after adjusting for covariates. Multiple logistic regression analyses showed that six risk factors (gender, age, physical activity, smoking, arthritis, and diabetes medicine intake) in Whites, three risk factors (age, arthritis, and diabetes medicine intake) in Latinos, four risk factors (age, binge drinking, arthritis, and diabetes medicine intake)

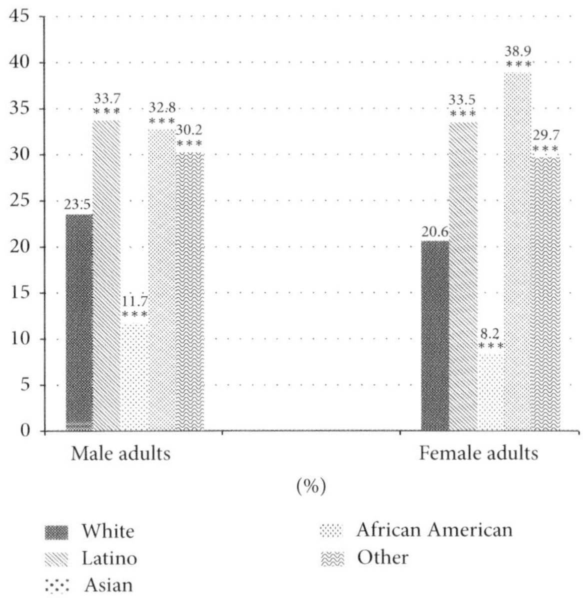

FIGURE 1: The prevalence (%) of obesity of adults in California in the United States, 2011-2012, by ethnicity and gender. *** $P < 0.001$ versus Whites. *Notes*. $P < 0.001$ for all ethnic groups versus Asians for both sexes. Not statistically significant (NS) for Latinos versus AAs, NS for the others versus AAs among men; $P < 0.01$ for Latinos versus AAs and $P < 0.001$ for the others versus AAs among women. NS for Latinos versus the others among men; $P < 0.01$ for Latinos versus the others among women.

in Asians, and five risk factors (gender, physical activity, smoking, binge drinking, and diabetes medicine intake) in AAs were associated with obesity, respectively.

The estimated ORs varied markedly across these ethnic groups. Females were more likely to be obese for AAs (OR = 1.43, 95% CI = 1.05–1.94), but less likely to be obese for Whites (OR = 0.80, 95% CI = 0.74–0.87); gender was not associated with obesity among Latinos and Asians. Whites and Asians who took diabetes medicine were more likely than Latinos and AAs to be obese (OR (95% CI): 3.74 (3.14–4.45) and 3.25 (2.14–4.96) versus 2.30 (1.79–2.95) and 2.24 (1.41–3.57)). The magnitude of differences in the association of risk factors with obesity also varied by ethnic group. The largest difference of OR was only 0.02 for the association of physical activity with obesity between Whites and AAs but was 1.17 for the association of arthritis with obesity between Asians and Whites.

Table 4 shows risk factors of BMI in different ethnic groups using multiple linear regression. Risk factors of BMI were the same as that of obesity for Whites and Latinos but varied for Asians and AAs. Five risk factors (gender, age, binge drinking, arthritis, and diabetes medicine intake) in Asians and six risk factors (age, physical activity, smoking, binge drinking, arthritis, and diabetes medicine intake) in AAs were associated with BMI, respectively. Specially, being female was associated with lower BMI for Whites and Asians ($\beta = -1.20, -1.59$, respectively, both $P < 0.0001$) and was not associated with BMI for Latinos and AAs. Whites and AAs with diabetes medicine intake had higher BMI than Latinos and Asians ($\beta = 4.42$ and 3.40 versus 2.01 and 2.12, respectively, all $P < 0.0001$). The magnitude of differences in the association between BMI and risk factors also varied by ethnic group. The largest difference of β was 0.39 for the association of gender with BMI between Whites and Asians but was 2.14 for the association of diabetes medicine intake with BMI between Whites and Latinos.

5. Discussion

This study sheds important light on ethnic differences in risk factors associated with obesity. This is one of the first studies to examine variation in risk factors for obesity prevalence across ethnic groups using a large representative sample in California, where large ethnic differences exist in obesity rates. We observed several key findings. First, we found considerable ethnic disparity in adult obesity prevalence: AAs (36.1%), Latinos (33.6%), Whites (22.0%), and Asians (9.8%). The prevalence in AAs was three times larger than that in Asians. The difference in females was even greater; for example, the prevalence in AAs was about 5 times that in Asians (38.9% versus 8.2%). A key strength of our study is that it had an adequate sample of Asians, while other national surveys, for example, National Health and Nutrition Examination Survey, do not include adequate numbers of Asians. It should be noted that several studies have recommended lowering the conventional BMI cutoff points for Asians by 2 to 3 points [18–20]. In 2000, the World Health Organization's (WHO) International Association for the Study of Obesity and the International Obesity Task Force published a report recommending that BMI cutoff of ≥23 and ≥25 for classifying overweight and obese for some Asian groups, respectively [20]. The WHO Expert Consultation have reviewed several publications on this issue and determined that the associations for health risk, BMI, and body fat percentage differ between European and Asian populations. The research shows risk for BMI of 22–25 kg/m^2 and high risk for ≥26 kg/m^2 for Asian populations [19]. Another study examined the relationship between BMI and mortality among Asians and showed that high BMI was significantly associated with increased risk of mortality among Asian Americans. The study also reported no significant increase in mortality for Asian Americans with a BMI between 20 and 25. The study is against lowering the cutoff points of overweight and obesity for Asians [21]. Given the apparent lack of consensus on use of lower obesity BMI cutoff points for Asians, we defined obesity as BMI ≥ 30, which may be indicative of the lower obesity percentage for Asians but may not necessarily mean that they are at lower health risk related to weight.

Another key finding is the considerable ethnic variation in the risk factors for obesity.

Only three (age, arthritis, and diabetes medicine intake), four (age, binge drinking, arthritis, and diabetes medicine intake), and five (gender, physical activity, smoking, binge drinking, and diabetes medicine intake) of the nine factors we examined were associated with obesity in Latinos, Asians, and AAs, respectively, while six (gender, age, physical activity, smoking, arthritis, and diabetes medicine intake) of the

TABLE 2: Risk factors for obesity and BMI in U.S. adults, the 2011-12 CHIS (n = 42,935).

Characteristics	Obesity (based on logistic regression)			BMI (based on linear regression)		
	OR	95% CI	*P* value	β	SE	*P* value
Race						
White (ref)						
Latino	**1.94**	**1.76–2.15**	**<0.0001**	**2.25**	**0.14**	**<0.0001**
Asian	**0.41**	**0.34–0.50**	**<0.0001**	**−1.82**	**0.14**	**<0.0001**
African American	**1.96**	**1.66–2.31**	**<0.0001**	**2.10**	**0.22**	**<0.0001**
Other	**1.51**	**1.34–1.71**	**<0.0001**	**1.46**	**0.17**	**<0.0001**
Gender						
Male (ref)						
Female	**0.91**	**0.85–0.98**	**0.0107**	**−0.74**	**0.08**	**<0.0001**
Age in years						
18–44 years (ref)						
45–64 years	**1.32**	**1.20–1.45**	**<0.0001**	**1.09**	**0.13**	**<0.0001**
65+	**0.73**	**0.66–0.82**	**<0.0001**	**−0.44**	**0.13**	**0.001**
Employment						
No (ref)						
Yes	0.97	0.88–1.06	0.494	0.01	0.11	0.932
Physical Activity						
No (ref)						
Yes	**0.82**	**0.75–0.89**	**<0.0001**	**−0.71**	**0.11**	**<0.0001**
Smoking status						
Never (ref)						
Current	1.00	0.87–1.14	0.956	−0.24	0.13	0.084
Past	**1.19**	**1.09–1.29**	**<0.0001**	**0.48**	**0.10**	**<0.0001**
Binge drinking						
No (ref)						
Infrequent	1.05	0.94–1.17	0.427	0.18	0.15	0.233
Frequent	0.99	0.85–1.16	0.906	−0.03	0.16	0.850
Arthritis						
No (ref)						
Yes	**1.66**	**1.52–1.82**	**<0.0001**	**1.50**	**0.12**	**<0.0001**
Diabetes medicine intake						
No (ref)						
Yes	**2.89**	**2.54–3.29**	**<0.0001**	**3.19**	**0.15**	**<0.0001**
Serious psychological distress						
No (ref)						
Yes	1.17	0.95–1.45	0.137	0.41	0.32	0.207

CHIS, California Health Interview Survey; OR, odds ratio; CI, confidence interval.
Notes. Sampling weights were used in analysis. Results in bold indicate to be statistically significant.

factors were associated with obesity in Whites. Further, although obesity prevalence was actually higher in AAs and Latinos, risk factors in the present study were more strongly associated with obesity in Whites. These disparate observations suggest that other underlying biological, sociocultural, and environmental mechanisms not accounted for in the present study may have contributed to the obesity prevalence in ethnic minorities. For example, the literature suggests that social context and cultural factors are possible explanations for obesity disparities [22, 23]. Other studies suggest that since the majority of health disparities in adulthood have their etiological origin in childhood [24], it is important to examine factors linked to an individual's childhood such as maternal socioeconomic position [23]. More recent findings suggest, however, that the effect of socioeconomic status on obesity may be diminishing due to the increasing rates of obesity across ethnic, geographic, and community factors [25, 26]. It is important to note that employment status (used

Table 3: Multiple logistic regression analysis of ethnic differences in risk factors for obesity, the 2011-12 CHIS.

Characteristics	Whites		Latinos		Asians		African Americans		Largest difference between the ORs
	OR	95% CI	OR	95% CI	OR	95% CI	OR	95% CI	
Gender									
Male (ref)									
Female	**0.80*****	**0.74–0.87**	1.02	0.85–1.22	0.74	0.52–1.04	**1.43***	**1.05–1.94**	0.63 (African Americans-Whites)
Age in years									
18–44 (ref)									
45–64	**1.39*****	**1.24–1.56**	**1.29****	**1.07–1.56**	0.84	0.58–1.22	1.42	0.97–2.08	0.10 (Whites-Latinos)
65+	**0.80****	**0.68–0.93**	**0.71***	**0.53–0.96**	**0.53***	**0.31–0.92**	0.65	0.41–1.04	0.27 (Whites-Asians)
Employment									
No (ref)									
Yes	0.96	0.84–1.09	0.95	0.78–1.15	1.24	0.84–1.83	1.08	0.78–1.50	—
Physical Activity									
No (ref)									
Yes	**0.70*****	**0.64–0.77**	0.97	0.81–1.16	1.32	0.95–1.83	**0.68***	**0.49–0.95**	0.02 (Whites-African Americans)
Smoking status									
Never (ref)									
Current	0.96	0.81–1.14	1.07	0.84–1.35	1.06	0.59–1.92	1.17	0.79–1.73	—
Past	**1.17****	**1.05–1.30**	1.24	0.99–1.55	0.91	0.61–1.35	**1.57***	**1.06–2.33**	0.40 (African Americans-Whites)
Binge drinking									
No (ref)									
Infrequent	0.92	0.81–1.04	1.11	0.90–1.38	**1.79***	**1.10–2.90**	1.00	0.64–1.56	—
Frequent	0.93	0.77–1.13	0.99	0.74–1.34	1.27	0.64–2.53	**1.73***	**1.02–2.92**	—
Arthritis									
No (ref)									
Yes	**1.60*****	**1.45–1.77**	**1.63*****	**1.28–2.07**	**2.77*****	**1.86–4.13**	1.32	0.92–1.90	1.17 (Asians-Whites)
Diabetes medicine intake									
No (ref)									
Yes	**3.74*****	**3.14–4.45**	**2.30*****	**1.79–2.95**	**3.25*****	**2.14–4.96**	**2.24*****	**1.41–3.57**	1.50 (Whites-African Americans)
Serious psychological distress									
No (ref)									
Yes	1.18	0.88–1.59	1.13	0.80–1.59	1.15	0.53–2.47	1.40	0.66–2.95	—

CHIS, California Health Interview Survey; AOR, adjusted odds ratio; CI, confidence interval.
Notes. Sampling weights were used in analysis. Results in bold indicate to be statistically significant.
$^{*}P < 0.05$, $^{**}P < 0.01$, and $^{***}P < 0.001$.

TABLE 4: Multiple linear regression analysis of ethnic differences in risk factors for body mass index (BMI).

Characteristics	Whites β (SE)	Latinos β (SE)	Asians β (SE)	African Americans β (SE)	Largest difference between the β's
Gender					
Male (ref)					
Female	**−1.20 (0.09)***	0.15 (0.27)	**−1.59 (0.27)***	0.61 (0.42)	0.39 (Whites-Asians)
Age in years					
18–44 (ref)					
45–64	**1.17 (0.12)***	**1.26 (0.29)***	**0.52 (0.26)***	**0.87 (0.43)***	0.74 (Latinos-Asians)
65+	−0.17 (0.14)	**−0.87 (0.42)***	0.29 (0.45)	**−2.00 (0.61)***	1.13 (Latinos-African Americans)
Employment					
No (ref)					
Yes	0.11 (0.12)	−0.09 (0.32)	0.54 (0.28)	−2.29 (0.44)	—
Physical activity					
No (ref)					
Yes	**−0.97 (0.09)***	−0.46 (0.29)	0.28 (0.23)	**−1.40 (0.40)***	0.43 (Whites-African Americans)
Smoking status					
Never (ref)					
Current	−0.28 (0.14)	0.20 (0.34)	0.20 (0.39)	−0.78 (0.50)	
Past	**0.41 (0.10)***	0.47 (0.26)	0.48 (0.37)	**1.17 (0.52)***	0.76 (African Americans-Whites)
Binge drinking					
No (ref)					
Infrequent	−0.02 (0.14)	0.10 (0.31)	**1.27 (0.41)***	0.63 (0.62)	—
Frequent	−0.20 (0.17)	0.001 (0.38)	0.62 (0.51)	**1.82 (0.75)***	—
Arthritis					
No (ref)					
Yes	**1.37 (0.11)***	**1.88 (0.36)***	**1.28 (0.31)***	**1.51 (0.51)***	0.60 (Latinos-Asians)
Diabetes medicine intake					
No (ref)					
Yes	**4.42 (0.22)***	**2.01 (0.33)***	**2.12 (0.44)***	**3.40 (0.71)***	2.41 (Whites-Latinos)
Serious psychological distress					
No (ref)					
Yes	0.30 (0.31)	0.13 (0.47)	−0.27 (0.47)	1.12 (1.24)	—

SE, standard error.
Notes. Sampling weights were used in analysis. Results in bold indicate to be statistically significant.
$^{*}P < 0.05$, $^{**}P < 0.01$, and $^{***}P < 0.001$.

as a proxy for socioeconomic status) was not associated with obesity in any ethnic groups.

In this study, age, arthritis, and diabetes medicine intake were the most consistently identified risk factors for higher BMI and obesity. In some cases, age (e.g., among participants who were 65+ years) played a protective role. However, middle age (i.e., 45–64 years) was associated with increasing BMI among all but one ethnic group. Arthritis was positively associated with BMI in all ethnic groups and positively associated with obesity in all ethnic groups except for AAs. Similarly, data from the 2003–2009 Behavioral Risk Factor Surveillance System reported that obesity prevalence in those with arthritis was 54% higher than in nonarthritis patients [27]. Rheumatoid arthritis is an autoimmune disease that causes chronic inflammation affecting multiple synovial joints [28]. This form of arthritis can trigger metabolic alterations [29] that degrade lean tissue especially muscle mass [30]. The most common form of arthritis is osteoarthritis, traditionally affecting more older adults (>60 years) [31, 32]. Combined with an inactive lifestyle, arthritis likely increases accumulation of body fat and body weight leading to reduced muscle mass [33].

On the other hand, research has shown that overweight/obese individuals are more likely to experience osteoarthritis in their knees, hips, and hands [34, 35], suggesting obesity is a risk factor for osteoarthritis, particularly knee osteoarthritis. Studies indicate that obesity increases the weight on a joint causing stress and the breakdown of cartilage that leads to knee and hip osteoarthritis [32, 36]. The cause of hand osteoarthritis has been linked to metabolic factors that are also associated with obesity such as adipocytokines [34]. More longitudinal studies are warranted to determine the potential pathways and interactions between arthritis and obesity.

Diabetes medicine intake was also positively associated with BMI and obesity in all ethnic groups. Adults with type 2 diabetes are more likely to report poorer health-related quality of life including limitations to daily activities thus increasing risk for obesity [37]. Given the increasing prevalence of arthritis (about 22%) and type 2 diabetes (about 10%) among U.S. adults [38, 39], clinicians should screen for chronic conditions to assess risk for obesity, particularly among adults between the ages of 45 and 64 years.

Lack of adequate physical activity is a key contributor of obesity in U.S. adults. Yet in the present study, we found that physical activity protected against obesity only among Whites and AAs. Interestingly, Whites are more likely to meet the federal guidelines for physical activity when compared to Asians and Hispanic/Latino populations (21.3% versus 17.8% and 14.4%, respectively). AAs are slightly less physically active than Asians but more active than Hispanics/Latinos [40]. Lifestyle behavior interventions focused on physical activity habits could result in weight loss in obese adults [5, 41] and reduce risk for obesity.

Our study has some limitations. First, the data are cross-sectional and cannot test causality. Second, data on other potential obesity risk factors such as dietary habits, built environment, and neighborhood level characteristics [22, 42, 43] were not collected. Third, we did not include other known predictors of obesity such as comorbidities, acculturation, and nativity. Moreover, this study utilized self-reported data, which may suffer from report errors and bias. Nevertheless, previous research has shown that such self-reported data can be reliable and are widely used [44]. With regard to BMI, self-report measures are used ubiquitously in large, population-based studies despite the potential for systematic misreporting [45]. Large sample sizes are critical in the epidemiologic examination of various public health issues such as obesity. When using large sample sizes, however, there can be various opportunities for potential bias, including sampling error, measurement error, multiple comparisons errors, aggregation error, and errors associated with the systematic exclusion of information [46]. For this particular study, for example, some participants may have underestimated their BMI. Studies have documented error in self-reported BMI (e.g., over or underestimates) [45]. While this is a potential limitation, a recent study provides promise. Racial/ethnic minorities (e.g., Blacks, Hispanics, and Native Americans) were found to more accurately report their BMI when compared to Whites [47].

Despite the limitations, the CHIS is the largest state health survey in the nation and one of the few to provide robust samples of many typically underrepresented racial and ethnic groups. Our study adds to the current literature by identifying ethnic variation in risk factors for obesity prevalence using a comprehensive state-level survey for adults. Variations by race underscore the influence of personal characteristics and contextual factors reported in previous studies [13, 14, 22]. There has been growing attention toward eliminating health disparities in the U.S. and toward improving the health of the population as a whole [7]. With the increasing diversity of America's population, it will be important for public health professionals and policy-makers to understand the determinants of obesity risk that are unique to ethnic groups when developing obesity prevention programming, a key target for eliminating health disparities.

6. Conclusion

Large disparities in the prevalence of obesity existed across ethnic groups in California. Risk factors for obesity also varied across ethnic groups. Understanding variations in risk factors is important for implementing effective obesity interventions in the increasingly diverse U.S. population. Public health practitioners and policy-makers cannot assume that obesity intervention programs and policies will impact ethnic groups uniformly. Therefore, public health and clinical interventions including communications on reducing obesity risk should be tailored to ethnic groups.

Competing Interests

The authors declare that they have no competing interests.

Acknowledgments

The authors thank the support of the 2011-2012 California Health Interview Survey, College of Public Health and Quillen College of Medicine of East Tennessee State University, and School of Public Health and Health Professions of University at Buffalo of State University of New York. Part of Dr. Youfa Wang's related effort was supported by research grants from the U.S. National Institutes of Health (NIH, 1R01HD064685-01A1, R01DK81335-01A1).

References

[1] Y. Wang, M. A. Beydoun, L. Liang, B. Caballero, and S. K. Kumanyika, "Will all Americans become overweight or obese? Estimating the progression and cost of the US obesity epidemic," *Obesity*, vol. 16, no. 10, pp. 2323–2330, 2008.

[2] Y. Wang and M. A. Beydoun, "The obesity epidemic in the United States—gender, age, socioeconomic, racial/ethnic, and geographic characteristics: a systematic review and meta-regression analysis," *Epidemiologic Reviews*, vol. 29, no. 1, pp. 6–28, 2007.

[3] C. L. Ogden, M. D. Carroll, B. K. Kit, and K. M. Flegal, "Prevalence of childhood and adult obesity in the United States, 2011-2012," *The Journal of the American Medical Association*, vol. 311, no. 8, pp. 806–814, 2014.

[4] M. A. Beydoun and Y. Wang, "Pathways linking socioeconomic status to obesity through depression and lifestyle factors among young US adults," *Journal of Affective Disorders*, vol. 123, no. 1–3, pp. 52–63, 2010.

[5] K. M. Flegal, M. D. Carroll, C. L. Ogden, and L. R. Curtin, "Prevalence and trends in obesity among US adults, 1999–2008," *The Journal of the American Medical Association*, vol. 303, no. 3, pp. 235–241, 2010.

[6] C. X. Romero, T. E. Romero, J. C. Shlay, L. G. Ogden, and D. Dabelea, "Changing trends in the prevalence and disparities of obesity and other cardiovascular disease risk factors in three racial/ethnic groups of USA adults," *Advances in Preventive Medicine*, vol. 2012, Article ID 172423, 8 pages, 2012.

[7] US Department of Health and Human Services, HealthyPeople.gov, Disparities; 2010, http://www.healthypeople.gov/2020/about/disparitiesAbout.aspx.

[8] US Centers for Disease and Control and Prevention (CDC), *Ethnic and Ethnic Minority Populations*, 2012, https://www.cdc.gov/minorityhealth/.

[9] S. L. Colby and J. M. Ortman, "Projections of the Size and Composition of the U.S. Population: 2014 to 2060," Current Population Reports P25-1143, U.S. Census Bureau, Washington, DC, USA, 2014.

[10] Nutrition, Physical Activity and Obesity Data, Trends and Maps, U.S. Department of Health and Human Services, Centers for Disease Control and Prevention (CDC), National Center for Chronic Disease Prevention and Health Promotion, Division of Nutrition, Physical Activity and Obesity, Atlanta, Ga, USA, 2015, http://www.cdc.gov/nccdphp/DNPAO/index.html.

[11] H. Lee, "Obesity among California adults: ethnic and ethnic differences," Public Policy Institute of California, 2006, http://www.ppic.org/content/pubs/report/R_906HLR.pdf.

[12] R. P. Lopez, "Neighborhood risk factors for obesity," *Obesity*, vol. 15, no. 8, pp. 2111–2119, 2007.

[13] J. Ludwig, L. Sanbonmatsu, L. Gennetian et al., "Neighborhoods, obesity, and diabetes—a randomized social experiment," *The New England Journal of Medicine*, vol. 365, no. 16, pp. 1509–1519, 2011.

[14] M. A. Papas, A. J. Alberg, R. Ewing, K. J. Helzlsouer, T. L. Gary, and A. C. Klassen, "The built environment and obesity," *Epidemiologic Reviews*, vol. 29, no. 1, pp. 129–143, 2007.

[15] C. E. Matthews, S. M. George, S. C. Moore et al., "Amount of time spent in sedentary behaviors and cause-specific mortality in US adults," *American Journal of Clinical Nutrition*, vol. 95, no. 2, pp. 437–445, 2012.

[16] California Health Interview Survey 2011-2012, *Adult Public Data File 2011*, UCLA Center for Health Policy Research, Los Angeles, Calif, USA, 2014, http://healthpolicy.ucla.edu/chis/design/Documents/chis2011-2012_method-1_2014-06-09.pdf.

[17] R. C. Kessler, G. Andrews, L. J. Colpe et al., "Short screening scales to monitor population prevalences and trends in non-specific psychological distress," *Psychological Medicine*, vol. 32, no. 6, pp. 959–976, 2002.

[18] W. C. Hsu, M. R. G. Araneta, A. M. Kanaya, J. L. Chiang, and W. Fujimoto, "BMI cut points to identify at—risk asian americans for type 2 diabetes screening," *Diabetes Care*, vol. 38, no. 1, pp. 150–158, 2015.

[19] WHO expert consultation, "Appropriate body-mass index for Asian populations and its implications for policy and intervention strategies," *The Lancet*, vol. 363, no. 9403, pp. 157–163, 2004.

[20] WHO, "The Asia-Pacific perspective: redefining obesity and its treatment," 2000, http://www.wpro.who.int/nutrition/documents/docs/Redefiningobesity.pdf.

[21] Y. Park, S. Wang, C. M. Kitahara et al., "Body mass index and risk of death in Asian Americans," *American Journal of Public Health*, vol. 104, no. 3, pp. 520–525, 2014.

[22] S. N. Bleich, R. J. Thorpe Jr., H. Sharif-Harris, R. Fesahazion, and T. A. LaVeist, "Social context explains race disparities in obesity among women," *Journal of Epidemiology and Community Health*, vol. 64, no. 5, pp. 465–469, 2010.

[23] L. J. Trotter, D. J. Bowen, and S. A. A. Beresford, "Testing for racial/ethnic differences in the association between childhood socioeconomic position and adult adiposity," *American Journal of Public Health*, vol. 100, no. 6, pp. 1088–1094, 2010.

[24] K. M. Ziol-Guest, G. J. Duncan, and A. Kalil, "Early childhood poverty and adult body mass index," *American Journal of Public Health*, vol. 99, no. 3, pp. 527–532, 2009.

[25] Q. Zhang and Y. Wang, "Trends in the association between obesity and socioeconomic status in U.S. adults: 1971 to 2000," *Obesity Research*, vol. 12, no. 10, pp. 1622–1632, 2004.

[26] Y. Wang and Q. Zhang, "Are American children and adolescents of low socioeconomic status at increased risk of obesity? Changes in the association between overweight and family income between 1971 and 2002," *The American Journal of Clinical Nutrition*, vol. 84, no. 4, pp. 707–716, 2006.

[27] Centers for Disease Control and Prevention (CDC), "Prevalence of obesity among adults with arthritis—United States, 2003–2009," *Morbidity and Mortality Weekly Report*, vol. 60, no. 16, pp. 509–513, 2011.

[28] K. Masuko, "Rheumatoid cachexia revisited: a metabolic co-morbidity in rheumatoid arthritis," *Frontiers in Nutrition*, vol. 1, article 20, 2014.

[29] G. S. Metsios, A. Stavropoulos-Kalinoglou, V. F. Panoulas et al., "New resting energy expenditure prediction equations for patients with rheumatoid arthritis," *Rheumatology*, vol. 47, no. 4, pp. 500–506, 2008.

[30] R. Roubenoff, R. A. Roubenoff, J. G. Cannon et al., "Rheumatoid cachexia: cytokine-driven hypermetabolism accompanying reduced body cell mass in chronic inflammation," *Journal of Clinical Investigation*, vol. 93, no. 6, pp. 2379–2386, 1994.

[31] D. T. Felson, "Weight and osteoarthritis," *The American Journal of Clinical Nutrition*, vol. 63, supplement, pp. 430S–432S, 1996.

[32] M. R. Sowers and C. A. Karvonen-Gutierrez, "The evolving role of obesity in knee osteoarthritis," *Current Opinion in Rheumatology*, vol. 22, no. 5, pp. 533–537, 2010.

[33] A. Stavropoulos-Kalinoglou, G. S. Metsios, Y. Koutedakis et al., "Redefining overweight and obesity in rheumatoid arthritis patients," *Annals of the Rheumatic Diseases*, vol. 66, no. 10, pp. 1316–1321, 2007.

[34] N. Arden and M. C. Nevitt, "Osteoarthritis: epidemiology," *Best Practice and Research: Clinical Rheumatology*, vol. 20, no. 1, pp. 3–25, 2006.

[35] D. T. Felson, "An update on the pathogenesis and epidemiology of osteoarthritis," *Radiologic Clinics of North America*, vol. 42, no. 1, pp. 1–9, 2004.

[36] A. T. Toivanen, M. Heliövaara, O. Impivaara et al., "Obesity, physically demanding work and traumatic knee injury are major risk factors for knee osteoarthritis—a population-based study with a follow-up of 22 years," *Rheumatology*, vol. 49, no. 2, pp. 308–314, 2010.

[37] Centers for Disease Control and Prevention (CDC), National Center for Health Statistics, Division of Health Interview Statistics, data from the National Health Interview Survey. Statistical analysis by the CDC, National Center for Chronic Disease Prevention and Health Promotion, Division of Diabetes Translation, http://www.cdc.gov/diabetes/statistics/mental/FigmentphyUS2008.htm.

[38] Centers for Disease Control and Prevention (CDC), "Prevalence of doctor-diagnosed arthritis and arthritis-attributable activity limitation—United States, 2007–2009," *Morbidity and Mortality Weekly Report*, vol. 59, pp. 1261–1265, 2010.

[39] Centers for Disease Control and Prevention (CDC), "National Diabetes Statistics Report," 2014, http://www.cdc.gov/diabetes/pubs/statsreport14/national-diabetes-report-web.pdf.

[40] V. L. Roger, A. S. Go, D. M. Lloyd-Jones et al., "Executive summary: heart disease and stroke statistics—2012 update: a report from the American Heart Association," *Circulation*, vol. 125, no. 1, pp. 188–197, 2012.

[41] B. H. Goodpaster, J. P. DeLany, A. D. Otto et al., "Effects of diet and physical activity interventions on weight loss and cardiometabolic risk factors in severely obese adults: a randomized trial," *Journal of the American Medical Association*, vol. 304, no. 16, pp. 1795–1802, 2010.

[42] P. A. Quatromoni, M. Pencina, M. R. Cobain, P. F. Jacques, and R. B. D'Agostino, "Dietary quality predicts adult weight gain: findings from the framingham offspring study," *Obesity*, vol. 14, no. 8, pp. 1383–1391, 2006.

[43] H. A. Beard, M. A. L. Ghatrif, R. Samper-Ternent, K. Gerst, and K. S. Markides, "Trends in diabetes prevalence and diabetes-related complications in older Mexican Americans from 1993-1994 to 2004-2005," *Diabetes Care*, vol. 32, no. 12, pp. 2212–2217, 2009.

[44] D. L. Paulhus and S. Vazire, "The self-report method," in *Handbook of Research Methods in Personality*, R. W. Robins, R. C. Fraley, and R. F. Krueger, Eds., pp. 224–239, Guilford Press, New York, NY, USA, 2007.

[45] A. Hattori and R. Sturm, "The obesity epidemic and changes in self-report biases in BMI," *Obesity*, vol. 21, no. 4, pp. 856–860, 2013.

[46] R. M. Kaplan, D. A. Chambers, and R. E. Glasgow, "Big data and large sample size: a cautionary note on the potential for bias," *Clinical and Translational Science*, vol. 7, no. 4, pp. 342–346, 2014.

[47] T. K. Richmond, I. Thurston, K. Sonneville, C. E. Milliren, C. E. Walls, and S. B. Austin, "Racial/ethnic differences in accuracy of body mass index reporting in a diverse cohort of young adults," *International Journal of Obesity*, vol. 39, no. 3, pp. 546–548, 2015.

27

The Association between Obesity and Cognitive Function in Otherwise Healthy Premenopausal Arab Women

Abdulaziz Farooq,[1,2] **Ann-Marie Gibson**,[2] **John J. Reilly**,[2] **and Nadia Gaoua**[3]

[1] *Athlete Health and Performance Research, Aspetar Orthopaedic and Sports Medicine Hospital, Doha, Qatar*
[2] *School of Psychological Sciences and Health, University of Strathclyde, Glasgow, UK*
[3] *School of Applied Sciences, London South Bank University, London, UK*

Correspondence should be addressed to Abdulaziz Farooq; mohammed.farooq@aspetar.com

Academic Editor: Sharon Herring

Objective. To examine the association between obesity and cognitive function in healthy premenopausal women. *Methods.* From a cohort of 220 women, 98 were randomly selected that provided complete data. Body composition was examined by dual-energy X-ray scan. All participants completed the Cambridge Neuropsychological Test Automated Battery (CANTAB) to assess cognitive performance in three domains: attention, memory, and planning executive function. The Reaction Time (RTI) test was used to assess motor and mental response speeds; the Stockings of Cambridge (SOC) test was used to assess planning executive function. For memory assessment, the Delayed Match to Sample (DMS), Pattern Recognition Memory (PRM), and Spatial Span (SSP) tests were used to assess forced choice recognition memory, visual pattern recognition memory, and working memory capacity, respectively. *Results.* 36 (36.7%) were morbidly obese, 22 (22.4%) obese, and 23 (23.5%) overweight. Performance on RTI and SOC planning ability were not associated with body mass index (BMI). DMS mean time to correct response, when stimulus is visible or immediately hidden (0 ms delay), was higher by 785 ± 302 ms (milliseconds) ($p = 0.011$) and 587 ± 259 ms ($p = 0.026$) in morbidly obese women compared to normal weight women. Memory span length was significantly lower in overweight (5.5 ± 1.3, $p = 0.008$) and obese women (5.6 ± 1.6, $p = 0.007$) compared to normal weight (6.7 ± 0.9). DEXA-assessed body fat (%) showed similar associations as BMI, and latency to correct response on DMS and PRM was positively correlated with percentage of body fat, but not with VO_2 max. *Conclusion.* In otherwise healthy premenopausal women, obesity did not impact accuracy on cognitive tasks related to attention, memory, or planning executive function, but morbid obesity was associated with higher latency to correct response on memory-specific tasks and lower memory span length.

1. Introduction

Cognitive function is a construct that represents an individual's ability to attain information and thus knowledge with constant application of memory, attention, and language skills [1]. While obesity is a well-known public health concern that leads to dyslipidemia, hypertension, type 2 diabetes, and cardiovascular diseases, there is limited research examining how it may influence cognitive function; however, several hypotheses have been put forward. These are pathophysiological changes with regard to vascular changes, insulin resistance, inflammation, reduced body fitness especially cardiovascular, and so on [2, 3]. Evidence suggests that the effect of obesity on cognitive function is not straightforward, rather obesity tends to affect the cognitive function of different people in different ways, specifically depending upon their age group. Lower body mass index (BMI) rather than higher BMI was found to be associated with increased incidence of dementia, especially in elderly people [4–8]. However, in midlife, the abovementioned findings were reversed; higher BMI was associated with increased incidence of dementia [9–11].

Some of the studies were observational, either longitudinal or cross-sectional studies, whereas some of them were designed to identify the underlying cellular processes [12–14]. Decrease in BMI in later years of life (postmenopausal women) is associated with poor cognitive performance. Driscoll et al. followed older postmenopausal women (65–79 years old) for an average of 3.5 years to examine the impact of weight gain on changes in cognition attributes. They found that women who maintained their weight or gained weight performed comparably on cognitive tests, but the women who lost weight during the study period had a poorer performance on cognitive tests, compared to either of the other two groups [15].

Conversely, studies have also concluded that there might not be any effect of obesity on cognitive function in females. For example, Elias et al. found that nonobese women and obese women scored comparably on various cognitive function tests (e.g., word fluency, visual reproduction, and digit span forward/backward), and the adverse outcome of obesity on cognitive function was limited to men only [16]. Some studies like that conducted by Kerwin et al. [17] were designed to explore the relationship between body fat distribution (measured by waist-to-hip ratio; WHR) and cognitive function. The researchers in this study classified older postmenopausal women by their BMI and found that the cognitive performance of women with a low waist-to-hip ratio decreased as their BMI increased, whereas the cognitive performance of women with a high waist-to-hip ratio increased as the BMI increased.

The majority of research is concentrated among menopausal women with underlying medical conditions. Therefore, further research is warranted especially in younger woman populations to explore the association between obesity and cognitive function by including more comprehensive and objective assessment of cognitive function as well as obesity. Again, BMI alone is an incomplete parameter to assess fatness; rather it should be supported by other parameters like fat distribution (assessed by dual-energy X-ray absorptiometry (DEXA) and computed tomography (CT) imagery) and cardiorespiratory fitness.

The aim of this study is to investigate the association between obesity and cognitive function in premenopausal healthy women.

2. Subjects and Methods

2.1. Subjects. We randomly recruited 220 women either from a gym (Aspire Active, Doha, Qatar) or by voluntary participation between February 2009 and December 2009. The study was conducted at Aspetar Qatar Orthopaedic and Sports Medicine Hospital. It was approved by the Institutional Research Ethics Committee, and all participants provided written consent prior to participation. The participants with diabetes mellitus, those who were pregnant or postmenopausal, or those receiving medical treatment for any chronic disease were excluded from the study; the only inclusion criterion was any willing healthy premenopausal women aged 18–50 years. The participants were clinically screened and excluded for the presence of diabetes mellitus, hypertension, or pregnancy. After 10-hour overnight fasting, the participants underwent a detailed clinical assessment, including body composition, fat distribution, and anthropometry measurements.

2.2. Anthropomorphic Assessment. Each participant's height was measured (without shoes) to the nearest 0.1 cm; weight was measured to the nearest 0.1 kg; and waist circumference was measured to the nearest 0.1 cm. A digital height-measuring device (Seca 242, Hamburg, Germany) and a portable stadiometer (Detecto, Webb City, Missouri, USA) were used to measure height and weight, respectively. Waist circumference was measured by a tape measurer horizontally at the smallest girth around the trunk. Two blood pressure readings were obtained 5 minutes apart with women in a relaxed seated position. The average systolic and diastolic blood pressures were calculated, and these values were used in subsequent analyses.

2.3. Body Composition Assessment. Fat mass (g), tissue (g), lean mass (g), and percentage of body fat were quantified by a DEXAD scanner XA (GE Medical Systems Lunar, Madison, Wisconsin, USA) uploaded with enCORE software (version 12.10; GE Medical Systems Lunar). CT scans were performed to obtain 5 CT axial images of each of the following regions: heart, liver, abdomen (at the L4-L5 level), and left and right midthighs. In the right thigh image, manual drawing was used to distinguish intramuscular adipose tissue from subcutaneous adipose tissue. For the abdominal region, cross-sectional axial images of the L4-L5 vertebral disc space were obtained. Manual drawing was used to differentiate omental adipose tissue from subcutaneous adipose tissue (which was further classified by manual drawing as superficial or deep). Two cross-sectional axial images of the left and right thighs at the femoral midpoint region were obtained. Intramuscular adipose tissue and subcutaneous adipose tissue in the thigh were distinguished by manual drawing using the right thigh image of adipose tissue. An upper limit of −30 Hounsfield units (HU) and a lower limit of −90 HU were used to differentiate adipose tissue from other tissue types on the CT images. All volumetric analyses were performed by an experienced radiologist by using the Somaris/5 Syngo CT2006A system (Siemens, Munich, Germany). The participants wore standard hospital gowns during the DEXA and CT scan procedures.

2.4. Fitness and Strength Assessment. The aerobic fitness of each participant was assessed by using the Bruce treadmill test. The starting speed was set to 2.74 km/h. The r and the intensity (speed and inclination) were increased by 2% at an interval of 3 minutes. The treadmill test was stopped once women requested to stop because of exhaustion. The peak heart rate (HR), percentage of predicted maximal HR, test duration, and peak oxygen uptake (i.e., VO_2 max) were measured. Subjects were also evaluated for hand grip strength using a dynamometer (Lode BV, Groningen, Netherlands) and the Biodex 3.0 system, version 3.4 (Biodex Medical Systems, Inc., Shirley, NY, USA). Leg strength was assessed by the same Biodex system used to measure hand grip strength, in terms of isokinetic knee flexion and extension concentrically (at 30°/second and 120°/second, resp.) and isometric extension at 90° on the dominant leg.

2.5. Cognitive Assessment. The Cambridge Neuropsychological Test Automated Battery (CANTAB; Cambridge, UK) is a validated computerized assessment tool used to measure cognitive function in adults [18].

In this study, it was used to administer the Delayed Match to Sample (DMS), Pattern Recognition Memory (PRM), Reaction Time (RTI), Stockings of Cambridge (SOC), and Spatial Span (SSP) tests. All cognitive tasks were performed in a closed room without any source of external disturbance. The investigator was only present to provide explanation of how to perform the tests. All participants attended familiarization sessions prior to the actual cognitive tests.

The DMS is a test of perceptual matching and immediate and delayed visual memory using a four-choice simultaneous and delayed recognition memory task. The participant is shown a complex visual pattern (i.e., the sample pattern). After a brief delay, the participant is shown four patterns (i.e., choice patterns). In some trials, the sample and the choice patterns are shown simultaneously. In other trials, the sample pattern is shown first, and then 0 seconds, 4 seconds, or 12 seconds later, the choice patterns are shown. A higher percentage of correct responses and shorter latency duration (ms) are indicators of better performance.

The PRM is a test that uses a visual pattern recognition memory in a two-choice forced discrimination task. In this test, a sequence of visual patterns is presented in the center of the screen. In the recognition phase, the participants must choose between a pattern they have already seen and a novel pattern. Lower reaction time and higher accuracy (%) indicate better performance.

The RTI is used to assess attention, based on reaction time. It comprises simple single and multiple-choice reaction time tasks. The participant is instructed to touch the screen when a yellow dot is displayed. For the multiple-choice reaction time task, the dot may appear in one of the five locations. Lower movement time, reaction time, and higher accuracy (%) indicate better performance.

The SOC test is used to assess planning and motor skill ability. The screen is divided into two halves. In the upper half, an image was shown containing three colored balls (red or green or blue). The balls were arranged randomly on three stockings. The CANTAB device displays the minimum number of moves needed to accomplish the task. On the lower display, the participant is required to try to copy the pattern in the top screen by using the touchscreen to move the balls. If the participant completes the problem without exceeding the number of minimum moves, the device records a success and the next problem is displayed. The level of complexity increases. The number of minimum moves for solving the problems randomly varies between two and five moves. The total number of problems the participant solves in the minimum moves out of maximum possible 12 is recorded by the CANTAB device. Generally, a higher number of problems solved in minimum moves and lower mean moves with each complexity indicate better performance.

The SSP is used to determine working memory capacity. The participants are shown 9 white squares arranged on the screen in a misaligned fashion. One at a time, a random square briefly changes color. The participant is required to memorize the sequence and then correctly identify the sequence by using the touchscreen. The sequence and color vary throughout the test, which starts with a span length of one to nine. The longest sequence a person correctly recalls is recorded. The participant can score 0–9, and a maximum score of 9 is indicative of higher memory span length.

2.6. Statistical Analysis. All data were coded and analyzed using SPSS (Statistical Package for the Social Sciences) v21.0. The data are presented as mean ± standard deviation (SD) for continuous variables and frequencies for categorical variables. The complex sampling method was applied to randomly selected women in different BMI categories to match them by age. One-way analysis of variance (ANOVA) was performed to determine any association of BMI with performance on the cognitive tasks. The post hoc Bonferroni comparisons were only done whenever a main effect was significant. Spearman's nonparametric correlation coefficient was computed for associations between performance on cognitive tasks with body fat (%) and the measure of cardiorespiratory fitness (VO_2 max). A p value < 0.05 was considered statistically significant.

3. Results and Discussion

Out of the 220 participants, 98 participants provided complete data on cognitive assessments. The average age of the participants was 36 ± 8.4 years and ranged from 18 to 50 years. The body fat (%) on average was 46.2 ± 6.6%, and the average determined VO_2 max was 23.6 ± 6.1 mL/kg/min (Table 1). From the 98 participants, 23.5% were classified as overweight, 22.4% as obese, and 36.7% as morbidly obese, and the rest were found to be included in the normal body weight group.

Table 2 shows the association of BMI categories with various cognitive outcomes like attention, memory, and planning ability. None of the attention parameters (outcomes for movement time and reaction times as well as accuracy for both simple and complex attention tasks) and planning ability tests showed (SOC) any significant difference among the various BMI categories. However, assessment of the association between memory testing parameters and cognitive function among different BMI categories using a one-way ANOVA revealed mixed results.

Although the accuracy on the memory tasks DMS and PRM was higher than 85% and comparable in all BMI categories, the time intervals for correct response expressed as mean correct latency in both DMS (simultaneously and 0 ms delay, $p = 0.005$ and 0.045, resp.) and PRM ($p = 0.044$) were significantly higher in the morbidly obese groups compared to normal participants. The memory span length on the SSP test was significantly lower among overweight and morbidly obese women compared to women with normal body mass index ($p = 0.011$). On the SOC task, the mean number of moves for tests that required only 4 moves was on average 5, and a total number of problems solved in minimum moves were similar across all BMI categories.

It was found in this study that cardiorespiratory fitness was not associated with any of the cognitive outcomes. In

Table 1: Characteristics of subjects.

	Number of subjects	Mean	Standard deviation	Median	Minimum	Maximum
Age (years)	98	36.00	8.44	37.00	18.00	50.00
Height (cm)	98	158.67	5.19	158.35	146.00	169.60
Weight (kg)	98	81.84	19.32	80.45	47.00	127.40
Body mass index (kg/m^2)	98	32.6	7.69	31.12	17.84	49.30
Waist circumference (cm)	91	96.68	14.67	94.00	64.00	135.00
VO_2 max (Bruce test)	74	23.67	6.12	24.46	9.24	41.07
Body fat (%)	96	46.16	6.56	46.80	29.00	56.90

Table 2: Association of BMI categories with cognitive outcomes (attention, memory, and planning ability).

Name of CANTAB test and cognitive outcomes	Body mass index category (kg/M^2) Normal ($n = 17$)	Overweight ($n = 23$)	Obese ($n = 22$)	Morbidly obese ($n = 36$)	p value*
Reaction Time (RTI) for attention					
Five-choice movement time (ms)	334.7 ± 103.8	371.5 ± 84.8	332.9 ± 70.6	338.8 ± 111.6	0.756
Five-choice reaction time (ms)	320.6 ± 43.6	342.1 ± 31.5	331.1 ± 42	351.4 ± 54.1	0.253
Five-choice accuracy (%)	98.8 ± 2.7	100 ± 0	100 ± 0	97.5 ± 5.4	0.175
Simple movement time (ms)	355.5 ± 134.9	408.4 ± 141.1	392.9 ± 172.3	340.6 ± 129	0.568
Simple reaction time (ms)	307.8 ± 76.7	305.5 ± 24.1	322.9 ± 86.9	323.6 ± 63.8	0.645
Delayed Match to Sample (DMS) for memory					
Mean correct latency (ms)	3163.1 ± 653.8	3321.5 ± 782.1	3473.5 ± 826.8	3715.4 ± 915.3	0.117
Mean correct latency (all delays) (ms)	3326.3 ± 627.7	3429.8 ± 822.9	3556.7 ± 853.7	3792.6 ± 1091.5	0.342
Mean correct latency (simultaneous) (ms)	2713.1 ± 939.8	3051.6 ± 876.5	3204.7 ± 1410.1	3498.2 ± 871.8*	0.005
Mean correct latency (0 ms delay) (ms)	2724.9 ± 767.4	2776.3 ± 650.1	2835.9 ± 561.4	3312.6 ± 1165.6*	0.045
Mean correct latency (4000 ms delay) (ms)	3219.7 ± 1013.5	3886 ± 1275.3	3518.9 ± 1068.4	3928.2 ± 1411	0.165
Mean correct latency (12000 ms delay) (ms)	4149.4 ± 644.9	3585.2 ± 953.9	4197.7 ± 1884.8	4092.6 ± 1460.2	0.228
Percent correct (%)	88.6 ± 12.1	85.4 ± 9	85.9 ± 9.5	86.6 ± 10.3	0.445
Percent correct (all delays) (%)	85.1 ± 15.6	81.7 ± 12.1	81.5 ± 12.3	82.6 ± 13.4	0.511
Percent correct (simultaneous) (%)	98.8 ± 4.9	96.5 ± 9.8	99.1 ± 4.3	98.3 ± 5.6	0.728
Percent correct (0 ms delay) (%)	85.6 ± 18.5	85.2 ± 16.2	79.8 ± 13.8	83.9 ± 19	0.436
Percent correct (4000 ms delay) (%)	87.1 ± 21.1	87 ± 14.3	89.4 ± 12.8	85.4 ± 14.9	0.679
Percent correct (12000 ms delay) (%)	83.5 ± 19	73 ± 23	75.5 ± 25.4	78.5 ± 24.4	0.476
Pattern Recognition Memory (PRM)					
Mean correct latency (ms)	2301.9 ± 824.2	2967.4 ± 1667.5	2629.9 ± 1034.6	2868.1 ± 995.5*	0.044
Percent correct (%)	92.2 ± 6.4	85.7 ± 12.7	88.6 ± 10.1	85 ± 14	0.182
Spatial Span (SSP) for memory					
Span length (1–9)	6.7 ± 0.9	5.5 ± 1.3*	6.1 ± 1.5	5.6 ± 1.6*	0.011
Total errors	17.6 ± 4.7	13.5 ± 5	14.6 ± 7.6	14.3 ± 6.5	0.082
Total usage errors	2.4 ± 1.9	2.4 ± 1.6	1.9 ± 1.3	2.7 ± 2.2	0.670
Stockings of Cambridge (SOC) for planning ability					
SOC mean moves (2 moves)	2.1 ± 0.2	2.2 ± 0.5	2.1 ± 0.2	2.2 ± 0.4	0.485
SOC mean moves (3 moves)	3.5 ± 0.9	3.7 ± 0.9	3.6 ± 0.7	3.6 ± 1	0.618
SOC mean moves (4 moves)	5 ± 1.1	5 ± 1	5.3 ± 1.4	5 ± 1.1	0.784
SOC problems solved in minimum moves (0–12)	5 ± 1.2	5 ± 1.5	4.7 ± 1.1	5.2 ± 1.5	0.549

ms: milliseconds; accuracy/correct (%) ranges from 0 to 100%. Span length is a discrete value (ranging from 1 to 9): the longest sequence participant correctly recalled. SOC parameters are all discrete. Mean move for 2, 3, or 4 is the average number of moves a participant takes to solve a problem that requires only 2, 3, or 4 moves, respectively. SOC: problems solved in minimum moves out of maximum possible 12. *Significantly different from Normal BMI group ($p \leq 0.05$).

addition to BMI, body fat assessed by CT scan and DEXA was tested for the presence of correlations with the cognitive outcomes. Body fat (%) showed similar associations as BMI, and there was a positive correlation of body fat (%) with latency to correct responses ($r = 0.232$ and $r = 0.229$ for DRM and PRM, resp.; $p < 0.05$) but no association with accuracy (Table 3). CT scan images describing the fat accumulation in the regions (heart, liver, abdomen, and thigh) showed no significant association of volume of fat in each region with any of the cognitive parameters (results not shown).

TABLE 3: Correlation of cognitive parameters assessed using CANTAB with body mass index, body fat (%), and VO_2 max.

Name of CANTAB test and cognitive outcomes	BMI (kg/m^2) r	VO_2 max r	Body fat (%) r
Reaction Time (RTI) for attention			
Five-choice accuracy score (%)	−0.04	0.06	−0.05
Five-choice movement time (ms)	−0.03	−0.08	−0.03
Five-choice reaction time (ms)	0.25	−0.28	0.27
Simple movement time (ms)	−0.03	−0.08	−0.14
Simple reaction time (ms)	0.18	−0.14	0.18
Delayed Match to Sample (DMS) for memory			
Mean correct latency (ms)	0.248*	−0.11	0.18
Mean correct latency (all delays) (ms)	0.17	−0.06	0.15
Mean correct latency (simultaneous) (ms)	0.377**	−0.17	0.232*
Mean correct latency (0 ms delay) (ms)	0.214*	0.02	0.15
Mean correct latency (4000 ms delay) (ms)	0.13	0.01	0.09
Mean correct latency (12000 ms delay) (ms)	0.01	−0.13	0.05
Percent correct (%)	−0.05	0.02	0.03
Percent correct (all delays) (%)	−0.06	0.05	0.02
Percent correct (simultaneous) (%)	0.03	−0.12	0.01
Percent correct (0 ms delay) (%)	−0.02	0.08	0.01
Percent correct (4000 ms delay) (%)	−0.13	0.13	−0.08
Percent correct (12000 ms delay) (%)	0.03	−0.09	0.09
Spatial Span (SSP) for memory			
Span length (1–9)	−0.16	−0.05	−0.08
Total errors	−0.14	0.02	−0.13
Total usage errors	0.06	0.15	0.04
Pattern Recognition Memory (PRM)			
Mean correct latency (ms)	0.209*	−0.16	0.229*
Percent correct (%)	−0.08	−0.02	−0.12
Stockings of Cambridge (SOC) for planning ability			
Mean moves (2 moves)	0.04	−0.23	0.04
Mean moves (3 moves)	−0.05	0.07	−0.06
Mean moves (4 moves)	0.06	0.05	−0.01
Problems solved in minimum moves (0–12)	0.06	0.05	0.04

r: correlation coefficient; **correlation is significant at the 0.01 level (2-tailed). *Correlation is significant at the 0.05 level (2-tailed). ms: milliseconds; accuracy/correct (%) ranges from 0 to 100%. Span length is a discrete value (ranging from 1 to 9): the longest sequence participant correctly recalled. SOC parameters are all discrete. Mean move for 2, 3, or 4 is the average number of moves a participant takes to solve a problem that requires only 2, 3, or 4 moves, respectively. SOC: problems solved in minimum moves out of maximum possible 12.

Similarly, DEXA-assessed lean body weight and lean mass % did not show any significant difference.

As discussed earlier, the association between obesity (measured by BMI) and cognitive function is not simple and is rather quite complex due to individual, possibly age-related differences. There are evidences from experimental, epidemiological, cross-sectional, and prospective studies that obesity is associated with cognitive decline [18]. Several studies have also confirmed that weight loss or low BMI can lead to decline in cognitive function in elderly population but can be beneficial in younger population in terms of improvement of cognitive function [4, 6–11]. In contrast to the above studies, Elias et al. have found no significant difference in cognitive function in obese and normal body weight female subjects [16].

In our study, the results indicate that obesity was not associated with accuracy on cognitive tasks with regard to attention or planning executive function; however, morbid obesity was significantly associated with a lower memory span and with higher latency to responses. The association of morbid obesity with greater loss of cognitive function is supported by evidences of improvement of cognitive function after bariatric surgery [19]. Moreover, between normal and morbidly obese women, statistical significant differences were found only on latencies that were less than 1 s, suggesting decrements in sensory memory rather than short-term memory. Previous studies demonstrated that obesity was negatively associated with visual acuity (VA) and other eye diseases among adults [20]. Although VA was not measured in the current study, it is possible that these differences observed in sensory memory were associated with decrements in VA in the morbidly obese group. In fact, studies from Henderson et al. [21] and Lindenberger and Ghisletta [22] reported correlations between measures of sensory functions and measures of cognitive functions at different ages.

Gunstad et al. examined attention and executive function among 408 healthy adult persons, aged 20 to 82 years [23]. Similar to our study, this study could not find any significant correlation between attention test performance and BMI. However, executive function test performances showed significant poor performance in overweight and obese that were apparent in the older adults.

Another factor that has been investigated is damage to the hippocampus, which is associated with memory (both short and long terms). Some investigators have found that people with an increased BMI have a reduced hippocampal volume. For example, Cherbuin et al. examined the magnetic resonance images of older individuals (60–64 years), who were followed for an average of 8 years to detect brain changes over time [24]. They assessed the relationship between BMI and hippocampal atrophy and found that BMI was negatively associated with hippocampal volume: people with a higher BMI tended to have greater hippocampal atrophy. A possible reason for this reduction is that excessive amounts of dietary saturated fats may induce changes in the integrity of the blood-brain barrier, which consequently may allow toxins to enter the brain and directly or indirectly impact the hippocampus [25].

In the current study, the volume of brain structures involved in memory was not measured. These factors nevertheless could have impacted our findings. However, DEXA- and CT scan-assessed body fat distribution provided some direct associations of body fat percentage and volume distribution with cognitive function parameters.

Aerobic fitness appears to have a positive effect on cognition [26, 27]. In our study, no association was seen between aerobic fitness and any of the cognitive functions tested. A possible reason for this finding may be related to the fact that the women had been recruited from a gym and were more active, although relatively not aerobically fit. The findings can be linked with practice of regular physical activity that can improve cognition [26]. However, we did not have a sedentary group of women for comparison.

In our study, BMI was negatively associated with some aspects of cognition. We therefore examined the possibility that an increased body fat percentage would similarly show negative impacts on cognition. In the morbidly obese women, body fat was negatively associated with a delayed response on the forced choice recognition memory task (i.e., DMS) and the visual pattern memory task (i.e., PRM). The extent that fat-related factors such as body fat distribution, percentage of body fat, and fat metabolism may be involved in this finding is unclear.

The findings of our study indicate that morbid obesity in otherwise healthy premenopausal women can have a negative impact on recognition memory and memory span length. Future studies are needed on different populations of premenopausal women (e.g., sedentary healthy premenopausal women).

3.1. Limitations. There are several limitations of our study: (1) cross-sectional design (assessments were done only once; no follow-up assessments were done to see the pattern of change in cognitive function with BMI over the years). (2) Besides BMI (which is measured in every participant), other parameters of obesity like body fat assessment (measured by CT scan and DEXA scan) were not measured in all the participants (measured only in morbidly obese and obese participants). Perhaps, due to insufficient sample size, CT-assessed body fat volume in various regions (heart, liver, abdomen, and thigh) did not show any significant correlations with cognitive parameters. (3) Visual acuity was not measured in this experiment although participants were allowed to use their glasses which therefore could not have affected our results; future studies investigating the link between obesity and cognitive performance should consider screening for potential decrements in sensory capabilities that may compromise the availability and encoding of relevant information (e.g., sight and hearing).

Our study is among few studies conducted on younger healthy obese and morbidly obese women. Along with BMI, we took into account body fat distribution and aerobic fitness status for any association with cognitive function which is otherwise lacking in literature. All cognitive tasks required finger/hand movements to touch the screen and provide responses. The high latency could be due to the arm movement speed that could be slow in morbidly obese women. The SSP memory span test assesses only short-term memory performance, and our study could not include other domains of memory performance.

4. Conclusion

Based on these findings, we conclude that obesity was not associated with cognitive performance related to attention and planning executive function in otherwise healthy premenopausal women; however, morbid obesity is associated with higher latency to correct response on memory-specific tasks and poorer short-term memory. These findings are similar to the findings of studies with similar age groups; however, the absence of link between cardiorespiratory fitness and cognitive function in this study suggests other pathways responsible for cognitive decline.

Disclosure

The authors declare that partial results of this study were presented as a poster presentation at the scientific conference of International Society of Behavioral Nutrition and Physical Activity, 3–6 June 2015, Edinburgh, UK [28].

Acknowledgments

The authors would like to extend their appreciation and gratitude for the contributions of Andrew McBride and Mahmooda Banu for the radiologic assessments and Ivana Girard in assisting with data entry.

References

[1] L. M. Hess and K. C. Insel, "Chemotherapy-related change in cognitive function: a conceptual model," *Oncology Nursing Forum*, vol. 34, no. 5, pp. 981–994, 2007.

[2] G. Shefer, Y. Marcus, and N. Stern, "Is obesity a brain disease?," *Neuroscience & Biobehavioral Reviews*, vol. 37, no. 10, pp. 2489–2503, 2013.

[3] K. Yaffe, "Metabolic syndrome and cognitive decline," *Current Alzheimer Research*, vol. 4, no. 2, pp. 123–126, 2007.

[4] C. K. Suemoto, P. Gilsanz, E. R. Mayeda, and M. M. Glymour, "Body mass index and cognitive function: the potential for reverse causation," *International Journal of Obesity*, vol. 39, no. 9, pp. 1383–1389, 2015.

[5] A. L. Fitzpatrick, L. H. Kuller, O. L. Lopez et al., "Midlife and late-life obesity and the risk of dementia: cardiovascular health study," *Archives of Neurology*, vol. 66, no. 3, pp. 336–342, 2009.

[6] T. F. Hughes, A. R. Borenstein, E. Schofield, Y. Wu, and E. B. Larson, "Association between late-life body mass index and dementia: the Kame Project," *Neurology*, vol. 72, no. 20, pp. 1741–1746, 2009.

[7] A. R. Atti, K. Palmer, S. Volpato, B. Winblad, D. D. Ronchi, and L. Fratiglioni, "Late-life body mass index and dementia incidence: nine-year follow-up data from the Kungsholmen Project," *Journal of the American Geriatrics Society*, vol. 56, no. 1, pp. 111–116, 2008.

[8] A. Singh-Manoux., S. Czernichow, A. Elbaz et al., "Obesity phenotypes in midlife and cognition in early old age: the Whitehall II cohort study," *Neurology*, vol. 79, no. 8, pp. 755–762, 2012.

[9] J. Gunstad, R. H. Paul, R. A. Cohen, D. F. Tate, and E. Gordon, "Obesity is associated with memory deficits in young and middle-aged adults," *Eating and Weight Disorders*, vol. 11, no. 1, pp. e15–e19, 2006.

[10] M. Cournot, J. C. Marquie, D. Ansiau et al., "Relation between body mass index and cognitive function in healthy middle-aged men and women," *Neurology*, vol. 67, no. 7, pp. 1208–1214, 2006.

[11] E. Kesse-Guyot, V. A. Andreeva, M. Touvier et al., "Overall and abdominal adiposity in midlife and subsequent cognitive function," *Journal of Nutrition, Health & Aging*, vol. 19, no. 2, pp. 183–189, 2015.

[12] M. E. Bocarsly, M. Fasolino, G. A. Kane et al., "Obesity diminishes synaptic markers, alters microglial morphology, and impairs cognitive function," *Proceedings of the National Academy of Sciences of the United States of America*, vol. 112, no. 51, pp. 15731–15736, 2015.

[13] J. M. Walker and F. E. Harrison, "Shared neuropathological characteristics of obesity, type 2 diabetes and Alzheimer's disease: impacts on cognitive decline," *Nutrients*, vol. 7, no. 12, pp. 7332–7357, 2015.

[14] S. A. Everson-Rose and J. P. Ryan, "Diabetes, obesity, and the brain: new developments in biobehavioral medicine," *Psychosomatic Medicine*, vol. 77, no. 6, pp. 612–615, 2015.

[15] I. Driscoll, M. A. Espeland, S. Wassertheil-Smoller et al., "Weight change and cognitive function: findings from the Women's Health Initiative Study of Cognitive Aging," *Obesity*, vol. 19, no. 8, pp. 1595–1600, 2011.

[16] M. F. Elias, P. K. Elias, L. M. Sullivan, P. A. Wolf, and R. B. D'Agostino, "Lower cognitive function in the presence of obesity and hypertension: the Framingham heart study," *International Journal of Obesity and Related Metabolic Disorders*, vol. 27, no. 2, pp. 260–268, 2003.

[17] D. R. Kerwin, Y. Zhang, J. M. Kotchen et al., "The cross-sectional relationship between body mass index, waist-hip ratio, and cognitive performance in postmenopausal women enrolled in the Women's Health Initiative," *Journal of the American Geriatrics Society*, vol. 58, no. 8, pp. 1427–1432, 2010.

[18] L. Haring, R. Mottus, K. Koch, M. Trei, and E. Maron, "Factorial validity, measurement equivalence and cognitive performance of the Cambridge Neuropsychological Test Automated Battery (CANTAB) between patients with first-episode psychosis and healthy volunteers," *Psychological Medicine*, vol. 45, no. 9, pp. 1919–1929, 2015.

[19] M. L. Alosco, R. Galioto, M. B. Spitznagel et al., "Cognitive function after bariatric surgery: evidence for improvement 3 years after surgery," *American Journal of Surgery*, vol. 207, no. 6, pp. 870–876, 2014.

[20] B. Bergman, H. Nilsson-Ehle, and J. Sjöstrand, "Ocular changes, risk markers for eye disorders and effects of cataract surgery in elderly people: a study of an urban Swedish population followed from 70 to 97 years of age," *Acta Ophthalmologica Scandinavica*, vol. 82, no. 2, pp. 166–174, 2004.

[21] R. D. Henderson, M. Allerhand, N. Patton et al., "Vision and intelligence at age 83 in the Lothian Birth Cohort 1921," *Intelligence*, vol. 39, no. 2-3, pp. 148–154, 2011.

[22] U. Lindenberger and P. Ghisletta, "Cognitive and sensory declines in old age: gauging the evidence for a common cause," *Psychology and Aging*, vol. 24, no. 1, pp. 1–16, 2009.

[23] J. Gunstad, R. H. Paul, R. A. Cohen, D. F. Tate, M. B. Spitznagel, and E. Gordon, "Elevated body mass index is associated with executive dysfunction in otherwise healthy adults," *Comprehensive Psychiatry*, vol. 48, no. 1, pp. 57–61, 2007.

[24] N. Cherbuin, K. Sargent-Cox, M. Fraser, P. Sachdev, and K. J. Anstey, "Being overweight is associated with hippocampal atrophy: the PATH Through Life Study," *International Journal of Obesity*, vol. 39, no. 10, pp. 1509–1514, 2015.

[25] S. E. Kanoski and T. L. Davidson, "Western diet consumption and cognitive impairment: links to hippocampal dysfunction and obesity," *Physiology & Behavior*, vol. 103, no. 1, pp. 59–68, 2011.

[26] C. L. Davis, P. D. Tomporowski, C. A. Boyle et al., "Effects of aerobic exercise on overweight children's cognitive functioning: a randomized controlled trial," *Research Quarterly for Exercise and Sport*, vol. 78, no. 5, pp. 510–519, 2007.

[27] H. Guiney, S. J. Lucas, J. D. Cotter, and L. Machado, "Evidence cerebral blood-flow regulation mediates exercise-cognition links in healthy young adults," *Neuropsychology*, vol. 29, no. 1, pp. 1–9, 2015.

[28] A. Farooq, A. M. Knowles, J. J. Reilly, and N. Gaoua, *The Association between Obesity and Cognitive Function in Healthy Premenopausal Women*, International Society of Behavioral Nutrition and Physical Activity, Edinburgh, UK, 2015.

28

Ferritin Is a Marker of Inflammation rather than Iron Deficiency in Overweight and Obese People

Abidullah Khan, Wazir Muhammad Khan, Maimoona Ayub, Mohammad Humayun, and Mohammad Haroon

KTH, Peshawar, Pakistan

Correspondence should be addressed to Abidullah Khan; dr.abidk@yahoo.com

Academic Editor: Philippe Gual

Background. In clinical practice, serum ferritin is used as a screening tool to detect iron deficiency. However, its reliability in obesity has been questioned. *Objectives.* To investigate the role of ferritin in overweight and obese people, either as a marker of inflammation or iron deficiency. *Methods.* On the basis of body mass index (BMI), 150 participants were divided into three equal groups: A: BMI 18.5–25 kg/m^2, B: BMI 25–30 kg/m^2, and C: BMI > 30 kg/m^2. Serum iron, total iron binding capacity (TIBC), transferrin saturation, ferritin, C-reactive protein, and hemoglobin (Hb) were measured for each participant and analyzed through SPSS version 16. One-way ANOVA and Pearson's correlation tests were applied. *Results.* Ferritin was the highest in group C ($M = 163.48 \pm 2.23$, $P < 0.001$) and the lowest in group A, ($M = 152.78 \pm 1.81$, $P < 0.001$). Contrarily to ferritin, transferrin was the lowest in group C, ($M = 30.65 \pm 1.39$, $P < 0.001$) and the highest in group A, ($M = 38.66 \pm 2.14$, $P < 0.001$). Ferritin had a strong positive correlation with both BMI ($r = 0.86$, $P < 0.001$) and CRP ($r = 0.87$, $P < 0.001$) and strong negative correlation with Hb, iron, TIBC, and transferrin saturation ($P < 0.001$). *Conclusion.* Ferritin is a marker of inflammation rather than iron status in overweight and obese people. Complete iron profile including transferrin, rather than serum ferritin alone, can truly predict iron deficiency in such people.

1. Introduction

Obesity is a global health problem. In 2014, 600 million adults and 42 million children, less than five years of age, were obese [1]. This is more common in women and is being considered as the most serious threat to human health by different authorities [2]. The normal body mass index (BMI) is 18–25 kg/m^2. Anyone with a BMI of 25–30 kg/m^2 is called overweight, while the term "obesity" is used, when BMI exceeds 30 kg/m^2. This most serious health problem was classified by the American Medical Association (AMA), as a "disease" in 2013 [3].

Overweight and obese people are at risk of developing certain serious complications like obstructive sleep apnea, cor pulmonale, ischemic heart disease, diabetes, and many others [4]. At the same time, it increases the likelihood of iron deficiency (ID) and iron deficiency anemia (IDA), leading to an escalating disease burden [5–9].

Obesity predisposes affected individuals to subclinical inflammation. Many studies have concluded that overweight and obese people are in a state of an ongoing subclinical inflammation that can secondarily lead to more catastrophic events like iron deficiency, malignancy, and so forth [10–13].

Ferritin is used a marker of iron deficiency in various healthcare facilities across the globe [14]. Being an acute phase reactant, serum ferritin level is prone to be higher in overweight and obese people, because of a state of subclinical, but generalized inflammation in them [15–17]. Due to this fact, using serum ferritin as a marker of ID or IDA in overweight or obese people is controversial [16, 17].

Obesity is an emerging health related concern in Pakistan and so are ID and IDA [18–20]. It is also worth mentioning that serum ferritin assay is the most commonly used blood test to diagnose ID or IDA, not only in Pakistan, but in other developing countries of the world also. This is so because there is a relative scarcity of more specific test for

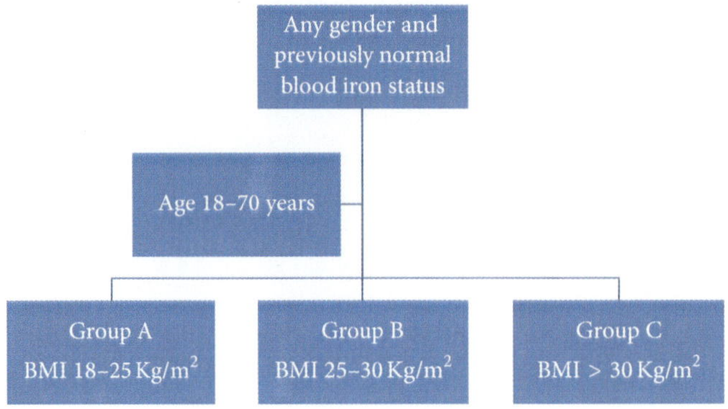

FIGURE 1: Inclusion criteria for suitability in the study sample.

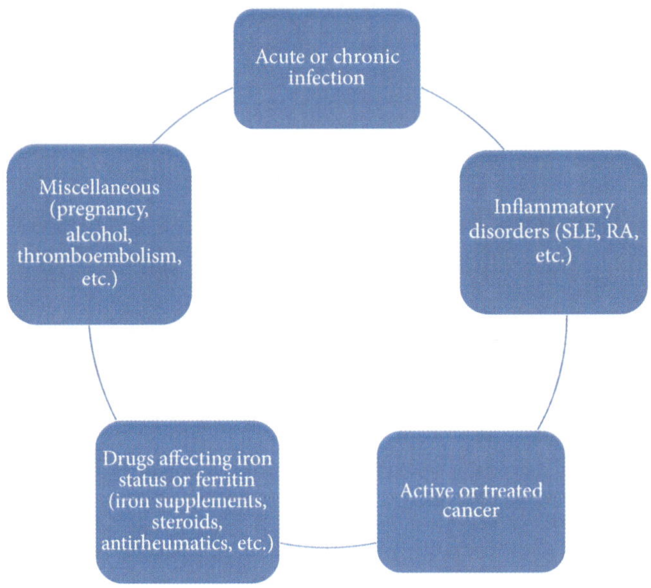

FIGURE 2: An overview of the chief exclusion criteria.

the diagnosis of ID or IDA like transferrin saturation or total iron binding capacity (TIBC) and so forth. Therefore, the use and interpretation of serum ferritin assay alone become challenging, because serum ferritin may not be a true measure of an underlying iron deficiency in overweight and obese people. Therefore, this study will focus on correlating serum ferritin with C-reactive protein (CRP) and its association with iron and BMI, and to find out whether, it is safe to keep using serum ferritin as a true measure of iron deficiency in overweight and obese people or not.

2. Material and Methods

This cross-sectional, observational study was conducted in the department of medicine of Khyber Teaching Hospital (KTH), Peshawar, Pakistan, between September 2015 and July 2016. This study was approved by the hospital's ethics review committee and included 150 otherwise healthy participants. Informed written consent was obtained from every participant individually.

A structured questionnaire including closed ended questions regarding demographic details, present and past medical/surgical history, any history of recent infections, recent or previous drug history, especially, iron tablets or injections, steroids or oral contraceptive pills, and chemotherapeutic medications like methotrexate, azathioprine, and so forth was used.

An overview of the inclusion and exclusion criteria is given below (Figures 1 and 2). The study included patients from both the genders in the age range of 18 to 70 years. Patients already diagnosed with iron deficiency or iron deficiency anemia were excluded from the study. Similarly, those diagnosed with iron overload were also excluded. Other exclusion criteria were set on the basis of medical conditions which could potentially affect the body iron stores or ferritin, such as pregnancy, alcoholism, hemoglobinopathies, diabetes mellitus, bleeding disorders, any acute or chronic inflammatory conditions like rheumatoid arthritis (RA) or systemic lupus erythematosus (SLE), and any acute illnesses during the preceding one month or chronic infections like

TABLE 1: Descriptive statistics of different study variables in each group.

Variable	Group A ($N = 50$)		Group B ($N = 50$)		Group C ($N = 50$)	
	Mean	SD	Mean	SD	Mean	SD
Age (years)	44.84	6.16	44.84	6.17	44.44	7.17
BMI (kg/m^2)	22.36	1.08	27.18	0.80	31.18	0.85
Hb (gm/dL)	14.13	0.83	12.68	0.68	11.86	0.88
Iron (μmol/L)	24.86	1.24	21.36	1.04	17.68	1.18
TIBC (μmol/L)	63.56	0.50	59.52	0.86	57.44	1.59
TSAT (%)	38.66	2.14	35.36	1.63	30.65	1.39
Ferritin (μg/L)	152.78	1.81	158.32	1.99	163.48	2.23
CRP (mg/L)	5.28	0.73	7.58	1.01	11.46	1.46

Group A: BMI 18.5–25 kg/m^2, group B: BMI 25–30 kg/m^2, and group C: BMI > 30 kg/m^2, Hb: hemoglobin, TIBC: total iron binding capacity, TSAT: transferrin saturation, CRP: C-reactive protein, and BMI: body mass index.

tuberculosis, brucellosis, and so forth. Patients on drugs which could influence serum iron or ferritin like any use of iron supplements, steroids, oral contraceptive pills (OCPs), nonsteroidal anti-inflammatory drugs (NSAIDS), disease modifying antirheumatic drugs like methotrexate, azathioprine, hydroxychloroquine, and so forth and those with cancer or on active treatment for it were also excluded from the study.

The final 150 individuals included in the study were divided into three groups, each group consisting of 50 participants as follows: group A: BMI 18.5–25 kg/m^2, group B: BMI 25–30 kg/m^2, and group C: BMI > 30 kg/m^2.

The BMI was calculated using the formula weight (kg)/height (meter^2). A weight scale with a built-in stadiometer was used to measure the weight and height of all the subjects in kilograms and meters, respectively. A morning sample of 5 mL of venous blood was drawn; 3 mL was put in gel tubes for the determination of serum ferritin, iron, total iron binding capacity (TIBC), transferring saturation, and C-reactive protein (CRP), while 2 mL was put in an EDTA tube for hemoglobin (Hb) determination. Serum ferritin and CRP were measured by using enzyme linked immunosorbent assay (ELISA) method, serum iron was measured using enzymatic colorimetric method, and Hb was measured on automated analyzer Sysmex. Transferrin saturation was determined by using the formula; iron/TIBC ×100. All these tests were done by the same technician in the main laboratory of Khyber Teaching Hospital (KTH), Peshawar.

All the data was entered into and analyzed by SPSS version 16. In order to compare the means of different study variables, one-way ANOVA with Turkey-HSD was used. Pearson's correlation test was run to analyze an association of BMI with serum ferritin, CRP, serum iron, TIBC, and transferrin saturation. P value of <0.05 was considered as significant.

3. Results

Amongst all the participants, 47.3% were males and 52.7% were females. The mean age, body mass index (BMI), and serum ferritin (μg/L) of all the participants were 44.71 ± 6.48, 26.91 ± 3.73, and 158.19 ± 4.82, respectively. Group specific descriptive statistics are given below (Table 1).

The data was tested for the assumptions of homogeneity of variances and normality. One-way ANOVA was used to compare the means of different dependent variables between the three groups, namely, group A, group B, and group C, to find out any impact of obesity on the dependent variables, namely, ferritin, Iron, TIBC, hemoglobin (Hb), and transferrin saturation. Ferritin was the highest in group C (M = 163.46, SD = 2.23, $P < 0.001$), higher in group B (M = 158.32, SD = 1.99, $P < 0.001$), and lowest in group A (M = 152–78, SD = 1.81, $P < 0.001$). However, despite the highest ferritin level in group C (the obesity group), transferrin saturation was the lowest (M = 30.65, SD = 1.39, $P < 0.001$). Similarly, along with transferrin, both Hb and iron were the highest in group A, intermediate in group B, and the lowest in group C (Table 1). The post hoc analysis for these variables was significant at $P < 0.001$ in each group (Table 2). There was a statistically significant difference between the three groups for ferritin ($F(2, 147) = 350.80$, $P < 0.001$), hemoglobin ($F(2, 147) = 101.90$, $P < 0.001$), and iron ($F(2, 147) = 644.54$, $P < 0.001$), respectively. The estimate of effect size (Partial Eta Squared) for the difference of ferritin, iron, and Hb between the three groups was 0.83, 0.86, and 0.58, respectively.

For both CRP and transferrin saturation (TSAT), the assumption of homogeneity of variances was not tenable ($P < 0.05$). However, robust tests for the equality of means were statistically significant ($P < 0.01$ for both Welch and Brown-Forsythe tests). Moreover, one-way ANOVA showed a statistically significant difference between the three groups with regard to CRP and TSAT. The results of one-way ANOVA for CRP and TSAT were $F(2, 147) = 396.87$, $P < 0.001$ and $F(2, 147) = 262.87$, $P < 0.001$, respectively. CRP was found to be highest in group C (M = 11.46, SD = 1.46, $P < 0.001$), higher in group B (M = 7.58, SD = 1.01, $P < 0.001$), and the lowest in group A (M = 5.28, SD = 0.73, $P < 0.001$).

Finally a correlation test was run between the BMI and the dependent variables, namely, ferritin, iron, transferrin, TIBC, and CRP (Table 3). It is worth mentioning that both ferritin and CRP correlated positively with BMI (r = 0.86,

Table 2: Results of post hoc analysis by Turkey HSD.

Dependent variable	(I) group	(J) group	Mean difference (I − J)	Std. error	Sig.	95% confidence interval	
						Lower bound	Upper bound
Hb	A	B	1.450*	.161	.000	1.07	1.83
		C	2.270*	.161	.000	1.89	2.65
	B	A	−1.450*	.161	.000	−1.83	−1.07
		C	.820*	.161	.000	.44	1.20
	C	A	−2.270*	.161	.000	−2.65	−1.89
		B	−.820*	.161	.000	−1.20	−.44
Iron	A	B	3.500*	.232	.000	2.95	4.05
		C	7.180*	.232	.000	6.63	7.73
	B	A	−3.500*	.232	.000	−4.05	−2.95
		C	3.680*	.232	.000	3.13	4.23
	C	A	−7.180*	.232	.000	−7.73	−6.63
		B	−3.680*	.232	.000	−4.23	−3.13
Ferritin	A	B	−5.540*	.404	.000	−6.50	−4.58
		C	−10.700*	.404	.000	−11.66	−9.74
	B	A	5.540*	.404	.000	4.58	6.50
		C	−5.160*	.404	.000	−6.12	−4.20
	C	A	10.700*	.404	.000	9.74	11.66
		B	5.160*	.404	.000	4.20	6.12

*The mean difference is significant at the 0.05 level.

TABLE 3: Pearson's correlation of BMI with test variables *(note a strong positive correlation with ferritin and CRP).*

Variable	Pearson's value (r)	P value
HB	−0.77	<0.001
Iron	−0.89	<0.001
TIBC	−0.87	<0.001
Transferrin	−0.84	<0.001
Ferritin	0.86	<0.001
CRP	0.89	<0.001

TABLE 4: Pearson's correlation of ferritin with the test variables *(note a strong positive correlation with CRP/BMI and an inverse correlation with transferrin).*

Variable	Pearson's value (r)	P value
Hb	−0.62	<0.001
Iron	−0.89	<0.001
TIBC	−0.84	<0.001
TSAT	−0.86	<0.001
CRP	0.87	<0.001
BMI	0.86	<0.001

$P < 0.001$ and $r = 0.89$, $P < 0.001$, resp.). However, there was a strong negative correlation between the BMI and the rest of the three variables, namely, iron ($r = -0.89$, $P < 0.001$), TIBC ($r = -0.87$, $P < 0.001$), and TSAT ($R = -0.84$, $P < 0.001$). It is also notable that ferritin had a strong positive correlation with CRP ($r = 0.87$, $P < 0.01$) but a negative one with iron ($r = -0.89$, $P < 0.001$), TIBC ($r = -0.85$, $P < 0.001$), and transferrin saturation ($r = -0.86$, $P < 0.001$). The detailed breakdown is given (Table 4). It must be noted that, for the falling values of iron, TIBC, and TSAT, as one moves upwards from group A to group C, there was a not only a corresponding decline in the level of hemoglobin (Hb), but also a significant increase in the level of ferritin ($P < 0.001$).

4. Discussion

Iron deficiency (ID) with or without anemia is common in obese people and has certain mechanisms involved in its pathogenesis mainly a state of subclinical inflammation. The low iron levels in overweight and obese subjects are most probably caused by the inflammatory mechanisms, which arrest iron in the reticuloendothelial system by releasing different inflammatory mediators like cytokines and so forth [21, 22]. Our study showed a positive correlation between ferritin and CRP, signifying an underlying low grade inflammation, leading to subsequent iron deficiency, most probably, because of inflammation mediated iron sequestration in the reticuloendothelial system.

Ferritin is an acute phase reactant and is potentially higher in any infective or inflammatory process, making its careful interpretation necessary in such situations. In a recent study, high levels of ferritin were positively correlated with the risk of metabolic syndrome and obesity [23]. In another study, ferritin was found to be positively associated with CRP [24]. Our findings are consistent with these results. However, in sharp contrast to our statistics, a study by Eftekhari et al. concluded that serum ferritin was lower in obese people [25].

Obesity is one of the biggest health challenges of the 21st century. Association of ID/IDA with obesity doubles the ill health effects of the obesity itself. Though chronic inflammation caused by excess adipose tissue, rather than dietary factors, offers a plausible explanation for ID or IDA in obese people, looking for the existence of both acute and chronic infections, and inflammatory conditions need to be considered as well. Moreover, treating IDA in obese people is another challenge itself, as they tend to respond poorly to iron supplementation [5, 26]. In another recent study, administering both oral iron and ascorbic acid as an enhancer of its absorption from the gut made little difference in correcting ID or IDA in overweight or obese individuals [27].

IDA is most commonly caused by nutritional deficiency. On the other hand, obesity is often caused by overnutrition. Hence, the coexistence of both IDA and obesity in the same person represents the opposite ends of the spectrum of under and overnutrition. However, amongst the different factors responsible for their mutual coexistence like dilutional hypoferremia, poor dietary iron intake, increased iron demands, and/or impaired iron absorption, a chemical called hepcidin was recently found to be the main culprit for ID or IDA in obesity. Hepcidin was found in higher titers in obese and overweight individuals. Hepcidin works by causing subclinical inflammation, decreases iron absorption from the gut, and blunts the effects of iron fortification [28, 29]. Reducing weight may lower hepcidin, which may in return improve the iron stores of the body. Treating obesity through surgical approaches like Roux-en-Y gastric bypass (RYGB) is unfortunately related to iron deficiency also. In a recent Chinese study, iron deficiency and IDA both were found to be extremely frequent after RYGB in obese patients with T2DM at 2-year follow-up [30]. It is therefore recommended to screen overweight and obese people for iron deficiency, both before and after any antiobesity surgical intervention is undertaken.

It is to be stated that the results of our study were according to the expectations of the authors. As is evident from our results, ferritin was not a true indicator of an underlying iron deficiency in our study population of overweight and obese individuals. Rather, ferritin correlated positively with the inflammatory marker, CRP, and BMI, making ferritin a marker of inflammation rather than iron status in overweight and obese people. However, we recommend further studies and would advocate a bigger sample size, in order to arrive at a more logical conclusion.

5. Conclusion

Ferritin is a marker of inflammation rather than iron status in overweight and obese individuals. Being an acute phase reactant, a high ferritin level secondary to subclinical inflammation in overweight and obese people may mask an underlying iron deficiency. It is therefore recommended to request a complete iron studies profile including transferrin saturation, ferritin, total iron binding capacity (TIBC), and serum iron, to confidently exclude ID in obese or overweight subjects.

Abbreviations

ID: Iron deficiency
IDA: Iron deficiency anemia
CRP: C-reactive protein
BMI: Body mass index
TSAT: Transferrin saturation
TIBC: Total iron binding capacity
Hb: Hemoglobin
RYGB: Roux-en-Y gastric bypass.

Competing Interests

The authors declare that there is no conflict of interests regarding the publication of this paper.

Authors' Contributions

Abidullah Khan, Mohammad Humayun, and Maimoona Ayub conceived the idea. All the authors contributed to the drafting, revising, and proofreading of this manuscript. All the authors approved the final manuscript.

References

[1] WHO, *Obesity and Overweight Fact Sheet N° 311*, WHO, Geneva, Switzerland, 2015.

[2] J. K. Dibaise and A. E. Foxx-Orenstein, "Role of the gastroenterologist in managing obesity," *Expert Review of Gastroenterology and Hepatology*, vol. 7, no. 5, pp. 439–451, 2013.

[3] https://en.wikipedia.org/wiki/Obesity.

[4] D. W. Haslam and W. P. James, "Obesity," *The Lancet*, vol. 366, no. 9492, pp. 1197–1209, 2005.

[5] C. Hutchinson, "A review of iron studies in overweight and obese children and adolescents: a double burden in the young?" *European Journal of Nutrition*, vol. 55, no. 7, pp. 2179–2197, 2016.

[6] A. C. Cepeda-Lopez, A. Melse-Boonstra, M. B. Zimmermann, and I. Herter-Aeberli, "In overweight and obese women, dietary iron absorption is reduced and the enhancement of iron absorption by ascorbic acid is one-half that in normal-weight women," *The American Journal of Clinical Nutrition*, vol. 102, no. 6, pp. 1389–1397, 2015.

[7] J. Baumgartner, C. M. Smuts, I. Aeberli, L. Malan, H. Tjalsma, and M. B. Zimmermann, "Overweight impairs efficacy of iron supplementation in iron-deficient South African children: a randomized controlled intervention," *International Journal of Obesity*, vol. 37, no. 1, pp. 24–30, 2013.

[8] L. Zhao, X. Zhang, Y. Shen, X. Fang, Y. Wang, and F. Wang, "Obesity and iron deficiency: a quantitative meta-analysis," *Obesity Reviews*, vol. 16, no. 12, pp. 1081–1093, 2015.

[9] H. L. Cheng, C. Bryant, R. Cook, H. O'Connor, K. Rooney, and K. Steinbeck, "The relationship between obesity and hypoferraemia in adults: a systematic review," *Obesity Reviews*, vol. 13, no. 2, pp. 150–161, 2012.

[10] A. Vehapoglu, S. Turkmen, N. Goknar, and Ö. F. Özer, "Reduced antioxidant capacity and increased subclinical inflammation markers in prepubescent obese children and their relationship with nutritional markers and metabolic parameters," *Redox Report*, vol. 21, no. 6, pp. 271–280, 2016.

[11] D. Herrera-Covarrubias, G. A. Coria-Avila, C. Fernández-Pomares, G. E. Aranda-Abreu, J. Manzo Denes, and M. E. Hernández, "Obesity as a risk factor in the development of cancer," *Revista Peruana de Medicina Experimental y Salud Pública*, vol. 32, no. 4, pp. 766–776, 2015.

[12] A. Kohlgruber and L. Lynch, "Adipose tissue inflammation in the pathogenesis of type 2 diabetes," *Current Diabetes Reports*, vol. 15, no. 11, article 92, 2015.

[13] J.-P. Bastard, M. Maachi, C. Lagathu et al., "Recent advances in the relationship between obesity, inflammation, and insulin resistance," *European Cytokine Network*, vol. 17, no. 1, pp. 4–12, 2006.

[14] P. Gupta Bansal, G. Singh Toteja, N. Bhatia et al., "Deficiencies of serum ferritin and vitamin B12, but not folate, are common in adolescent girls residing in a slum in Delhi," *International Journal for Vitamin and Nutrition Research*, vol. 85, no. 1-2, pp. 14–22, 2015.

[15] H. T. O'Brien, R. Blanchet, D. Gagné, J. Lauzière, and C. Vézina, "Using soluble transferrin receptor and taking inflammation into account when defining serum ferritin cutoffs improved the diagnosis of iron deficiency in a group of Canadian preschool Inuit children from Nunavik," *Anemia*, vol. 2016, Article ID 6430214, 10 pages, 2016.

[16] J.-W. Kim, D. H. Kim, Y. K. Roh et al., "Serum ferritin levels are positively associated with metabolically obese normal weight: a nationwide population-based study," *Medicine*, vol. 94, no. 52, Article ID e2335, 2015.

[17] Y.-F. Huang, T.-S. Tok, C.-L. Lu, H.-C. Ko, M.-Y. Chen, and S. C. Chen, "Relationship between being overweight and iron deficiency in adolescents," *Pediatrics & Neonatology*, vol. 56, no. 6, pp. 386–392, 2015.

[18] S. A. Patel, M. K. Ali, D. Alam et al., "Obesity and its relation with diabetes and hypertension: a cross-sectional study across 4 geographical regions," *Global Heart*, vol. 11, no. 1, pp. 71.e4–79.e4, 2016.

[19] M. Khaskheli, S. Baloch, A. S. Baloch, S. Baloch, and F. K. Khaskheli, "Iron deficiency anaemia is still a major killer of pregnant women," *Pakistan Journal of Medical Sciences*, vol. 32, no. 3, pp. 630–634, 2016.

[20] M. A. Habib, K. Black, S. B. Soofi et al., "Prevalence and predictors of iron deficiency anemia in children under five years of age in Pakistan, a secondary analysis of national nutrition survey data 2011–2012," *PLOS ONE*, vol. 11, no. 5, Article ID 0155051, 2016.

[21] A. Lecube, C. Hernández, D. Pelegrí, and R. Simó, "Factors accounting for high ferritin levels in obesity," *International Journal of Obesity*, vol. 32, no. 11, pp. 1665–1669, 2008.

[22] S.-B. Chen, Y.-C. Lee, K.-H. Ser et al., "Serum C-reactive protein and white blood cell count in morbidly obese surgical patients," *Obesity Surgery*, vol. 19, no. 4, pp. 461–466, 2009.

[23] R. F. Gillum, "Association of serum ferritin and indices of body fat distribution and obesity in mexican american men—the third national health and nutrition examination survey," *International Journal of Obesity*, vol. 25, no. 5, pp. 639–645, 2001.

[24] F. Alam, F. Fatima, S. Orakzai, N. T. Iqbal, and S. S. Fatima, "Elevated levels of ferritin and hs-CRP in type 2 diabetes," *Journal of the Pakistan Medical Association*, vol. 64, no. 12, pp. 1389–1391, 2014.

[25] M. H. Eftekhari, H. Mozaffari-Khosravi, and F. Shidfar, "The relationship between BMI and iron status in iron-deficient adolescent Iranian girls," *Public Health Nutrition*, vol. 12, no. 12, pp. 2377–2381, 2009.

[26] C. Jericó, I. Bretón, A. García Ruiz de Gordejuela et al., "Diagnosis and treatment of iron deficiency, with or without anemia, before and after bariatric surgery," *Endocrinologia y Nutricion*, vol. 63, no. 1, pp. 32–42, 2016.

[27] A. C. Cepeda-Lopez, A. Melse-Boonstra, M. B. Zimmermann, and I. Herter-Aeberli, "In overweight and obese women, dietary iron absorption is reduced and the enhancement of iron absorption by ascorbic acid is one-half that in normal-weight women," *American Journal of Clinical Nutrition*, vol. 102, no. 6, pp. 1389–1397, 2015.

[28] A. C. Cepeda-Lopez, I. Aeberli, and M. B. Zimmermann, "Does obesity increase risk for iron deficiency? a review of the literature and the potential mechanisms," *International Journal for Vitamin and Nutrition Research*, vol. 80, no. 45, pp. 263–270, 2010.

[29] H. P. Villarroel, O. M. Arredondo, and G. M. Olivares, "Hepcidin as a central mediator of anemia of chronic diseases associated with obesity," *Revista Medica de Chile*, vol. 141, no. 7, pp. 887–894, 2013.

[30] H. Yu, R. Du, N. Zhang, M. Zhang, Y. Tu, and L. Zhang, "Iron-Deficiency Anemia after Laparoscopic Roux-en-Y gastric bypass in chinese obese patients with type 2 diabetes: a 2-Year Follow-Up Study," *Obesity Surgery*, vol. 26, no. 11, pp. 2705–2711, 2016.

Trends and Disparities in the Prevalence of Childhood Obesity in South Texas between 2009 and 2015

Byron A. Foster,[1] Trevor M. Maness,[2] and Christian A. Aquino[1]

[1]*Department of Pediatrics, University of Texas Health Science Center at San Antonio, San Antonio, TX, USA*
[2]*School of Public Health, University of Texas Health Science Center at Houston, Houston, TX, USA*

Correspondence should be addressed to Byron A. Foster; fosterba@uthscsa.edu

Academic Editor: David H. St-Pierre

Background. Recent reports have highlighted possible decreases over time in obesity, particularly among children aged 2–5 years. Hispanic children experience significantly higher obesity rates, and less is known about trends for Hispanic children. *Methods.* A large healthcare system-based dataset from south Texas was used to analyze body mass index (BMI) values obtained clinically from 2009 through 2015. Age and race/ethnicity specific prevalence of overweight and obesity were calculated using CDC standards and trends were examined over time using regression analyses, and mapping software was used to identify geographic variation. *Results.* Hispanic children in south Texas experience levels of obesity (25.3%, 95% CI: 25.1–25.6) significantly higher than their white (16.6%, 95% CI: 16.0–17.2) or black (18.2%, 95% CI: 17.3–19.1) peers. Obesity in Hispanic children aged 2–5 years decreased from 18.5%, 95% CI: 16.6–20.5, in 2009 to 15.1%, 95% CI: 14.3–15.9, in 2015. Obesity in Hispanic adolescents was stable at 30.4%, 95% CI: 28.5–32.4, in 2009 and 31.3, 95% CI: 30.3–32.2, in 2015. *Conclusions.* While obesity decreased in the youngest age group of Hispanic children, south Texas continues to experience high levels of obesity that exceed national averages with significant disparities.

1. Introduction

Multiple analyses of nationally representative data show an overall increase in obesity from the 1980s through the 1990s followed by a more recent plateau with no significant increase in the prevalence of obesity since the late 2000s [1–3]. These data also suggest a decrease in the prevalence of obesity for children aged 2–5 years [1, 2]. This decrease is primarily in white children while Hispanic children continue to experience a higher rate of obesity [1]. This disparity is particularly concerning given our understanding of weight trajectories [4] and the higher risk of both liver disease and diabetes seen in the Hispanic population [5]. For children aged 6–11 years, national data showed a recent plateau and, for adolescents, a continued increase in the prevalence of obesity across racial and ethnic groups [1].

A large, healthcare-based cohort in southern California showed a significant reduction in the prevalence of overweight, obesity, and extreme obesity from 2008 to 2013, in both the white and Hispanic populations [6]. Also, a recent study from Ohio using an academic medical center's records showed a similar plateau in overweight and obesity prevalence from 2011 to 2014 [7]. These data from individual localities and regions are valuable in both substantiating national trends and identifying important differences that may help identify policy-level effects or environmental changes driving regional differences. For example, a recent report from the Centers for Disease Control and Prevention examining participants in the Special Supplemental Nutrition Program for Women, Infants, and Children (WIC) identified important differences in prevalence between Los Angeles and New York [8], and another report using WIC data from Oklahoma showed no decline in obesity prevalence from 2005 to 2010 [9].

San Antonio, Texas, is the seventh largest city in the United States with 55% of the population being Hispanic making it an important potential indicator of obesity trends for Hispanic children. Data from the local Health District indicate that 65% of the adult population are overweight or obese, and 30% of the high school students population are overweight or obese [10].

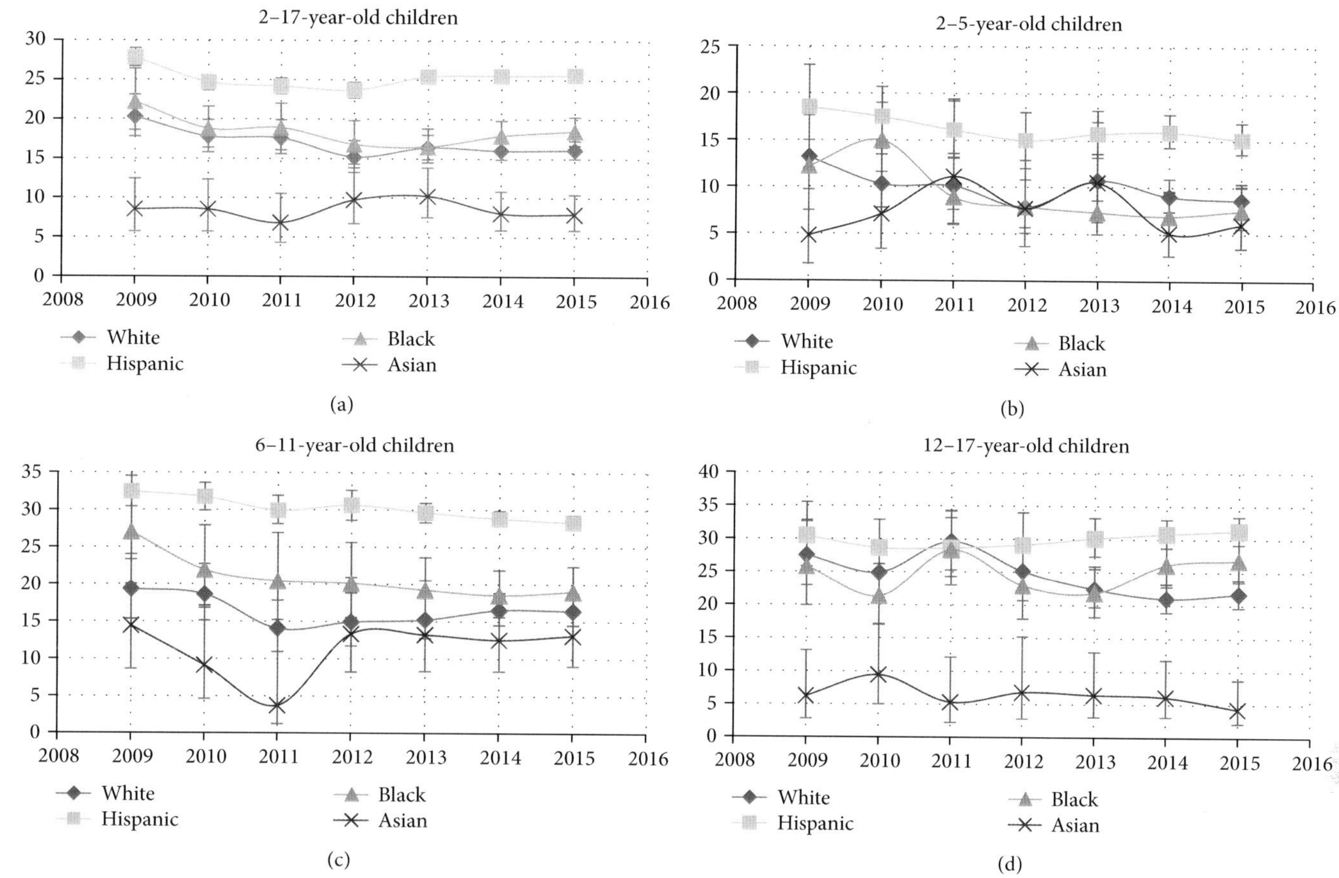

FIGURE 1: Prevalence of obesity in children in San Antonio over time, 2009 through 2015, with point estimates of percent of obese population shown with 95% CI as error bars. (a) All age groups; (b) 2–5-year-old children; (c) 6–11-year-old children; (d) 12–17-year-old children.

Here we describe trends in obesity prevalence for children aged 2–17 years using a healthcare dataset. The health system is one of the three largest providers of children's healthcare in San Antonio.

2. Methods

2.1. Data Source. A dataset from a healthcare system (University Health System) in San Antonio, Texas, was used to generate the estimates. Height and weight are measured during clinic or hospital encounters by clinical staff. Race and ethnicity categories are based on self-reported data.

Biologically implausible values were removed from the dataset (BMI z-scores < -5 and >8). From 2009 to 2015, there were 114,406 individuals with 352,744 visits for children between 2 and 17 years of age with height and weight entered. Individuals had between 1 and 110 visits with a biologically plausible BMI in the record over the seven years of data with a mean of 2.4 and a median of 2 measurements per year (Supplemental Table 1, in Supplementary Material available online at https://doi.org/10.1155/2017/1424968).

2.2. Statistical Analysis. EpiInfo (Centers for Disease Control) was used to generate BMI z-scores using the CDC 2000 criteria. BMI z-scores were categorized for this analysis as normal weight: >-2 through 1.03; overweight: ≥ 1.04 (equivalent to $\geq$85th percentile); obese: ≥ 1.65 (equivalent to $\geq$95th percentile) [11].

Each individual is represented once per year. The median of each individual's BMI z-scores for the year was calculated and used to categorize that individual in that year to minimize the effect of any outlying measurements.

Absolute changes over time were calculated using the absolute difference between estimates and relative changes over time calculated using the absolute change divided by the baseline estimate (2009 data). Generalized linear models were used to account for an individual child occurring in more than one year with thus repeated measures of their weight status. We examined trends over time with the binary dependent outcome of obesity and calendar year, sex and race/ethnicity included as independent variables. SPSS 23.0 (IBM, USA) was used for analyses.

Maps were created using Tableau (version 10.0) and individuals were only counted once per year. Zip codes having less than 10 observations in a year were censored (excluded from the map data).

2.3. Ethics. The Institutional Review Board for the University of Texas Health Science Center at San Antonio approved the data collection.

Table 1: Prevalence of overweight (≥85th and <95th percentile) and obesity (≥95th percentile) by age group, race, and ethnicity, data from all years (2009–2015) combined.

	Age 2–17 years	Age 2–5 years	Age 6–11 years	Age 12–17 years
Overweight				
All groups	16.2 (16.0–16.5)	13.4 (13.1–13.8)	16.7 (16.3–17.0)	18.5 (18.1–18.9)
Male	15.2 (14.9–15.5)	13.4 (12.9–13.9)	15.5 (15.0–16.0)	16.5 (16.0–17.0)
Female	17.4 (17.1–17.7)	13.5 (13.0–14.0)	17.9 (17.3–18.4)	20.4 (19.9–21.0)
Hispanic	17.0 (16.7–17.2)	14.2 (13.8–14.6)	17.2 (16.7–17.6)	19.4 (19.0–19.8)
Male	15.7 (15.4–16.1)	14.1 (13.5–14.6)	15.9 (15.3–16.5)	17.2 (16.6–17.8)
Female	18.2 (17.9–18.6)	14.4 (13.8–14.9)	18.5 (17.8–19.1)	21.5 (20.9–22.1)
White	14.0 (13.5–14.6)	10.7 (9.8–11.6)	15.3 (14.3–16.4)	15.9 (14.9–16.9)
Male	13.3 (12.5–14.1)	11.0 (9.8–12.4)	14.4 (13.1–15.9)	14.3 (13.0–15.8)
Female	14.8 (14.0–15.7)	10.3 (9.1–11.6)	16.2 (14.8–17.8)	17.3 (15.9–18.8)
Black	14.3 (13.5–15.1)	11.7 (10.5–13.1)	15.3 (13.9–16.8)	15.8 (14.5–17.2)
Male	13.5 (12.5–14.7)	12.0 (10.3–13.9)	14.7 (12.8–16.8)	13.9 (12.2–15.9)
Female	15.1 (14.0–16.4)	11.4 (9.6–13.3)	16.0 (13.9–18.3)	17.6 (15.7–19.7)
Asian	9.9 (8.8–11.1)	7.9 (6.3–9.8)	12.4 (10.4–14.8)	9.4 (7.5–11.7)
Male	11.0 (9.4–12.9)	9.2 (6.9–12.2)	13.6 (10.6–17.4)	10.6 (7.8–14.2)
Female	8.8 (7.3–10.5)	6.4 (4.4–9.2)	11.4 (8.7–14.6)	8.4 (6.1–11.5)
Obese				
All groups	23.4 (23.2–23.7)	14.5 (14.2–14.9)	26.8 (26.4–27.3)	28.6 (28.1–29.0)
Male	24.8 (24.5–25.2)	15.1 (14.6–15.6)	29.1 (28.5–29.8)	30.3 (29.7–30.9)
Female	22.0 (21.6–22.3)	13.5 (13.0–14.0)	24.4 (23.8–25.1)	27.0 (26.4–27.6)
Hispanic	25.3 (25.1–25.6)	15.9 (15.5–16.4)	29.5 (29.0–30.0)	30.3 (29.8–30.8)
Male	27.1 (26.7–27.5)	16.6 (16.0–17.2)	32.3 (31.5–32.0)	32.4 (31.7–33.1)
Female	23.6 (23.2–24.0)	15.2 (14.6–15.8)	26.6 (25.9–27.3)	28.4 (27.7–29.1)
White	16.6 (16.0–17.2)	9.6 (8.7–10.5)	16.3 (15.3–17.4)	23.1 (22.0–24.3)
Male	17.5 (16.6–18.3)	9.8 (8.7–11.1)	17.5 (16.0–19.1)	24.7 (23.0–26.5)
Female	15.8 (14.9–16.6)	9.2 (8.1–10.5)	15.0 (13.6–16.6)	21.6 (20.1–23.2)
Black	18.2 (17.3–19.1)	8.9 (7.8–10.1)	19.8 (18.3–21.5)	24.9 (23.3–26.6)
Male	16.8 (15.6–18.0)	9.2 (7.7–10.9)	18.1 (16.0–20.3)	22.7 (20.5–25.0)
Female	19.6 (18.4–21.0)	8.6 (7.1–10.4)	21.9 (19.5–24.5)	27.1 (24.8–29.5)
Asian	8.5 (7.4–9.6)	7.2 (5.7–9.1)	11.9 (9.8–14.2)	6.2 (4.7–8.1)
Male	10.8 (9.2–12.7)	9.6 (7.3–12.6)	15.1 (12.0–19.0)	7.5 (5.2–10.7)
Female	6.2 (5.0–7.7)	4.5 (2.9–7.0)	8.9 (6.6–11.9)	5.0 (3.2–7.5)

3. Results

There were 352,744 data points evaluated representing 114,406 individual children (see Supplemental Table 1) in the final sample with measurements from January 2009 through December 2015 with 50.3% being male and 78.9% of Hispanic ethnicity. Overall, 16.2% (95% CI: 16.0–16.5) of children were overweight and 23.4% (95% CI: 23.2–23.7) of children were obese. Hispanic children had the highest proportion of overweight or obesity compared with other racial and ethnic groups (Tables 1 and 2).

Examining trends over time among Hispanic children (Figure 1, Table 3), overall there was an absolute reduction in obesity of 2.2% (relative reduction of 7.9%) from 2009 to 2015. In the multivariable model including time, Hispanic children had an odds ratio of 1.71 (95% CI: 1.61–1.82) compared with white children of being obese (Table 2). For 2–5-year-olds, an absolute reduction of 3.4% (relative reduction of 18.4%) was observed between 2009 and 2015, with every year starting in 2011 showing a significant reduction compared with 2009 (Table 3). In contrast, there was no difference over time for the 12–17-year-old age group ($p > 0.05$), for all years examined (Table 3). There was a significant decrease seen over time in the unadjusted model for 6–11-year-old Hispanic children that was not sustained after accounting for sex in the final model (Table 3).

White children experienced overall reductions in obesity from 20.3% in 2009 to 16.1% in 2015 for an absolute reduction

Table 2: Regression results of year on obesity (dependent variable) accounting for repeated measures within individuals, with covariates of sex, race/ethnicity, and age group, presented as odds ratios (95% CI), p value, in San Antonio, Texas.

Variable	Estimate
Year	
2015	0.93 (0.88–0.97), 0.002
2014	0.91 (0.87–0.96), <0.001
2013	0.90 (0.85–0.95), <0.001
2012	0.91 (0.87–0.96), 0.004
2011	0.90 (0.85–0.94), <0.001
2010	0.95 (0.91–1.00), 0.03
2009	1.00 (reference)
Gender	
Male	1.00 (reference)
Female	0.84 (0.81–0.87), <0.001
Race/ethnicity	
White	1.00 (reference)
Hispanic	1.71 (1.61–1.82), <0.001
Black	1.09 (0.99–1.20), 0.08
Asian	0.44 (0.36–0.53), <0.001
Age	
2–5 years	1.00 (reference)
6–11 years	1.79 (1.73–1.86), <0.001
12–17 years	1.99 (1.92–2.07), <0.001

of 4.2% (relative reduction of 20.7%) (Figure 1, Table 3). Similar to the findings for Hispanic children, the most consistent decrease comparing years was in the 2–5-year-old age group (Table 3).

For black children in this sample, a similar reduction in obesity in the 2–5-year-old population was observed though the differences between baseline (2009) and subsequent years were less consistent than in the Hispanic group with only 2013 and 2014 having a significant reduction compared with 2009 (Table 3). The changes in other age groups of black children were not significant. Notably, black 12–17-year-olds were the only subgroup where females were more likely to be obese than males (OR = 1.30 (95% CI: 1.04–1.62)). No significant trends for Asian children in obesity were found.

Figure 2 shows a graphical representation of the proportion of children by zip code who are obese. Comparing 2009 (panel (a)) to 2015 (panel (b)), there are fewer zip codes with 30% or greater children who were obese in 2015 compared with 2009 with significant heterogeneity across the mapped region (Figure 2). Panels (c) and (d) show the distribution of white and Hispanic obese children, respectively, with striking differences in the prevalence of obesity by ethnicity across the San Antonio metropolitan area.

4. Discussion

In south Texas where adult obesity rates are higher than the national average [12], there have been limited data on the prevalence and trends over time in Texas for children. The data presented here show a higher prevalence of obesity overall (23.4%, 95% CI: 23.2–23.7) compared with both recent national estimates (17.0%, 95% CI: 15.5–18.6) [2] and an estimate from a healthcare-based dataset from southern California (17.5%) [6]. The overall prevalence of obesity is also higher than the overall prevalence in the study from Ohio (19.5%) that also used a healthcare dataset, though the prevalence among Hispanics was 26.3% in that study, and the relatively small proportion of Hispanics in the population explains that difference [7]. Data from the WIC population which has a lower income and it is more similar to our population in socioeconomic status have a more similar estimate of 14.9% for obesity in Texas in 2014 for children aged 2–4 years [13].

The finding of a decrease among children aged 2–5 years is consistent with recent national reports [2]. Two different groups examining Massachusetts school-based data [14] and healthcare-based data similar to this dataset [15] found a decline in obesity among the youngest children [14, 15]. One notable outlier is the Ohio report which found a significant recent increase for 2–5-year-old girls [7]. The decreases in the youngest children are encouraging given the strong correlation between weight at that age and weight status in both adolescence and early adulthood [4, 16, 17].

In San Antonio, there have been multiple recent efforts to address obesity. The local health department with the city led an effort to improve the built environment and facilitate physical activity programs. Additionally, Head Start and PreK4SA, programs for early childhood education, have focused their efforts on making their menus healthier and promoting physical activity at a younger age, and recent studies have found that Head Start participation can lead to a healthier weight [18]. Most of the efforts outlined above are focused on prevention of obesity; however, there are limited resources for treating obesity in children in San Antonio. This may explain why we see a decrease in the youngest age group while also observing a potential increase or at least no change in obesity for adolescents, working under the rubric that more intensive therapies are required for treatment of obesity [19–21]. The disparities seen by race/ethnicity are striking with Hispanic children at much higher risk of obesity compared with their white peers.

For 2–5-year-old children, Hispanic children in this sample have a prevalence of obesity that is 5% higher than all other racial or ethnic groups. National data [2] have found an even larger gap with an estimate of 15.6% (95% CI: 12.5–19.2) in Hispanic 2–5-year-olds and 5.2% (95% CI: 3.1–8.3) in white children; data from Massachusetts showed a similar gap to the national data with an estimate of 11.8–12.9% for Hispanic children less than 6 years old compared with 6.2–8.5% for white children [15].

The map data demonstrate the variation in obesity across San Antonio and suggest a decrease between 2009 and 2015 in areas of San Antonio with very high levels of obesity; however,

TABLE 3: Regression results of year on obesity (dependent variable) accounting for repeated measures within individuals and adjusted for sex, stratified by race/ethnicity, presented as odds ratios (95% CI), p value, in San Antonio, Texas. Odds ratios indicate the value for the independent variable of year of measurement with 2009 for that race/ethnicity and age stratum as the reference.

	All ages[1]	2–5 years	6–11 years	12–17 years
Hispanic				
2015	0.94 (0.89–0.99), 0.02	0.85 (0.75–0.97), 0.02	0.98 (0.90–1.06), 0.57	1.00 (0.92–1.09), 0.98
2014	0.92 (0.88–0.97), 0.003	0.84 (0.73–0.96), 0.009	0.93 (0.85–1.01), 0.10	1.00 (0.92–1.08), 0.94
2013	0.91 (0.87–0.97), 0.001	0.78 (0.68–0.90), 0.001	0.93 (0.85–1.01), 0.09	1.00 (0.92–1.09), 0.99
2012	0.94 (0.88–1.00), 0.04	0.81 (0.70–0.94), 0.005	1.02 (0.92–0.85), 0.76	0.97 (0.88–1.06), 0.50
2011	0.90 (0.85–0.96), <0.001	0.83 (0.72–0.95), 0.009	0.95 (0.87–1.04), 0.24	0.96 (0.88–1.05), 0.39
2010	0.94 (0.90–0.99), 0.03	0.91 (0.80–1.04), 0.17	0.98 (0.91–1.06), 0.60	0.97 (0.90–1.05), 0.45
Female (reference = male)	0.82 (0.79–0.85), <0.001	0.89 (0.82–0.95), 0.001	0.76 (0.71–0.81), <0.001	0.83 (0.79–0.88), <0.001
White				
2015	0.80 (0.68–0.94), 0.008	0.68 (0.47–1.00), 0.05	0.98 (0.75–1.28), 0.88	0.84 (0.66–1.06), 0.13
2014	0.80 (0.68–0.94), 0.006	0.69 (0.47–1.01), 0.06	0.97 (0.74–1.27), 0.83	0.82 (0.65–1.03), 0.09
2013	0.77 (0.65–0.92), 0.003	0.72 (0.48–1.09), 0.12	0.86 (0.65–1.15), 0.31	0.81 (0.64–1.02), 0.08
2012	0.81 (0.67–0.96), 0.02	0.66 (0.43–1.02), 0.06	0.78 (0.57–1.08), 0.13	0.89 (0.69–1.16), 0.39
2011	0.85 (0.72–1.01), 0.06	0.67 (0.43–1.03), 0.07	0.85 (0.65–1.12), 0.24	0.99 (0.77–1.27), 0.93
2010	0.95 (0.81–1.12), 0.054	0.87 (0.59–1.29), 0.49	0.96 (0.76–1.21), 0.74	1.02 (0.82–1.28), 0.83
Female (reference = male)	0.89 (0.79–0.99), 0.04	0.92 (0.73–1.15), 0.46	0.85 (0.70–1.03), 0.09	0.87 (0.74–1.02), 0.08
Black				
2015	0.92 (0.74–1.14), 0.45	0.61 (0.36–1.03), 0.07	0.88 (0.61–1.28), 0.51	1.30 (0.91–1.85), 0.15
2014	0.84 (0.67–1.04), 0.11	0.47 (0.28–0.82), 0.007	0.88 (0.61–1.27), 0.51	1.24 (0.88–1.75), 0.22
2013	0.79 (0.63–0.99), 0.04	0.55 (0.32–0.97), 0.04	0.82 (0.56–1.20), 0.30	1.02 (0.72–1.44), 0.93
2012	0.81 (0.64–1.03), 0.09	0.61 (0.34–1.08), 0.09	0.82 (0.54–1.24), 0.35	1.05 (0.72–1.54), 0.80
2011	0.84 (0.67–1.05), 0.13	0.65 (0.37–1.16), 0.15	0.78 (0.52–1.15), 0.21	1.31 (0.91–1.90), 0.15
2010	0.96 (0.79–1.17), 0.67	1.15 (0.73–1.82), 0.54	0.91 (0.73–1.29), 0.84	0.95 (0.68–1.34), 0.77
Female (reference = male)	1.12 (0.96–1.30), 0.16	0.85 (0.62–1.18), 0.33	1.13 (0.88–1.46), 0.34	1.30 (1.04–1.62), 0.02
Asian				
2015	1.07 (0.64–1.79), 0.80	1.47 (0.51–4.27), 0.48	0.90 (0.45–1.82), 0.77	0.91 (0.30–2.79), 0.87
2014	0.97 (0.57–1.65), 0.91	1.16 (0.37–3.58), 0.80	0.99 (0.50–1.97), 0.97	1.02 (0.31–3.37), 0.97
2013	1.23 (0.72–2.10), 0.45	2.24 (0.78–6.45), 0.13	0.90 (0.43–1.88), 0.77	1.15 (0.34–3.85), 0.82
2012	1.07 (0.61–1.87), 0.83	1.74 (0.53–5.70), 0.36	0.72 (0.34–1.54), 0.40	1.12 (0.33–3.83), 0.85
2011	0.75 (0.39–1.44), 0.39	1.68 (0.53–5.38), 0.38	0.29 (0.12–0.70), 0.006	1.02 (0.29–3.57), 0.98
2010	1.00 (0.56–1.80), 1.00	1.15 (0.37–3.59), 0.82	0.62 (0.26–1.50), 0.29	1.49 (0.47–4.75), 0.50
Female (reference = male)	0.59 (0.41–0.86), 0.005	0.47 (0.24–0.93), 0.03	0.58 (0.35–0.95), 0.03	0.82 (0.41–1.63), 0.57

[1] Multivariable generalized linear model with all age groups included but adjusted for age.

the only decreases noted in the regression analysis were in the youngest children. The higher prevalence zip codes generally correspond to lower reported income zip codes in San Antonio [22]. These maps also highlight areas of significant disparity by ethnicity, highlighting the complex drivers of obesity with both environmental and cultural components.

A strength of this study is its sheer size with over 300,000 measurements representing over 100,000 children. A limitation is the nonrandom nature of the sample. While the health system does have clinics spread throughout San Antonio, it is also a major academic center with a large referral population which may select for a more morbid population, potentially with higher obesity rates than the population of children at large. Utilization of these local, nonrandom data in comparison with the few random samples available nationally, with appropriate limitations, can allow for a better understanding of obesity trends and variation. Another limitation is the lack of a specific measure of socioeconomic status which would have allowed for examination not only by race/ethnicity but accounting for disparities by socioeconomic status as well. Variations in obesity prevalence have also been observed across countries of origin for adults of Hispanic ethnicity [23], and our study did not have that information available to compare.

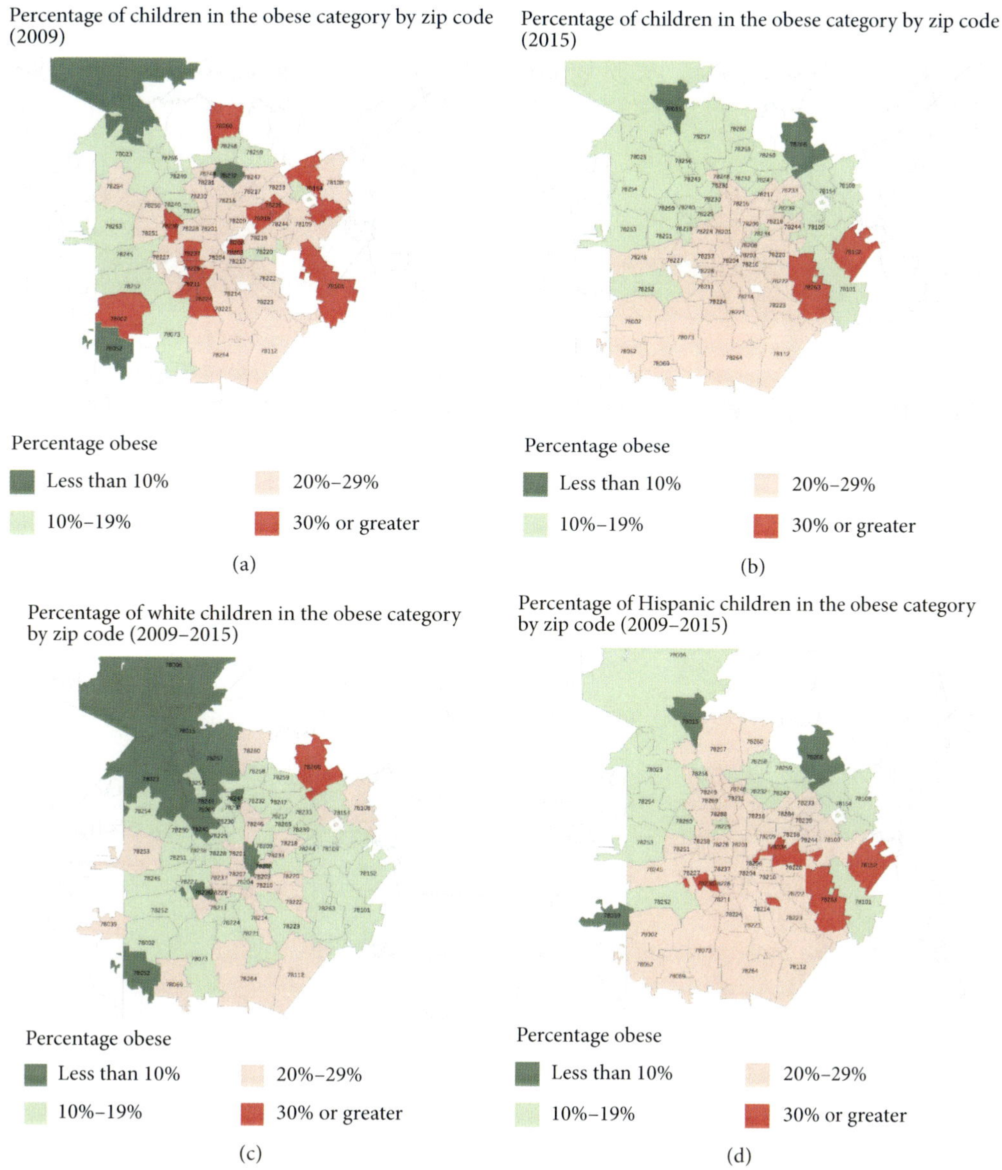

FIGURE 2: Percentage of children with obesity showing (a) 2009 and (b) 2015 distributions over San Antonio by postal zip code and (c) percentage of white children with obesity from all years (2009–2015) and (d) percentage of Hispanic children with obesity from all years (2009–2015). Dark green indicates less than 10% obese, light green 10–19% obese, light red 20–29% obese, and dark red 30% or greater obese in the indicated zip code. *Note.* zip codes with less than 10 observations were censored (in all figures).

Acknowledgments

The authors acknowledge the hard work of Tracy Jeffers, Sunrise Data Analyst & System Administrator, in obtaining the data. Author Byron A. Foster was supported by the National Institute of Diabetes and Digestive and Kidney Diseases, National Institutes of Health (NIH), through Grant K23DK109199.

References

[1] C. L. Ogden, M. D. Carroll, B. K. Kit, and K. M. Flegal, "Prevalence of childhood and adult obesity in the United States, 2011-2012," *The Journal of the American Medical Association*, vol. 311, no. 8, pp. 806–814, 2014.

[2] C. L. Ogden, M. D. Carroll, H. G. Lawman et al., "Trends in obesity prevalence among children and adolescents in the United States, 1988–1994 through 2013-2014," *Journal of the American Medical Association*, vol. 315, no. 21, pp. 2292–2299, 2016.

[3] A. C. Skinner and J. A. Skelton, "Prevalence and trends in obesity among children in the United States, 1999–2012," *JAMA Pediatrics*, vol. 68, no. 6, pp. 561–566, 2014.

[4] A. S. Singh, C. Mulder, J. W. R. Twisk, W. van Mechelen, and M. J. M. Chinapaw, "Tracking of childhood overweight into adulthood: a systematic review of the literature," *Obesity Reviews*, vol. 9, no. 5, pp. 474–488, 2008.

[5] M. Lazo, U. Bilal, and R. Perez-Escamilla, "Epidemiology of NAFLD and Type 2 Diabetes: Health Disparities Among Persons of Hispanic Origin," *Current Diabetes Reports*, vol. 15, no. 12, article no. 116, 2015.

[6] C. Koebnick, Y. D. Mohan, X. Li, and D. R. Young, "Secular Trends of Overweight and Obesity in Young Southern Californians 2008-2013," *The Journal of pediatrics*, vol. 167, no. 6, pp. 1264–1271, 2015.

[7] R. Y. Kharofa, J. A. Klein, P. Khoury, and R. M. Siegel, "Severe Obesity Decreasing in Children in Cincinnati, Ohio," *Clinical Pediatrics*, vol. 56, no. 8, pp. 752–758, 2016.

[8] Centers for Disease Control and Prevention (CDC). Obesity prevalence among low-income, preschool-aged children—New York City and Los Angeles County, 2003–2011. MMWR Morb Mortal Wkly Rep. 2013;62: 17–22.

[9] A. E. Weedn, J. J. Hale, D. M. Thompson, and P. M. Darden, "Trends in obesity prevalence and disparities among low-income children in Oklahoma, 2005-2010," *Childhood Obesity*, vol. 10, no. 4, pp. 318–325, 2014.

[10] Obesity in Bexar County. In: City of San Antonio Metropolitan Health District [Internet]. 2013, https://www.sanantonio.gov/Portals/0/Files/health/HealthyLiving/FactSheet-Obesity.pdf.

[11] K. M. Flegal, R. Wei, C. L. Ogden, D. S. Freedman, C. L. Johnson, and L. R. Curtin, "Characterizing extreme values of body mass index-for-age by using the 2000 Centers for Disease Control and Prevention growth charts," *The American Journal of Clinical Nutrition*, vol. 90, no. 5, pp. 1314–1320, 2009.

[12] J. Levi, L. Segal, J. Rayburn, and A. Martin, State of Obesity 2015. In: Robert Wood Johnson Foundation [Internet]. 2015, http://stateofobesity.org/files/stateofobesity2015.pdf.

[13] L. Pan, D. S. Freedman, A. J. Sharma et al., "Trends in Obesity Among Participants Aged 2–4 Years in the Special Supplemental Nutrition Program for Women, Infants, and Children—United States, 2000–2014," *MMWR. Morbidity and Mortality Weekly Report*, vol. 65, no. 45, pp. 1256–1260, 2016.

[14] W. Li, J. H. Buszkiewicz, R. B. Leibowitz, M. A. Gapinski, L. J. Nasuti, and T. G. Land, "Declining trends and widening disparities in overweight and obesity prevalence among Massachusetts public school districts, 2009-2014," *American Journal of Public Health*, vol. 105, no. 10, pp. e76–e82, 2015.

[15] X. Wen, M. W. Gillman, S. L. Rifas-Shiman, B. Sherry, K. Kleinman, and E. M. Taveras, "Decreasing prevalence of obesity among young children in Massachusetts from 2004 to 2008," *Pediatrics*, vol. 129, no. 5, pp. 823–831, 2012.

[16] K. Tilling, N. M. Davies, E. Nicoli et al., "Associations of growth trajectories in infancy and early childhood with later childhood outcomes," *American Journal of Clinical Nutrition*, vol. 94, no. 6, pp. 1808s–1813s, 2011.

[17] U. Ekelund, K. Ong, Y. Linné et al., "Upward weight percentile crossing in infancy and early childhood independently predicts fat mass in young adults: the Stockholm Weight Development Study (SWEDES)," *American Journal of Clinical Nutrition*, vol. 83, no. 2, pp. 324–330, 2006.

[18] J. C. Lumeng, N. Kaciroti, J. Sturza et al., "Changes in body mass index associated with head start participation," *Pediatrics*, vol. 135, no. 2, pp. e449–e456, 2015.

[19] K. D. Hesketh and K. J. Campbell, "Interventions to prevent obesity in 0-5 year olds: an updated systematic review of the literature," *Obesity*, vol. 18, no. S1, pp. S27–S35, 2010.

[20] E. Waters, A. de Silva-Sanigorski, B. J. Burford et al., "Interventions for preventing obesity in children," *Cochrane Database of Systematic Reviews*, no. 12, Article ID CD001871, 2011.

[21] H. Oude Luttikhuis, L. Baur, H. Jansen et al., "Interventions for treating obesity in children," *Cochrane Database of Systematic Reviews*, no. 1, Article ID CD001872, 2009.

[22] Internal Revenue Service [Internet]. 2014, https://www.irs.gov/uac/soi-tax-stats-individual-income-tax-statistics-zip-code-data-soi.

[23] M. L. Daviglus, G. A. Talavera, M. L. Avilés-Santa et al., "Prevalence of major cardiovascular risk factors and cardiovascular diseases among Hispanic/Latino individuals of diverse backgrounds in the United States," *JAMA: Journal of the American Medical Association*, vol. 308, no. 17, pp. 1775–1784, 2012.

Permissions

All chapters in this book were first published in JO, by Hindawi Publishing Corporation; hereby published with permission under the Creative Commons Attribution License or equivalent. Every chapter published in this book has been scrutinized by our experts. Their significance has been extensively debated. The topics covered herein carry significant findings which will fuel the growth of the discipline. They may even be implemented as practical applications or may be referred to as a beginning point for another development.

The contributors of this book come from diverse backgrounds, making this book a truly international effort. This book will bring forth new frontiers with its revolutionizing research information and detailed analysis of the nascent developments around the world.

We would like to thank all the contributing authors for lending their expertise to make the book truly unique. They have played a crucial role in the development of this book. Without their invaluable contributions this book wouldn't have been possible. They have made vital efforts to compile up to date information on the varied aspects of this subject to make this book a valuable addition to the collection of many professionals and students.

This book was conceptualized with the vision of imparting up-to-date information and advanced data in this field. To ensure the same, a matchless editorial board was set up. Every individual on the board went through rigorous rounds of assessment to prove their worth. After which they invested a large part of their time researching and compiling the most relevant data for our readers.

The editorial board has been involved in producing this book since its inception. They have spent rigorous hours researching and exploring the diverse topics which have resulted in the successful publishing of this book. They have passed on their knowledge of decades through this book. To expedite this challenging task, the publisher supported the team at every step. A small team of assistant editors was also appointed to further simplify the editing procedure and attain best results for the readers.

Apart from the editorial board, the designing team has also invested a significant amount of their time in understanding the subject and creating the most relevant covers. They scrutinized every image to scout for the most suitable representation of the subject and create an appropriate cover for the book.

The publishing team has been an ardent support to the editorial, designing and production team. Their endless efforts to recruit the best for this project, has resulted in the accomplishment of this book. They are a veteran in the field of academics and their pool of knowledge is as vast as their experience in printing. Their expertise and guidance has proved useful at every step. Their uncompromising quality standards have made this book an exceptional effort. Their encouragement from time to time has been an inspiration for everyone.

The publisher and the editorial board hope that this book will prove to be a valuable piece of knowledge for researchers, students, practitioners and scholars across the globe.

List of Contributors

Jacynthe Lafrenière, Jessica McNeil and Éric Doucet
Behavioural and Metabolic Research Unit, School of Human Kinetics, University of Ottawa, Ottawa, ON, Canada

Véronique Provencher
Institute of Nutrition and Functional Foods, Laval University, Quebec City, QC, Canada

Joshua H. F. Cooper, Blake E. G. Collins, David R. Adams and Cheyne E. Donges
School of Exercise Science, Sport and Health, Charles Sturt University, Bathurst, NSW, Australia

Robert A. Robergs
Queensland University of Technology, Brisbane, QLD, Australia

Charlotta Pisinger
Research Centre for Prevention and Health, Glostrup Hospital, Building 84/85, 2600 Glostrup, Denmark

Helle Øster Nielsen and Caroline Kuhlmann
Faculty of Health and Medical Sciences, University of Copenhagen, 1123 Copenhagen K, Denmark

Susanne Rosthøj
Section of Biostatistics, Institute of Public Health, University of Copenhagen, 1014 Copenhagen, Denmark

Ryan D. Burns, Timothy A. Brusseau and Yi Fang
Department of Health, Kinesiology, and Recreation, University of Utah, 250 S. 1850 E.,HPER North, RM241,Salt Lake City, UT 84112, USA

You Fu
School of Community Health Sciences, University of Nevada, Reno, 1664 North Virginia Street, Reno, NV 89557, USA

James C. Hannon
College of Physical Activity and Sport Sciences, West Virginia University, P.O. Box 6116, 375 Birch St., Morgantown, WV 26505-6116, USA

Gabrielle Araujo do Nascimento, Lupe Furtado-Alle, Mayza Dalcin Teixeira and Ricardo Lehtonen Rodrigues de Souza
Department of Genetics, Centro Politécnico, Setor de Ciências Biológicas, Federal University of Paraná, Francisco H. dos Santos, 210 Jardim das Américas, 81531-970 Curitiba, PR, Brazil

Neiva Leite, Gerusa Eisfeld Milano, Larissa Rosa da Silva, Juliana Pizzi, Maria de Fátima Aguiar Lopes and Ana Cláudia Kapp Titski
Department of Physical Education, Federal University of Paraná, Coração de Maria, 92 Jardim Botânico, 80215-370 Curitiba, PR, Brazil

Wendell Arthur Lopes
Department of Physical Education, State University of Maringa, Av. Colombo 5790, 87020-900 Maringa, PR, Brazil

Luciane Viater Tureck
Department of Genetics, Centro Politécnico, Setor de Ciências Biológicas, Federal University of Paraná, Francisco H. dos Santos, 210 Jardim das Américas, 81531-970 Curitiba, PR, Brazil
Academic Department of Education, Federal University of Technology–Paran´a, Av. Monteiro Lobato Km 04, 84016-210 Ponta Grossa, PR, Brazil

Bolaji Fatai Oyeyemi
Integrative Biology Unit, Transcriptional Regulation Group, International Centre for Genetic Engineering and Biotechnology, New Delhi, India
Department of Science Technology, The Federal Polytechnic Ado-Ekiti, Ado-Ekiti, Nigeria

Charles Ayorinde Ologunde
Department of Science Technology, The Federal Polytechnic Ado-Ekiti, Ado-Ekiti, Nigeria

Ayonposi Bukola Olaoye
Department of Science Technology, The Federal Polytechnic Ado-Ekiti, Ado-Ekiti, Nigeria
Institute of Biological, Environmental and Rural Sciences, Aberystwyth University, Aberystwyth, UK

Nanfizat Abiket Alamukii
Cell Biology and Genetics Unit, Department of Zoology, University of Ibadan, Ibadan, Nigeria

Emilie Rune Hegelund
Section of Environmental Health, Department of Public Health, University of Copenhagen, Øster Farimagsgade 5A, 1353 Copenhagen K, Denmark

Cathrine Lawaetz Wimmelmann, Emilie Just-Østergaard, Erik Lykke Mortensen and Trine Flensborg-Madsen
Section of Environmental Health, Department of Public Health, University of Copenhagen, Øster Farimagsgade 5A, 1353 Copenhagen K, Denmark

Center for Healthy Aging, Faculty of Health and Medical Sciences, University of Copenhagen, Copenhagen, Denmark

Anna Paldam Folker
National Institute of Public Health, University of Southern Denmark, Øster Farimagsgade 5A, 1353 Copenhagen K, Denmark

Merete Osler
Research Center for Prevention and Health, Glostrup Hospital, Glostrup, Denmark
Danish Aging Research Center, University of Aarhus, Aarhus, Denmark
Danish Aging Research Center, University of Southern Denmark, Odense, Denmark
Danish Aging Research Center, University of Copenhagen, Copenhagen, Denmark
Section of Social Medicine, Department of Public Health, University of Copenhagen, Øster Farimagsgade 5A,1353 Copenhagen K, Denmark

Kristin E. Finn
School of Education and Human Services, Canisius College, 2001 Main Street, Buffalo, NY 14208, USA

Myles S. Faith and Young S. Seo
Department of Counseling, School, and Educational Psychology, University at Buffalo–State University of New York,420 Baldy Hall, Buffalo, NY 14260-1000, USA

Sarah Nutter, Shelly Russell-Mayhew, Nancy Arthur, Anusha Kassan, Monica Sesma-Vazquez and Emily Williams
Counselling Psychology, Werklund School of Education, University of Calgary, Calgary, AB, Canada

Angela S. Alberga
Werklund School of Education, University of Calgary, Calgary, AB, Canada

Darren E. Lund
Curriculum and Learning, Werklund School of Education, University of Calgary, Calgary, AB, Canada

Jumanah Albeeybe, Tasneem Alahmari, Nawal Asiri, Reema Alajaji and Reem Almassoud
College of Medicine, King Saud University

Abdulaziz Alomer
Department of Orthopedics, King Saud University Medical City, King Saud University

Hazzaa M. Al-Hazzaa
Lifestyle and Health Research, Health Science Research Center, Princess Nourah Bint Abdulrahman University

Thirumagal Kanagasabai, Ramandeep Dhanoa, Jennifer L. Kuk and Chris I. Ardern
School of Kinesiology and Health Science, York University, Toronto, ON, Canada

Stella Maris Honoré, Maria Virginia Grande, Jorge Gomez Rojas and Sara Serafina Sánchez
Instituto Superior de Investigaciones Biol´ogicas (INSI-BIO), Consejo Nacional de Investigaciones Cient´ıficas y Técnicas-Universidad Nacional de Tucumán (CONICET-UNT), Chacabuco 461, T4000ILI San Miguel de Tucum´an, Argentina

Janna D. Stephens, Alai Tan and Bernadette Mazurek Melnyk
The Ohio State University College of Nursing, Columbus, OH, USA

Andrew Althouse
Heart and Vascular Institute, University of Pittsburgh Medical Center, Pittsburgh, PA, USA

Cézane P. Reuter and Silvia I. R. Franke
Physical Education and Health Department, Postgraduate Program in Health Promotion, University of Santa Cruz do Sul (UNISC), 96.815-900 Santa Cruz do Sul, RS, Brazil

Elza D. de Mello
Postgraduate Program in Child and Adolescent Health, Federal University of Rio Grande do Sul (UFRGS), 90.035-003 Porto Alegre, RS, Brazil

Priscila T. da Silva and Elisa I. Klinger
Postgraduate Program in Health Promotion, University of Santa Cruz do Sul (UNISC), 96.815-900 Santa Cruz do Sul, RS, Brazil

Tássia S. Borges
School of Dentistry, Lutheran University Center of Palmas (CEULP-ULBRA), 77.019-900 Palmas, TO, Brazil

Andréia R. de M. Valim
Biology and Pharmacy Department, Postgraduate Program in Health Promotion, University of Santa Cruz do Sul (UNISC), 96.815-900 Santa Cruz do Sul, RS, Brazil

Abigail M. Pauley and Krista S. Leonard
Exercise Psychology Laboratory, Department of Kinesiology, e Pennsylvania State University, University Park, State College, PA, USA

Emily Hohman and Jennifer S. Savage
Center for Childhood Obesity Research, Department of Nutritional Sciences, College of Health and Human Development, e Pennsylvania State University, University Park,PA, USA

Daniel E. Rivera and Penghong Guo
School for Engineering of Matter, Transport, Energy, Arizona State University, Tempe, AZ, USA

Danielle Symons Downs
Exercise Psychology Laboratory, Department of Kinesiology, e Pennsylvania State University, University Park, State College,PA, USA
Department of Obstetrics and Gynecology, College of Medicine, e Pennsylvania State University, Hershey, PA, USA

Jenna Taylor, Shelley E. Keating, David J. Holland, Jeff S. Coombes and Michael D. Leveritt
School of Human Movement and Nutrition Sciences, e University of Queensland, St. Lucia, Brisbane, QLD 4072, Australia

Jessica Rieder, Agnieszka Cain, Erica Carson, Andrea Benya, Neal Hoffman, Colleen Kelly, Ellen J. Silver and Laurie J. Bauman
Department of Pediatrics, Children's Hospital at Montefiore, e Pediatric Hospital for Albert Einstein College of Medicine, Bronx, NY, USA

Paul Meissner
Department of Family and Social Medicine, Albert Einstein College of Medicine, Bronx, NY, USA

Carmen R. Isasi and Judith Wylie-Rosett
Department of Epidemiology and Population Health, Albert Einstein College of Medicine, Bronx, NY, USA

Scott V. Monte, Kristen M. Russo and Esra Mustafa
University at Buffalo School of Pharmacy and Pharmaceutical Sciences, 213 Kapoor Hall, Buffalo, NY 14214, USA

Joseph A. Caruana
Synergy Bariatrics, A Department of ECMC, University at Buffalo School of Medicine, Buffalo, NY 14214, USA

Asma Deeb and Salima Attia
Pediatric Endocrinology Department, Mafraq Hospital

Samia Mahmoud
Pediatric Clinic, Police Health Services, Abu Dhabi, UAE

Ghada Elhaj
Primary Health Care Center, BaniYas, Abu Dhabi, UAE

Abubaker Elfatih
Biochemistry Department, Shaikh Khalifa Medical City, Abu Dhabi, UAE

Moonseong Heo, Judith Wylie-Rosett and Sarah N. Martin
Department of Epidemiology and Population Health, Albert Einstein College of Medicine, Bronx, NY, USA

Singh R. Nair
Department of Anesthesiology, Montefiore Medical Center, Bronx, NY, USA

Myles S. Faith
Department of Counseling, School, and Educational Psychology, Graduate School of Education, University at Buffalo-SUNY, Buffalo, NY, USA

Angelo Pietrobelli
Department of Pediatrics, University of Verona, Verona, Italy
Pennington Biomedical Research Center, Baton Rouge, LA, USA

Nancy R. Glassman
D. Samuel Gottesman Library, Albert Einstein College of Medicine, Bronx, NY, USA

Stephanie Dickinson and David B. Allison
Department of Epidemiology and Biostatistics, School of Public Health, Indiana University-Bloomington, Bloomington, IN, USA

Nisha Hariharan, Carolina B. Livi and Desiree Wilson
Department of Cell Systems and Anatomy, University of Texas Health Science Center, San Antonio, TX 78229, USA

Keith A. Ashcraft, Robert S. Svatek, Dharam Kaushik and Teresa L. Johnson-Pais
Department of Urology, University of Texas Health Science Center, San Antonio, TX 78229, USA

Robin J. Leach
Department of Cell Systems and Anatomy, University of Texas Health Science Center, San Antonio, TX 78229, USA
Department of Urology, University of Texas Health Science Center, San Antonio, TX 78229, USA

Byron A. Foster
Departments of Dermatology and Pediatrics, Oregon Health and Science University, Portland, OR, USA
Center for Research to Advance Community Health, University of Texas Health San Antonio, San Antonio, TX, USA

Christian A. Aquino and Sharol Mejia
School of Medicine, University of Texas Health San Antonio, San Antonio, TX, USA

Barbara J. Turner
Center for Research to Advance Community Health, University of Texas Health San Antonio, San Antonio, TX, USA
School of Medicine, University of Texas Health San Antonio, San Antonio, TX, USA

Arvind Singhal
Department of Communication, é University of Texas at El Paso, El Paso, TX, USA
Inland University of Applied Sciences, Elverum, Norway

Samuel N. Forjuoh
Department of Family and Community Medicine, Baylor Scott and White Health, College of Medicine, Texas A and M Health Science Center, Temple, TX, USA
Department of Health Promotion and Community Health Sciences, School of Public Health, Texas A&M University, College Station, TX, USA

Marcia G. Ory and Samuel D. Towne Jr.
Department of Health Promotion and Community Health Sciences, School of Public Health, Texas A&M University, College Station, TX, USA

Jaewoong Won and Chanam Lee
Department of Landscape Architecture and Urban Planning, College of Architecture, Texas A and M University, College Station, TX, USA

Suojin Wang
Department of Statistics, College of Science, Texas A&M University, College Station, TX, USA

Roger Figueroa
University of Illinois at Urbana-Champaign, 905 South Goodwin Ave., 230 Bevier Hall MC-180, Urbana, IL 61801, USA

Jaclyn Saltzman and Jessica Jarick Metcalfe
University of Illinois at Urbana-Champaign, 904W. Nevada St., #1014, MC-081, Urbana, IL 61801, USA

Angela Wiley
University of Illinois at Urbana-Champaign, 904W. Nevada St., #2004, MC-081, Urbana, IL 61801, USA

Simin Mouodi, Seyed Reza Hosseini, Ali Bijani, Hassan Ashrafian Amiri, Fatemeh Bayani and Shima Sum
Social Determinants of Health Research Center, Health Research Institute, Babol University of Medical Sciences, Babol, Iran

Reza Ghadimi
Health Research Institute, Babol University of Medical Sciences, Babol, Iran

Robert Graham Cumming
School of Public Health, University of Sydney, Sydney, NSW, Australia

Liang Wang, Beth A. Bailey, Arsham Alamian and Marc A. Stevens
Department of Biostatistics and Epidemiology, College of Public Health, East Tennessee State University, Johnson City, TN, USA

Jodi Southerland
Department of Community and Behavioral Health, College of Public Health, East Tennessee State University, Johnson City, TN, USA

Kesheng Wang
Department of Family Medicine, Quillen College of Medicine, East Tennessee State University, Johnson City, TN, USA

Youfa Wang
Fisher Institute of Health andWell-Being, Systems-Oriented Global Childhood Obesity Intervention Program, Department of Nutrition and Health Sciences, College of Health, Ball State University, Muncie, IN, USA

Abdulaziz Farooq
Athlete Health and Performance Research, Aspetar Orthopaedic and Sports Medicine Hospital, Doha, Qatar
School of Psychological Sciences and Health, University of Strathclyde, Glasgow, UK

Ann-Marie Gibson and John J. Reilly
School of Psychological Sciences and Health, University of Strathclyde, Glasgow, UK

Nadia Gaoua
School of Applied Sciences, London South Bank University, London, UK

Abidullah Khan, WazirMuhammad Khan, Maimoona Ayub, Mohammad Humayun and Mohammad Haroon
KTH, Peshawar, Pakistan

Byron A. Foster and Christian A. Aquino
Department of Pediatrics, University of Texas Health Science Center at San Antonio, San Antonio, TX, USA

Trevor M. Maness
School of Public Health, University of Texas Health Science Center at Houston, Houston, TX, USA

Index